P9-EEM-201

POINT LOMA NAZARENE COLLEGE
WITHDRAWN
Ryan Library
3900 Lomaland Drive, San Diego, CA 92106-2899

Perioperative Patient Care

610.7367
p445k

Third Edition

Perioperative Patient Care
The Nursing Perspective

Julia A. Kneedler, R.N., M.S., Ed.D.
Director, Education Services
Education Design, Inc.

Nursing Faculty
University of Phoenix
Denver, Colorado

Gwen H. Dodge, R.N., M.S.
Education Consultant
Education Design, Inc.
Denver, Colorado

Jones and Bartlett Publishers

Boston   London

POINT LOMA NAZARENE COLLEGE
WITHDRAWN
RYAN LIBRARY

Editorial, Sales, and Customer Service Offices
Jones and Bartlett Publishers
One Exeter Plaza
Boston, MA 02116
1-800-832-0034
617-859-3900

Jones and Bartlett Publishers International
PO Box 1498
London W6 7RS
England

Copyright © 1994, 1987, 1983 by Education Design, Inc.

All rights reserved. No part of the material protected by this copyright
notice may be reproduced or utilized in any form, electronic or mechanical,
including photocopying, recording, or by any information storage and
retrieval system, without written permission from the copyright owner.

Library of Congress Cataloging-in-Publication Data
Perioperative patient care: the nursing perspective / [edited by]
  Julia A. Kneedler, Gwen H. Dodge. — 3rd ed.
    p. cm.
  Includes bibliographical references and index.
  ISBN 0-86720-642-X
  1. Surgical nursing.   I. Kneedler, Julia A.
II. Dodge, Gwen H.
  [DNLM: 1. Surgical Nursing—methods. 2. Intraoperative Care.
3. Preoperative Care. 4. Postoperative Care. WY 161 P445 1994]
RD99.P43 1994
610.73´677—dc20
DNLM/DLC
for Library of Congress   93-31156
                                                        CIP

Printed in the United States of America

97 96 95 94 93   10 9 8 7 6 5 4 3 2 1

This book is dedicated to the members of the Association of Operating Room Nurses, who have a commitment to excellence in the practice of perioperative nursing.

Contents

Foreword

Anyone reading this book will have to agree that that branch of nursing concerned only with the operating room no longer exists. The phrase operating room nursing is replaced by the term perioperative nursing and the use of this new name is a conscious attempt to change the conception of this field of nursing and to promote a truly professional practice.

Thoughts that this branch of nursing is "technical," "mechanical," a "physician's assistant role," or "just not nursing," are dispelled by this book. Perioperative nursing is presented with all its complexities as a professional and specialized field of nursing. The authors describe and stress the rights of patients and the corresponding responsibilities of the nurse, thereby depicting the social contract of professional nursing practice.

The intellectual, clinical, decision-making nature of nursing is described as part of every nurse–patient encounter. Autonomy within the scope of perioperative nursing and the profession's role in regulating that practice are clear. One additional characteristic of the professional nature of perioperative nursing, namely a practice that generates from a distinct knowledge base, is presented by these authors. In addition to being an encyclopedia of perioperative nursing, this book delivers a message on the nature of professional nursing in the 1990s. It is a valuable contribution to the literature.

To label this book incredible is an understatement. The authors have combined in one volume an intensive and extensive presentation of both the art and the science of nursing relevant to the practice of perioperative nursing. The authors deal with the entire scope of perioperative nursing from a perspective that emphasizes psychosocial factors to the same degree as physiological and environmental factors. They have been successful in conveying the need to approach all types of patient cues with equal concern and rigor.

It is obvious that the authors have the experience and academic backgrounds relevant to perioperative nursing. The ease with which they move from the abstract to the concrete, with enough intermediate steps that the novice can track the logical flow, is impressive. Only experts in the field could have such command of both the art and the science. Only truly seasoned, knowledgeable nurses would be able to conceptualize the scope of practice and present nursing actions and the nuances of practice in the detailed manner of these authors.

This book is a valuable contribution to the nursing literature. It will serve as a useful guide for those in practice, as a text for those entering this field of practice, and as a helpful reference for those concerned with the scope and complexity of nursing practice.

Carol A. Lindeman, R.N., Ph.D., F.A.A.N.
Dean, School of Nursing
The Oregon Health Sciences University

Preface

The third edition of *Perioperative Patient Care: The Nursing Perspective* is written in response to the rapid changes in U.S. health care since publication of the second edition in 1987. Escalating health care costs with their associated difficulties are the driving force behind these changes. This third edition hopes to address these changes as well as the following concerns and issues facing the perioperative nurse today.

- The shift from a primarily hospital-based setting to one that includes ambulatory surgery centers and/or one-day surgery units.
- New and expanded technical skills associated with these settings.
- The increasing emphasis on rapid patient assessment with identification of desired outcomes, implementation of nursing activities and evaluation of outcome attainment.

Obviously, the nursing and medical communities, which are exquisitely sensitive to health care indicators, have had to be responsive to changes in technology, assessment and cost containment. We hope this new edition will help perioperative nurses respond effectively to these new demands.

This text presents an innovative approach to the care of patients having surgery. Its intent is to show the progression of the patient, from the decision for surgery until discharge from care. Integrated throughout are the professional and technical roles and functions of the perioperative nurse.

The role of nursing in the healthcare matrix is constantly adapting to society's expectations, scientific and medical advancement, and social change. It is imperative that a nursing resource such as this text operationalize the concept associated with the term *perioperative* as applied to patient care and nursing activities. A complete analysis of the concept of perioperative patient care is given to assist nurses as they strive to fulfill their expanding responsibilities to surgical patients. The content adds to the theory base in nursing and provides a framework for further exploration of concepts underlying perioperative nursing practice. Associated with such a purpose is the intent to furnish a reference point for investigative research to validate the practice described in the text.

We have written this text with practicing registered nurses in mind, in order to guide them in developing their unique role in caring for the perioperative patient. Because students of nursing have limited exposure to perioperative nursing during their formal education, we also hope that nursing faculty will use this text as an adjunct to curriculum content. The text furnishes the novice with a wealth of information about providing care to the surgical patient through the use of the nursing process and implementation of perioperative standards of practice. Other members of the healthcare team will find the text useful in increasing their understanding of the patient's surgical experience. Team members will be able to grasp professional nurses' perioperative functions as well as how they

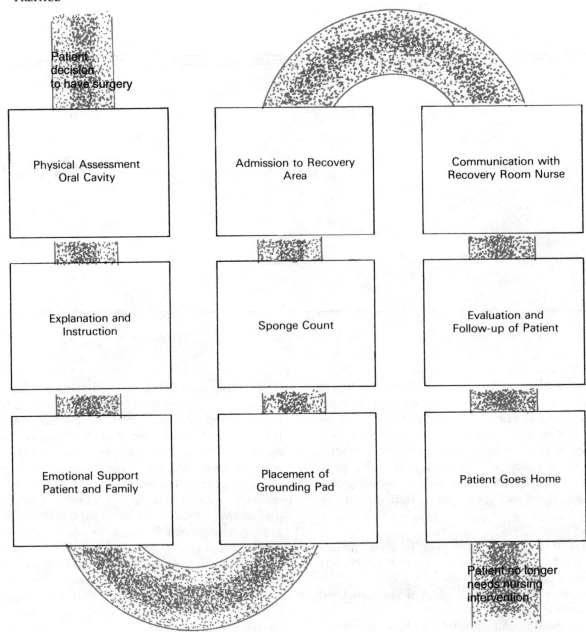

FIGURE 1. Following the patient's surgical intervention.

interrelate as members of a team whose primary goal is to return patients to their highest level of wellness.

Readers of this textbook, whether nurses, students, faculty, or other members of the healthcare team, can readily visualize the organizational framework used to present the content. There are two major focuses throughout—the surgical patient who is the recipient of care and the professional nurse who provides that care during the patient's surgical experience.

We have used an organizational framework that is based on the needs and experiences of the patient having surgery. Preoperatively, it begins with the decision to have surgery, continues through the intraoperative experience, and ends postoperatively when the patient no longer needs nursing care associated with surgery. The text focuses on the patient's surgical intervention as the nurse applies the nursing process through implementation of standards of practice. (See Figure 1.)

The camera lens used as the graphic design at the beginning of each chapter represents the dual focus of the text. (See Figure 2.) Because a camera lens enables one to change focal points without phasing out an image entirely, it was chosen as the model to

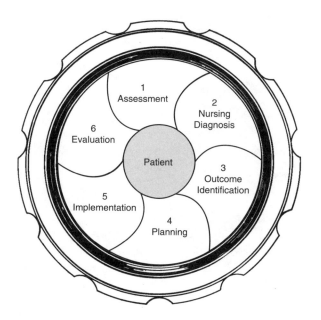

FIGURE 2.   The focal point of nursing practice is the patient.

provide continuity to the text. Throughout perioperative practice, the focal point or center of the lens is the patient.

The nursing process is the framework the nurse uses in providing care. Standards of care and the nursing process are represented as the various lens settings that permit a sharper emphasis on one image without eliminating the central focus. Throughout the text, the reader is visually reminded of the predominant perioperative nursing standard or standards that are specific to that chapter. We have made every attempt to present material in a manner that is practical.

The first three chapters of the third edition include a philosophical discussion of the nurse's approach to perioperative care, a historical review of operating room nursing, and a view of the changing focus of perioperative nursing practice.

Chapter 4 covers the first phase of the nursing process—physiological, psychological, and sociocultural assessment. The second phase—nursing diagnosis—forms the basis for Chapter 5. Chapter 6 reviews the process of outcome identification; it is followed by six chapters analyzing specific outcomes that apply to surgical patients.

The planning and implementation phases of the nursing process are the focus of Chapters 13 and 14. Chapters 15 through 23 deal with specific nursing actions that are performed in the implementation phase, beginning with transporting the patient to the operating room and ending with postanesthesia care.

Evaluating the extent to which expected outcomes are attained and measuring the effectiveness of nursing care through the integration of quality improvment actions are the subjects of Chapters 24 and 25.

We believe that AORN's *Standards of Nursing Practice* are guides to practice and should be used daily. To reinforce this approach, an actual patient situation is used throughout the text. This patient had a left hemiglossectomy, left hemimandibulectomy, and a temporary tracheostomy. The patient's case example starts in Chapter 4, which details his assessment, and ends with evaluation of his care in Chapter 24. A plan of care is included in appropriate chapters to illustrate application of content.

Acknowledgments

The framework described in this text was conceived in 1976 during two intense evenings while the authors were staff employees in the Education Department of the Association of Operating Room Nurses. The individual contributors have added the content and examples which provide a workable model that can easily be implemented by perioperative nurses. Their contributions are a matter of historical record. It was the dozens of practitioners performing patient care in the operating room, however, who made the concept a living reality. Fired with the true pioneer spirit, commitment to quality surgical patient care, and enthusiasm for a broader professional focus, they sallied forth to put the concept into practice. They welcomed the challenge and responded to it. Although individual recognition is not possible here, the authors salute those early advocates and acknowledge the credit they so richly deserve. Without them, the concept would have been just another idea.

Our gratitude to the writers who contributed to the manuscript is profound. Although the material of specific contributing authors has not been credited directly due to editorial considerations, their expertise was essential for a book of this nature. Many of them are nurses practicing perioperative patient care and all of them are busy people. For some, the translation of their expertise into the written word was an arduous and time-consuming task they undertook with some trepidation. We hope their experience positively reinforced their own professional images and helped them to grow. For those for whom writing was easier, we acknowledge the responsibility a commitment of this kind requires and respect the sacrifice of personal time involved. We extend our deepest appreciation for each and every effort.

We are especially indebted to our editor, Linda Sexton, who reviewed the manuscript for consistency and content omissions, suggested organizational revisions, and made sure the level of writing corresponded with the target audience's level of understanding.

Jack Milne, of Denver, and his wife, Florence, were our photographic models for the surgical patient and his family pictured throughout the book. Their concentration on what was being discussed or was supposed to be happening produced photographs of remarkable realism. Mr. Milne's ability to identify with the patient role contributed a great deal to the effectiveness of our planning. Lilly Nelson, a nurse in perioperative patient care, portrayed that role in the photographs. She practices what she modeled and was therefore an effective catalyst in creating the realistic atmosphere for the photographic sessions.

The patient situation, or case study, that illustrates application of content throughout the book is a real one. Although some alteration in certain data was made, we are indebted to Ralph Pfister, who let us share his surgical experiences with the readers and gave us access to his hospital records for that purpose.

Porter Memorial Hospital, Denver, Colorado,

granted permission for us to use its operating room suite for photographs as well as some of its forms and materials. Staff at the hospital critiqued some of the content for accuracy and currency. No institution could have been more supportive or caring.

Steve Nazario, medical illustrator for Porter Hospital, produced several of the graphics. Charles Pfister was responsible for the drawings depicting the standards-camera model. His ability to draw from a verbal description is uncanny.

Last, but certainly not least, we acknowledge the support of our Education Design colleagues, who wrote for the book, did word processing, copying, and all other tasks that are essential in preparing a manuscript for printing. To them, our friends, and family we say thank you for being there when we needed you and for giving us the time to do what had to be done.

Contributors

Carol J. Alexander, MS(N), RN
Director of Nursing Education, Research and
  Resources
Presbyterian/St. Luke's Medical Center
Denver, Colorado

Carol D. Applegeet, MSN, RN, CNOR, CNAA,
  FAAN
Director, Center for Nursing Practice
Association of Operating Room Nurses, Inc.
Doctoral Student, University of Colorado
Denver, Colorado

Margaret A. Camp, MSN, RN
Director of Education
Association of Operating Room Nurses, Inc.
Denver, Colorado

Louise A. Coburn, MS, RN
Manager, Professional Education and Services
Johnson and Johnson Medical, Inc.
Arlington, Texas

Mary E. Craig, RN, CNOR
Staff Development Coordinator, Operating Room
  Nursing
Thomas Jefferson University Hospital
Philadelphia, Pennsylvania

Gwen H. Dodge, MS(N), RN
Education Consultant
Education Design
Denver, Colorado

Julia S. Garner, MN, RN
Nurse Consultant, Hospital Infections Program
National Center for Infectious Diseases
Centers for Disease Control
Atlanta, Georgia

Julian M. Goldman, MD
Assistant Professor of Anesthesiology
University of Colorado School of Medicine
Denver, Colorado

Patricia A. Hercules, MS(N), RN
Manager, Department of Nursing Education
The Methodist Hospital
Houston, Texas

Susan H. Hicks, BSN, RN
Perioperative Nurse
Rose Medical Center
Denver, Colorado

Julia A. Kneedler, MS, EdD, RN
Director, Education Services
Education Design
Nursing Faculty, University of Phoenix
Denver, Colorado

Rose Marie McWilliams, MA, RN
Operating Room Consultant
Administrator, Archdiocese of Denver
Denver, Colorado

Ellen K. Murphy, MS, JD, FAAN
Associate Professor, School of Nursing
University of Wisconsin/Milwaukee
Milwaukee, Wisconsin

Lillian Seene Nelson, MHS, RN, CNOR
Clinical Director of the Operating Room
Providence Medical Center
Seattle, Washington

Paul S. Nelson, MD
Assistant Professor of Anesthesiology
University of Colorado School of Medicine
Denver, Colorado

Annette Parsons, MS, RN, CNOR
Perioperative Practitioner
Medical Practice of Dr. Bruce Baker
Denver, Colorado

June C. Persson, BSN, RN, CNOR
Evening Charge Nurse, Operating Rooms
Methodist Hospital
Sacramento, California

Judith I. Pfister, BS, MBA, RN
President/Laser Consultant
Education Design
Denver, Colorado

Mark Phippen, MN, RN, CNOR
Manager, Main/Dunn Operating Room/PACUs
The Methodist Hospital
Houston, Texas

Janet K. Schultz, MSN, RN
Vice President for Professional Affairs
American Sterilizer Company
Pittsburgh, Pennsylvania

Roma Schweinefus, RN, CCRN, CPAN
Clinical Nurse IV Educator
Rose Medical Center
Denver, Colorado

Linda R. Sexton, BS
Consultant
Education Design
Denver, Colorado

Sharon Sibal, MS, MT(ASCP)SH
QA/QI Consultant
Education Design
Denver, Colorado

Ann Tibbs Thayer, MSN, RN
Staff Nurse, Medical Intensive Care
Veterans Administration Medical Center
Doctoral Candidate, Florida International
    University
Miami, Florida

Elaine Thomson-Keith, BSN, RN, CNOR
Manager, Neurosensory Operating Rooms,
    Postanesthesia Care Unit, Admission,
    Observation, Discharge
The Methodist Hospital
Houston, Texas

Linda A. Tollerud, RN
Head Nurse
The Methodist Hospital
Houston, Texas

Perioperative Patient Care

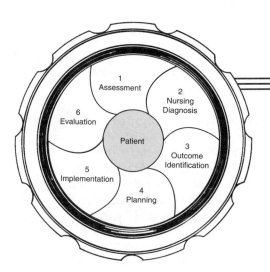

A Philosophical Approach to Perioperative Nursing

Philosophical approaches are reflected in nursing care focused on the patient.

The practice of a perioperative nurse stems from philosophical beliefs about the value of human beings, human life, and general perioperative nursing. The cornerstones of such a philosophy are the cultural and social mores to which the nurse subscribes. A philosophy is the general beliefs, concepts, and attitudes of an individual or group. It reflects the values and general perception of reality based on reasoning. Nursing as a profession has a philosophical basis, and nurses as individuals have philosophies.

Some nurses may be uncomfortable with the intellectual connotation of the word *philosophy*. But whether or not they recognize it as such, all nurses have a philosophy of nursing based on their personal beliefs, values, and attitudes acquired through their professional education. These are then shaped and redefined almost daily by nursing practice and life experiences.

Beliefs about nursing formed while still a nursing student or recent graduate, or even before, change as a nurse gains experience and begins to put theory into practice. Interaction with colleagues and patients, professional practice, and continuing education all constantly reaffirm or reshape each nurse's philosophy. A personal philosophy helps give meaning to the nurse's practice and provides a rational basis for nursing actions.

For the nurse who intends to practice perioperative nursing, an examination of the ideological basis for the role will demonstrate its values and concepts. With only superficial comprehension of the role,

there is danger that the role of the perioperative nurse will remain what it was in the past—a skilled manipulation of equipment and supplies. The contemporary role of the perioperative nurse is patient-oriented—not environment- or physician-oriented.

Examining the philosophical foundations and acquiring concrete awareness of this philosophy have tangible benefits for the nurse. A philosophy is helpful in several ways: it helps define the major beliefs held by an individual; it establishes a direction for action; it determines the level or quality of care; and it is the reference point for evaluation of practice.

Writing down a philosophy helps clarify the concepts underlying nursing practice as well as values and beliefs. A written philosophy need not be lengthy, but should cover the basic components. Once written, a philosophy should not be shelved. It is a working tool, providing guidance for practice and professional behavior.

As a statement of the major beliefs and values of an individual, a philosophy makes short, clear statements that are action-oriented. Take, for example, the statement, "Human beings are holistic individuals with physical, intellectual, emotional, and spiritual needs." This covers a number of separate but related beliefs that direct the nurse's behavior. The nurse who believes in the patient as a whole person with a broad spectrum of needs will attempt to help meet patients' intellectual, emotional, and spiritual needs as well as immediate physical needs.

A philosophy establishes direction for action. For the nurse, a philosophy guides short- and long-term planning and career decisions. A nurse who views the patient holistically would be frustrated in a work environment that did not permit time for caring about individual patient needs and would soon seek other employment. Nurses who have consciously noted their values and beliefs use that self-knowledge to determine whether or not their behavior is in alignment with them. Providing both processes have been honest, the outcomes will furnish the bases for modifying future activity. The aim is to have the value system (philosophy) reflect thinking, feeling, and acting behaviors insofar as is humanly possible.

THE PERIOPERATIVE PERSPECTIVE OF THE PATIENT

The perioperative role of nurses caring for surgical patients is a natural extension of the operating room nurse's traditional role. Before the advent of anesthesia and antiseptic technique, surgery was performed only under dire circumstances, and the specialty of operating room nursing did not exist. Nurses assisted in the operating room and also cared for patients preoperatively and postoperatively. As surgery became safer and more common in the late 1800s, nurses began to specialize in intraoperative patient care, often losing personal contact with patients. Such specialization was instigated by physician specialization in surgery as well as expanding knowledge of asepsis and its application in the field of surgical therapy. Surgeons' demand for skilled surgical nurses and nurses' assumption of responsibility for managing the operating room environment confined nurses to the operating room. They rarely left the surgical suite to communicate with conscious patients. Premedicated patients were often unaware that professional nurses were involved with their care during surgery.

The perioperative patient care concept has made that limited technical role obsolete. The perioperative role is constantly evolving. Nursing has changed so much that the surgical patient's needs have become the focus of practice.

The well-being of patients is the primary concern of all nurses. Nursing consists of a service directed toward alleviating untoward responses to existing or anticipated health problems so that an individual may attain a state of optimal wellness relative to a particular condition. The concept of optimal well-being does not necessarily imply that the patient is restored to health. In the extreme, it may mean that the nurse assists the patient to achieve a peaceful,

natural death. In certain instances, the psychological comfort of human contact may be more important than any material or physiological comforts provided by technology.

Perioperative nurses recognize that a patient's needs are not likely to be satisfied by being connected to the latest machine or by their own understanding of the newest surgical procedure. They realize that the patient may need personal contact, help in coping with fears and anxiety, and explanations other than those provided by the surgeon and anesthetist. They acknowledge their professional and legal accountability for making nursing judgments and decisions within their area of expertise for the optimal well-being of the surgical patient.

For perioperative nurses, the patient is an individual—not a disease, a symptom, or a case. Patients have interdependent physiological, psychological, and social needs and are capable of rational, mature behavior. Nursing views the patient as a total entity and interacts with that whole rather than with one or more of the various parts.

Nurses have not always had such positive views of patients. A strong concept of Western civilization has been that human beings are naturally bad. They are born that way and the aim of designated mentors was to force them into the paths of righteous or good behavior. Education was based on the idea that children need strong discipline imposed by an authoritarian teacher. In healthcare, physicians and nurses replaced the teacher, and the patient assumed the role of the ignorant schoolchild. Patients were expected to obey these authorities without question. Much of the authoritarian behavior of nurses stems from this theory of human nature. Such behavior may annoy or antagonize contemporary patients, producing uncooperative responses or encouraging childish rather than adult reactions.

Healthcare professionals are now influenced by more modern theories of human nature that portray each person as aspiring or evolving. The adaptation model of human nature, based on the theories of Charles Darwin and Sigmund Freud, shows human beings continually adapting to an ever-changing physical and social environment. Calista Roy's model of nursing uses this framework. Maslow's hierarchy of human needs is based on the idea of striving human beings whose basic needs for physiological essentials, safety, and belonging must be partially met before they can look toward satisfying self-esteem needs. Once esteem needs are met to some degree, each person aspires to achieve self-actualization or his own potential (1).

Nurses who believe Maslow's theory feel that a

patient's physiological and psychological needs must be met, not just a gallbladder removed or a cancerous tumor excised. Maslow's theory has come to be a widely accepted basis for contemporary nursing practice.

Perioperative nurses consider the patient as an individual because treating patients in such a way is beneficial to their well-being. The assessment phase of the diagnostic process in nursing is important not only to acquire a data base for health-problem identification but to reduce the patient's anxiety by providing information. By listening to patients' concerns and answering their questions, the nurse shows respect for patients and reaffirms their self-worth.

In the operating room, the nurse continues to treat the patient as an individual. Special needs will have been identified by preoperative assessment data. If the patient is extremely heavy, the necessary special equipment for the patient's safety and comfort will be immediately at hand. In addition, the nurse acts as a patient advocate in the operating room when the patient is incapacitated. For instance, the nurse makes certain the Mayo stand is not resting on the patient's toes or reminds assistants not to lean on the patient's chest. The nurse monitors physiological responses and, if the patient is awake, endeavors to bolster healthy coping mechanisms during the surgical procedure. In some situations, if the surgeon must make an intraoperative decision, the nurse's opinion of the patient's preference, based on preoperative assessment data, may be sought.

The perioperative nurse's view of the patient as a rational and mature individual recognizes and encourages the patient's ability to learn because the patient's cooperation is necessary. In most cases, the patient is internally motivated, recognizing how this is beneficial. Through learning, patients assume a responsibility for their own healthcare. Maturity is recognized by involving patients in planning their own care and giving them the freedom to make choices when feasible. In same-day surgery units, perioperative nurses have a vested interest in applying their belief in a patient's maturity. Brief preoperative and postoperative encounters require all of a nurse's talents and resources to promote a smooth postoperative course. Authoritarian approaches, including scare tactics, are unlikely to encourage compliance with therapy once the patient escapes the authority's presence.

Values discussed above concerning the perioperative patient stem from American cultural and social systems. Additional concepts could have been mentioned that refer to views held about human beings, their lives, and environments. Professional nursing and the healthcare system in the United States obviously incorporate the predominant values of American society. A unique facet of the American values system, however, concerns the number of subcultures to which many citizens belong. Members of such groups subscribe to many components of American cultural and social systems and may additionally hold other or different beliefs particular to their ethnic or national origins. In accordance with American philosophy, perioperative patient care recognizes the cultural beliefs of all segments of society.

THE PERIOPERATIVE PERSPECTIVE OF THE NURSE

Perioperative practice is patient-oriented nursing, benefiting both patient and nurse. For the nurse the role emphasizes the professional, intellectual, and human aspects of nursing and increases responsibility to the patient and his or her family. The patient benefits from direct communication with the perioperative nurse as well as from individualized care. Because the nurse sees the role as significant and gains greater personal satisfaction, better nursing care may be given, which also directly benefits the patient.

As a specialty, perioperative patient care is based on general definitions and concepts of nursing. Nursing has been and still is predominantly a woman's profession. Nurses are still expected to demonstrate so-called feminine characteristics. They are expected to be caring and compassionate, even self-sacrificing. With the women's movement and the shifting role of women in society, the women and men entering the nursing profession bring to it different characteristics. These nurses are no longer willing simply to carry out medically related activities. They clearly see the independent functions of nursing as well as the different focus nursing has in contrast to medicine. Perioperative nursing reflects this perspective. Although perioperative nurses perform medically related activities during surgical procedures, they also give direct nursing care in collaboration with physicians and other healthcare personnel.

As professionals, nurses have become more assertive. Although they still value the caring characteristics of nursing, they expect to be compensated fairly for their work and acknowledged for their professional skills. For both men and women the challenge is not to discard what might be considered feminine—the caring and compassion—but to combine these characteristics with professional knowledge-based nursing.

A philosophy of perioperative patient care from the nursing perspective is predicated upon a philosophy of nursing. Technically, one cannot have a philosophy without a definition of the defining entity. Lack of a commonly accepted definition of nursing is one of the profession's problems identified in *Study of Credentialing in Nursing: A New Approach* (2). Consequently, there are almost as many definitions of nursing as there are nurses. One of the first efforts at defining nursing was made by Florence Nightingale in *Notes on Nursing: What It Is and What It Is Not* (3). She wrote that the knowledge of nursing was "how to put the constitution in such a state as that it will have no disease, or that it can recover from disease" (3). It was her belief that health nursing involved "charge of the personal health of somebody, whether child or invalid" (3). She distinguished in this work between the nursing provided by women in general and the trained nurse. Nightingale described nursing as an art with a specific body of knowledge. According to another of her writings, nursing consists of two types: the "art of nursing proper," involving direct care to the sick, and health nursing for the purpose of keeping people healthy. "Nursing proper is therefore to help the patient suffering from disease to live—just as health nursing is to keep or put the constitution of the healthy child or human being in such a state as to have no disease" (4). This two-pronged belief of nursing as care of the sick and of the healthy persists in modern definitions.

The American Nurses' Association, in *Nursing: A Social Policy Statement*, defined nursing as "the diagnosis and treatment of human responses to actual or potential health problems" (5). Note the term *human responses*. Although the definition has not gained popular acceptance, it contains considerable food for thought.

In developing the perioperative role concept, the Association of Operating Room Nurses Task Force, composed of operating room nurses and other nursing leaders, adopted Rozella Schlotfeldt's definition of nursing in which she holds that nursing is an independent, autonomous, self-regulating profession with the primary function of helping each person attain the highest possible level of general health (6). Furthermore, she believes the practice of nursing focuses

on assessing people's health status, assets, and deviations from health, and on helping

sick people to regain health, and the well or near-well to maintain or attain health through selective application of nursing science and the use of available nursing strategies (6,7).

This statement provides a framework for perioperative nursing practice.

A common theme in all these definitions is that nursing addresses health-related human responses; that is, nursing focuses on the reactions of individuals or groups to actual or potential health problems. In so doing nurses diagnose and treat these responses. For instance, a perioperative nurse who observes signs of anxiety in a patient endeavors to discover the threat to the patient's safety causing the anxiety and, if appropriate, plans strategies for helping the patient cope.

All the definitions fail to acknowledge that there are certain health problems that nurses are qualified and licensed to treat. Such problems include self-care limitations, impaired functioning in areas such as rest and sleep, and stresses related to birth, death, growth, and development.

Nurses use a set of concepts to guide general decisions about what to assess and diagnose, how to intervene, and what to evaluate. This set, in nursing language, is called a conceptual framework. Perioperative practice is based on the nursing process. This six-step process of assessment, nursing diagnosis, outcome identification, planning, implementation, and evaluation is an adaptation of problem-solving theory and widely used in nursing practice. This book will go through the nursing process as it applies to perioperative nursing. In perioperative practice, intellectual activities predominate over technical skills. Although technical skills will always be important in the operating room, technical mastery most often is necessary for tasks that can be delegated to less prepared personnel. Nurses functioning in the perioperative role must value and consciously carry out activities that require intellectual skills and professional preparation. Professional nursing education prepares practitioners for arriving at nursing diagnoses, making data-based decisions, and evaluating outcomes related to patient health problems. Nurses who devote time to technical functions while patient health needs are unmet are wasting professional expertise. They are not fulfilling professional accountability to patients.

Nurses should be able to ascertain what activities they alone can accomplish and concentrate attention in that direction, assigning other activities to nonprofessional personnel. Nurses who demonstrate proficiency and expertise in cleaning and caring for general surgical instruments only make the nonprofessional person wonder why professional nurses are needed in the operating room. For too long, nurses have believed and acted as if they personally had to do everything in the operating room—or elsewhere—otherwise it would not be done properly or safely. The perioperative role is not for nurses who prefer technical to professional activities. Nurses who do not have the inclination, warmth, and skill to work directly with patients have no place in a role emphasizing those qualities.

Perioperative nursing requires a strong philosophical belief that the role is a nursing function in a specialized area. Nurses are nurses before they engage in any of the other roles they are called upon to fulfill. Although the perioperative nurse may have to perform tasks as surgeon's assistant, epidemiologist, or mechanic, these functions are only transitory. Perioperative nurses must see themselves first as nurses before they see themselves as specialists. What influences nursing affects them; what concerns nursing should also concern nurses in a specialist nursing role.

Recognition of the professional activities inherent in the perioperative role and the desire to fulfill them requires commitment. Perioperative nurses have encountered some opposition from nursing colleagues and physicians who see the role as encroaching on their territory. Administrators have argued that perioperative nursing requires more time—an expensive commodity in a cost-conscious era.

Through good communication and documentation by published research findings, nursing colleagues in other areas, as well as physicians, can be shown that perioperative nursing assessment and postoperative evaluation do not detract from the roles of other healthcare professionals but complement them in ways important to the patient. Perioperative nurses must recognize the limits of their role and refrain from infringing on those of others. It is the surgeon's legal responsibility, for instance, to explain to the patient the location, direction, and length of the incision through which the surgical procedure will be performed, just as it is the anesthesiologist's responsibility to discuss the anesthetic agent and its administration. Administrators must be persuaded of the value of quality patient care in attracting patients and surgeons to the hospital and the merit of better communications with patients in preventing complaints and even lawsuits.

Although nurses from the operating room have sometimes met with opposition in implementing the perioperative role, they have also been welcomed with enthusiasm as they have moved into the mainstream of nursing. Nurses in the past have judged colleagues from the operating room as technicians rather than professional nurses. But as perioperative nurses have come to the units to care for patients and demonstrated their knowledge of the nursing process, they have shown colleagues that they are indeed professionals. As they interact with nurses on patient care units and in other areas of the hospital, they are recognized as professional peers.

CODE FOR NURSES

Nursing ethics are an integral part of any nursing philosophy and perioperative patient care. Professional behavior of nurses is guided by the American Nurses' Association *Code for Nurses* (Fig. 1.1). Ethics is a system of moral principles—the rights and wrongs of human behavior and the underlying values. These principles prescribe generally how reasonable human beings should behave in relation to other human beings. Professional ethics are the rules of conduct expected of practitioners to whom society entrusts certain functions. They presuppose the presence of a moral value system of rightful behavior upon which professional rules of conduct can be built. The *Code for Nurses* addresses the professional duties of nursing. Constantly reviewed, the *Code* remains current and applicable to nursing practice as nursing adjusts to social and technological change.

In the first and principal statement, the *Code* establishes the basic responsibility of all nurses to provide services with respect for the human dignity of the patient regardless of social or economic status, personal attributes, or the nature of the health problems. *This is an absolute duty, and there can be no moral justification for any exception. To act otherwise is failure to act as a professional nurse.*

Inherent in this statement, however, is the nurse's right to refuse to participate in the management of health problems or procedures that he or she holds to be morally wrong. In exercising this right, the nurse must give sufficient warning that a certain treatment or procedure constitutes a moral conflict. This may be established at time of employment. Also, adequate and competent nursing care must be available for the patient. These two conditions imply that the patient's right to care supersedes the nurse's right to refuse to give care. Consider the following situation: On emergency call, a nurse is called in for a cesarean section on a 30-year-old woman with a footling presentation.

Preamble

A code of ethics makes explicit the primary goals and values of the profession. When individuals become nurses, they make a moral commitment to uphold the values and special moral obligations expressed in their code. The Code for Nurses is based on a belief about the nature of individuals, nursing, health, and society. Nursing encompasses the protection, promotion, and restoration of health; the prevention of illness; and the alleviation of suffering in the care of clients, including individuals, families, groups, and communities. In the context of these functions, nursing is defined as the diagnosis and treatment of human responses to actual or potential health problems.

Since clients themselves are the primary decision makers in matters concerning their own health, treatment, and well-being, the goal of nursing actions is to support and enhance the client's responsibility and self-determination to the greatest extent possible. In this context, health is not necessarily an end in itself, but rather a means to a life that is meaningful from the client's perspective.

When making clinical judgments, nurses base their decisions on consideration of consequences and of universal moral principles, both of which prescribe and justify nursing actions. The most fundamental of these principles is respect for persons. Other principles stemming from this basic principle are autonomy (self-determination), beneficence (doing good), nonmaleficence (avoiding harm), veracity (truth-telling), confidentiality (respecting privileged information), fidelity (keeping promises), and justice (treating people fairly).

In brief, then, the statements of the code and their interpretation provide guidance for conduct and relationships in carrying out nursing responsibilities consistent with the ethical obligations of the profession and with high quality in nursing care.

Code for Nurses

1. The nurse provides services with respect for human dignity and the uniqueness of the client, unrestricted by considerations of social or economic status, personal attributes, or the nature of health problems.
2. The nurse safeguards the client's right to privacy by judiciously protecting information of a confidential nature.
3. The nurse acts to safeguard the client and the public when healthcare and safety are affected by the incompetent, unethical, or illegal practice of any person.
4. The nurse assumes responsibility and accountability for individual nursing judgments and actions.
5. The nurse maintains competence in nursing.
6. The nurse exercises informed judgment and uses individual competence and qualifications as criteria in seeking consultation, accepting responsibilities, and delegating nursing activities to others.
7. The nurse participates in activities that contribute to the ongoing development of the profession's body of knowledge.
8. The nurse participates in the profession's efforts to implement and improve standards of nursing.
9. The nurse participates in the profession's effort's to establish and maintain conditions of employment conducive to high quality nursing care.
10. The nurse participates in the profession's effort to protect the public from misinformation and misrepresentation and to maintain the integrity of nursing.
11. The nurse collaborates with members of the health professions and other citizens in promoting community and national efforts to meet the health needs of the public.

FIGURE 1.1. *Code for Nurses.* (Copyright © by the American Nurses' Association, 1985. Reprinted with permission of the American Nurses' Association.)

One of the infant's legs has been delivered, but the other is crossed upon its upper abdomen, and the obstetrician cannot grasp the ankle and straighten the leg to deliver the infant vaginally. The infant is showing signs of distress. While the nurse is setting up for the procedure, the physician informs the nurse that he also intends to perform a tubal ligation at the patient's request. The nurse is opposed to any form of birth control on moral grounds and does not want to participate in the procedure. But there is no other nurse available who has the necessary knowledge and skills to provide nursing care. The nurse in this situation cannot refuse to participate in the patient's care because delay would further compromise the infant and could endanger the mother's life. Under no circumstances is it permissible to abandon the patient.

The first three statements of the *Code* outline the nurse's obligation to protect patient rights and safety. Patients' right to control what is done to their

persons is also addressed in the first statement. The right to privacy, spoken to in the second statement, requires constant vigilance. In the operating room these rights are protected by preventing unnecessary exposure of the patient and excluding all but essential personnel from the room. Patient records are of course confidential, but the patient's privacy is also considered in conversations that might be overheard or when posting surgical schedules.

Research indicates that under general anesthesia some patients are able to recall conversations among surgical team members (8). Discussion of anatomical characteristics of patients, off-color jokes, and other non-health-problem-related comments might be remembered by a patient and considered a violation of the privacy right.

Under the third statement, the nurse acts as an advocate to protect the patient from incompetent, unethical, or illegal practice. Especially in the operating room, where patients are unable to defend themselves, this is an important nursing responsibility. The nurse has the responsibility to bring any substandard or improper care to the attention of the person providing that care. If corrective measures are not taken, the next highest person in the chain of command must be informed. In a 1981 lawsuit that involved a surgeon removing nineteen feet of a patient's small bowel through a perforated uterus, the operating room nurses were asked whether they should have stopped the surgeon. They believed they could question the surgeon if their observations clearly indicated something was wrong, but they could not stop him or interrupt the procedure (9). The nurses were found liable by the court based on the testimony of expert witnesses who stated that professional ethics and hospital procedure demand that nurses stop a doctor's action if in their judgment it is incorrect. This decision was appealed to a higher court, but is illustrative of the seriousness of the nurse's responsibility as outlined in this segment of the *Code*.

Nurses have a responsibility to act if aware of negligence, and failure to do so constitutes negligence on their part if harm is sustained by the patient. Nurses have encountered hostility and resistance from physicians, administrators, and their nursing peers when they have raised questions about patient care or the competency of caregivers. At least one state, Oregon, passed a law protecting nurses and others who report questionable practice. Hospitals should also have written policies and procedures for reporting substandard or questionable practice.

The next three statements of the *Code* address nurses' qualifications in giving patient care. The fourth concerns nurses' responsibility and accountability for nursing judgments and actions. Perioperative nurses comply with this principle, for example, by documenting care in the patient's record, completing incident reports, making nursing diagnoses based on facts, and performing postoperative evaluations. They also participate in hospital or departmental quality-assurance programs and peer review processes for measuring the effectiveness of care and correcting deficiencies.

The fifth statement obligates nurses to maintain competency in nursing. Although the merits of mandatory continuing education for nursing license renewal are debatable, most nurses believe continuing education is essential for maintaining competency. They regularly attend workshops, seminars, courses, and national meetings to update their knowledge and skills. Accountability for continued competency is evidenced by the number of nurses who voluntarily seek certification as a generalist or specialist.

The sixth statement encourages nurses to use expert judgment and awareness of their own competence and qualifications in accepting responsibility, seeking help, and delegating nursing activities to others. Nurses in the operating room, for instance, are sometimes asked to staff the postanesthesia care unit. If they lack knowledge and skills in caring for patients recovering from anesthesia, they should not accept the assignment until the needed education has been acquired. Nurses also should exercise judgment in delegating nursing activities to nonprofessionals. Although technicians have been well accepted in the operating room in the scrub position, their training prepares them to perform only technical tasks, not professional functions. In perioperative patient care, nurses perform supervisory functions, circulating duties, and other activities that require professional nursing education and skills. These activities include collecting data from patients, making nursing diagnoses, developing patient care plans, and evaluating patient care. Delegating professional responsibilities to personnel who are not qualified to meet them is ethically wrong and, in several states, illegal.

Although the last five statements refer to nurses' responsibility to the profession and society, many nurses overlook these obligations. All nurses benefit from the activities of professional organizations. Yet of the more than 1 million working nurses, less than 25 percent belong to the American Nurses' Association (ANA). The Association of Operating Room Nurses (AORN) estimated that about 50 percent of nurses working in the operating room belong to it. Statement number seven of the *Code* indicates that nurses should contribute to the profession's body of knowledge. This means they have an obligation to conduct or participate in nursing research, to write for publication, or to develop speaking skills so knowledge may be shared with colleagues. Developing and testing nursing diagnoses is a professional arena likely to profit from perioperative nurse involvement. Designing workshops and acting as preceptors in the perioperative role are other activities.

The eighth statement refers to nurses' obligation to implement and improve standards of nursing. The ANA and AORN originally jointly published standards for perioperative nursing, and AORN has published standards for perioperative nursing practice plus a number of recommended technical practices. Nevertheless, some nurses resist using these practice references, preferring to rely on ritualistic practice—"the way it has always been done." But most nurses welcome the opportunity to base their practice on generally accepted standards and research findings.

The ANA has been active for many years in upgrading the economic and general welfare of nurses. Through its state associations, it now represents nurses in collective bargaining units working toward conditions of employment conducive to high-quality healthcare, as mandated in the ninth statement. The ANA also is deeply involved in national healthcare legislation and, through its Washington office, monitors federal government activities of concern to nurses and nursing. Constituent state associations carry on these activities at the state level. Although not registered as a union and not involved in collective bargaining, AORN has supported the registered nurse as supervisor and circulator in the operating room when regulatory agencies attempted to downgrade these positions. Members participated in these efforts by writing letters to agencies, members of Congress, and newspapers.

Nurses, also have an obligation to participate in the profession's efforts, as stated in the tenth proposition of the *Code*, to protect the public from misinformation and misrepresentation. Because nurses teach and provide information about healthcare, they are cautioned against endorsing or implying endorsement of any commercial products or services in advertising through public media. Intentional or implied endorsement of a product or service by a nurse in public advertising may be interpreted by the public as professional approval. Nursing is also frequently misrepresented in public media (10, 11). Nurses are working to correct the false image and establish in the public's mind a truly professional image of nursing.

Nurses are expected to have concerns about society's health in general. The final statement of the *Code* speaks to nurses' obligation to work with other healthcare professionals and citizens to support community and national efforts to meet healthcare needs of the public. Their concern should go beyond individual patients to include participation in local or national health goals. Nurses carry out this obligation by volunteering their services for hypertension, cancer, and other screening programs, blood and United Way contribution drives, and health fairs. They act as first-aid counselors for scout troops and teach Red Cross lifesaving classes. They are active in promoting public awareness of health problems, such as multiple sclerosis and sudden infant death syndrome, and through participation in voluntary health groups. Nurses have also become increasingly aware and active politically in recent years.

The *Code* provides a framework for making ethical decisions as well as a yardstick for measuring ethical conduct. Since it is impossible to address all the situations in which nurses may have to make ethical decisions, the *Code* considers in general the major ethical issues confronting nurses. Representing the moral values held by the profession, the *Code* indicates to both nurses and the public the responsibilities and expectations required by the profession. It is the profession's response to the trust invested by society in nursing. For amplification, see *The Code for Nurses with Interpretative Statements* (12).

Although the *Code for Nurses* is not a legally binding document, in malpractice cases it is cited as the standard of conduct for the profession. Some of its values have been incorporated into nursing practice acts or rules and regulations governing the practice of nursing. Most nurses comply voluntarily with the *Code's* precepts. Failure to abide by its principles erodes the public trust, threatening nursing's control over professional matters and affairs.

IDEALS VERSUS REALITY

The ideals acquired in school sometimes are threatened when nurses begin to practice. Nurses may find their philosophy of nursing conflicts with that of their employer, and they find that society's expectations for healthcare cannot always be met.

Making the transition from the educational setting to the practice setting can be difficult. Basic education provides nurses with facts, principles, values, and beliefs. These are obtained through contact with faculty, student peers, and practicing nurses as well as through nursing courses. The type of education they receive influences their philosophy of nursing. Associate degree programs are geared to produce nurses proficient in technical and clinical skills. Four-year programs are designed to prepare nurses with greater depth in understanding a patient's physiological and psychosocial responses. Regardless of basic preparation, moving into the work setting will shake and test each nurse's ideals. Ideals may survive and grow stronger, or they may be abandoned.

Nurses talk about reality shock. Later they talk about burnout. Many become disillusioned and leave nursing. Baccalaureate nurses feel they have wasted expensive college educations when their knowledge is denigrated by physicians and even other nurses. Many nurses are frustrated when they are unable to practice the nursing they learned in school. During students' clinical experience, for example, they may have cared for one or two surgical patients at a time. Their learning experience with these patients probably allowed adequate opportunity to diagnose health problems, write outcomes and plans of care, and evaluate care. But now that they are in practice, life is much more hectic. They are so busy managing the care of many patients, they can only spend a brief time with each patient, completing a minimal assessment.

As a result of different educational and personal backgrounds, nurses vary in their philosophies. In the operating room, some are patient-oriented while others are more concerned with technical aspects of care. For instance, a common problem for surgical patients is anxiety. The patient-oriented nurse learns ways to help patients cope with anxiety and, as part of his or her philosophy of practice, helps them alleviate their anxiety. A technically oriented nurse might not have the skills to recognize the problem, particularly if the patient has disguised it, or might not feel capable of helping the patient.

The healthcare facility's philosophy may also influence how nursing is practiced. In a cost-conscious environment, the quality of patient care may suffer. This is not only frustrating but presents a moral dilemma for nurses who cannot, because of staffing and time, meet their own standards of patient care. The facility might discourage perioperative nursing care because it requires additional staffing. But if the philosophy is oriented to a high level of patient care, it might see preoperative assessment by a nurse from the operating room as an important component of patient care.

The institution's philosophy will also dictate the proportion of professional nurses to patients and the ratio of nurses to paraprofessionals. If it believes in the best individual care for patients, it will have a high number of professional nurses to patients and a low number of paraprofessionals. In the operating room where patient care is given a high priority, there will be a high proportion of nurses to technicians. In purchasing, nurses and physicians will participate in decisions about supplies and equipment. Patient safety will be more important than cost alone.

While the facility's philosophy affects nursing practice, nurses also influence the facility's philosophy. Nurses are gaining stronger representation in management, where they can make the importance of their philosophy of care known. They are serving on committees and interacting with administrators and physicians. Through collective bargaining, nurses are negotiating contracts that establish working conditions with sufficient staffing to provide good nursing care. Although at one time nurses saw themselves as powerless against administrators and physicians, they are now realizing their importance in the institutions' structure and are being more assertive in working toward what they believe is important to patient care.

COSTS OF CARE

Nurses feel that they are caught in the dilemma of society's expectations for healthcare and the decreasing ability to pay for it. One of nursing's basic beliefs is that everyone is entitled to healthcare regardless of ability to pay. Healthcare is one of the primary social needs of any society. The World Health Organization adopted the goal of "healthcare for all by the year 2000." Many countries have instituted national health insurance or socialized medicine as the way to provide healthcare for all its citizens. But the United States, despite its wealth and sophisticated medical technology, is seeing a widening gap between healthcare for those who can afford it and those who cannot. Once a burn patient was turned away from more than 40 medical centers because he had no insurance and no way to pay for his care. In the past, hospitals were able to absorb costs of indigent patients through charges to private patients, or local agencies paid the bills. Then with the Great Society of the 1960s, Medicare and Medicaid were enacted to pay for healthcare of the elderly and the poor. National health insurance was a goal. Everyone would have equal access to healthcare regardless of ability to pay.

That was the ideal, but now we face the reality. Healthcare costs have risen so drastically that they are a drain on the national economy. The causes are multiple. Medicare and Medicaid as well as tax incentives for private medical insurance are blamed. Since most healthcare costs are paid by insurers, the consumer is not cost conscious. Lawsuits and the availability of high technology encourage expensive diagnostic testing, and treatments which then may be followed by sophisticated care such as that offered in intensive care units.

Paying for and providing access to healthcare is one of our most critical social problems. The government, private insurers, and the healthcare industry are looking for ways to solve the problem. Like the causes, the solutions will also be multiple. It seems unlikely, however, that we will be able to return to the past. Cost containment and cost consciousness now and in the future will be constraints on healthcare. People may be willing to accept a lower level of care. One poll indicated that 54 percent of the respondents were willing to accept cheaper and more limited insurance coverage. The implication is that they might be willing to consult with a nurse practitioner rather than a physician; that they might be willing to go to a clinic rather than to a private office. Ambulatory surgery will continue to be used for many surgical procedures, while hospital-stay surgery will decrease.

In this last decade of the twentieth century, multiple philosophical and ethical issues associated with the cost of providing healthcare must be faced in this country. Every nurse, as a citizen, has a responsibility to know what these issues are, to take a position on them, and to participate in the decisions made about them. When confronting the ever-escalating cost of providing healthcare, professional nurses may be required to modify their patient advocacy position in the general sense, if not in the individual sense. This, in itself, will constitute a philosophical change of major proportions in the nursing community.

A strong philosophy will give the nurse direction when faced with the demands of society, the expectations of patients and of the nursing profession, and even self-imposed demands. As the nurse learns and gains experience, this philosophy will continue to evolve, but its base will be the values and beliefs acquired early in life. With experience, a nurse's philosophy of nursing practice will be strengthened or, if necessary, changed. Experience will either validate existing beliefs or indicate where they need to be reexamined. A philosophy gives essential strength and support to a nurse's practice.

REFERENCES

1. Maslow, A. H. *Motivation and Personality.* New York: Harper and Row, 1954.
2. American Nurses' Association. *Study of Credentialing in Nursing: A New Approach.* Kansas City: ANA, 1979.
3. Nightingale, F. *Notes on Nursing: What It Is and What It Is Not.* London: Harrison and Sons, 1859.
4. Nightingale, F. "Sick nursing and health nursing." In: I. Hampton, ed. *Nursing the Sick 1893.* New York: McGraw-Hill, 1949.
5. American Nurses' Association. *Nursing: A Social Policy Statement.* Kansas City: ANA, 1980.
6. Schlotfeldt, R. M. "Planning for progress." *Nurs Outlook* 21:766–769, 1973.
7. Schlotfeldt, R. M. "Operating Room Nursing: Perioperative Role" *AORN Journal* 27:1156–1175, 1978.
8. Guerra, F., and Aldrete, A. J., eds. *Emotional and Psychological Responses to Anesthesia and Surgery.* New York: Grune and Stratton, 1980.
9. Cushing, M. "A matter of judgment." *Am J Nurs* 82(6):992, 1982.
10. Kalisch, P., and Kalisch, B. "Nurses on prime-time television." *Am J Nurs* 82(2):262–270, 1982.
11. Kalisch, P., and Kalisch, B. "The image of the nurse in motion pictures." *Am J Nurs* 82(4):605–611, 1982.
12. American Nurses' Association: *The Code for Nurses with Interpretative Statements.* Kansas City: ANA, 1985.

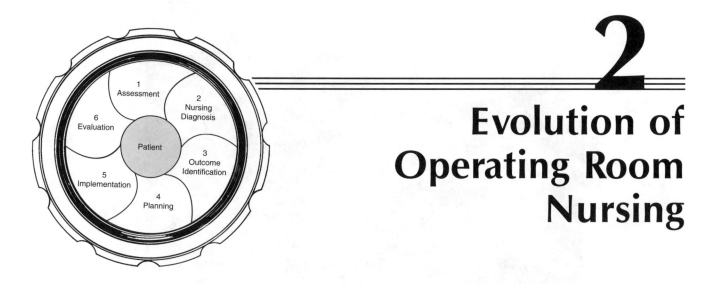

Evolution of Operating Room Nursing

Operating room nursing has continued to progress.

The specialty of operating room nursing emerged in the late 1880s as the number of operations increased and surgeons recognized the important assistance nurses provided. According to Eva C. E. Luckes, an English nurse in the late nineteenth century, nurses were shadow figures in the operating room who handed and wrung out sponges and kept the operating theater "fresh" (Fig. 2.1). Luckes added, "Nurses are not there to *see* the operation . . . but to make their presence realized by the perfectly quiet way in which all wants are foreseen or supplied" (1). Care of the patient and preparation of the operating room were not considered nursing responsibilities until later. Instrument care was not a duty, but Luckes did advise nurses, "It is well for you to notice them as you have the opportunity. They should be covered with a towel, that the patient may be spared the sight of them" (1).

EARLY SURGERY

In the mid-nineteenth century, surgery was a new specialty making some remarkable advances. Although surgeons had adequate knowledge of surgical anatomy and physiology, surgical mortality was high. "Pain, hemorrhage, infection, and gangrene were rife in the hospital wards and mortality from surgical instruments was as high as ninety and even one hundred percent" (2). Concepts of antisepsis were vague, and many surgeons thought infections in surgical wounds should be encouraged. Surgeons

were also careless, frequently operating in their street clothes, using the same instruments on patient after patient, and only washing their hands *after* surgery. In fairness to the surgeons and hospitals of this era, their cities and towns were also unsanitary and dirty, and personal hygiene was poor. Accident victims frequently arrived at hospitals for surgery with an infection already started.

As a result, surgery was usually performed as a last resort. Most operations were limited to "the removal of superficial tumors of various sorts, drainage of infection, traumatic surgery, removal of stone in the bladder, and operations about the head and face . . . operations upon the contents of the peritoneal and pleural cavity were practically unknown" (3).

Antiseptic techniques and anesthesia changed the course of surgery and the role of the operating room nurse. Antisepsis and, later, asepsis dramatically reduced surgical mortality from infection. Anesthesia not only made surgery painless, but made it possible for the surgeon to perform longer procedures. Gradually, surgery became a means to improve and prolong life instead of a last resort. Most important for operating room nurses, "Lister's revolutionary discovery of the value of antisepsis in surgery . . . made it absolutely necessary that nurses should be of such an intellectual calibre and development as would permit them to be trained in the prevention of infection through absolute cleanliness" (4).

As surgery became more complex and demand-

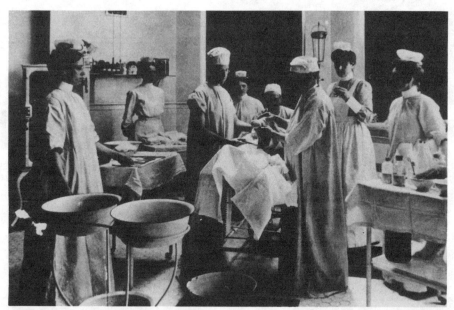

FIGURE 2.1.   During the early years of surgery, nurses came from patient care units to perform technical tasks needed by surgeons. They donned coverups to protect uniforms and wore nursing caps. Surgery was performed without gloves, and hands were cleansed by washing in an antiseptic solution. Anesthesia consisted of open-drop ether or chloroform administered through a gauze-covered, cone-shaped mask. Windows in every operating room provided natural daylight for surgical visibility and could be opened on warm days for air circulation. Upon completion of the operation, the same nurses accompanied the patient back to the surgical ward, providing care until discharge. One junior nurse or nursing student was left behind to clean the room and equipment. There might be one highly skilled nurse permanently assigned to the operating room to supervise tasks performed by transient nurses and to prepare sponges, linen, instruments, pans, and sutures needed in the future. (Photograph c. 1890–1900, courtesy of Porter Memorial Hospital Audiovisual Department, Denver.)

ing, nurses acquired new and broader responsibilities. For example, the Scottish physician Joseph Bell (c. 1888) required nurses to prepare patients, instruments, table sponges, dressings, and the patient's bed. He suggested that nurses prepare checklists of the instruments they used. Because nurses in the operating room had new responsibilities, Bell said they needed "very special training . . . for certain important surgical cases and operations. You must try to get this from the senior staff nurses, from the residents, and even a few most precious hints from the acting surgeon" (5).

EARLY TRAINING PROGRAMS AND NURSING EDUCATION

General training programs for nurses were first established in hospitals, using the model developed by Florence Nightingale in England. In 1873 three Nightingale schools were opened in the United States: Bellevue in New York City, the Connecticut Training School in New Haven, and the Massachusetts General Hospital Training School in Boston. These schools were among the first in the U.S. to change the existing concept of nursing as a subservient and menial profession. They were established to improve the care of the sick and to educate nurses. These goals, plus Nightingale's belief that nursing schools should be controlled and run by qualified nursing staff, ruffled many physicians' feathers. Others criticized the Nightingale programs for overtraining nurses.

Today, when we look back on nurses' training programs of the late 1800s and early 1900s, these concerns seem inappropriate. The early Nightingale programs were usually only one year long, with student nurses committed to another year's employment with the hospital upon completion of the program. Curriculum was dictated by services offered by the hospital. There were no real classes and few formal lectures, and faculty did not follow standards or use curriculum guides. Instruction was usually carried out at the patient's bedside, where daily nursing functions were conducted at the same time. There was a variety of instructors—physicians, staff nurses, and other nursing students. Student nurses also took on housekeeping and cooking chores at their hospital, and during their first year of training, they were generally paid—sometimes $4 to $10 a month (6)!

Operating room nursing education began at Massachusetts General Hospital in 1876 when student nurses were first allowed in the operating room for clinical instruction (6). By the 1880s many hospitals were integrating specialty instruction, such as operating room nursing, into their nurses' training. By the early 1900s student nurses were regularly placed in operating rooms for daily clinical experience, and it would be safe to say that nurses' training programs identified specific content for preparing OR nurses. For example, the National League of Nursing Education incorporated a section on operating room technique into its standard curriculum in 1919. The content included the nurse's duties in relation to equipment, the sterilizing room, the instrument and supply room, preparation of dressings and supplies, and duties during surgery (6).

Clinical experience in the operating room could vary widely. For example, a student nurse could be required to prepare surgical patients and operating rooms:

> She sterilized supplies and made sterile salt solutions. . . . The gas pipe railing around the rising rows of wooden seats in the amphitheatre had to be wiped with carbolic and the seats were damp-dusted with bichloride of mercury. She had already soaked towels and bandages in bichloride the night before and hung them to dry. She had to consider the needs of the anesthetist and be prepared to handle instruments or sponges. Natural sea sponges were prepared for use in the operation after sand and shell were beaten from them. Boric acid crystals were used in the abdominal cavity; packing was iodized gauze. The pupil nurse would spend the whole day in the operating room, which was airtight as could be, and her dinner was brought in on a tray (6).

Students were also required to know the properties and uses of anesthetics, to hold the patient's jaw and sponge out mucus during anesthetization, and to administer artificial respiration if necessary.

EMERGENCE OF OR NURSING AS A SPECIALTY

The actual specialty of operating room nursing emerged in 1888 at Johns Hopkins Hospital in Baltimore, partly the result of an attempt to pacify two feuding nurses. A graduate of Bellevue Hospital School of Nursing, Isabel Hampton came to Johns Hopkins in 1889 as its director of nursing. She was also charged with organizing a school of nursing for the hospital. Caroline Hampton (no relation to Isabel) arrived in 1889 as head nurse of the hospital's surgical division. There is disagreement about what happened between them.

One report says that "an intense animosity" existed between the nurses because Caroline, a Southerner, disliked taking orders from Isabel, a Canadian. Hopkins' chief of surgery, William S. Halsted, appointed Caroline operating room supervisor to relieve some of the tension that existed between the women (7). A second version has Isabel appointing Caroline head nurse of the surgical wards in an attempt to relieve an apparent shortage of nurses. There are those, however, who believe the appointment was made "to limit Caroline Hampton's activities to the operating room" (8).

In 1894 Hunter Robb, an associate in gynecology at Johns Hopkins, suggested that a team be used in the hospital's operating rooms. His recommendation that a surgeon, the head nurse, a second nurse, and five assistant surgeons be present at every operation was quickly adopted. The head nurse became the scrub nurse; the second nurse performed "all duties which involve the handling of any articles which have not been rendered aseptic" and watched for "any opportunity to be of service to the surgeon and his assistants" (9). By the turn of the century, the operating room team concept was being used in hospitals throughout the United States, and nurses became permanent and necessary members of every surgical team.

The specialty of operating room nursing had evolved: operating room technique had become a recognized part of nursing education curricula, and operating room nurses had become integral members of the operating room team. All this was accomplished during the last 50 years of the nineteenth century. The twentieth century would see growth and refinement of operating room nursing.

It took two world wars to project nursing in general into a position of national interest and importance. Operating room nursing naturally benefited from this national attention. By the end of the Spanish-American War in 1900, Dr. Anita Newcomb

McGee saw a critical need to organize and improve healthcare delivery in the armed forces. Hospital corpsmen had been trained to care for the sick and wounded, but in wartime, there were too few corpsmen and too little time to train them. McGee proposed that fully accredited graduate nurses be enlisted for military nursing service. Within 10 years the fledgling Army Nurse Corps had 233 regular nurses and 170 reserve nurses (7).

During World War I, nurses' roles were primarily limited to caring for the sick and wounded recuperating at base and auxiliary hospitals. About 10,000 nurses served overseas. Because most were women, none was stationed at field hospitals, which were on or near the front. Goodnow wrote, "Most wounds were from shrapnel, a few were from bombs, still fewer from bullets. Wounds of the head and face were common and terrible" (10). Most surgeons took a somewhat conservative approach to surgery because of the serious threat of infection. Wounds were generally stabilized and the patients sent to a base hospital for further treatment. Most patients arrived at the base hospital with an infection raging— not because of poor surgical or medical treatment but because of the poor hygienic conditions in the trenches. Goodnow added, however, that "dental and plastic surgery was perfected; the Carrel-Dakin treatment for infected wounds was developed. All these new methods needed expert nurses" (10).

The global nature of World War II created new roles and responsibilities for women and for nurses in particular. Nurses in the armed forces as well as those serving in volunteer agencies such as the Red Cross found themselves working at the battlefront, in prisoner-of-war camps, and in the midst of air, land, and sea attacks. In the face of personnel shortages, both military and civilian nurses were required to take on new administrative roles and expand their nursing functions in many areas. The operating room team, including the nurse, performed in a variety of environments and conditions. With the development of sulfa and penicillin and the subsequent reduction in postoperative infection, wartime surgery became more aggressive. Larger, more specialized teams were required to handle heavier surgical loads, and operating room nurses were required to perform a wider range of duties. In fact, an operating room nurse's responsibilities frequently included anesthesia, asepsis, and sanitation; preparation of the surgical patient, instruments, and the operating area; supervision of other OR personnel; and under special circumstances, surgical assistance.

Nurses returning from military service wanted to retain many of these new responsibilities in civilian hospitals and in operating rooms. By the late 1940s, operating room nurses managed the care of patients in the operating room and assisted surgeons. Many OR nurses also believed it was time to organize the members of their specialty to pool professional knowledge and exchange new ideas. In January 1949, seventeen operating room supervisors in the New York City area met to discuss forming an independent association of operating room nurses. A month later, officers and a board of directors were elected from a group of fifty-six staff and administrative operating room nurses. These nurses appointed a committee to work with the American Nurses' Association (ANA) and the National League for Nursing (NLN) in forming an independent organization solely for operating room nurses.

FORMATION OF AORN

The first national conference of the Association of Operating Room Nurses (AORN) was held in 1954. At this meeting, ANA and NLN officers joined AORN members to look at the question posed by the association: "Where do we belong?" (among nursing organizations). Although the panel discussion was inconclusive, the program led to an agreement to explore the issue further. By 1956 AORN's officers and board of directors felt the association was ready for "a special affiliation with ANA permitting it to hold an annual national meeting and develop the specialty of nursing in the operating room" (11). The ANA disagreed and countered the board's proposal, stating that its programs already met OR nurses' needs. Nevertheless, the AORN board of directors presented the plan to the House of Delegates at the association's annual meeting in 1956. The plan was enthusiastically accepted, a constitution and bylaws were adopted, and officers and a board of directors elected. Edith Dee Hall, a driving force behind the advancement of operating room nursing who strongly promoted the idea of an independent OR nursing organization, was appointed executive secretary. Her New York City apartment became the association's first national headquarters.

By 1960 organized groups or chapters of AORN existed throughout the United States. The primary purpose of the newly formed association was to exchange ideas, gain new knowledge, and explore methods of improving nursing care of patients undergoing surgery. At first, the association's goals were (11):

1. to stimulate operating room nurses in other parts of the country to form similar groups.
2. to be a specific group to pool and share nursing knowledge and technology.
3. to provide surgical patients with optimal care through a broad educational program.
4. to make a body of knowledge available to operating room nurses.
5. to motivate experienced operating room nurses to share their expertise with others.
6. to be an association for the benefit of all professional operating room nurses.

CLINICAL PRACTICE DEFINED

In the early 1960s AORN faced one of its first great challenges. The nature of nursing education was changing, with increasing emphasis placed on the college- or baccalaureate-prepared nurse. The focus was shifting from hospital-based programs that offered student nurses maximum experience in the operating room, to four-year college programs that stressed a broader psychosocial approach to patient care. In these programs, operating room nursing was sometimes overlooked as less patient-oriented and more technical in practice. In 1969, concerned for the future of professional nurses, the Association adopted a "Definition and objectives for clinical practice of professional operating room nursing." It was AORN's first attempt at defining nursing care in the operating room.

The organization was concerned with the nature of operating room practice, the means for improving that practice, standards for practice, and the appropriate education for operating room nurses. The 1969 statement provided guidelines for nursing educators and administrators who wanted to incorporate concepts of OR nursing into their curriculum or daily patient care. Operating room staff nurses could use the statement in developing a professional role that included providing nursing care to their patients before, during, and after surgery.

Further clarification of the operating room nurse's role was required in the 1970s. Nurses in other specialties based their practice around the nursing process: they assessed patients' physical and emotional needs and then planned, implemented, and evaluated the care they performed in terms of these needs. Nurses argued that the nursing process could not be applied in the operating room. They also said that nursing in general had outgrown the "handmaiden" image that OR nurses seemed to retain. Still other health professionals suggested that nursing care was no longer necessary in the operating room since nonnursing personnel, such as operating room technicians, had been trained to perform scrub and other duties previously performed by nurses.

These challenges prompted delegates at the Association's 1973 congress to approve a statement on the necessity for the registered nurse in the operating room. The statement showed that professionals with a nurse's training and background were necessary for the optimal care of surgical patients. Unlike OR nurses, personnel trained only to carry out certain technical duties could not adequately care for patients physically and emotionally. The statement also maintained that operating room nurses used the nursing process in their care of surgical patients: they assessed the needs of patients coming to surgery; planned and implemented preoperative, intraoperative, and postoperative care to meet these needs; and then documented their care.

DEVELOPMENT OF STANDARDS OF PRACTICE

Many AORN members believed that more was needed to keep their specialty viable. In the late 1960s the nursing community began to look at the need to establish standards that would guide the practice of nursing. It was thought that such standards would demonstrate nursing's concern for the patient and the quality of care being provided. The first standards, developed by the American Nurses' Association in 1973, became the model for standards in specialty nursing. These were generic standards that focused on the nursing process. In 1975, Standards of Nursing Practice: OR (12) were published jointly by the AORN and ANA. These standards later became the Standards of Perioperative Nursing Practice (13). The Association encouraged nurses to use the standards in their daily practice and to incorporate them into the existing philosophy and objectives of their operating rooms.

During the next fifteen years many nursing groups and organizations had developed nursing standards, some in conjunction with the ANA and others on their own. The proliferation of standards raised concerns as to consistency, intent, format, and the divergent approaches used in developing them. The outcome was that the ANA appointed a task force that involved all nursing specialties to take another look at the "nature and purpose of standards of practice for nursing and the relationship of quality assurance activities and standards of practice to specialization in nursing practice, credentialing, and implications for nursing information systems" (14). The ANA task force differentiated standards and guidelines in terms of their scope and intent: standards were defined as being broad in nature and applying to care provided to all patients, whereas guidelines were considered to be more narrow and focused on managing specific patients.

In 1992, the Association of Operating Room Nurses revised the process standards and called them "Standards of Perioperative Clinical Practice" (15). These standards continue to be based on the nursing process and to serve as a model by which the quality of care can be evaluated. In addition, AORN continues to have structure for nurses with administrative roles, as well as outcome standards that reflect desirable outcomes for patients having surgical intervention.

PERIOPERATIVE NURSING ROLE

In conjunction with developing standards of practice it became evident that nurses in the operating room needed to more clearly define their role and practice. Standards were in place to guide practice, but these were general in nature and provided the framework without actually delineating the practice. In 1978 AORN's Project 25 task force presented the following definition of operating room nursing, entitled "Statement of the Perioperative Role" (16):

> The perioperative role of the operating room nurse consists of nursing activities performed by the professional operating room nurse during the preoperative, intraoperative, and postoperative phases of the patient's surgical experience. Operating room nurses assume the perioperative role at the beginning level dependent on their expertise and competency to practice. As they gain knowledge and skills they progress on a continuum to an advanced level of practice.

With standards of practice and a redefined statement of their role, nurses begin to expand the scope of their nursing practice. Use of the prefix *peri*, which means "around or surrounding," reflected a desire to look at roles other than the intraoperative role. The term *perioperative* referred to the time and activities in the period surrounding the patient's surgical experience. This was important because, for the first time in the history of operating room nursing practice, there were no geographic boundaries. Perioperative nursing would take place wherever the patient might be—in the clinic, the physician's of-

fice, the nursing unit and, of course the operating room.

In an attempt to stay current with changes in the practice setting and the scope of nursing practice, the AORN board of directors charged the nursing practices committee with reviewing the *Statement of Perioperative Nursing Practice*. The committee believed the original definition was too restrictive and focused on the individual nurse's role rather than on the scope of practice in the operating room. In 1985, the following revised statement was published (17):

> Statement of Perioperative Nursing Practice. The registered nurse in the operating room is responsible for providing nursing care to surgical patients. *Perioperative* is used as an encompassing term to incorporate the three phases of the surgical patient's experience. This includes the preoperative, intraoperative, and postoperative time periods. Practice refers to expected behavior patterns reflecting professional activities, which include the range of clinical activities performed during the preoperative, intraoperative, and postoperative phases. Perioperative practice incorporates both technical and professional components of nursing practice. The perioperative nurse delivers care through the use of the nursing process as reflected in the *Standards of Perioperative Nursing Practice* in a manner that is cost effective without compromising quality of care.

In reality, the concepts incorporated into the perioperative statements have barely touched the universe of operating room nurses. The concept of perioperative nursing was not internalized by grassroots nurses. Nurses continued to see themselves as "operating room nurses" practicing in operating rooms rather than as "perioperative nurses" practicing wherever the patient might be. Once again, in 1992, AORN has commissioned a task force to redefine and reconceptualize perioperative nursing. The question that must be asked is, When will perioperative nursing truly become the practice model for this group of nurses?

RN AS FIRST ASSISTANT

The registered nurse performing the role of a first assistant was another critical issue debated by AORN members in the early 1980s. This role had traditionally been performed by a qualified surgeon or a resident in an approved surgical training program. Although this was ideal in theory, a surgeon or resi-

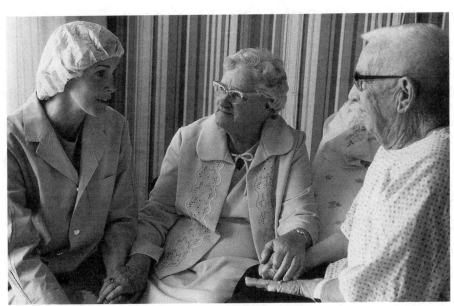

FIGURE 2.2. Perioperative nurses assess a surgical patient's health status and identify special needs pertinent to the patient's safety and comfort.

dent was not always available in practice. Because the safety and welfare of the patient is of primary importance when performing surgery, operating room nurses believed that they had the knowledge and technical skills to serve as first assistant if a qualified surgeon or resident was not available. An official statement on RN first assistants (18) was developed by AORN in 1984. The RN first assistant was defined as a nurse performing the first assistant role during a surgical procedure. While functioning in this role, the nurse practices under the direct supervision of the surgeon and must demonstrate acquisition of the knowledge, skills, and judgment necessary to assist the surgeon. An important element of this definition is that the nurse acting as first assistant functions within the framework of perioperative nursing practice.

The first assistant role has continued to be accepted as a viable component of perioperative nursing. State Boards of Nursing have incorporated this role into Nurse Practice Acts. Hospitals are credentialing nurses to perform services that were performed by physician assistants in the past. The Association of Operating Room Nurses has developed a core curriculum to be used as a guide by hospitals or schools offering curricula to prepare first assistants. Efforts are now underway to develop a certification process that will recognize individuals whose practice incorporates the first assistant role.

CREDENTIALING MECHANISMS

Methods of granting credentials to healthcare personnel have been discussed at all levels of the government, in hospitals, and by professional asso-

ciations since the early 1970s. The impetus behind this concern has been the quality of services provided to patients and the qualifications of individuals providing those services.

Credentialing encompasses licensure, certification, and accreditation. Perioperative nurses are required by law to be licensed. Some states have mandated that continuing education is a component of demonstrating continued competency and have required a certain number of hours for relicensure. In 1979, AORN developed a certification process. This is a voluntary process whereby an individual nurse demonstrates professional achievement in providing care to patients during surgical intervention. There are two components of the program: a self-assessment of the applicant's current practice; and the successful completion of a written examination.

AORN as a professional organization provides education as a benefit of membership. Educational activities award continuing education credit to nurses who participate. These credits are then used to meet requirements for relicensure as well as recertification.

In 1985, the Joint Commission on Accreditation of Hospitals (JCAH) in the *Accreditation Manual for Hospitals* (19) required hospitals to establish a mechanism to assure that all individuals who provide patient care are competent to provide such services. In response to this statement, AORN developed a perioperative nursing credentialing model (20). This model depicts a method for annually documenting specific data on each perioperative nurse practicing in the hospital setting. It is hoped that this mechanism will be beneficial in monitoring employee performance and competency.

Determining perioperative nurse competency was a logical outgrowth of defining practice. In 1982 the original Basic Competency statements were developed and have since been revised to make them more precise, objective, and measurable. The competency statements are defined as knowledge, skills, and abilities necessary to fulfill the professional role of the registered nurse caring for surgical patients (15).

Today the perioperative nurse performs nursing functions in a variety of healthcare settings. With the advent of less invasive procedures patients are coming into the hospital for ambulatory surgery the same day of surgery and leaving within a day or so. This has revolutionized the approach to patient care and has continued to create a challenge for the future practice of perioperative nursing (Fig. 2.2).

REFERENCES

1. Luckes, E. C. E. *Lectures on General Nursing.* London: Kegan Paul and Co., 1887.
2. MacEachern, M. T. *Hospital Organization and Management.* Chicago: Physician's Record Co., 1935.
3. Finney, J. M. T. *A Surgeon's Life: The Autobiography of J. M. T. Finney.* New York: G. P. Putnam's Sons, 1940.
4. Walsh, J. J. *History of Nursing.* New York: P. J. Kennedy, 1929.
5. Bell, J. *Notes on Surgery for Nurses.* Edinburgh: Simpkin Marshall, 1888.
6. Metzger, R. S. "The beginnings of OR nursing education." *AORN J* 24(July):73–90, 1976.
7. Robinson, V. *White Caps: The Story of Nursing.* Philadelphia: J. B. Lippincott, 1946.
8. Johns, E., and Pfefferkorn, B. *The Johns Hopkins School of Nursing.* Baltimore: The Johns Hopkins Press, 1954.
9. Robb, H. *Aseptic Surgical Technique.* Philadelphia: J. B. Lippincott, 1894.
10. Goodnow, M. *Nursing History in Brief.* Philadelphia: W. B. Saunders, 1950.
11. Driscoll, J. "1949–1957: AORN in retrospect." *AORN J* 24(July):140–148, 1976.
12. *Standards of Nursing Practice: OR.* Kansas City: Association of Operating Room Nurses and American Nurses' Association, 1975.
13. *Standards of Perioperative Nursing Practice.* Kansas City: Association of Operating Room Nurses and American Nurses' Association, 1981.
14. American Nurses' Association. "Task Force on Nursing Practice Standards and Guidelines: Working paper." *J Nurs Qual Assur* 5(3):1–17, 1991.
15. Association of Operating Room Nurses. *AORN Standards and Recommended Practices for Perioperative Nursing—1992.* Denver: AORN, 1992.
16. Association of Operating Room Nurses. "Operating room nursing: Perioperative role." *AORN J* 27 (May):1165, 1978.
17. Association of Operating Room Nurses. "A model for perioperative nursing practice." *AORN J* 41 (January):188–194, 1985.
18. Association of Operating Room Nurses. "Task force defines first assisting." *AORN J* 39(February):403, 1984.
19. Joint Commission on Accreditation of Hospitals. *AMH/85: Accreditation Manual for Hospitals.* Chicago: JCAH, 1984.
20. Association of Operating Room Nurses. "Perioperative credentialing model." *AORN J* 43(January):262, 1986.

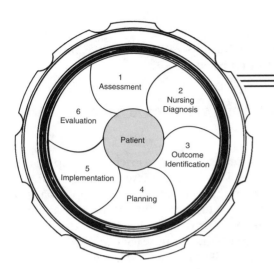

3

The Changing Focus of Perioperative Nursing Practice

The patient is the primary concern of the perioperative nurse.

Perioperative nursing is no longer a new concept. For the past twenty years nurses providing care to patients having surgery have been striving to implement the prescribed perioperative role. This role originally specified that nurses should be concerned about the patient from the time a decision is made for surgical intervention until the patient no longer requires nursing intervention. Patient needs were delineated into three time periods—preoperative, intraoperative, and postoperative. Typically, perioperative nurses believed they could provide for all of the needs of these patients during all three phases.

In the past, operating room nurses were nurses who provided for the needs of the patient in the operating room suite. The nurse's domain was defined geographically. The operating room nurse would not think of leaving this area to provide care to patients in other parts of the hospital. Therefore, operating room nursing was defined as care provided to patients while they were in the surgical suite.

Now, the focus of perioperative nursing practice is changing in response to the social, economic, environmental, political, and technological trends that impact healthcare and the practice of nursing. The nurse must recognize that the practice setting is constantly expanding. Technology has revolutionized surgery. For instance, patients are coming directly from their homes to outpatient surgery centers for removal of cataracts and returning home within a short period of time. Hospitals are becoming critical care centers that treat patients with increased acuity over a decreased length of stay. Less acute patients are being cared for at home. Alternative care centers, such as ambulatory care and recovery centers, are competing with hospitals for patients with less acute, less intensive needs. Less invasive surgical procedures are becoming more commonplace, including laparoscopic cholecystectomy, hernia repair, hysterectomy, and bowel resection. Procedures requiring technology such as lithotripsy, lasers, and ultrasound are considered noninvasive.

With the changes that are already occurring and those we know will take place within the next twenty years, healthcare in general, and perioperative nursing practice in particular, will change even more rapidly than in the past. The perioperative nurse will continue to be more specialized. He or she will be responsible for managing the care of groups of patients having surgical and/or noninvasive procedures. The nurse will demonstrate clinical competency through certification in perioperative nursing. Computers will be used for documenting patient care and providing databases for measuring quality of care. Perioperative nurses will assume more of a voice in the practice setting and will become even more important in decisions regarding care of patients having invasive, less invasive, and noninvasive procedures.

DEFINING PERIOPERATIVE NURSING PRACTICE

Perioperative nursing practice encompasses those activities performed by the professional nurse for the patient experiencing surgical intervention. The prefix *peri* means "around or surrounding." Linked with *operative*, the term takes on the meaning of "around the surgical procedure." Thus, perioperative nursing activities are based on the needs of the patient around the time of surgery.

In the past, the time frame for perioperative nursing practice was distinctly divided into the preoperative, intraoperative, and postoperative phases. This arbitrary delineation was more useful in determining who cared for patients' needs than in defining when and where nursing activities were performed. Instead, the scope of perioperative nursing practice should be viewed as any activity performed for the patient and family, beginning with the decision to have surgery and ending with the resolution of surgical sequelae (1). The family continues to be an integral part of the surgical patient's care.

Perioperative nursing encompasses the entire nursing process. The perioperative nurse performs a patient assessment before surgery and evaluates the nursing care given in the operating room after the patient has returned to the nursing unit, the outpatient department, or the home. In addition to assessing the patient's physical and social needs, nurses instruct their patients on complex procedures, such as open heart surgery. For example, a staff nurse and cardiovascular coordinator at a Wisconsin hospital attended the weekly cardiovascular conferences with the surgeons, cardiologists, and pump technicians. After discussing individual patients with other members of the healthcare team, the nurse would go to the unit and see patients who were scheduled for surgery the next day. From these interviews, the nurse was able to predict whether the procedure would go well or whether it would be difficult.

In a major Texas hospital, patients having eye procedures come in prior to their procedure for preoperative preparation and preadmission. Information obtained about patients and their families determines the care provided and the amount of teaching needed. It is a well-documented fact that patients who know what to expect during surgery are usually more cooperative and less anxious than uninformed patients. Recovery is also quicker for well-informed patients. Figure 3.1 illustrates the full scope of practice, as the nurse performs an assess-

ment, assists intraoperatively, and evaluates the results of care provided.

THE PERIOPERATIVE PRACTICE SETTING

Perioperative practice is not restricted to hospital operating rooms. The setting where the surgical procedure occurs might be an eye center, outpatient surgery area, obstetrical unit, endoscopy department, or any number of other locations. Assessment may begin in the clinic or physician's office and continue after the patient is admitted to the surgical unit or outpatient area. Assessment continues at every step in the patient's experience, including the holding area, surgical suite, postanesthesia care unit (PACU), and the patient's home. Planning activities such as establishing expected outcomes and outlining a plan of care also occur throughout the patient's experience, regardless of where the patient is physically located. In other words, the needs of the patient during this time period have no geographic boundaries. If a surgical procedure is being performed, the perioperative nurse will be providing care.

A FRAMEWORK FOR PERIOPERATIVE NURSING PRACTICE

At one time, nursing might have been defined in terms of performing skills and nurturing the sick. Today the practice of nursing is based on scientific principles. These principles are derived from theories that are used to explain, predict, and provide an understanding and framework for practice. In turn, these theories have been derived from scientific inquiry or investigation, which is the basis of problem solving used in all scientific fields. There are basically four steps in the scientific method:

1. Identifying a problem
2. Collecting data
3. Devising and implementing a solution
4. Evaluating the solution

These four steps are expanded in the traditional problem-solving process to include gathering data, analyzing data, devising a plan, carrying out the plan, and evaluating the results. Both the scientific method and the problem-solving method have been used to describe what we call the nursing process

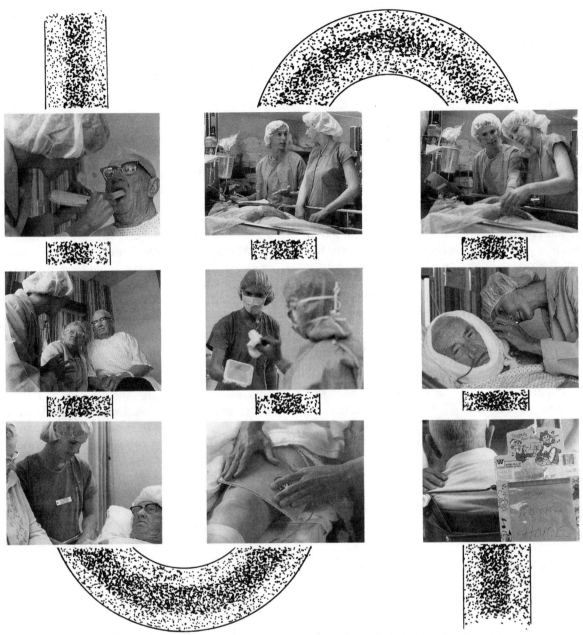

FIGURE 3.1. Perioperative role diagram shows the scope of the perioperative role, the geographical locations in which nursing activities occur, and the three phases of the patient's surgical experience.

(2). The nursing process comprises the intellectual and physical activities a professional nurse performs in giving patient care. The word *process* indicates a systematic movement in a forward direction that involves a series of steps, operations, or phases. The progression is planned and controlled by the nurse, based on the data collected and the expected outcome. A process should be viewed as an action, as it implies deliberate efforts to solve a problem. It is progressive and successive, with each step building

on and being influenced by the previous step. The nursing process is a vehicle through which the nurse applies knowledge and skills in a systematic, goal-directed manner in order to obtain the desired outcome.

The nursing process is flexible and can be used in any nursing situation, with patients of varying ages, health statuses, and cultural backgrounds (3). The nursing process consists of six concurrent, interrelated steps:

1. Assessment
2. Nursing diagnosis
3. Outcome identification
4. Planning care
5. Implementing care
6. Evaluation

Assessment is a continuous activity by which the nurse collects data in order to identify the patient's existing needs and problems or potential problems. During assessment, the nurse might interview the patient to identify any physical problems that would relate to the patient's care in the operating room or immediate postoperative period. If the data reveal that the patient has arthritis in the cervical spine that would affect positioning during the procedure, the nursing diagnosis might be, "Potential for injury due to positioning." The expected patient outcome is that the patient would have no evidence of harm related to positioning. The nurse would outline a plan of care to ensure that care was taken in positioning the patient. This would include consideration of positioning devices, as well as communicating with other members of the healthcare team. It would also require that the nurse document the findings and what actions will be taken to ensure the desired outcome. Evaluation would determine whether the action taken proved successful in averting harm to the patient.

NURSING PROCESS AND STANDARDS OF PERIOPERATIVE CLINICAL PRACTICE

Standards of practice have been established as authoritative statements that describe the responsibilities of nursing practitioners. Standards are developed by professional organizations and reflect the values and priorities of a particular group—in this case, perioperative nurses. Standards for perioperative nurses are developed by the Association of Operating Room Nurses (AORN). They are congruent with the Standards of Clinical Practice published by the Executive Committee of the American Nurses' Association (ANA) Division on Medical-Surgical Nursing Practice (4). The AORN *Standards of Perioperative Clinical Practice* (5) are process standards that focus on what the nurse should do in providing individualized care for patients experiencing surgical intervention. They describe a level of practice that encompasses assessment, nursing diagnosis, outcome identification, planning, implementation, and evaluation.

AORN's *Standards of Perioperative Clinical Practice* are broad in scope and consistent with the nursing process. They are written in measurable terms and provide a means to direct and evaluate professional perioperative nursing practice.

Assessment

Assessment, the first step in the nursing process, involves collecting data relevant to the health status of the patient having surgery. The nurse obtains this information through a patient interview, physical assessment, review of patient records and reports, and consultation with other members of the healthcare team. The patient, significant others, and family all contribute to data collection. Pertinent information might include the current medical diagnosis, previous hospitalizations and responses to those hospitalizations, as well as occupational, financial, educational, social, and spiritual data that relate to the patient's work role and habits. Physical and psychosocial status relative to the proposed surgery might also be relevant.

These data are collected systematically on a continuous basis and are documented on the patient record and plan of care. Documentation permits assessment data to be retrieved as needed and serves as a means of communicating with others involved in the patient's care.

In collecting and analyzing data, the nurse applies nursing theory and prior knowledge and experience to the individual patient. The nurse observes what is happening to the patient and uses communication skills to obtain information from the patient and to relay that information to other members of the healthcare team.

Nursing Diagnosis

Once the information is gathered, the nurse sorts, interprets, and analyzes the data and then formulates a nursing diagnosis. Based on the data collected, one or more nursing diagnoses may be identified for any given patient.

A nursing diagnosis is an explicit, concise statement of the patient's health status. It is based on assessment and forms the basis for nursing intervention. Using established norms and the patient's previous condition, the nurse identifies the patient's health problem(s). For example, if a patient is thrashing about in bed, is disoriented to time and place, and does not respond appropriately to the nurse's questions, the nursing diagnosis might be, "Patient confused" or "Patient disoriented."

In order to make a nursing diagnosis, the nurse reviews the data collected to determine if the patient's problems are consistent with the data. The intellectual process of combining, interpreting, and analyzing is essential in every patient situation.

Once a nursing diagnosis is formulated, it is documented and used to facilitate the identification of patient outcomes and development of the plan of care.

Outcome Identification

After determining the nursing diagnosis, the perioperative nurse identifies expected patient outcomes. These outcomes direct the activities of the nurse and will be reflected in the plan of care. Outcomes must be stated in terms that can be measured. An outcome that cannot be measured is inappropriate and not consistent with a realistic approach to providing continuity of care. Patient outcomes are measurable in many ways: patients verbalize and demonstrate behavior patterns or signs and symptoms; they state, explain, or describe what they know, what they understand, and how they feel about their illness, treatment, or expectations.

The patient, the family, significant others, and members of the healthcare team should cooperate in establishing realistic outcomes. A patient who is involved and cooperative will participate in achieving the expected outcome.

Outcomes must be congruent with the data, realistic, and attainable. An example of an unrealistic outcome is, "The patient will not experience the phantom limb phenomenon after an amputation." It would be unrealistic to expect an amputee to be free of the phantom limb phenomenon. A more realistic outcome might be "The patient will have minimal pain at the surgical site." For an elderly patient, it might be, "The patient will ambulate 6 hours postoperatively."

As the nurse reviews the nursing diagnoses, outcomes are prioritized according to the needs of the patient and the sequence of events that the patient will experience related to surgery. Since patients undergoing surgery generally have multiple problems, the perioperative nurse must be realistic in determining which of these problems the nurse can alleviate or provide supportive care for. If material or personnel resources are inadequate, the nurse has to consider this in establishing outcomes.

Every outcome statement should include a time frame that can be used to ascertain the extent to which it has been reached. If the desired outcome is, "Patient will be free of pain at the incision site," a

time of 48 to 72 hours might be appropriate. A time outcome is based on two factors: the norm and other data relative to the patient. As an example, the norm will not be applicable to a patient who is a narcotic addict. Research and current nursing knowledge enable the nurse to determine appropriate time periods in which outcomes should be attained. Time periods are influenced by the patient's condition, so they will have to be determined individually.

In establishing outcomes, the nurse must consider the cost of services and the time available. The nurse influences the course of action by identifying all possible alternative nursing actions that could help the patient achieve the expected outcomes and then selecting the best options for a particular patient.

Planning Care

The next step in the nursing process is to develop a plan of care. The plan of care is a guide for the nurse to help the patient attain the identified outcomes. In it, the nurse lists nursing actions sequentially, which, if carried out according to the plan, should result in achievement of the desired outcome. The plan should be documented so that information is communicated to all members of the healthcare team. The priorities the nurse has established will be reflected in the sequence of actions. For example, in positioning a patient who is in pain on the operating table, the nurse determines a sequence of actions that will minimize the patient's pain. For a patient in the supine position, nursing actions might be:

1. Place body in resting alignment.
2. Place pillow under head.
3. Apply knee straps in position of comfort.
4. Pad and secure arms and legs.
5. Extend arm on arm rest in comfortable position.

The plan should be realistic, reflecting available personnel and material resources. The nurse assigned this activity should also have the knowledge and skills to carry it out.

The patient is always the focus of the plan. In consideration of the patient's right to information, the nurse includes in the plan ways to assure that the patient is informed of what is happening and what is planned. The patient, family, and other members of the healthcare team also should know what the plan contains. The nurse must discuss the plan of care with the patient and family and involve them to the greatest extent possible in its development. The patient and family should know what is expected of them and how they can participate in the patient's care. The plan is relayed to other personnel through the plan of care and the patient's record.

The plan of care specifies what nursing actions are performed, how they are to be done, when and where they will be performed, and who is to do them. For a patient with a fractured hip, the plan of care might include the following information:

What?	Transferred to operating room with minimal pain, maintaining continuous traction.
How?	In unit bed, with portable intravenous (IV) pole attached to bed. Note: (1) secure Foley catheter drainage system; (2) raise bed to highest position before unplugging from electrical outlet.
When?	Thirty minutes before surgery is scheduled to begin.
Where?	From room to surgical suite holding area.
Who?	Two transport personnel—one to push bed, one to pull and guide the bed and stabilize the weights if traction not secured prior to transfer.

When developing the plan of care, the nurse uses the assessment data to ensure that the plan is consistent with the information obtained from the patient.

Implementing Care

The next step in the nursing process is implementation—putting the plan of care into action. As planned nursing actions are performed, the plan becomes a reality. Will the activities planned result in the expected patient outcomes? In this step of the process, the nurse relies on intellectual, interpersonal, and technical skills to carry out nursing activities. Success of the nursing actions depends upon the nurse's level of competency, as well as skills in decision making, observation, and communication.

The two elements of implementation are nursing activities and their documentation. Each nursing action performed should be consistent with the written plan of care. For example, the nurse from the operating room has documented a plan for transporting a patient with a fractured femur to the surgical suite, keeping the femur in alignment with minimal pain for the patient. If the plan is not communicated to the transport personnel or is not accessible for use, the nursing activities identified may not be followed. In this situation the transport per-

sonnel will make decisions about how the patient should be transported without the knowledge and data about the patient that the nurse who developed the plan had and used when planning nursing activities.

Another important factor related to implementing nursing actions according to the plan of care has to do with providing continuity. Preparation of the patient includes assessing and determining problems, either actual or potential. The plan is developed to provide consistency throughout the perioperative period. Therefore it is essential that nursing actions be based on the identified problems and expected outcomes.

In performing the nursing actions that make up implementation, it is essential that the nurse be proficient in technical as well as intellectual skills. In other words, the nurse must know how to do specific tasks that will result in the desired patient outcome. For example, during the surgical procedure the nurse continuously monitors the patient's position. Damage to the skin, nerves, and muscles may result if the nurse does not carefully monitor the devices and the people that can cause harm to the patient during the operation. Demonstrating knowledge that provides safety for the patient is also a factor in carrying out nursing activities. Scientific principles guide the nurse in performing nursing actions.

The second element of implementation is recording the nursing actions performed. This necessitates that the nurse monitor the patient's response to the nursing actions. Monitoring can be accomplished by observing the care as it is given or by obtaining feedback from the patient. Patients can tell the nurse how they are feeling, if their pain has subsided, or if they are warm and comfortable. Members of the family may also give input regarding the effectiveness of care. Documentation provides a method for measuring attainment of expected outcomes. It serves as proof that the care was given. It also demonstrates the nurse's recognition of accountability. The nurse should be factual in documenting the patient's response and report only observations and signs that accurately reflect the patient's reaction.

Evaluation

The final step in the nursing process is evaluation of the quality and results of care provided to the patient. Documentation is reviewed to evaluate the extent to which the specified outcomes were met and to assess the consistency of care. Were the prescribed nursing actions implemented? To determine the extent of outcome achievement, the nurse observes the patient's signs and symptoms or asks the patient to demonstrate a behavior. For the patient with a fractured hip, the nurse evaluates by observing whether the patient's leg is in physiological alignment on admission to the operating room. The nurse also asks the patient about any pain and observes body language to determine if there is evidence of pain. The nurse then records that the patient arrived in surgery with the fractured leg in alignment, with continuous traction applied, and that there was no evidence of pain at the time.

In evaluating care, the nurse reviews the expected outcomes and judges the degree to which they are attained. Did nursing care make a difference? To do this, the nurse reviews each outcome and evaluates whether the patient expresses, demonstrates, or shows signs and symptoms that indicate that the expected outcome was achieved. The nurse compares current data to the initial information from the assessment.

Each outcome is measured by criteria. If the expected outcome is, "Patient will be free from reaction to blood transfusions," the criteria to measure achievement are:

• Patient is free of rash on skin.
• Patient demonstrates no evidence of sudden elevation of temperature.
• Patient has no evidence of chills.

Because the patient, family, significant others, and healthcare personnel are all intrinsically involved in the patient's care, the nurse should consult them regarding their perceptions of the results. How do they feel about their progress toward mutually established outcomes? What observations do they have? What are their suggestions for future considerations when dealing with patients having similar problems?

When the nurse has made a judgment about the extent to which outcomes have been achieved, it should be communicated to others involved in the patient's care. Nursing care that results in positive outcomes should be shared with others, as should care that results in deficiencies.

Evaluation also entails constant review and revision of the entire nursing process. The perioperative nurse gathers information continually. New data are used to identify problems, revise or create new outcomes, and set forth a new or revised plan. The nurse asks if the outcomes are appropriate for the present situation. If not, new deadlines are set and priorities are restructured. The plan is modified, and

nursing actions are selected to meet the revised outcomes. The nurse should also examine why the original plan did not result in the outcomes expected.

For example, a patient undergoing surgery may go into a malignant hyperthermia crisis. When this occurs, the nurse must reassess the patient's condition. New outcomes are formulated and nursing actions implemented that are consistent with managing the patient's problem and decreasing his or her temperature to a safe margin.

To demonstrate that the nursing process and standards provide an organized progression of activities and at the same time are fluid and constantly in motion, consider the following situation:

Mr. Miller is admitted for a lumbar laminectomy. The perioperative nurse conducts an assessment to plan for individualized care during surgery. In assessing his psychological status, the nurse perceives that Mr. Miller is frightened about the possibility of being paralyzed from the surgery. The nurse determines a plan to assist Mr. Miller in working through this fear and immediately implements nursing strategies. In doing this, the nurse also collects additional data and continues the physical assessment. In this situation, the nurse is performing more than one activity simultaneously.

FROM STANDARDS TO PRACTICE

The extent to which standards of practice can be implemented depends on the individual nurse and his or her level of expertise. The individual's values and belief systems influence the philosophy of nursing and the perception of the perioperative role. The nurse's educational background may be a factor, depending on amount of clinical experience and the willingness to be guided by the standards.

A nurse who believes that nursing activities include autonomous independent nursing as well as carrying out physicians' orders will include such activities in practice. The nurse's personal commitment to the professional role also influences the extent to which the standards will be implemented. Professional growth will be accompanied by increased knowledge, as well as increased proficiency in the use of intellectual skills.

The philosophy of the employing institution may also dictate perioperative nursing practice. If the hospital is dedicated to excellence in patient-oriented care, it will encourage perioperative nurses to carry out their prescribed role. The standards of performance and nursing philosophy of the surgical suite also set expectations for the level of care. A surgical suite with established high standards of care will stimulate nurses to implement the nursing process. Nurses will be aware of the institution's expectations and the way in which they must perform to maintain their positions.

If perioperative nurses are unable to perform preoperative assessments prior to surgery, the nurse assigned to the patient during the procedure will not have sufficient information to plan care for the patient. The plan devised may not be completely accurate or may have some data missing. For example:

Mrs. Carson was having a total abdominal hysterectomy. She did not have a preoperative assessment by a perioperative nurse prior to admission to the surgical suite. Upon arrival in the operating room, the nurse became aware that the urologist was planning to insert ureteral catheters. The nurse quickly made adjustments in the plan and set up for a cystoscopy. When it was time to place the patient in the lithotomy position, the nurse discovered that the patient had a fused right hip. Consequently, the nurse was unable to raise Mrs. Carson's right leg to place it in the leg holder.

The above situation demonstrates the interruption of continuity that takes place when the sequential steps of the nursing process as outlined in the standards are not put into action.

AORN has also developed *Standards of Perioperative Professional Performance* (6). These standards set forth an expected level of behavior for the perioperative nurse. They differ from the *Standards of Perioperative Clinical Practice* in that they deal with the professional aspects of nursing, including such behaviors as evaluating the quality and appropriateness of nursing practice. The criteria for evaluating this standard follow the ten-step model for monitoring and evaluating care devised by the Joint Commission on Accreditation of Healthcare Organizations (JCAHO).

Other professional performance standards include individual evaluation of practice as it relates to compliance with practice standards, relevant rules, and regulations; staying abreast of developments in practice and demonstrating accountability for maintaining competency; supporting and advancing the practice of perioperative nursing through role modeling, mentoring, and providing instruction; protecting the rights of patients through advocacy and ethical decision making; collaborating with patients, families, healthcare members, physicians and others who are directly or indirectly involved with patient care; applying research to practice; and conserving human and material resources.

The extent to which the above standards are internalized and operationalized is determined by the environment where the nurse practices. The question of education is sometimes considered; however, any nurse who has been prepared in a nursing program should be able to put these professional standards into practice at some level. For the beginning practitioner, it may be at the entry level, whereas the nurse who has had advanced education and years of experience will be more adept at implementing professional standards. The perioperative nurse who demonstrates commitment to caring for the surgical patient will seek the knowledge and skills needed to meet the patient's needs.

Many practice settings have encouraged perioperative nurses to be self-governed and creative in establishing centers for excellence or other types of programs that reward the nurse for competence in clinical practice. For the perioperative nurse, the incentive for providing competent care comes from within and brings with it a sense of satisfaction and self-worth.

REFERENCES

1. Association of Operating Room Nurses. "A model for perioperative nursing practice." *AORN Standards and Recommended Practices for Perioperative Nursing—1992.* pp. I:1–1 to I:1–5. Denver: AORN, 1992.
2. Sunberg, M. C. *Fundamentals of Nursing* 2nd ed. Boston: Jones and Bartlett, 1989.
3. Bellack, J. P., and Bamford, P. A. *Nursing Assessment: A Multidimensional Approach.* Boston: Jones and Bartlett, 1987.
4. American Nurses' Association. *Standards of Medical-Surgical Nursing Practice.* Kansas City, Mo.: ANA, 1974.
5. Association of Operating Room Nurses. "Standards of perioperative clinical practice." *AORN Standards and Recommended Practices for Perioperative Nursing—1992.* pp. II:4–1 to II:4–4. Denver: AORN, 1992.
6. Association of Operating Room Nurses. "Standards of perioperative professional performance." *AORN Standards and Recommended Practices for Perioperative Nursing—1992.* pp. II:5–1 to II:5–3. Denver: AORN, 1992.

SUGGESTED READINGS

American Nurses' Association "Task force on nursing practice Standards and Guidelines: Working paper." *Journal of Nursing Quality Assurance* 5(3):1–17, 1991.

Reeder, J., and Kapsar, P. "Perioperative nursing competencies: The process and study." *AORN J* 43(January):215–227, 1986.

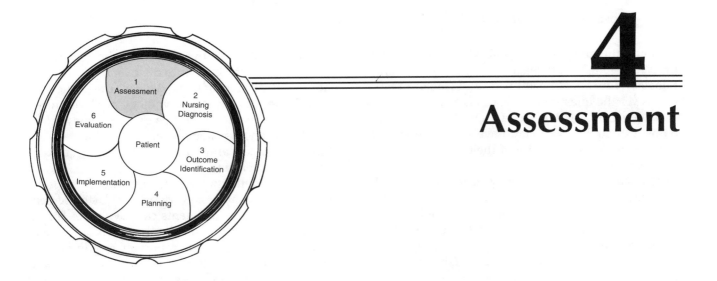

Assessment

Assessment involves gathering physiological, psychological, and sociocultural data.

The perioperative nurse plays a major role in ensuring safe care for surgical patients. Accomplishing this goal requires using the nursing process as it pertains specifically to patients who are undergoing surgery. Assessment, the first step in the six-step nursing process, is also the most crucial step. Without the collection of data through assessment, a nursing diagnosis cannot be made, desired outcomes cannot be identified, and the plan of care cannot be formulated, implemented, or evaluated.

In an institutional setting, the perioperative nurse must rely heavily on other nurses' assessment data. In an outpatient or freestanding surgery unit, however, the perioperative nurse may be the nurse performing the initial assessment, unless the surgeon employs a professional nurse in the office to perform this function. The following discussion is intended to review the entire assessment process for professional nurses working in any location where surgery is performed.

In order to be valid, assessment must be continual. Just as the patient's vital signs change continually, so do physiological and psychosocial factors. The nurse must use all five senses and must be alert to the patient's verbal and nonverbal communication (1).

Like the detective who pursues every clue, no matter how seemingly insignificant, the nurse must carry out a thorough "investigation," or assessment, of the total patient. Assessment enables the nurse to identify existing as well as potential problems and facilitates the formulation of a plan of care.

A FRAMEWORK FOR DATA COLLECTION: FUNCTIONAL HEALTH PATTERNS

Effective data collection involves knowing what information to collect and how it should be collected. Thoughtful nurses may ask such questions as, "What areas should I assess?" "How can I structure the data collection process so my search for information will result in identification of health problems?"

Since a common conceptual framework used in nursing is human or basic needs, healthcare institutions often use an inventory-type format based on needs as reflected in functional health patterns. The nurse uses the inventory format to question the patient about health patterns related to rest, sleep, food and fluid intake, elimination, and the like. All too often, these inventory formats do not consider such important assessment areas as a patient's home situation and conditions, exercise habits, sexual relationships, and coping strategies.

Some nurses have a tendency to pursue data related to medical problems instead of nursing problems. For example, if the patient reports having had one hard stool a week, the nurse might immediately think of a medical problem. Questions would be directed toward tentative verification of that medical problem rather than identification of a problem that the nurse can treat, such as a problem with diet or fluid intake.

Any structural format used should enable the nurse to collect comprehensive data about the patient for the purpose of identifying and treating problems. Gordon (2) suggests that using the functional/dysfunctional health patterns structure helps to answer the question of what data to collect.

Patients engage daily in activities that promote or damage their health. They have an awareness of those activities and an idea of their health status. If problems are to be identified, assessment of a patient's health perceptions and practices is essential. Looking at and talking about a patient's health status by using a structural format (functional health patterns) is an appropriate way to begin the assessment process.

The nurse constructs patterns using data obtained by reviewing the patient's chart, interviewing the patient, and conducting a physical examination. A comparison of past and current practices may uncover changes that can be indicative of a problem. A patient might say, "I used to go to bed at 11 o'clock every night and sleep soundly until 7 o'clock the next morning. Now I find myself having trouble getting to sleep and wake up about 4 o'clock." Since the statement indicates both past and current patterns as well as a change, the nurse can explore when the change was first noted, any other changes the patient can say happened at the same time and what, if anything, the patient has tried to help restore his or her former sleeping patterns.

The overall objective of using the functional health patterns structure is to discover dysfunctional patterns (health problems) within the structural areas. Table 4.1 provides a typology of eleven functional health problems. In this case, typology refers to a classification system for areas in which assessment takes place, and a pattern refers to sequences of behavior over time (2).

Nurses often say they do not have time for a complete assessment of every patient. Using screening questions and statements can save time. For instance, the nurse might say, "Let's talk a moment about the things that are important to you in your life. You mentioned that you read the paper and magazines or books every day [patient nods], so keeping up with current events must be important. What are some of the other things?" A patient's response to screening comments and questions often permits the nurse to determine that no dysfunctional pattern exists. However, if the patient's response in one functional area conflicts with or reinforces a suspected problem in another, further investigation may be necessary. Should a patient respond to the above value-belief screening question by saying, "I read the papers to find out all I can about the crooked politicians and police in this country," it could be important to find out why this is the focus of the patient's interest. Cues of this

TABLE 4.1.   Typology of eleven functional health patterns.

Health Pattern	Description
Health perception–health management pattern	Describes client's perceived pattern of health and well-being and how health is managed
Nutritional–metabolic pattern	Describes pattern of food and fluid consumption relative to metabolic need and pattern indicators of local nutrient supply
Elimination pattern	Describes pattern of excretory function (bowel, bladder, and skin)
Activity–exercise pattern	Describes pattern of exercise, activity, leisure, and recreation
Cognitive perceptual pattern	Describes sensory-perceptual and cognitive pattern
Sleep–rest pattern	Describes patterns of sleep, rest, and relaxation
Self-perception/self-concept pattern	Describes self-concept pattern and perceptions of self (e.g., body comfort, body image, feeling state)
Role–relationship pattern	Describes pattern of role engagements and relationships
Sexuality–reproductive pattern	Describes client's patterns of satisfaction and dissatisfaction with sexuality pattern; describes reproductive pattern
Coping–stress tolerance pattern	Describes general coping pattern and effectiveness of the pattern in terms of stress tolerance
Value–belief pattern	Describes patterns of values, beliefs (including spiritual), or goals that guide choices and decisions

Reprinted by permission from Gordon, Marjorie, *Nursing Diagnosis: Process and Application.* New York: McGraw-Hill, 1982, p. 81.

nature may be the first indication of another dysfunctional area. Nurses experienced in diagnosing are aware that a problem in one health pattern is commonly related to problems in other patterns. The functional health pattern format also provides a scheme or framework for an organized information search. (For more details, consult Gordon's material on functional health patterns [2]).

Types of Data to Collect

What types of information are necessary to complete an initial assessment of a surgical patient? A nurse needs baseline data about the patient's home and work situation; current and previous physiological, psychological, and sociocultural status; and current and past medical problems and treatments. Without that information, nurses cannot identify health problems they can treat independently.

Data collection involves a mental process of sorting information; that is, keeping and discarding cues. For example, getting-to-know-you chitchat may elicit kernels of useful data. What data to collect depends upon the nature of the available information, the circumstances surrounding data collection, and the psychological set (beliefs and attitudes) of the nurse/data gatherer.

Nurses collect both subjective and objective information about a patient. Objective data include those things that can be ascertained directly through the senses: color, appearance, temperature, blood pressure, heart rate, observation of behavior, and the like. Subjective data consist of things reported by the patient or secondarily by a family member or friend. The patient's perception of his or her health status is important, because it reflects what is real and true to the patient.

Accuracy of Assessment Data

It is imperative that data collected during the assessment process be as accurate as possible. Without an accurate assessment, nursing diagnoses, expected outcomes, and implementation strategies will not be valid.

A nurse must consider the reliability and accuracy of each cue. For instance, the reliability of a hospitalized patient's report of his or her regular sleeping pattern is quite possibly good. Better accuracy and quality cannot be obtained since regular sleep-rest patterns in the hospital are often disrupted. Conversely, a patient may be reluctant to provide accurate information about alcohol consumption patterns. The quality of a cue can be ascertained by validating it with other data, by checking other sources, or by obtaining additional information.

The accuracy of a cue often can be judged by its source. For example, a hospital admission reading of blood pressure is often taken to be accurate, while a patient's own blood pressure reading may require verification. Sometimes cues with less than desirable validity and reliability have to be acted upon because better data are not available—for an unconscious patient, for example.

A perioperative patient may tell the nurse that the surgeon has not fully explained the anticipated procedure. If the nurse has read in the record a full description of what the surgeon told the patient, should the patient's statement be ignored as bad information in favor of the surgeon's report? Certainly not. The report given by the patient must be accepted as an accurate perception of the patient's understanding. Further questioning may provide cues that the patient understands everything that will happen physiologically, but does not know what to expect regarding induction of anesthesia.

Psychological Set

The psychological set of the nurse is another determining factor in how information is collected. Psychological set refers to the tendency to respond to certain cues in a specific way because of attitudes or internal motives. For example, a nurse who responds to a patient's crying by saying, "Don't cry, everything will be all right," is responding, not to the patient's distress cue, but to the uncomfortable feelings triggered in the nurse by the patient's behavior. Focusing on the nurse's feelings and behavior fails to accomplish the aim of the assessment process, which should be focused on the patient.

As an individual and as a member of society, each nurse is entitled to hold personal opinions and attitudes, as long as those personal opinions and attitudes do not influence the assessment process. It is not unusual for a nurse to encounter a patient whose attitudes and behaviors conflict with those held by the nurse. For example, individual nurses may disapprove of women with illegitimate children on state aid, homosexuals, smokers, or obese individuals. It is up to the nurse to keep these personal biases out of the assessment process.

The nurse must assume a psychological set that relates to his or her role as a healthcare professional motivated to work with the patient to discover problems. That set is not a social one, a self-maintenance one, or judgmental one; it is a perceptive–interpretive set. Without it, the end result of the assessment process—a nursing diagnosis—can be faulty.

SOURCES OF ASSESSMENT INFORMATION

Collection of assessment data involves the application of various techniques. Most nurses who graduate from nursing programs today have at least beginning skills in the use of these techniques. However, practice is required to refine skills and maintain proficiency. The following content is offered for perioperative nurses who may feel the need for review of concepts underlying the application of such techniques.

Patients become impatient and frustrated with people who repeatedly ask the same questions or behave in a rote manner when a little preparation could have prevented such behavior. For example, providing detailed explanations of routine medical procedures to a patient who happens to be a medical professional can be insulting and demeaning to the patient. It is best to begin the assessment process by consulting any and all sources of written information before interviewing and examining the patient.

For the perioperative nurse, data collection begins with a check of the surgical schedule, followed by a review of the patient's chart. The nurse then interviews the patient, performs a physical examination, and often confers with other members of the healthcare team. All of this is done to establish a presurgical baseline for setting realistic goals relative to the impending surgery.

Surgical Schedule

The surgical schedule provides information regarding the patient's age, sex, planned operative procedure, type of anesthesia, surgeon, anesthesiologist, and estimated length of time of surgery. The perioperative nurse begins to analyze this information before even seeing the patient, because the type of procedure scheduled will influence the nurse's assessment. For example, before a tonsillectomy, the perioperative nurse must check the patient's bleeding time as well as hemoglobin and hematocrit levels, because this procedure may result in large amounts of blood loss. Because the neck may be hyperextended in positioning for the tonsillectomy, the nurse also will have to check the patient's range of motion.

The Patient's Chart

The patient's chart contains data that have already been obtained by other members of the healthcare team, including:

- The *admission information sheet*, which includes patient's legal name, address, and telephone number; Social Security number; birth date; sex; marital status; religious preference; place and type of employment; type of insurance and policy number; and information on next of kin and an emergency contact person. The admission file should also include the patient's current medical diagnosis and hospital or case number and a signed admission agreement.
- Although it is the physician's responsibility to provide explanations and to obtain *informed consent*, it is the nurse's responsibility to confirm that the chart includes a valid informed consent before taking the patient to surgery. The perioperative nurse also must verify that risks and alternative procedures have been adequately explained to the patient (Figure 4.1).

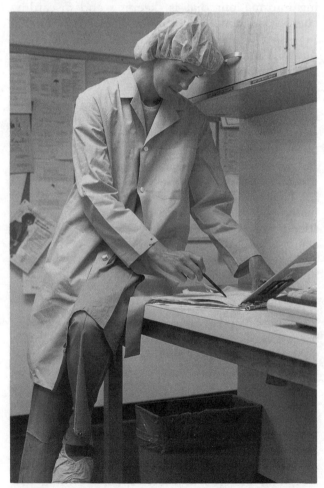

FIGURE 4.1. Careful review of the operative consent is necessary to protect the patient's right to informed consent. Consent forms also prevent operative errors and protect personnel and hospitals from lawsuits.

- On the *medical history and physical examination* record the primary physician notes the patient's chief complaint and the reason for the surgery. The physician's physical examination record also provides information about the patient's physical condition and a description of the area or body part where the pathology is located. The perioperative nurse can use these notes to supplement or validate data obtained from other sources.
- *Medical records* may be in the form of the traditional source-oriented medical record, where each person or department makes notations in a specific section; or in the form of a problem-oriented medical record (POMR) where data about the patient are recorded and arranged according to the problems the patient has, rather than according to the source of the information.
- It is critical that the perioperative nurse review the *medication sheet* in the patient's chart in order to determine what drugs the patient is currently taking.
- The patient's chart should also include reports of *diagnostic tests,* including any blood tests and urinalysis, bacterial cultures, diagnostic imaging, electrocardiograms, ultrasound, or endoscopic procedures. Table 4.2 lists blood and urine tests of particular importance to the perioperative nurse.
- The *nursing notes* constitute a daily record of the patient's progress. A review of body systems

through the nursing notes allows the nurse to collect information that could affect perioperative nursing activities, such as transportation to the OR or intraoperative positioning. The nurse should also note records of vital signs and intake and output.

- The *nursing history* consists of a written or computerized compilation of data accumulated by any and all professional nurses who have come in contact with the patient, including the admitting nurse. Perioperative nurses should review the entire history, paying particular attention to the admission notes, any patient directives, allergies, time and nature of last food/fluid intake, possibility of pregnancy, medical history, sociocultural background, physical nursing observations, the patient's emotional state, and any nursing diagnoses formulated by other nurses.
- It has become customary to include *patient directives* that specify the patient's wishes in regard to certain medical procedures, especially transfusions, resuscitation, prolongation of life, organ donation, and autopsy. Patients have a right to expect that the healthcare team will act in accordance with such directives.
- Additional patient data may be obtained from reports of *other members of the healthcare team,* such as medical specialists, other nurses, the anesthesiologist, physical and occupational therapists, respiratory therapists, dietitians, and social workers (Figure 4.2).

TABLE 4.2. Diagnostic Tests of Importance to the Perioperative Nurse

CBC (complete blood count)	**SMAC (sequential multiple analyzer)**
(WBC) white blood cells)	Glucose
Hgb (hemoglobin)	BUN
Hct (hematocrit)	Creatinine
Platelets	Electrolytes
Polys	CO_2
Bands	Uric acid
Monos	Total protein
Eos	Albumin
Lymphs	A:G ratio
Reticulocytes	Globulin
UA (urinalysis)	Cholesterol
Protein	Triglycerides
Glucose	Total bilirubin
WBC	Indirect bilirubin
RBC (red blood cells)	Alkaline phosphatase
Coagulation studies	CPK
APTT (activated partial thromboplastin time)	LDH
PROTIME (used to determine dosages of anticoagulant drugs)	SGOT
FSP (fibrin split product, indicates fibrinolysis triggered by clotting)	

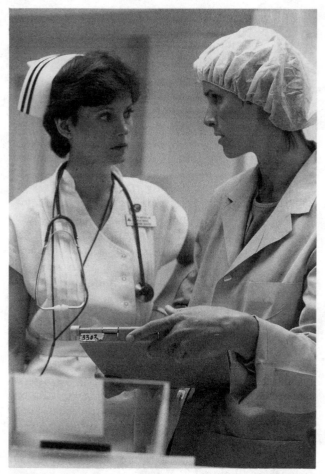

FIGURE 4.2. Professional consultation with nursing colleagues is an important part of assessment and planning for the perioperative patient's care during the surgical procedure. All nurses share a common concern and interest in the patient's well-being.

A thorough chart review provides the nurse with a preliminary understanding of the physiological, psychological, and sociocultural aspects of the patient.

The Patient Interview

In the patient interview, the perioperative nurse utilizes communication and interviewing skills to obtain objective and subjective data that will influence operative nursing care. Information is obtained about the patient's past and present physical and psychological health, including any history of headaches, hypertension, anemia, diabetes, lung/breathing problems, blood transfusions or reactions, use of alcohol or tobacco, current medications, physical abnormalities, previous surgeries, use of internal and external prostheses, and sensory deficits. The inter-

view process also helps the nurse identify what the patient needs to be taught in order to manage the present illness or disability.

In addition to interviewing the patient, the perioperative nurse can obtain important data by interviewing significant others, including family members, friends, neighbors, and/or members of the clergy. The nurse uses significant others to verify information provided by the patient or to obtain information when the patient is incapable of or unwilling to communicate. It is important to note, however, that information provided by significant others may be subject to bias and misinterpretation and that the presence of significant others during the interview may cause the patient to withhold vital information.

Whether interviewing the patient personally or relying on information provided by significant others, it is important that the nurse be aware of the skills required for effective interpersonal communication and successful interviewing.

Communication Skills

Effective verbal and nonverbal communication is an essential part of the nurse–patient relationship. The quality and amount of information the nurse is able to obtain from a patient is directly related to the ability to facilitate communication. The nurse can readily perceive the verbal message that is communicated, but it is important to recognize that gestures, facial expressions, body language, and appearance can also be used to set the mood and to help elicit the desired response from the patient (Figure 4.3).

The key to good communication is fusing the verbal and nonverbal messages. For the patient to receive the correct message, the nurse's body and words must send the same signal. The nurse who says to the patient, "I'm here to spend time with you," but frequently glances at the clock, is sending out a conflicting nonverbal message. Although the nurse might want to spend time with the patient, the subconscious message delivered is that the nurse is in a hurry. In response, the patient might attempt to end the interview quickly by giving short answers. The astute nurse is able to interpret the patient's verbal and nonverbal behavior to determine if the patient received the message that was intended.

The patient may also misinterpret the nurse's words, especially if they are ambiguous, vague, or highly technical. The nurse delivers the message in such a way that it is clear and understood by the patient. Depending on the patient's level of understanding, explanations may take different degrees of time and patience. Even with a complex subject, a

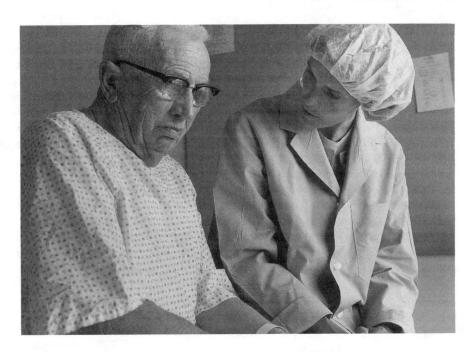

FIGURE 4.3. Feeling tones and cues are given through body language as well as verbally. Empathy on the part of the nurse gives a patient the freedom to express his feelings.

relatively simple explanation can often allay the patient's fears.

The nurse must also keep in mind that there is both one-way and two-way communication. In one-way communication, what the patient receives determines whether communication occurs. The receiver (patient) chooses whether or not to continue listening to the words of the transmitter (nurse). Two-way communication, by contrast, involves direct feedback—give and take between sender and receiver. When possible, two-way communication should take place. The nurse should recognize that two-way communication takes longer, but results in greater mutual understanding. In one-way communication the sender often feels frustrated or angry; the receiver relatively confident (3).

Interviewing Skills

In addition to communication skills, it is important that the nurse have good interviewing skills. Interviewing requires an open attitude as well as basic curiosity—a desire to know more about another person. The interview situation provides the nurse with the opportunity to establish a relationship with the patient and to assess the patient's needs from a physiological, psychological, and sociocultural perspective. Interviewing is perhaps one of the most difficult parts of the assessment, but it becomes easier with practice.

For interviewing to be effective, "it is essential for the nurse to systematically observe his or her own verbal and nonverbal behavior. In this way the nurse's effect on the client and the interaction can be assessed" (1). Nursing students often assume that the interview is simply a series of questions designed to elicit specific information from the patient. Although following a list of questions seems easier, it can result in the patient's omitting important information.

In order to encourage an open interview where the patient spontaneously offers information, the nurse should allow the patient to give as thorough a history as possible, with few interruptions. When taking a nursing history, the nurse needs the patient's own story, not what the nurse wants or expects to hear.

Interviewing skills are learned by trial and error, but certain guidelines help to make an interview more successful. As in any encounter with a patient, the nurse must introduce him- or herself by name and title. Before the interview starts, the nurse should also verify the identity of the patient by wristband and verbal acknowledgment. After proper introductions, the nurse should explain the purpose of the visit and the value that can come from the interview.

Ideally, the interview should take place before the day of surgery; if this is not feasible, the interview should be conducted in such a way that the patient will not feel rushed. The atmosphere must be conducive to open communication. If the patient does not have a private room, the nurse should draw the curtain or close the door to create privacy and prevent distraction from other patients or visitors. It may be necessary to turn off the radio or television, or to ask nonessential persons to leave the room temporarily. Comfort is a factor: Is the patient warm? Is he or she comfortable? Does the patient appear to have acknowledged nonverbally (e.g., by a smile) that the interview is a nonthreatening experience?

The nurse can also encourage open communication by using simple nonverbal cues, such as sitting close to the patient, which shows that the patient has the nurse's undivided attention. A standing position implies that the nurse is in a hurry. Crossing the arms on the chest implies an unwillingness to open up. Taking notes or looking at a list is distracting and interferes with the patient's responses.

Above all, the nurse should listen, indicating recognition of the value of the other person and what the other person has to say. The nurse also should be alert to unspoken thoughts or feelings. One way of demonstrating interest in the patient is to summarize or repeat the patient's statements.

Most interviewers use an open-ended interview style. Other techniques that can be used to gain greater insight into the patient include silence, facilitation, confrontation, questions, direction, support, and reassurance. The first three techniques are the least controlling.

Silence. In normal conversation, especially between strangers, silence often seems awkward and uncomfortable. In an interview situation, silence allows the patient time to gather his or her thoughts and gives the interviewer time to reflect on what was said. The nurse can follow certain cues to determine the need to break the silence. If the patient has come to a natural pause or if the nurse needs clarification of a previous statement, it may be appropriate for the nurse to speak up. If the patient continues to go off on tangents, the nurse can take advantage of silent moments to bring the conversation back to the topic at hand.

Facilitation. In order to get the patient to elaborate on something, the nurse can employ such actions as a nod of the head or verbal statements such as "Mmm-hmm," "I see," or "I understand." Questions such as, "Really?" or "Why is that?" may be effective. A puzzled look or even a change in position communicate to the patient that the nurse is encouraging the patient to continue.

Confrontation. What can the nurse do when the interview comes to an impasse? The patient does not seem willing to discuss the topic, and both verbal and nonverbal communication indicate that the patient's emotions are preventing further conversa-

tion. At this point, the nurse should assess the patient's emotional state and confront the patient with it. The nurse can pick up on the patient's anger, depression, or sadness and reflect it back onto the patient. By saying, "You seem angry," or "You look sad," the nurse will usually promote further conversation. Confrontation can have a detrimental effect if the patient senses hostility or criticism, or if the patient feels forced to continue an uncomfortable discussion. The use of confrontation should be limited.

Questions. Direct questioning can be useful when the answers are brief but yield good information. Care should be taken, however, when asking questions that require yes or no answers. The patient tends to feel that it is not necessary to elaborate and will depend upon the interviewer to imply the kind of information required.

Direction and Suggestion. The nurse can encourage the patient to elaborate on a previous statement by asking, "Tell me more about that." Asking a direct question, however, limits the amount of information to be gained. Also, making suggestions in the assessment interview can subconsciously encourage the patient to adopt the nurse's own thoughts and attitudes. For example, saying to a patient scheduled to undergo a cystoscopy, "You have probably been experiencing burning upon urination," could cause the patient to imagine the expected symptom, thus biasing the report.

Support and Reassurance. To encourage a patient to relate intimate personal details, the nurse must establish trust. Trust can be brought about by providing support and reassurance. A patient will naturally respond more readily and willingly to an individual who creates a secure environment and who demonstrates honesty, warmth, and interest. A touch to the shoulder or elbow may provide support and reassurance, restoring a patient's confidence and sense of well-being. On the other hand, the nurse must be careful to avoid becoming overly sympathetic and unrealistically reassuring. Statements such as "Everything will be all right," or "There's nothing to worry about," will only undermine the relationship if the patient learns that the nurse was wrong.

The Physical Examination

After completing the patient interview, the nurse conducts a brief physical examination, which is discussed in greater detail in the section Collecting Physiological Data, below.

Consultation with Other Healthcare Professionals

If necessary, the nurse may seek further clarification from the physician or from other members of the healthcare team regarding the patient's medical diagnosis, progress, and plans to meet medically oriented goals that are designed to eliminate or ease the patient's illness or disability.

Other nurses, in particular, provide continuity of care by communicating information to the oncoming shift nurses with the same patient assignments. Nurses rely upon one another for information when the patient is transferred to another unit or healthcare facility. The perioperative nurse uses data obtained from the unit nurse to plan for the surgical patient.

Nurses on the surgical unit contribute significantly to the collection of data and the validation of information already collected. These nurses have obtained the initial patient information, and the perioperative nurse uses their knowledge to complete the collection of patient data.

COLLECTING PHYSIOLOGICAL DATA

Physiological assessment should incorporate the cardiovascular, integumentary, respiratory, gastrointestinal, genitourinary, skeletal, and nervous systems. Observations on the patient's height; weight; skin color, temperature, and turgor; and vital signs should be included. Any abnormalities, injuries, or previous surgeries that may affect the current surgical experience should be noted. The patient's use of internal or external prostheses and any sensory deficits should also be noted.

A physical examination is the classic process used to obtain data relating to the patient's physical condition. In performing a physical assessment the perioperative nurse utilizes the techniques of inspection, palpation, percussion, and auscultation.

- In *inspection* the nurse uses his or her eyes to observe the patient. The nurse who is skillful at inspection concentrates on what to look *at* rather what to look *for*. For example, the nurse must correlate visual perceptions with previous knowledge to create an observation; the observation becomes a recordable image.
- In *palpation*, the nurse uses the hands and fingertips to distinguish temperature variations, hard and soft, rough and smooth, and stillness and vibration. The fingertips are the most sensitive to touch. The palmar and ulnar regions of the hands are the most sensitive to vibration. In detecting temperature variations, the dorsal and ulnar parts of the hands are the most sensitive. Light palpation is best because sensitivity can be dulled by pressure.
- *Percussion* is used to detect tenderness or pain in the underlying surfaces, which could indicate pathology. The nurse lays an outstretched middle finger over the area to be percussed and taps the distal part using the tip of the middle finger of the opposite hand.
- For *auscultation*, the nurse employs a stethoscope to listen to the quality and quantity of the patient's respiratory, heart, and bowel sounds.

There are two approaches to physical examination, the cephalocaudal (head-to-toe) approach and the major systems (cardiovascular, respiratory, digestive) approach. The nurse should experiment with both approaches and choose the method that is most comfortable. Table 4.3 covers areas in which physiological assessment pertinent to perioperative nursing must occur.

In an effort to save time, the nurse might try to categorize the patient according to the physician's medical diagnosis. It is easy for a nurse to rely on previous experience in dealing with a certain disease and to formulate a plan of care based on that experience. But doing this circumvents the assessment process, replacing assessment with assumption. No matter what the medical diagnosis, each patient is first and foremost an individual who will respond to life situations in an individual way. In the long run, nurses who make assumptions without first assessing their patients are using time inefficiently and compromising the quality of care those patients receive. The nurse's previous experience does have value, but it is important to recognize that it can also contaminate the assessment process by creating preconceived ideas about the patient.

COLLECTING PSYCHOLOGICAL DATA

In order to plan and implement comprehensive care for surgical patients, perioperative nurses must evaluate the patient's coping mechanisms, level of anxiety, fear, self-image, mental capabilities, and the presence of psychopathology, if any.

TABLE 4.3. Physiological Data, Validating Information, and Nursing Response

Data	Validating Information	Nursing Response
Allergies	Medications (antibiotics, narcotics, etc.)	Confirm allergy or sensitivity with patient and communicate to other members of healthcare team (surgeon, anesthesiologist, scrub nurse, relief personnel, etc.).
	Soap (povidone-iodine, hexachlorophene, baby shampoo).	Check with patient as to what type of reaction occurs and with what agents.
		Have alternate prepping solutions available.
		Note reaction, if any, to prep solution and handle necessary documentation and communication to appropriate personnel (i.e., postanesthesia care unit [PACU]).
	Tape (adhesive, plastic, paper, Elastoplast, ribbon).	Check with patient as to what type of reaction occurs and communicate to surgeon, anesthesiologist, and PACU.
Previous problems with surgery or anesthesia	Patient or family member has a history of excessive blood loss during surgery.	Check current hemoglobin and hematocrit levels.
		Check for coagulation studies (i.e., APTT); communicate history of blood loss to surgeon and anesthesiologist and check to see if coagulation studies will be required. Monitor blood loss carefully.
	Patient or immediate family member has a history of hyperthemia under anesthesia.	Communicate to anesthesiologist.
		Have supplies available for possible malignant hyperthermia reaction, including new anesthesia machine tubes, mask, and bag.
		Have IV Dantrium available.
		Observe hospital protocol to be followed in the event of such a reaction.
	Patient or immediate family member with history of pseudocholinesterase (low level of enzyme necessary for reversal of anesthetic paralyzing agents—Anectine).	Communicate to anesthesiologist potential need for nerve stimulator.
		Communicate to PACU and/or ICU possibility of postop mechanical ventilation.
	History of postop nausea and vomiting.	Communicate to anesthesiologist and PACU potential need for antiemetic drugs.
		Communicate to surgeon that IV therapy may have to be maintained until patient is able to tolerate oral intake of fluids.
Skin integrity	Rash.	Presence preoperatively will rule out a reaction to anesthetic agents, as well as other medications given in the intraoperative period.
	Decubitus ulcer.	Will require positioning devices to keep pressure off, such as a foam ring, air or flotation mattress.
	Poor turgor.	Potential dehydration and electrolyte imbalance will require careful monitoring of intake and output, and ECG monitoring (potential cardiac arrhythmias).
	Bruising.	Potential bleeding problems will require careful monitoring of blood loss and increased need for replacement.
		Avoid placement of electrocautery grounding pad over ecchymotic areas to prevent further injury.
		Use care in moving bruised areas due to possibility of associated tenderness or pain.
	Excoriation secondary to colostomy, ileo-loop conduit, etc.	Increased risk for reaction to prepping solution. Increased risk for infection.
Limited range of motion and physical handicaps	Rheumatoid arthritis.	Potential need for positioning devices to maintain body alignment (i.e., wrist and finger rolls, sandbags, foot board).
		Potential difficulty with IV and Foley insertion.
		Potential difficulty with stirrup positioning.
		Quads.

TABLE 4.3. *(continued)*

Data	Validating Information	Nursing Response
	Paralysis (secondary to stroke trauma, disease—MS, myasthenia gravis, polio, etc.).	Presence should be noted preoperatively to rule out neuro-muscular damage due to positioning and length of procedure postoperatively. Need for extra assistance in moving patient. Avoid placement of electrocautery grounding pad over desensitized areas. Increased safety needs of the patient.
	Decreased range of motion of cervical spine.	Potential difficulty with endotracheal intubation. Potential problems with positioning. Increased safety needs.
	Total joint replacement (i.e., total hip, knee, wrist, metacarpal, etc.).	Move joint slowly and carefully. Increased safety needs.
Prosthetic devices	Glass eye, artificial limb, orthopedic hardware (i.e., traction device, internal fixation devices, total joint replacement prostheses).	Potential need for removal. Awareness of internal prosthetic devices with regard to positioning. Plan for extra time when transporting patients with external fixation devices.
Medications	Heparin or coumadin.	Check for blood coagulation studies. Check for Hemoglobin and Hematocrit. Assess skin for bruising. Potential need for blood replacement. Monitor blood loss carefully.
	Dilantin.	Be aware that other drugs may potentiate serum drug levels (alcohol, anticoagulants). Presence of liver and/or kidney disease can also potentiate the serum drug level.
Tubes, drains, IVs, monitoring lines	NG tube.	Potential abnormality of electrolyte levels that could in turn produce cardiac arrhythmias. Increased risk of dehydration.
	Arterial line.	Risk of air embolus. Have essential equipment ready for monitoring intraoperatively.
Height and weight	Obesity.	Need for additional positioning equipment to maintain proper body alignment. Be aware of increased risk for infection, cardiovascular problems, respiratory disturbance, etc.
	Excessive height.	Need for table extension to maintain proper body alignment.
Vital signs	Tachypnea.	Assess normalcy for patient. Check pulmonary tests and/or arterial blood gases for abnormal gas concentrations (if not ordered, check with anesthesiologist).
History and presence of chronic illness	Hyptertension.	Be aware of medical regimen of patient (meds., exercise, etc.). Potential need for vasopressor drugs (availability of equipment—IVAC, etc.). Check electrolyte levels, esp. K and Na. Potential need for electrolyte replacement.
	Asthma.	Be aware of date and severity of last attack. Be aware of medical regimen (meds., exercise tolerance, etc.). Potential need for bronchodilator drugs. Check pulmonary tests and/or arterial blood gases for abnormal gas concentrations. Potential needs for oxygen therapy during transport to OR.
	Congestive heart failure.	Check CXR for pleural effusion, degree of cardiac enlargement, etc., and plan care accordingly.

(continued)

TABLE 4.3.   *(continued)*

Data	Validating Information	Nursing Response
		Potential for confusion due to cerebral hypoxia.
		Be aware that restraint may agitate patient and increase cardiac workload.
		Need for bladder catheterization due to potential need for diuresis.
		Potential need for cardiac drugs, equipment, etc.
		Monitor ECG.
		Potential need for transport to OR on oxygen and life-support system (LifePack).
	Diabetes mellitus.	Assess for peripheral vascular disease and peripheral neuropathy.
		Check pedal pulses; check for ulcerations and presence of infection in feet and legs.
		Note impaired sensation of feet, fingers, and toes; avoid placement of bovie over insensitive area).
		Be alert for changes in visual acuity (alteration in glucose levels will produce blurring).
		Assess presence of lesions of mouth that could interfere with intubation.
		Check medical regimen (type of meds., dosage, and frequency).
		Potential for evaluation of blood sugar levels intraop, with subsequent intervention if abnormality presents.
	Myocardial infarction.	Assess patient's current cardiac status by checking ECG, lab, medical clearance for surgery, etc.
		Increased risk for thromboembolus and potential need for antiembolus stockings.
		Be aware that cold temperatures can cause vasoconstriction.
		Need for careful monitoring of ECG if recent: patient may have to be transported on oxygen and life-support system.
		Check arterial blood gases for abnormal acid/base concentrations.
		Potential need for cardiac emergency drugs and equipment.
		Be aware that noxious stimuli (loud noises, cold environment, sudden movement or touch, etc.) as well as increased anxiety levels may produce angina and lead to MI.

Source: Linda Rooney Pajank, RN, BSN, CNOR.

Surgery can precipitate an emotional crisis in individuals who are vulnerable due to a distorted perception of the situation, lack of a support system, or inadequate coping mechanisms. A period of mental disorganization may occur during which customary methods of problem solving fail. Because surgery can precipitate a psychological crisis for the patient, it is imperative that the perioperative nurse understand crisis intervention theories and methodologies.

The nurse must also be able to assess mental health status effectively. This knowledge and these skills allow the nurse to help patients manage anxiety. Nursing interventions can also promote wellness, prevent pathology, and enable adaptive resolution of crises.

MENTAL STATUS ASSESSMENT

The major focus of a mental status assessment is the determination of an individual's strengths, capabilities, and resources for environmental, social, and intrapsychic adjustment. Such an assessment requires nurses to identify physical, behavioral, and conversational cues relative to the patient's ability to achieve an optimal level of functioning. Among the items that should be considered are attitudes and motivation, affective responses and feelings, speech characteristics, thought processes, sensorium and reasoning, self-concept, and support from significant others. Table 4.4 depicts four concise mental health assessment checklists dealing with appearance, behavior, conversation and crises. (4)

TABLE 4.4. Mental Health Assessment Checklists

Checklist for Mental Health Assessment: Appearance

This table presents a *range* of signs and symptoms that *may suggest* dysfunction. They are not in themselves necessarily reflective of mental illness, nor are they all necessarily confined to a specific area of appearance, but may overlap with behavior and conversation.

Mental functions	Appearance	Mental functions	Appearance

1. Attitude
   a. Cooperativeness
   b. Interpersonal
      relationships
	Client is aloof, unclean, disheveled, indifferent	4. Thought processes
		   a. Logical
		   b. Coherent
		   c. Perceptual
			Client is inattentive, easily distracted, preoccupied

2. Affect/mood
   a. Appropriate
   b. Harmony
   c. Swings
	Client has masklike face; is apathetic, flat, rigid, labile, euphoric, depressed, suspicious, hostile; displays inappropriate affect; shows physical signs of anxiety (flushing, sweating, tremors, respirations)	5. Sensorium and reasoning
		   a. Levels of consciousness
		   b. Orientation
		   c. Memory (recent, remote)
		   d. Calculation
		   e. Abstract thinking
		   f. Judgment/insight
		   g. Intelligence
			Client displays decreased or absent physiologic reflexes, disinterest, peculiarity of dress, bewilderment

3. Speech characteristics
   a. Description
   b. Speed
   c. Quantity
	Client is soft-spoken, loud, boisterous, has monotonous, slow, or rapid speech	6. Potential for danger
		   a. Self-concept
		   b. Harm to self/others
			Client is docile, sad, hostile, angry, apathetic

		7. Client's psychologic assets	Few or no physical assets

Checklist for Mental Health Assessment: Behavior

This table presents a *range* of signs and symptoms that *may suggest* dysfunction. They are not in themselves necessarily reflective of mental illness, nor are they all necessarily confined to a specific area of behavior but may overlap with appearance and conversation.

Mental functions	Behavior	Mental functions	Behavior

1. Attitude
   a. Cooperativeness
   b. Interpersonal
      relationships
	Client is negativistic, uncooperative, hostile, belligerent, passive, drooping, withdrawn, impulsive, has slow gait	4. Thought processes
		   a. Logical
		   b. Coherent
		   c. Perceptual
			Client avoids anxiety, displays phobic behavior, compulsiveness, echopraxia

2. Affect/mood
   a. Appropriate
   b. Harmony
   c. Swings
	Client is overactive, underactive; cries or laughs easily; wrings hands; paces floor; strikes head with hands; holds fixed posture for prolonged periods; has silly smile	5. Sensorium and reasoning
		   a. Levels of consciousness
		   b. Orientation
		   c. Memory (recent, remote)
		   d. Calculation
		   e. Abstract thinking
		   f. Judgment/insight
		   g. Intelligence
			Client displays stupor, lethargy, coma, confusion, agitation, delirium panic, twilight state, behavior problems, conduct disorder

3. Speech characteristics
   a. Description
   b. Speed
   c. Quantity
	Client grimaces, stammers, stutters; displays uncoordinated or exaggerated movement, mutism, echolalia	6. Potential for danger
		   a. Self-concept
		   b. Harm to self/others
			Client has made suicide attempts; is malingering, withdrawn, assaultive, combative, violent; lacks temper control; displays antisocial or criminal behavior (arrests), irritability, explosiveness, excitability, maladaptive coping

		7. Client's psychologic assets	Few or no behavioral assets

(continued)

TABLE 4.4.   *(continued)*

Checklist for Mental Health Assessment: Conversation

This table presents a *range* of signs and symptoms that *may suggest* dysfunction. They are not in themselves necessarily reflective of mental illness, nor are they all necessarily confined to a specific area of conversation but may overlap with appearance and behavior.

Mental functions	Conversation	Mental Functions	Conversation
1. Attitude a. Cooperativeness b. Interpersonal relationships	Client avoids topics; is pessimistic	4. Thought processes a. Logical b. Coherent c. Perceptual	Client displays phobias, obsessions, paranoid ideas, illogical flow; has feeling of strangeness, depersonalization, hallucinations, delusions (somatic, grandeur, persecution, alien control)
2. Affect/mood a. Appropriate b. Harmony c. Swings	Client displays disharmony with thought processes, talks of guilt, sin, or unworthiness		
3. Speech characteristics a. Description b. Speed c. Quantity	Client displays exaggeration, confabulation, blocking of thought, circumstantiality, tangentiality, autistic speech, incoherence, flight of ideas; is overtalkative; uses neologisms	5. Sensorium and reasoning a. Levels of consciousness b. Orientation c. Memory (recent, remote) d. Calculation e. Abstract thinking f. Judgment/insight g. Intelligence	Client displays aphasia, memory defect, disorientation, poor judgment, lack of insight, inability of abstract thinking and calculations
		6. Potential for danger a. Self-concept b. Harm to self/others	Client has ideas of self-accusation and condemnation, self-depreciation, suicidal ideations
		7. Client's psychologic assets	Few or no conversational assets

Checklist for Assessing Crisis

1. Is the client's chief complaint indicative of internal discomfort?
2. Did the symptoms appear rapidly?
3. Will the situation take time to resolve?
4. Can you identify an event leading up to or contributing to the situation?
5. Does the client show any physical or behavioral signs of disturbance?

If the answers are yes, the client may be facing a crisis. Many times the client may only need support, someone to talk to who will listen and reflect both the content and feeling of the client's statements. In some cases, however, the crisis may become intense and referral for therapy may be warranted.

Source: Grimes, Jorge and Burns, Elizabeth. *Health Assessment in Nursing Practice.* 2nd ed. Boston: Jones and Bartlett, 1987, pp. 76, 78, 80, 81.

The nurse analyzes these data and makes inferences about the patient's psychological state that allow him or her to formulate nursing diagnoses and to plan, implement, and evaluate nursing care throughout the patient's surgical experience.

Attitudes and Motivation

The perioperative nurse should explore the patient's attitudes toward the impending surgery and whether the patient appears to be complying with suggested treatment or prevention regimens in a responsible, informed manner. Does the patient appear to have a rational understanding of his or her health/illness status? How will surgery and hospitalization affect the patient's current lifestyle? Does he or she trust the caregivers to provide quality care throughout the perioperative period? Is the patient motivated to engage in self-care practices? If necessary, will the patient adopt lifestyle modifications that will enhance wellness?

Affective Responses or Feelings

The nurse should focus on the patient's feelings or affective responses. How does the patient feel about having surgery? Is the patient anxious, apprehensive, angry, sad, or relatively calm? Is the patient's emotional state appropriate to the situation? Are any of the patient's fears irrational? Is there a discrepancy between how the nurse perceives the person's affect and how the patient describes his or her mood? Does surgery threaten the patient's self-image?

Because these are complex issues, four of these areas are addressed in greater depth: anxiety, powerlessness, anger, and despair.

Anxiety

Anxiety is a state of apprehension, tension, concern, or uneasiness in response to a real or imagined danger that is often nonspecific (5). During a mental status assessment, the nurse first observes physiological reactions to anxiety, such as pallor; cold, clammy skin; muscular tension; rapid pulse; diarrhea; and increased urination. Noted next are behavioral manifestations of anxiety, such as restlessness, wringing of hands, difficulty maintaining eye contact, general irritation, sullenness, withdrawal, crying, and defensiveness.

Next, the nurse evaluates the intensity, appropriateness, and duration of the symptoms of anxiety. The degree of anxiety has implications for the patient's ability to learn:

- During mild anxiety, the patient's alertness is heightened; learning can occur at this time.
- Moderate anxiety causes selective inattention and a diminished ability to perceive events accurately; learning must be directed.
- During severe anxiety, the ability to perceive and communicate details is limited and events may be distorted; learning is blocked.

The nurse should determine if the anxiety appears to be provoked by a realistic or imaginary threat or danger. The plan of care should focus on identifying internal and external sources of anxiety, providing information about current and future events, and teaching the patient new ways of overcoming anxiety and effectively managing its behavioral manifestations.

The nurse should ascertain what coping devices or defense mechanisms the patient has used in the past to manage anxiety and maintain psychological integrity. How does the patient usually resolve tension, nervousness, or apprehension? Has the patient tried any of these methods this time? If not, why not? If the patient's usual coping methods are not working, why does the patient think they are ineffective at this time? What new methods might reduce the patient's anxiety?

Powerlessness

When patients experience loss of control over their behavior and environment, or feel a lack of knowledge regarding their illness or life predicament, feelings of powerlessness often result (6). When these feelings occur, the nurse and the patient must work together to define what factors cause the patient to feel powerless or helpless.

The administration of anesthesia heightens a patient's concerns about being out of control. Patients may fear they will say something inappropriate during induction, or feel modest about nudity.

The nurse must determine what behaviors would enhance the patient's sense of power and control. It may be helpful to describe the temperature, general appearance, and noise in the surgical suite; to permit the patient to keep dentures or a particular piece of clothing until reaching the operating room; or to encourage patients to participate actively in their care.

Anger

One common means of handling perceived danger and feelings of powerlessness is to get angry and become aggressive. If a patient is verbally abusive, the nurse must remember that the patient needs to vent this anger, and must not take it personally. It is important that the nurse allow the patient time to blow off steam and then help the patient recognize the cause of the anger. Often a patient who directs anger at the nurse is testing to see just how much the nurse is capable of handling. By listening to both positive and negative feelings, the nurse shows interest in every aspect of the patient, helps to establish a trusting relationship, and helps the patient recognize underlying problems and participate in solving them.

For the most part, hospitalized patients tend to use passive-aggressive methods of expressing anger, such as sulking or refusing to talk, rather than active, direct forms. This may make assessment of aggressive behavior more difficult, since passive-aggressive behavior is more subtle and harder to recognize.

Despair

To some patients and family members, surgery may involve a loss of something of great value, thus triggering despair. Examples include amputation; changes in sexual identity related to mastectomy or prostatectomy; and loss of self-respect because of alterations in the capacity to perform desired family or career roles.

Sometimes perceptions of failure and punishment haunt surgical patients, precipitating feelings of remorse and guilt. Anger may be repressed and introjected, intensifying feelings of sadness and pessimism, and culminating in helplessness and depression, a psychophysiological response to real or perceived failure or significant loss (7).

Psychological assessment must include observing the patient for behavioral manifestations of depression, grief, and mourning.

Speech Characteristics

The nurse assesses the pace and volume of the patient's speech activity. For example, does the patient monopolize the conversation, share little information in response to inquiries, or keep up a balanced dialogue? Evasive replies should be noted. What is the quality of the speech activity in terms of loudness, pitch, tone, inflection, and clarity? Are unusual words or phrases used? Is there evidence of self-coined words or autistic speech? Are words misused or transposed, thus suggesting aphasia?

Thought Processes

The nurse should assess the attention and concentration capabilities of the patient. Often, attention span is one of the first cognitive functions to be disturbed (8). Attentiveness to external conditions can be evaluated to a great degree by the quality of the patient's response to questions, directives, and comments. Also, is the patient aware of surrounding people and objects without being inappropriately distracted or confused? Is the patient able to maintain interest in the interview process and to concentrate enough to provide thorough answers? Does the patient have any illusions, misinterpretations of sensory stimuli, or hallucinations?

Evaluate the patient's ability to be logical, coherent, and relevant. Is there continuity among ideas? Does conversation flow in an orderly sequence, or does the patient ramble and skip from subject to subject? If the nurse interjects a new idea into the interview, does the patient comprehend it and respond appropriately? How negative or pessimistic are the patient's thoughts? Are the thoughts rational or irrational? Finally, the nurse assesses for evidence of delusions, obsessions, errors of reference, ruminations, and suspicious or paranoid reasoning.

Sensorium and Reasoning

Usually sensorium and reasoning are evaluated within the context of the patient's total health history. The perioperative nurse probably gathers most of these data from the patient's record or other team members. During the preoperative interview, however, it is critical that the nurse assess any deviations from the patient's reported normal level of functioning.

The items assessed under the broad category of sensorium and reasoning include level of consciousness; orientation to person, place, and time; recent and remote memory; ability to calculate and reason abstractly; judgment and insight; and intelligence (based on fund of general information and vocabulary).

Self-Esteem/Self-Concept

What is the patient's self-concept? Does he or she feel capable, significant, and successful; or useless, inept, and unlovable (9)? Is the patient able to identify both assets and limitations? Is there a correlation between physical appearance and the patient's self-esteem? Does the patient value most aspects of the self without harsh censorship or self-hate? How might the patient's self-concept affect adaptation to surgery? What impact does the perioperative experience have on the patient's body image and self-concept?

Surgery may raise a patient's concerns regarding body image. Specifically, what impact will surgery have on physical appearance? Will scarring be a probable outcome? The patient may worry about coping with the anticipated loss of a body part or its usual functioning during and/or after surgery. Some patients fear mutilation, even if surgical outcomes are basically viewed as corrective. Radical procedures trigger anxieties about dismemberment, major alterations in body structure, paralysis, and possible death.

The nurse should note the patient's physical appearance prior to the surgical intervention and then determine what body image alterations the patient perceives will result from surgery (Figure 4.4). The nurse should give positive reinforcement about the patient's ability to adapt and allow expressions of denial, anger, or sadness.

Sexuality is also an integral part of a patient's self-concept. Allowing surgical patients to vent their concerns surrounding sexuality is imperative. Drugs, procedures, and conditions that can alter either physical or psychological aspects of sexuality should be discussed with patients and significant others. Guidance and emotional support may be

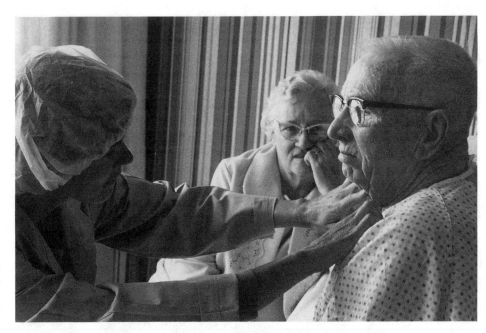

FIGURE 4.4. The periopera-tive nurse determines whether the patient understands that sur-gery has the potential to disfig-ure. This patient is scheduled for a radical neck dissection.

necessary to reassure patients that techniques exist to enable individuals to cope with sexual dysfunc-tions resulting from disease processes or surgical procedures.

Coping and Defense Mechanisms

The nurse should ascertain coping devices or de-fense mechanisms the patient has used in the past to manage anxiety and maintain psychological in-tegrity. How are tension, nervousness, or appre-hension usually resolved? Have any of these methods been tried this time? If not, why? If the usual methods are not working, why does the pa-tient think they are ineffective at this time? What new methods might reduce the patient's anxiety? How can any threat to self-image be overcome? Are defense mechanisms, such as rationalization, pro-jection, displacement, denial, and introjection, be-ing used to manage stress? Are the coping devices and defense mechanisms appropriate to the situa-tion? Are addictive coping habits used that might adversely affect the patient's recovery, such as smoking, alcohol, drug abuse, or excessive food in-take?

Support from Significant Others

The nurse should ask the patient about support available from significant others. Who is capable of providing the patient with emotional support, espe-cially preoperatively and postoperatively? Are there family members to whom the patient feels particu-larly close (Figure 4.5)? Is there someone outside

the immediate family who is meaningful to the pa-tient, such as a friend, teacher, pastor, or colleague? Whom does the patient trust? How can members of the healthcare team effectively render emotional support? What support would the patient like dur-ing the intraoperative phase?

Assessment of a surgical patient's mental status allows the perioperative nurse to collect critical data relative to psychological functioning. Such informa-tion is essential if the nurse is to help the patient and family maintain emotional equilibrium in a haz-ardous situation or regain it in a crisis state. Effec-tive psychological assessment helps the nurse capitalize on a patient's strengths to maximize effec-tive adaptation and prevent pathology.

COLLECTING SOCIOCULTURAL DATA

The patient's sociocultural background, including level of education, religious affiliation, position in the family and community, and lifestyle, must also be explored. Collecting cultural information about patients is a task nurses tend to ignore or disregard. There are probably a number of reasons why this is so, but two reasons immediately come to mind: (1) the nurse is acting out of his or her own cultural val-ues and believes that all patients hold, or should hold, the same values; or (2) the nurse knows so little about other cultures and subcultures that he or she tends to ignore this aspect of assessment. Most nurses have some knowledge about subcultures, but often their own values prevent them from devis-

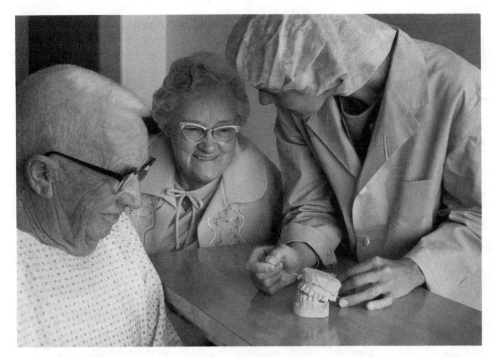

FIGURE 4.5. The patient's wife participates in the preoperative preparation by listening attentively and being interested in what will happen to her husband. Thus she provides emotional support.

ing and implementing effective nursing interventions. The intent of this discussion is to raise the consciousness of practicing nurses regarding the importance of cultural assessment in their everyday nursing practice rather than to provide specific information about different cultural groups.

Culture, in the anthropological sense, broadly refers to the learned, shared, and transmitted values, beliefs, norms, and practices of a particular group that guide thinking, decisions, actions, and patterned ways (10). Subcultures constitute groups of people who have cultural values similar to a larger society but hold additional values particular to certain patterns of living. Thus, in the United States we have subcultures that are defined by age, profession, or educational attainment, in addition to perhaps an ethnic group of origin. Cultures of subgroups may, or may not, be transmitted to succeeding generations without alteration. In essence, culture encompasses the behaviors, values, world view, and lifestyles particular to a specified group of people.

Why is it so necessary that nurses obtain a cultural assessment? Leininger (11) maintains that caring is a universal characteristic of human behavior regardless of cultural orientation. She further contends that caring is essential for human development and that a caregiver should seek out information about a person's culture in order to implement care that will most satisfactorily meet the expectations of the recipient. Health–illness appraisal should lead to the discovery that people are

not alike in their values and should begin to lead to culturally congruent care.

Leininger (11) also cautions that a cultural assessment should be done in the environment in which the patient is most comfortable (usually the patient's home). Some guiding principles in obtaining data are applicable: (1) the nurse should have an objective, open attitude; (2) the nurse should consciously avoid perceiving all people as being alike; (3) the nurse should examine both subtle and gross cultural differences; (4) the assessor should focus initially on only one individual before considering significant others and the family group; (5) the nurse should be aware that his/her own culture creates cultural blindness and ethnocentrism; (6) the nurse should examine the reasons for any and all behavior rather than discarding some parts and keeping others (10).

Nine domains for cultural assessment are defined by Leininger (11). Some of the domains are primarily for the benefit of nurse anthropology researchers. Obviously, the practicing nurse usually has neither the cultural knowledge, the research experience, nor the time to engage in serious cultural research. However, the nurse should assess the following culture-specific factors when planning appropriate nursing interventions:

- How wellness or general health is perceived
- How illness is perceived, or what constitutes illness in the patient's perception
- How the patient's illness is perceived

- How the patient wishes to be helped
- The ways in which healthcare personnel can help

In order to obtain such data, the nurse can ask the individual to describe a typical day in his/her life and the length of time a dysfunctional health pattern has existed. Because food and eating patterns provide cultural clues, the nurse should pursue them. Daily activities, if reviewed over a period of time, furnish clues to the physical and social aspects of a person's life.

Values and norms provide additional clues to cultural information. A value is a summarizing statement or observation that refers to a desirable or undesirable state of affairs. A norm is a rule that guides human behavior and expresses a cultural value. Values and norms can be determined from observation of behavior, from verbal and emotional expressions, and from children's attitudes toward, and actions following, value-laden communications from their parents.

Every culture has proscribed ways of behaving in order to prevent actual or possible harm to self and others, as well as stories that explain the reasons for behaving in a prescribed manner. Finding out what these proscribed behaviors (taboos) are and the accompanying stories (myths) will assist nurses in relating to patients of other cultures. For example, the "evil" or "bad eye" taboo is fairly common among individuals of Latin and Greek origin. It involves giving extraordinary—or what is interpreted as extraordinary—verbal admiration for someone, especially a child. The myth says this admiration constitutes envy and, if not immediately alleviated by touching the person, illness (a curse) can result. Removal of the curse requires special knowledge and skills (12, 13). To an Anglo-American nurse, the "mal ojo" may be difficult to comprehend; but failing to take it into consideration can lead to complete estrangement from a patient and his or her family.

Nursing itself is full of taboos and myths. Not allowing parents to be with their children in the postanesthesia recovery room is only one example. The rationale for such a taboo is that staff can control the recovering child better and more effectively without the parents' presence. Obviously, the child's and parents' emotional well-being is given a low priority by nurses who subscribe to this taboo and myth. Limiting hospital visiting hours is another example that fails to consider patient and family needs to support one another during illness. Taboos and myths make complete sense to people within a culture but seem senseless to individuals outside it.

Various cultures have a particular way of looking at their own world and at the outside world. This is called the world view. Investigating a patient's world view helps the nurse determine how an individual within a cultural group perceives life, health, illness, and death, as well as caregivers and care recipients. Questions about how a patient views these entities provide valuable information upon which to base nursing interventions. But this is true only so long as the nurse comprehends his or her own world view. Conflict results when the world views of the patient and the nurse are different. For example, many people believe that human beings are evil and are born as sinners. Others believe that human beings control their own destinies in life and are born free of sin. Thus, the former feel that evil must be overcome and only God can really help a person survive illness, while the latter feel that what happens to them is a consequence of their own decisions.

Ethnocentrism refers to the belief and feeling that one's own world view and life are desirable and probably superior to others (11). Ethnocentrism is evident in the ways in which other cultures are labeled "Third World," "aboriginal," or "backward." People in Anglo-American cultures who do not meet general behavioral standards are called a variety of derogatory names. National health insurance is politically decried as socialism, and the U.S. healthcare and medical systems are felt to be the best in the world despite the numbers of people without access to care. Ethnocentrism is, as a consequence, a major deterrent in the cultural assessment and care of patients. Nurses must know their own biases and prevent them from impinging on others of a different culture in the effort to obtain objective assessment data.

Determining the folk healthcare systems available to and used by peoples of different cultures is an important area of cultural assessment. Benefits of folk healthcare systems are: their immediate availability and accessibility; folk practitioners know the people; generally lower cost for services; use of medicine and caring behaviors familiar to the patients; and availability of local support and follow-up services (11). Satisfaction and problems experienced with professional (as we know them) services and caregivers are also important to determine.

In summary, the nurse assessor should obtain the patient's views in relation to nursing care services; medical and other professional services; support services such as dietary or laboratory; emergency and long-term care services; financial costs; cultural norms of the caregiving institution; effectiveness and flexibility of the agency in accommodating cultural needs; and location and accessibility of the caregiving institution (11). Finally, the nurse should review the individual's values in relation to caring behaviors, norms, beliefs, and practices, as well as the degree to which acculturation into a different or predominant cultural group has taken place.

Cultural assessments are critically important to modern nursing care in the United States. Leininger (11) reminds perioperative nurses that the "more dependence nurses have upon technological tasks and activities, the greater the interpersonal distance and the fewer the client satisfactions." Although cultural nursing knowledge is as yet fairly sparse and practicing nurse cultural anthropologists relatively few, most practicing nurses can complete basic, simplified cultural assessments providing they have the patient's interests at heart.

SUMMARY

Collecting data enables the perioperative nurse to make a nursing diagnosis, identify expected outcomes, and plan intraoperative care for the patient. With comprehensive information about the patient, the perioperative nurse is better prepared to assist in meeting a patient's needs, including any crisis situations.

Just as the patient's blood pressure, pulse, and respirations are the vital signs of life, so assessment is one of the vital elements of the nursing process. It is inconceivable that a patient's vital signs would be taken only once during the length of a hospital stay. The assessment process also must be continuous. Based on their professional experience, nurses have the analytical capability to sort the data, categorize it, and recognize what is pertinent. Documentation of these findings helps promote continuity of care.

The current emphasis on cost containment has resulted in a shorter hospital stay than in the past for many patients. The challenge is to fine-tune nursing skills without compromising quality of care so as to reap the maximum benefits from each patient contact. In order to facilitate data acquisition, for example, preadmission packets have been developed. The assumption is that patients can be given and receive information in a nonthreatening environment at their own speed. Patients' questions can be discussed with designated nursing personnel by telephone or at the time of admission. Preadmission calls made to the patient are reassuring, provide individual attention, and set the tone for a positive perioperative experience. A preadmission/preassessment form (Figure 4.6) provides a basis for a more in-depth assessment, can be completed at home when the patient is not maximally stressed, and is usually more accurate than the in-hospital interview, particularly in the area of medication history.

The preoperative processes described are often implemented simultaneously; therefore, systems should be put in place that optimize nursing contact. Each interaction, when concisely recorded, contributes to the total experience and plan of care. This is essential to eliminate redundancy.

Assessment provides the perioperative nurse with information about the surgical patient that has direct implications for patient safety and well-being throughout the surgical experience. Once data collection is complete, the nurse sorts out the pertinent information and proceeds to the next phase of the nursing process, the nursing diagnosis.

Case Example

A case example is used here and in Chapters 5, 6, 13, 14, and 24 to illustrate to the nurse how theory might be applied to practice. An intraoperative plan of care, used in conjunction with the patient situation, provides additional emphasis when needed. The following details refer to the assessment initially obtained on Mr. Fischer.

Mr. Ralph Fischer is a 79-year-old man admitted for possible surgery with a medical diagnosis of recurrent squamous cell carcinoma of the left lateral tongue and floor of the mouth, with possible mandibular involvement. Physically, he appears well and is well nourished. Mr. Fischer weighs 182 pounds and is 5 feet, 7½ inches tall. Upon admission, his vital signs are: blood pressure, 120/70; respiration, 20; and oral temperature, 99° F.

Mr. Fischer is energetic and active. He and his wife, who is also 79, live in a ground-level home in a friendly, upper-class neighborhood. Their chief support is Social Security, supplemented by Mr. Fischer's part-time work.

Mrs. Fischer is in frail health. She does not drive and must rely on neighbors to transport her to and from the hospital so that she can be with her husband. The couple have five sons and two daughters. Both daughters are nurses and live in the immediate area. The sons reside in other cities. Mr. Fischer has one brother and two sisters, all living. A sister was recently diagnosed as having breast carcinoma, but the other siblings are in good health. Mr. Fischer's mother died of carcinoma of the liver; his father, of "old age." None of the Fischers' children has been diagnosed with cancer.

TO HELP US KNOW YOU BETTER, WE WOULD LIKE YOU TO PLEASE FILL THIS OUT AT HOME AND BRING IT TO THE HOSPITAL WITH YOU WHEN YOU COME IN FOR SURGERY.

PATIENT'S NAME _____ HT. _____ WT. _____ SEX _____ AGE _____

PROPOSED OPERATION _____ DATE _____

CHECK THE APPROPRIATE BOXES AND ANSWER ALL QUESTIONS:

1. **DISEASE HISTORY:** DO YOU HAVE OR HAVE YOU HAD ANY OF THE FOLLOWING?

LUNG	VASCULAR	SYSTEMIC	
☐ BRONCHITIS	☐ HIGH BLOOD PRESSURE	☐ DIABETES	☐ HEADACHES
☐ EMPHYSEMA	☐ HEART ATTACK: WHEN _____	☐ GLANDULAR TROUBLE	☐ GLAUCOMA
☐ ASTHMA	☐ HEART MURMUR	☐ KIDNEY OR BLADDER TROUBLE	
☐ TB	☐ CIRCULATORY PROBLEM	☐ STOMACH OR BOWEL PROBLEM	
☐ SINUSITIS	☐ HEART DISEASE	☐ JAUNDICE	
☐ COLDS OR RESPIRATORY INFECTIONS	☐ SICKLE CELL	☐ HEPATITIS	
☐ PNEUMONIA	☐ BLEEDING PROBLEM	☐ CONVULSIONS	
☐ SHORTNESS OF BREATH	☐ STROKE	☐ FAINTING	

2. **DRUG HISTORY:** IN THE LAST SIX MONTHS HAVE YOU TAKEN ANY OF THE FOLLOWING DRUGS?

☐ STEROIDS	☐ ASPIRIN	☐ THYROID
☐ BIRTH CONTROL PILLS	☐ ARTHRITIS OR JOINT MEDICATION	☐ BLOOD PRESSURE MEDICATION
☐ ANTIBIOTICS	☐ TRANQUILIZERS	☐ HEART MEDICATION
☐ ANTI-COAGULANTS (BLOOD THINNERS)	☐ NARCOTICS	☐ OTHER
☐ WATER PILLS	☐ INSULIN OR DIABETIC MEDICATION	

3. **ALLERGY AND REACTION:**

☐ NARCOTICS _____   ☐ ANTIBIOTICS _____

☐ LOCAL ANESTHETICS _____   ☐ OTHER DRUGS _____

☐ NON MEDICAL _____

4. PLEASE LIST YOUR CURRENT MEDICATIONS _____

5. HAVE YOU HAD ANY OPERATIONS IN THE LAST SIX MONTHS? _____

6. PLEASE LIST THE OPERATIONS YOU HAVE HAD DURING YOUR LIFE _____

7. HAVE ANY FAMILY MEMBERS HAD PROBLEMS WITH ANESTHESIA? _____

8. PLEASE LIST THE MAJOR ILLNESSES YOU HAVE HAD DURING YOUR LIFE _____

9. DO YOU SMOKE? _____ HOW MUCH? _____ HOW OFTEN DO YOU DRINK ALCOHOL? _____

10. DO YOU HAVE ANY LOOSE TEETH? ____ FALSE TEETH? ____ DENTURES? ____ BRIDGES? ____ CAPPED TEETH? ____ CHIPPED TOOTH? ____

11. DO YOU WEAR GLASSES? _____ CONTACT LENSES? _____ HEARING AIDS? _____

12. HAVE YOU HAD ANY PROBLEMS WITH GENERAL ANESTHESIA? _____

13. DO YOU HAVE ANY PHYSICAL LIMITATIONS? EXPLAIN: _____

ALLERGIES AND REACTIONS _____

_____	/ /	_____	/ /
PATIENT OR AUTHORIZED SIGNATURE	DATE	INTERVIEWER'S SIGNATURE	DATE

MERCY MEDICAL CENTER
Toward a century of caring. †
DENVER, COLORADO

DAY SURGERY A.M. ADMIT
PRE ASSESSMENT

OR 1003*

FIGURE 4.6.   A preassessment form used to obtain medical history for day surgery and morning admission. (Form used with permission of Mercy Medical Center, Denver, Colorado.)

Although Mr. Fischer has not smoked in twenty years, he smoked heavily for forty years. During World War II he worked in an explosives plant. After the war, he managed a business consisting of a grain elevator, a lumberyard, and a fertilizer operation. For two years he was employed in a position that required daily contact with acids. Six years ago, that company discovered that a number of its previous and current employees had been diagnosed with cancer. They contacted Mr. Fischer and scheduled him for a complete physical examination at the company's expense.

Before this examination took place, Mr. Fischer was diagnosed with carcinoma of the transverse colon and had a subtotal colectomy. The examination was rescheduled, and the company continues to monitor Mr. Fischer.

In addition to the colectomy, Mr. Fischer's medical history includes a cholecystectomy at age 51 and a subtotal gastrectomy at age 60. Recovery from these procedures progressed normally.

The original diagnosis of an epidermoid carcinoma of the tongue and buccal mucous membrane was made three years ago. A laser vaporization was performed, and a month later a recurrent lesion was vaporized by laser. A year after that procedure, a squamous cell carcinoma of the left alveolar ridge was excised. Since then, lesions of both left tongue, alveolar ridge, and the floor of the mouth have reappeared. Mr. Fischer is now scheduled for a possible left hemiglossectomy, left mandibulectomy, and neck dissection. His surgeon has discussed with him the need for a postoperative tracheostomy and nasal tube feedings while his jaw is wired. He is apparently unaware that the extent of the lesions may indicate a total glossectomy and radical neck dissection.

During the preoperative interview, Mr. Fischer explained that he was scheduled for surgery because of recurrent cancer of the left part of his tongue and possibly surrounding tissue and jaw bone. He understood that part of his tongue and jaw bone would be removed, together with the lymph nodes.

During the preoperative interview, Mr. Fischer's knowledge of the scheduled surgical procedure appeared excellent. He viewed the disease as life-threatening, but was optimistic that he could be helped medically. He mentioned that he occasionally felt sad to be in poor health, but he had basically lived a very happy, productive 79 years.

As the conversation proceeded, several concerns emerged. First, Mr. Fischer would not sign the surgical consent form unless the results of his whole-body computerized tomography (CT scan) showed no evidence of metastatic cancer. It was apparent that this judgment was based upon personal insight and logical, coherent thought processes. The perioperative nurse made arrangements to ensure that communication regarding the final outcome of the CT scan was clearly conveyed to appropriate nursing

personnel. If the decision was to proceed with surgery, intraoperative nursing care could then continue to be planned, implemented, and evaluated.

Second, Mr. Fischer was aware that his daughters had had a serious argument about whether he should have the surgery. Although they were controlled in his presence, he was aware of their tension and anger. He reported that the situation made him feel slightly guilty and depressed, because he could not assure his daughters that everything would be alright. The perioperative nurse reassured Mr. Fischer that he could not realistically prevent the anxiety and conflict his daughters were experiencing, but she assured Mr. Fischer that all of the surgical team members would be encouraged to provide emotional support to his entire family.

Third, Mr. Fischer talked about some of the "unknowns" associated with his surgery. For example, what would he look like after the partial removal of his tongue and jaw? How much speech would he lose? How would the surgery affect his eating habits? Would he be able to wear dentures again? Would he be able to withstand the pain? How would he communicate with a tracheostomy? Would his family, especially his wife, be able to accept physical changes in his appearance? He anticipated that most family members would ultimately be able to accept any permanent disfigurement.

Fourth, Mr. Fischer was concerned that he would have to be more dependent upon others, particularly on his wife. Because of his wife's precarious health, he did not want to become a burden to her, but he definitely did not want to be placed in a nursing home for recovery.

Fifth, Mr. Fischer had some financial concerns, since Medicare probably would not cover all of the costs of his care. Some of the extensive dental reconstruction would be in addition to normal allowable hospitalization expenses and surgery would prevent him from working for awhile. He knew that his family would help him if necessary, but he took pride in being financially independent.

Finally, Mr. Fischer recognized that his age and condition required him to "face the possibility of his death." He planned to discuss his feelings about dying with his family that evening, along with his personal preferences regarding the management of his death. He expressed that it was imperative that he recover, so he would be able to care for his wife.

Throughout the interview, Mr. Fischer's anxiety level ranged from mild to moderate. For the most part, he was able to talk about his apprehensions. Occasionally, he minimized the seriousness of his condition. Mr. Fischer said that he saw himself coping by becoming more introverted, quiet, withdrawn, and silent. He appeared to be struggling with depressive behavior. The interviewer acknowledged that he was facing a number of losses, even though some were anticipated to be temporary and that feelings of sadness and powerlessness were normal given

MENTAL HEALTH ASSESSMENT

Identifying Data

Date of Admission _____

Date of Interview _____

NAME *Ralph Fischer* _____

SEX __*M*__ AGE __*79*__ BIRTHDATE __*7/17/02*__   SOCIAL SECURITY NUMBER *351-13-9167* _____

MARITAL STATUS __*M*__ RELIGION *Protestant* ___   RACE/CULTURE *Caucasian* _____

OCCUPATION *P.T. worker at collection agency* ____   EDUCATIONAL BACKGROUND *High school - grade 10* ___

DIAGNOSIS *Recurrent squamous cell carcinoma of the left lateral tongue*   FINANCIAL STATUS *$25,000+ / yr. / S.S. after 65* ___

and alveolar ridge _____   ALLERGIES *Ethanol; penicillin* _____

CHIEF COMPLAINT (IN QUOTES) *"Mass on left side of jaw, plus tenderness"* _____

_____

1. **Physical Appearance** (a brief description including height, weight, bodily functions, energy level, sleep patterns, and dress)
   5'7" 182 lbs well-groomed, elderly gentleman; pale, cold, clammy skin; c/o stiff neck due to tension and fatigue due to stress associated with illness; averaging 5 hrs. of sleep at night; wearing pajamas and robe from home.

2. **Motor Ability** (posture, gait, gestures)
   Posture erect and straight; proud bearing; some agitation of hands; general restlessness; slow gait; mild mannered.

3. **Sensory Ability** (see, hear, touch, taste, smell)
   Limited vision in both eyes due to cataracts and macular degeneration. Other senses intact. Responsive to touch.

4. **Level of Consciousness**
   Responsive to:

   Verbal stimuli __*X*__ Noxious stimuli _____

   Touch _____ Unresponsive _____

5. **Orientation**   Person __*X*__ Place __*X*__ Time __*X*__

6. **Memory**   Recent __*X*__ Past __*X*__

7. **Intelligence** (cite supporting data)
   Good - well read; 10th grade high school education only but regards self as committed to taking advantage of ongoing adult continuing-education opportunities.

8. **Fund of Information**
   General _____
   About illness (state specifics) Very well informed about his cancer, scheduled surgery, possible postoperative complications, anticipated surgical outcomes, and possible negative consequences as well as positive. Previous surgical experiences provided him with a good knowledge base of what to expect intraoperatively. Seeks additional data when questions arise.

9. **Judgment/Insight** (cite supporting data)
   Good judgment relative to changes in lifestyle that might result as consequence of surgery. Won't have surgery if positive indicators of metatastic cancer are found on CT scan. Realizes death might be an outcome due to age and condition. Has insight as to historical events that might have contributed to current health status. Also, aware of specific concerns that precipitate current emotional and behavioral patterns.

10. **Thought Process**
    Logical __*X*__ Coherent __*X*__ Relevant __*X*__

    Unusual patterns (cite supporting data) No gross distortion noted. Is not evasive or guarded. Occasional evidence of irrational thinking, especially in relation to need to protect wife and daughters and exaggerated concerns about loss of control or being left alone, including being abandoned in a nursing home.

11. **Speech Pattern** (speed, comprehensiveness, spontaneity)
    Rapid pace but quality of speech activity good in terms of clarity, pitch, loudness, and tone. No unusual words or phrases. No evidence of made-up language. Words were not misused or transposed.

FIGURE 4.7.   Mental health assessment. (Reprinted by permission from the August issue of *Nursing 79.* Copyright © 1979, Intermed Communications Inc. All rights reserved.)

the circumstances. He was encouraged to vent such feelings, as well as any anger or guilt he might experience.

Upon conclusion of the interview, the nurse completed a mental health assessment form. In many institutions, these data are combined on a form with physiological information in order to expedite documentation. Figure 4.7 concisely illustrates many of the components that must be examined within the context of performing a mental status assessment.

The surgery schedule was posted. The nurse preparing to do the perioperative assessments noted Mr. Fischer's room number and his age. The schedule described the operative procedure, including the fact that general anesthesia would be administered.

12. **Ideation** (cite supporting data)
No self-destructive or suicidal thoughts were noted.
Realistic regarding desire to enhance quality of remaining life, yet accepts death as a possible outcome. Recognizes impact of surgery on self-concept/body image but believes his age mitigates some of negative impact of disfigurement. No suspicious/paranoid thinking.

Self-destructive/suicidal _____
Suspicious/paranoid _____

13. **Affect** (cite supporting data)
Feelings of sadness, frustration, powerlessness, guilt, helplessness manifested through anxious, depressive-dependent and withdrawn behavioral patterns - feelings of anger denied - affect appears realistic, for most part, given circumstances.

14. **Family and Significant Others**
A. Position in family *Oldest son of 4 children, 2 sisters and 1 brother are living*

B. Others in family *5 sons and 2 daughters, plus wife are living*

C. Living arrangements *home in upper middle class neighborhood in large, metropolitan city.*

D. Role/roles in family *husband, father, breadwinner*

E. Significant others *Neighbors, work colleagues*

F. Other Support systems *none mentioned*

G. Interactional ability *good, very authentic, strong sense of honesty, aware that anxious and depressive behaviors are affecting his spontaneity in terms of volume of conversation, responsive to others but initiating fewer interactions.*

15. **Addictive/Coping Habits and Amounts** (positive and negative)
A. Smoking *prior to 1955*   Amount *2 packs x 19 yrs, plus cigars and pipe*

B. Alcohol ___*0*___ Amount ___*0*___ Frequency ___*0*___

C. Medications (list all: over the counter, legal, illegal)

_____

D. Food intake *Normal*   Amount *Appropriate quantities*   When *Regular meals some snacks*
E. Other _____

16. **Sexual Functioning**
Does not perceive that his masculinity will be negatively impacted due to his close relationship with wife and family. Realizes that serious disfigurement or disability could make him feel less of a man if he allowed such thoughts to dominate his thinking processes. Believes his wife will be affectionate and nurturing in many ways, including sexual intimacy. Verbalized that sexual intercourse had decreased during past 8 years due to many factors and that surgery would not adversely affect present patterns of sexual intimacy.

17. **Need Level**
Physiological, safety, love and belonging, and esteem

18. **Developmental Level**
Mature, elderly man with minimal regression

19. **Coping Devices and Defense Mechanisms** (assess for effectiveness, usefulness, and appropriateness)
Ventilation of feelings. Use of touch. Appropriate increase in dependent behavior. Stoicism. Quiet time to allow introspection about illness. Protective behavior toward wife and daughters. Use of repression and introjection in terms of defense mechanisms.

20. **Assets, Resources, Interests**
Supportive wife and family. Realistic view of cancer and his specific diagnosis. Open discussion of concerns. Willingness to be an active participant in his care. Excellent rapport with physician and nursing staff. Desire to live a full, productive life, including returning to work on a part-time basis. Acceptance of limitations.

21. **Impression/Nursing Diagnoses**
Impression: 79 year old white male responding with depressive behavior to pending changes in lifestyle and altered body image due to anticipated surgical intervention for recurrent cancer.

Other behavioral patterns (anxious, dependent and withdrawn) appear related to possible losses associated with illness, hospitalization, surgery, and unknown outcomes.

NGS DX: Psychological disequilibrium (depressive behavior) related to anticipated changes in body image and self-concept, ↑ powerlessness and dependency, ↑ anxiety associated with the absence of known surgical outcomes, pending lifestyle changes, and possibility of death.

FIGURE 4.7.   *(cont.)*

After writing this information on the patient plan of care, the nurse went to the surgical unit where Mr. Fischer had been admitted. Here, the perioperative nurse reviewed his record and verified the presence of a signed surgical consent form.

The patient's history and physical examination stated the chief complaint as being recurrent squamous cell carcinoma of the left lateral tongue and alveolar ridge. His medical history was described in detail.

The nurse noted that Mr. Fischer had a present allergy to ethanol and possibly to penicillin as well. Reviewing the systems, the nurse found no further pertinent information, with the exception of the present node in his jaw. The patient had trace edema in both legs, which the nurse noted on the data collection form.

Diagnostic data included a chest X-ray with no significant abnormalities and a panorex of the mandible. There was no evidence of bone destruction to suggest invasion of *the mandible by the existing tissue neoplasm. Admission laboratory data showed the patient's blood chemistry and urinalysis to be within normal limits. Blood had been ordered, and the type and cross-match was compatible for Type O positive.*

From the nursing history, the nurse entered information on vital signs and information about Mr. Fischer's glasses and dentures on the plan of care. Other data included in the nursing history did not seem pertinent to the surgery. The unit nurse offered information regarding the relationship of Mr. and Mrs. Fischer.

With this information, the perioperative nurse approached Mr. Fischer's room and found his wife sitting on the bed. Upon entering, the nurse noted that Mr. Fischer was a well-developed, well-nourished white male who was not in acute distress. He wore glasses and had a pleasant manner. Mrs. Fischer appeared healthy, if somewhat overweight. The nurse asked Mr. Fischer to explain, in his own words, the reason for his hospitalization and his understanding of the surgical procedure. The nurse determined that Mr. Fischer will have a communication problem postoperatively due to the surgical resection, jaw wiring, and tracheostomy.

The nurse continued to gather physical data through observation, interview, and physical examination. She noted that Mr. Fischer had minimal edema in both lower extremities. This indicated the need for him to wear elastic stockings during the procedure. She also determined that the length of the procedure and the required position might necessitate positioning devices and padding of various areas interoperatively. An assessment of the skin showed that the patient has relatively good turgor and no areas of rash or excoriations, and that the skin was not impaired in any area. He had no evidence of physical limitations and his range of motion seemed normal. Mr. Fischer demonstrated moderate anxiety.

The nurse completed obtaining data from Mr. Fischer and told him she will see him in the operating room. After leaving the room, the nurse completed documenting the data collected and continued to develop the plan of care.

REFERENCES

1. Werger-Ryan, Nancy M. "A nursing process methodology." *Nursing Outlook* 4 (July/August):191, 1990.
2. Gordon, Marjorie. *Nursing Diagnosis: Process and Application* 2nd ed. New York: McGraw-Hill, 1987.
3. Griffin, Kim, and Patton, Bobby. *Fundamentals of Interpersonal Communication* 2nd ed. Lanham, MD: University Press of America, 1986.
4. Grimes, Jorge, and Burns, Elizabeth. *Health Assessment in Nursing Practice* 2nd ed. Boston: Jones and Bartlett, 1987.
5. Bowlby, John. *Separation, Anxiety, and Anger.* New York: Basic Books, 1976.
6. Neal, Margo. *Nursing Diagnosis Care Plans for Diagnosis-Related Groups.* Boston: Jones and Bartlett, 1990.
7. Arieti, S., and Bemporad, J. *Severe and Mild Depression.* New York: Basic Books, 1978.
8. Malasanos, L., et al. *Health Assessment* 4th ed. St. Louis, MO: C.V. Mosby, 1989.
9. Elkins, Dov P., ed. *Self-Concept Sourcebook: Ideas and Activities for Building Self-Esteem.* Rochester, N.Y.: Growth Associates, 1989.
10. Alexander, Sr., Judith, Beagle, Carolyn, Butler, Pan, et al. "Cultural care theory." In: A. Marriner-Tomey, ed., *Nursing Theorists and Their Work* 2nd ed. St. Louis, MO: C.V. Mosby, 1989.
11. Leininger, M. *Transcultural Nursing: Concepts, Theories, and Practices* 2nd ed. New York: John Wiley & Sons, 1988.
12. Saunders, L., *Cultural Difference and Medical Care: The Case of the Spanish-Speaking People of the Southwest.* New York: Russell Sage Foundation, 1954.
13. Bellack, Janis P., and Bamford, Penny A. *Nursing Assessment: A Multidimensional Approach.* Boston: Jones and Bartlett, 1987.

SUGGESTED READINGS

Association of Operating Room Nurses. *Standards and Recommended Practices for Perioperative Nursing—1992.* Denver: AORN, 1992.

Aguilera, D., and Missick, J. *Crisis Intervention: Theory and Methodology* 6th ed. St. Louis, MO: C.V. Mosby, 1990.

Bleich, Michael R. "Clinical judgements: Essential elements of the nursing process." *Quality Assurance* 4 (August):2, 1990.

Carpenito, Lynda J. *Nursing Diagnosis: Application to Clinical Practice* 3rd ed. New York: J. B. Lippincott, 1989.

Derenge, Sara, and Rupp, Monica. "The nursing process." *Preparing for Certification* February:35, 1991.

Haselfeld, Danne. "Patient assessment: Conducting an effective interview." *AORN J* 52(September):551–557, 1990.

Kozier, Barbara, Erb, Glenara, and Buffalino-McKay, Patricia. *Introduction to Nursing.* Reading, MA: Addison-Wesley, 1989.

Leuze, M., and McKenzie, J. "Preoperative assessment using the Roy adaptation model." *AORN J* 46 (December):1122–1134, 1987.

Rothrock, J. "Perioperative nursing research (part 1): Preoperative psychoeducational interventions." *AORN J* 49(February): 597–619, 1989.

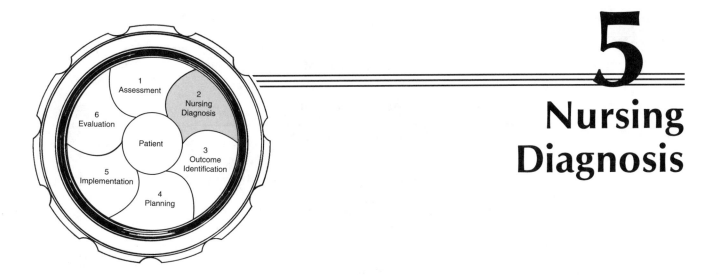

5

Nursing Diagnosis

Nursing diagnoses are derived from health status data.

In the nursing process, the outcome of assessment is one or more nursing diagnoses. While assessing a patient's health status to discern actual or potential problems, the nurse engages in a diagnostic process similar to the one physicians use to diagnose disease or pathology. The diagnostic process involves a systematic search for information that will lead to discovery of a problem or problems. The search in both professional groups initially takes a broad approach followed by reduction of possible causes for a problem until one becomes reasonably certain the difficulty has been located. Figure 5.1 outlines the sequence of diagnostic steps in nursing.

Although both nurses and physicians use the same diagnostic process for the purpose of treating problems, the focus for each is different. Physicians use a body systems approach; nurses a functional-dysfunctional health patterns approach. Physicians focus on discovering and treating pathophysiological and pathopsychological problems. Realizing that health management and health conditions influence the quality of human life, nurses have turned their attention to the actions and reactions that take place among individuals, families, and their environments. (Environment refers to the internal physical and psychological conditions of human beings as well as the external conditions of the surroundings in which human beings live, work, and play.) Unmet health needs create problems, many of which nurses can treat. Identification of these problems is

the thrust of the diagnostic process in nursing, and the end products are nursing diagnoses.

WHAT IS A NURSING DIAGNOSIS?

A nursing diagnosis is a clinical judgment about an individual, family, or community response to actual or potential health problems/life processes which provides the basis for definitive therapy toward achievement of outcomes for which the nurse is accountable (1). Actual problems are real difficulties that prevent an individual or family from responding in a normal, healthy fashion. Potential health problems are those situations in which there are enough symptoms to indicate a high degree of probability that actual problems could occur in the future.

Only professional nurses can make nursing diagnoses. In most states, professional nurses are accountable by law for directing and supervising the delegated nursing activities of other healthcare workers. The judgment and decision making involved in determining nursing diagnoses, however, cannot be delegated since the process is primarily mental. Although nonprofessional nursing personnel can make valuable contributions to treatment by carrying out planned interventions and observing patient reactions, they do so after diagnoses have been made.

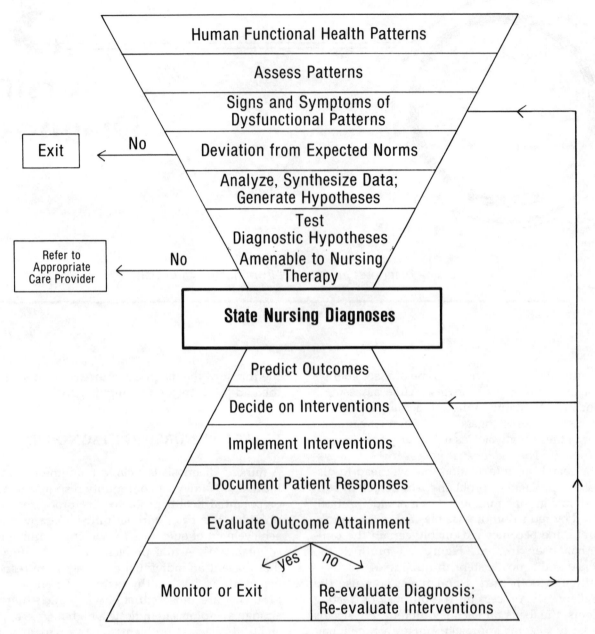

FIGURE 5.1.   Diagnostic steps in nursing process. (Adapted and reprinted by permission from *Nursing Diagnosis: Process and Application,* by Marjorie Gordon. Copyright 1982, McGraw-Hill Book Co.)

Standards of practice and many state nursing practice rules and regulations encourage registered (professional) nurses to make nursing diagnoses. These guidelines and the American Nurses' Association (ANA) *Code for Nurses* (2) are frequently used in courts of law to establish the usual conduct of professional nursing practice.

A nursing diagnosis can also represent a class of health problems. It is a label given to a cluster of associated factors. Within such a class, there may be subcategories of related but different health prob-

lems. For instance, the diagnostic class "Potential for injury" comprises the subcategories (1) potential for poisoning, (2) potential for suffocation, (3) potential for trauma, (4) potential for aspiration, and (5) potential for disuse syndrome (2). Classifying and labeling phenomena is a human way of making sense out of the environment to facilitate understanding and communication. Naming health problems treated by nurses serves this purpose. It is a kind of shorthand. A nursing diagnosis, "Impaired physical mobility (level 2) related to postoperative pain," enables a nurse to understand several things about a patient that would otherwise require extensive verbal or written explanation. The nurse recognizes that a patient with this diagnosis requires assistance or supervision to turn physically in bed or move about his or her hospital room (Table 5.1). Level 2 in the diagnosis signifies that the patient can move, although movement causes additional pain. The need for assistance or supervision implies that there is a potential for injury if the patient gets out of bed without another person standing by. The cause of the impaired physical mobility is stated, and in the absence of other contrary diagnoses, either nursing or medical, indicates that the patient can be expected to achieve independent movement. The nurse understands that the signs and symptoms of pain with movement are present. Experience with other patients and recall of signs and symptoms of impaired physical mobility and of pain and levels of functional activity enable the nurse to understand what responses can be expected without even seeing the patient.

In a recent needs assessment survey, using nursing diagnoses in the operating room setting was a priority learning need. The above information illustrates how nursing diagnoses made by others can be used in that location during transporting and moving functions.

Having determined what a nursing diagnosis is, attention will now be directed toward the structured elements of a nursing diagnosis.

STRUCTURAL ELEMENTS OF NURSING DIAGNOSES

A nursing diagnosis consists of three structural elements: (1) the problem statement, (2) its etiology, and (3) the defining cluster of signs and symptoms. The problem statement should be clear, precise, and succinct: "Impaired physical mobility (level 2)" and "Impaired verbal communication" are two examples. Certain diagnoses require additional clarifying words so the problem area can be located more precisely. If impaired daily living activities, such as physical mobility and self-care, are the problem, it is necessary to designate the level of impairment using a standard and accepted scheme. Table 5.1 provides such a framework. Other diagnoses not related to daily living activities need other clarifying words to indicate the area in which the problem lies. Noncompliance is one of these. Since noncompliance is a person's informed decision not to adhere to a therapeutic regimen, the diagnosis, "Noncompliance (diabetic diet)," helps nurses understand that the area of difficulty is not in care of the skin or prescribed medication, but in the area of diet.

The second structural component is the etiology or cause of the problem. Etiological indicators consist of patient behaviors, factors in the environment, or an interaction between them. For instance, with the diagnosis, "Knowledge deficit," possible etiological factors are as follows: (1) lack of exposure, (2) lack of recall, (3) information misinterpretation, (4) cognitive limitation, (5) lack of interest in learning, and (6) unfamiliarity with information sources. Without causative reasons, therapy is likely to be hit-and-miss, involving unnecessary time and effort for both patient and nurse. Efficient, effective therapy should focus on the precise need. Table 5.2 gives two other diagnoses with etiological factors and further illustrates the need to narrow the diagnostic focus for adequate planning and interaction.

The final structural part of a nursing diagnosis is the cluster of signs and symptoms characteristic of the category. Just as medical diagnoses have charac-

TABLE 5.1.   Classification of Functional Activity Level

Score	Activity Level
0	Total independence.
1	Requires use of equipment or assistive device.
2	Requires assistance or supervision from another person.
3	Requires assistance or supervision from another person and equipment or device.
4	Dependent and does not participate in self-care.

Reprinted by permission from *Nursing Diagnosis: Process and Application*, p. 88, by Marjorie Gordon. Copyright 1982 by McGraw-Hill Book Co.

TABLE 5.2.   Two Nursing Diagnoses with Etiological Factors

Nursing Diagnosis	Etiological Factors
Impaired physical mobility	Therapy/medical regimen Pain/discomfort Fatigue/decreased strength and endurance Trauma Lack of physical support Neuromuscular impairment Psychosocial/depression
Impaired verbal communication	Circulatory impairment to brain Physical barrier (brain tumor, tracheostomy, intubation) Anatomical deficit (cleft palate) Psychological barrier (psychosis, lack of stimuli) Developmental (age-related)

teristic signs and symptoms, so do nursing diagnoses. The diagnosis, "Altered nutrition: more than bodily requirements," has several signs and symptoms (Table 5.3). It also has two critical defining characteristics without which the diagnosis cannot be made. If the critical characteristics are absent but other noncritical characteristics are present, additional data may indicate that the diagnosis is, "Altered nutrition: potential for more than body requirements."

Nurses have just begun naming nursing diagnoses, determining etiological factors, and defining signs and symptoms of diagnostic categories. The examples cited and others have been accepted for validation in clinical practice; however, they have not been published in a taxonomy of diagnoses such as physicians use. Diagnoses published in books on nursing diagnoses often need additional work and refinement to be standardized. Consequently, the field is open for new labels, additional signs and symptoms for diagnoses already identified, and refinement of causative factors. Some nursing diagnoses already accepted for testing may be discarded or placed in other diagnoses as etiological factors.

Defining Nursing Diagnoses

Could a nurse recognize a nursing diagnosis in a patient's record without its being identified as such? Certainly, the presence of the structural components would help to identify a nursing diagnosis. Dispelling a few common misconceptions about nursing diagnoses may also be of benefit.

Statements about a patient's therapeutic needs

TABLE 5.3. Defining Characteristics of the Nursing Diagnosis "Altered Nutrition: More Than Body Requirements"

Related Factors	Defining Characteristics
Intake exceeds metabolic needs	*Weight 10–20% over ideal body weight
Stress	*Triceps skinfold > 15 mm in males and > 25 mm in females
Low self-concept	
Medical problems, e.g., hypertension, polycythemia, hypercholesterolemia, non-insulin dependent diabetes mellitus, thyroid hormone insufficiency	Sedentary lifestyle
	Dysfunctional patterns of eating
	Majority of intake at bedtime
	Eating in response to specific activities, emotions, and/or feelings

*Critical defining characteristic

are not diagnoses. "Needs emotional support" and "Turn every two hours" fail to identify the health problem or its cause , although such statements may indicate ways of treating a problem.

Maslow's hierarchy of human needs and Henderson's basic needs classification furnish nurses with theoretical frameworks for their approach to nursing, but they fail to specify patient-oriented health problems. Both frameworks are too general. Every human being, for example, has a need for sleep and rest. Unmet human needs can produce actual or potential health problems, and human needs underlie the functional health patterns approach to assessment; but they in themselves are inadequate to serve as diagnoses.

Just as therapeutic and human needs are not nursing diagnoses, neither are therapeutic nursing or patient goals. Statements such as "to alleviate pain" or "to experience minimal pain" do not tell us anything about the problem causing the pain. Therapeutic goals are derived from nursing diagnoses and, as outcomes, help nurses plan therapeutic measures and evaluate achievement of therapy (Figure 5.1).

Staff difficulties experienced in treating a patient or managing patient care are not nursing diagnoses. For instance, personnel may unethically label a patient as uncooperative, demanding, or stubborn. Such labels applied to patients have no meaning in terms of health problems. In fact, uncooperative, demanding behaviors can be a way of expressing undiagnosed problems and inadequate planning. Such problems are the staff's, not the patient's.

Nursing diagnoses are not medical diagnoses, tests, treatments, procedures, or equipment. "On respirator," "cholecystectomy," "continuous intravenous therapy" have all been mistakenly referred to as nursing diagnoses. While nurses do make tentative medical diagnoses, these are referred to physicians for affirmation and treatment. Certain secondary problems arising from medical diagnoses, complications, tests, and the like, for example, "Fear of death related to surgery," can be treated by nurses. Sometimes symptoms of a medical diagnosis are the same as health problems that nurses treat. For instance, colitis is associated with persistent, copious diarrhea. As a result, the patient with this disease has a high potential for fluid and electrolyte imbalance. Both diarrhea and fluid imbalance are among nursing problem areas. In colitis, however, the symptoms are caused by the pathology. Causative factors are often the source for distinguishing problems treatable by nurses from those treatable by physicians.

Just as with medical diagnoses, one or two signs

and symptoms do not make a nursing diagnosis—a cluster of related signs and symptoms is necessary. Among the cluster must be those that are considered critical, or "defining," signs and symptoms, An actual problem cannot be determined unless the defining characteristics are present. Assumptions based on one or two symptoms are likely to be erroneous and misleading. In the extreme, such assumptions can result in harm to the patient; minimally, they can waste time without patient benefit. A patient might state that he is not concerned with his physical appearance. The nurse cannot automatically think, "Probably a self-image problem," because the statement is only one cue that must be considered in relation to others. (A cue is an indicator that triggers action on the part of the person noting it.) But if the patient is an elected public official, is scheduled for a radical neck dissection, is meticulous in dress, and keeps himself lean and fit, the cluster of cues might perhaps indicate a potential problem in self-image or coping, depending on other cues available.

The diagnostic process is not a series of consecutive, forward steps. It can be separated, however, into four major activities: (1) collecting data, (2) interpreting data, (3) clustering data, and (4) naming the cluster or the problem. These activities may occur simultaneously when the diagnostician is experienced. The nurse may note a cue and almost before the patient is finished speaking or the reading finished, process the information mentally. After blood pressure has been taken, for example, the nurse knows instantaneously whether the systolic and diastolic pressures are within the expected range.

Collecting Assessment Data

Since the collection of data has been addressed in the chapter on assessment, it will not be discussed further unless the subject is necessary to illustrate a point.

Interpreting Assessment Data

As the nurse collects clinical health data, the information is interpreted using a number of mental processes that eventually permit the nurse to reduce possible diagnoses from a great many to a few and finally to as many as or few as necessary to identify problems. A general term for these thought processes is hypothesizing. Hypothesizing is formulating an explanation for the occurrence of related events, conditions, or behavior. The explanation is a conjecture used to guide the search for additional cues. It is an educated guess, based initially on one

or two cues. Hypothesizing involves clinical reasoning and retrieval from memory of theory and experiential data. The process is one that human beings use constantly every day.

Human beings grow up asking the questions, "What is it?" "Why?" and "What is it used for?" We learn from these questions to distinguish among similar objects in our environment, to identify the unknown from the known, and to predict (hypothesize) an event, condition, or object on the basis of cues. For instance, a young child learns the word *chair.* He or she may associate the word first with a high chair where food is consumed in a sitting position, or with a chair in which the mother holds and rocks the child. The child notes the appearance and purpose of both chairs. Eventually, the child learns that there are many types of chairs and can distinguish between the different types. This is a purely discriminatory mental process that all human beings have and use constantly.

Nurses take this line of reasoning during the diagnostic process. In reviewing functional patterns and observing the patient, they evaluate cues by asking, "What does this mean? Why is he or she saying this?" A conscious decision is made to explore some cues and not others. Perhaps nurses do not follow up a cue immediately but return later to it. What is the meaning of a blood pressure of 160/90 in a 20-year-old male athlete? When a patient says, "I'm not concerned with what I look like," what does that mean and what is causing him to say that? A hypothesis is made that the cue is an indicator of a problem. The nurse might even make a tentative hypothesis about the nature of the problem—a tentative explanation. Sometimes there is no need for this because the cues are obvious. The cause of that problem, however, must be investigated.

Nurses reason from one or two cue clusters to hypothesize a problem (inductive reasoning). For example:

1. This patient is scheduled for surgery tomorrow (cue).
2. This patient has the signs and symptoms of anxiety (observation cue cluster).
3. This patient's anxiety might be related to the proposed surgery (inductive hypothesis).

Nurses also use clinical inferences in inductive reasoning. Inferences can be equated with hypotheses, although there is a slight difference. One infers something that goes beyond the data base. In making an inference, the nurse takes a known principle and applies it to the situation under consideration.

Reasoning by inductive inference proceeds as follows:

1. The patient belongs to the class, partially physically dependent (inductive inference).
2. The patient once belonged to the class, physically independent (inductive inference).
3. Therefore the change in status from independence to dependence might produce a self-concept disequilibrium (tentative problem hypothesis).

(Dependent and independent in this sense refer to the patient's need or lack of need for support in the activities of daily living, i.e., dressing, toileting, etc.) Inferences 1 and 2 go beyond the actual data to infer circumstances so that the hypothesis in 3 can be reached. Inference 2 must be substantiated and more information is required to support the hypothesis.

Deductive reasoning is also used to make clinical inferences. In deductive reasoning, a general premise believed to be true in a large number of instances is used to infer a possible individual problem:

1. Surgical patients experience anxiety (verified by research and experience).
2. This is a surgical patient (cue).
3. Therefore this patient might be anxious (deductive inference or hypothesis).

A deductive inference is a prediction about the nature of a problem and must be supported by careful collection of additional data to avoid a diagnostic error. The general premise must also fit the circumstances. One could not use the premise, "Surgical patients experience anxiety" as the proposition to support anxiety for a nonsurgical patient. The premises used in deductive reasoning are drawn from the nurse's knowledge of concepts acquired from education and experience.

Data interpretation also involves generating two or more possible explanations for a group of related cues. Because the chances of identifying human problems are always less than 100 percent, the element of uncertainty stimulates the diagnostician to consider all possible explanations. Multiple hypotheses enable the nurse to concentrate the search for additional cues. The cue cluster might be: Mrs. Kelso, who is five months pregnant, is admitted for an appendectomy. She is a para 0, gravida 3. She says, "I can't believe this is happening—just when I thought everything was going so well!" What are some possible hypotheses to be made in Mrs. Kelso's situation?

- Hypothesis 1: knowledge deficit
- Hypothesis 2: psychological disequilibrium (guilt? depression?)
- Hypothesis 3: anticipatory grieving related to premature delivery of nonviable infant

The separation of data collection and interpretation is artificial because the two activities occur simultaneously. The objective of the diagnostic process is to reduce the number of possible problems as rapidly, efficiently, and accurately as possible. For this reason, hypotheses are generated and serve as a focus for the search for additional data. Clinical reasoning also furnishes predictive hypotheses that serve the same function.

Clustering the Data

After data collection and interpretation, clustering information is the third activity of the diagnostic process. Clustering is the realignment of related cues—a mental sorting of data pertaining to hypotheses and inferences. Use of a data-gathering tool based on the functional pattern typology assists in obtaining partially clustered data. As the nurse investigates the meanings of cues, however, the information may fit with another pattern or hypothesis.

Clustering involves judgmental tasks. One must be aware of inconsistencies among cues—data that refute other cues—and decide which inconsistencies should be held for further study and which discarded. Awareness of these difficulties should open the nurse's thinking to include all the possibilities so that the diagnostic errors can be prevented.

Once the cues have been clustered, two or three probable diagnoses with probable causes for each cluster are predicted. These are then tested one by one through a search for critical defining characteristics that differentiate one diagnosis from another. The presence of the defining characteristics confirms a diagnosis. If all the critical defining characteristics of a diagnosis are not present but other characteristics are, the patient is at risk for the actual problem to occur and has a potential problem.

Naming the Diagnosis

The final task in the diagnostic process is to record the diagnosis, its etiologies, and the cues. Only those diagnoses for which critical defining characteristics are present should be recorded. If no currently accepted diagnosis is available, the nurse should record the diagnosis in his or her own words as briefly and concisely as possible. If adequate supporting data for a diagnosis are not present, signs and symptoms or tentative hypotheses can be recorded.

EFFORTS TO DEVISE AND CLASSIFY NURSING DIAGNOSES

The current work in generating and classifying nursing diagnoses began as an outgrowth of a project initiated at St. Louis University by Kristine Gebbie and Mary Ann Lavin. These two faculty members were attempting to identify the nurse's role in their ambulatory care unit. Difficulties in naming problems treated by nurses made them aware of the need for a classification of nursing diagnoses similar to the medical classification system used by physicians. St. Louis University school of nursing hosted a conference on the subject in 1973, at which the National Conference Group for Classification of Nursing Diagnoses was formed. In 1982 the conference group chose a new name, North American Nursing Diagnosis Association (NANDA).*

The association is made up of nurse practitioners, educators, researchers, and theorists. The group meets every 2 years to generate new diagnoses, refine or discard others, identify etiologies and characteristics, and formulate an overall framework for nursing diagnoses. Regular meetings of the association membership are required by the bylaws.

At the first conference, a national task force was appointed to carry out the developmental work between meetings. Marjorie Gordon, a recognized authority on nursing diagnosis, chaired the task force from 1973 to 1982. The national task force as the interim board of directors of NANDA was initially responsible for organizing the newly formed association. Much work is yet to be accomplished if the goal of NANDA is to be reached—the publication of an international classification system of nursing diagnoses with a standardized nomenclature. Usually, within a year, the proceedings of the most recent meeting of NANDA are published. Information about purchasing the proceedings can be obtained by contacting the Association. They are valuable for nurses because they contain not only the most recent proceedings but also papers presented during the meeting and the most recent developments in naming and classifying nursing diagnoses.

It seems appropriate to reiterate that acceptance

by NANDA does not imply that diagnoses generated and published by the group are finished, final, or valid. Questions have been raised about the appropriateness of physiological diagnoses as *nursing diagnoses* (3). Although the published diagnoses represent the educational and clinical expertise of their originators, all must be subjected to research for validation. Testing of many diagnoses is ongoing.

Perioperative nurses have not yet given much attention to using diagnostic labels, to researching proposed diagnoses, or to generating new ones. Are there nursing diagnoses germane only to the intraoperative phase of perioperative nursing care? Roy (4) suggested that perioperative nurses may become specialists in helping patients cope with fears associated with surgery. As the perioperative role develops and expands, these nurses may be more involved in defining and treating patients' actual and potential health problems related to surgery.

A brief discussion of one approach to defining nursing diagnoses was provided in this chapter. The beginning practitioner or nurse who is unfamiliar with the concept will have to flesh out this skeleton of information in detail and depth. Too many nurses fail to perceive the rigorous intellectual discipline, depth of knowledge, and lengthy clinical experience necessary to apply the concept for true patient benefit. To them, nursing diagnoses are a kind of fad, and as such, will soon be replaced by something else to occupy their attention. Yet making nursing diagnoses is one, and probably the only, function that distinguishes the professional nurse from all other healthcare workers.

Case Example
The data collected on Mr. Fischer revealed several nursing diagnoses. Because of the extensive nature of his surgery, only a few problems are illustrated (Fig. 5.2). Mr. Fischer was asked in an interview to explain his understanding of the proposed procedure. The perioperative nurse was attempting to determine Mr. Fischer's knowledge base. The premise was that coping with the unknown is more likely to produce psychological disequilibrium than coping with the known. The nurse could also be thinking of other predictive hypotheses, such as the alteration in self-concept, ineffective individual coping strategies, and fear. These would all be appropriate considering the potentially mutilating surgery proposed for Mr. Fischer. All the predictive hypotheses are changed to predictions of potential problems.

When the nurse learned that Mr. Fischer was unaware

*Membership in NANDA is available to all licensed nurses on payment of an annual fee. Inquiries should be directed to: Executive Director, NANDA, 3525 Caroline Street, St. Louis, MO 63104.

PATIENT CARE PLAN
Mr. Ralph Fischer

Nursing Diagnosis	Expected Outcome	Plan	Implementation	Evaluation
PREOPERATIVE				
Knowledge deficit; lack of specific information regarding phenomena that might affect level of functioning				
Communication impaired; verbal, resulting from tracheostomy, wired jaw, and possible impaired anatomical structure (tongue)				
INTRAOPERATIVE				
Potential for neuromuscular damage due to required positioning and length of surgical procedure				
POSTOPERATIVE				
Respiration; alteration in, due to tracheostomy				
Increased risk for postoperative (respiratory) complications due to history of bronchitis, history of smoking, exposure to environmental irritants				

FIGURE 5.2. Beginning patient care plan for Mr. Fischer.

of the possible total glossectomy and that extensive jaw resection might be necessary, the nursing diagnoses was identified as, "Knowledge deficit, lack of specific information regarding phenomena that might affect level of functioning." The second preoperative nursing diagnosis was, "Communication impaired; verbal, resulting from tracheostomy, wired jaw, and possible impaired anatomical structure (tongue)." The nature of the proposed surgery and the wired jaw with associated tracheostomy were the cues and inferences from which inductive reasoning generated this diagnosis. The probability for the problem to occur was 100 percent.

Because of the extensive nature of the surgery and the reconstructive and plastic work scheduled for the patient's mandible and mouth floor as well as the tongue and mandibular resection, the procedure would probably take 10 to 12 hours. Artificial maintenance of neck, head, arm, and other body parts in an abnormal position for a lengthy period of time would cause pressure on nerves that could result in muscular weakness or paralysis. As a consequence, there was a potential in this patient for neuromuscular damage during the operative period. The diagnosis was based on the nurse's knowledge of positioning for the procedure and physiological concepts, an inference about the length of the procedure, and experience. It was a predictive hypothesis and had a high risk factor associated with it.

The perioperative nurse predicted two potential problems for Mr. Fischer during the postoperative phase, but had difficulty naming the diagnosis. Because nursing diagnoses are as yet undefined, and because the validity of those in the physiological category is being questioned, the nurse finally settled on the diagnosis, "Respiration; alteration in, due to tracheostomy." However, the nurse was aware that perhaps the problem was not a nursing diagnosis in the true sense but rather a statement of medically prescribed therapy that involved specific nursing responsibilities, observations, and tasks. Although there were no specific data to warrant another prediction, the nurse's knowledge and experience indicated that patients who have airway alterations and are dependent on someone else for clearing secretions show varying degrees of anxiety. In Mr. Fischer's case, the airway alteration would be complicated by a wired jaw, swollen tongue, and perhaps glossectomy, making his ability to control salivary secretions difficult. While this would not interfere with respiration, he would have to experience and adapt to the reality before some of his probable anxiety dissipated. Although not indicated on the care plan, the nurse formulated another diagnosis, "Anxiety; potential, due to alteration in physiological airway path (tracheostomy)." The nurse believed this to be a difficulty nurses can treat and predicted the possibility of its occurrence as fairly high in the immediate postoperative period.

The second postoperative problem identified, "Increased risk for postoperative (respiratory) complications," further illustrates the question of separating problems nurses can treat from those for which they have traditionally observed and reported the presence or absence of signs and symptoms to physicians. Nevertheless, the nurse left the problem on the care plan based on cues such as history of smoking, history of exposure to noxious gaseous inhalants, and tracheostomy.

REFERENCES

1. Gordon, Marjorie. *Nursing Diagnosis: Process and Application.* New York: McGraw-Hill, 1982.
2. American Nurses' Association. *The Code for Nurses with Interpretative Statements.* Kansas City, MO: ANA, 1985.
3. Crowell, R. M., ed. *Classification of Nursing Diagnoses: Proceedings of the Ninth Conference. North American Nursing Diagnosis Association.* Philadelphia: J. B. Lippincott, 1991.
4. Roy, C. "The impact of nursing diagnosis." *AORN J* 21:1023, 1975.

SUGGESTED READINGS

Carnevali, D., and Blainey, C. *Diagnostic Reasoning in Nursing.* Philadelphia; J. B. Lippincott, 1984.

Carpenito, L. K. *Nursing Diagnosis: Application to Clinical Practice* 3rd ed. Philadelphia: J. B. Lippincott, 1989.

Gordon, M. *Nursing Diagnosis: Process and Application.* 2nd ed. New York: McGraw-Hill, 1987.

Happ, M. B., and Kerr, M. E. "Nursing effort and the exchanging human response pattern." *Nursing Diagnosis* 2(4):155–161, 1991.

Iyer, P., Taptich, B., and Bernocchi-Losey, D. *Nursing Process and Nursing Diagnosis.* Philadelphia: W. B. Saunders, 1986.

Kelly, M. *Nursing Diagnosis Source Book: Guidelines for Clinical Application.* Norwalk, CT: Appleton-Century-Crofts, 1985.

Kolcaba, K. Y. "A taxonomic structure for the concept comfort." *Image* 23(4): 237–240, 1992.

LeMone, P. "Analysis of a human phenomenon: Self concept." *Nursing Diagnosis* 2(3):126–130, 1991.

Loomis, M. E., and Conco, D. "Patients' perceptions of health, chronic illness, and nursing diagnosis." *Nursing Diagnosis* 2(4):162–170, 1991.

McFarland, G. K., and McFarlane, E. A. *Nursing Diagnosis and Intervention: Planning for Patient Care.* St. Louis, MO: C. V. Mosby, 1989.

Mehmert, P. A., and Delaney, C. W. "Validating impaired physical mobility." *Nursing Diagnosis* 2(4):143–154, 1991.

Minton, J. A., and Creason, N. C. "Evaluation of admission nursing diagnoses." *Nursing Diagnosis* 2(3):119–125, 1991.

Mitchell, G. J. "Nursing diagnosis: An ethical analysis." *Image* 23(2):99–103, 1992.

Ouellet, L. L., and Rush, K. L. "A synthesis of selected literature on mobility: A basis for studying impaired mobility." *Nursing Diagnosis* 3(2):72–80, 1992.

Popkiss, S. "Diagnosing your patient's strengths." *Nurs 81* 11(7):34, 1981.

Roberts, C. "Identifying the real patient problems." *Nurs Clin North Am* 17:481, 1982.

Smith, A. R. "Examination of nursing diagnosis for adults hospitalized with acquired immunodeficiency syndrome." *Nursing Diagnosis* 2(3):111–117, 1991.

Summers, S. "Hypothermia: One nursing diagnosis or three?" *Nursing Diagnosis* 3(1):2–11, 1992.

Summers, S. "Inadvertent hypothermia: Clinical validation in postanesthesia patients." *Nursing Diagnosis* 3(2):54–64, 1992.

Whitley, G. G. "Concept analysis of anxiety." *Nursing Diagnosis* 3(3):107–116, 1992.

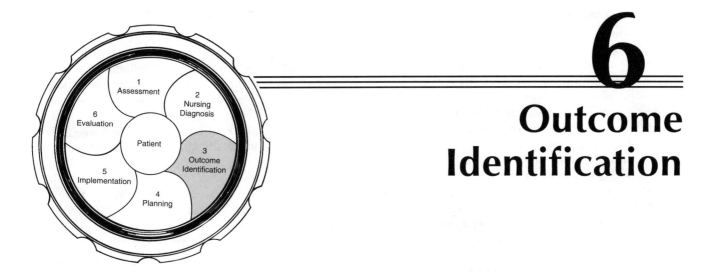

6

Outcome Identification

The perioperative nurse deliberately plans care for the patient.

Perioperative nurses demonstrate a commitment to assist surgical patients to return to their level of wellness by following through on each step of the nursing process. In chapter 5 we discussed the formulation of a nursing diagnosis or what is often referred to as the patient problem. These diagnoses are derived from the data collected and form the basis for determining the expected outcome or the end result of the care provided. Expected outcomes direct the plan of care and subsequent nursing interventions. The nursing interventions selected should produce the desired outcomes.

This chapter provides the perioperative nurse with information on how to develop and evaluate outcome statements. It also introduces six patient outcomes that are specifically related to the perioperative patient. Each of these six outcomes is discussed in detail in a subsequent chapter. The patient situation will further explain outcomes as they relate to total care.

WHAT ARE PATIENT OUTCOMES?

In its *Patient Outcomes: Standards of Perioperative Care,* the Association of Operating Room Nurses (AORN) defines patient outcomes as the "observable and/or measurable physiological, psychosocial, and psychological responses to perioperative nursing intervention" (1). Outcomes are the desired end result of carefully planned and orchestrated care. Achievement of these outcomes requires that the peri-

operative nurse be knowledgeable regarding current nursing concepts and skilled in practice and application of new technology. The expected outcomes can only be achieved by implementing care as outlined in the plan.

ESTABLISHING PATIENT OUTCOMES

Planning care for the perioperative patient starts with collection of data through assessment, and proceeds through formulation of a nursing diagnosis, identification of expected outcomes, and prescribing nursing actions to achieve these outcomes. Patient outcomes are an end toward which action is taken.

Outcomes are patient-centered. They enable the perioperative nurse to measure the effectiveness of nursing care and provide a guide for evaluating the extent to which intervention was effective.

Outcomes are stated in measurable, behavioral terms. The patient may indicate progress toward an expected outcome by verbalizing, demonstrating, or exhibiting certain signs and symptoms.

- In verbalizing, the patient states, explains, or describes what he or she knows, understands, or feels about illness, treatment, or expectations. Such an outcome might be, "The patient will openly discuss feelings about having a radical neck dissection prior to receiving his preoperative medication."
- An example of an outcome in which the patient

demonstrates an expected behavior might be, "The patient will demonstrate coughing and deep-breathing exercises prior to receiving the preoperative medication."

- Some outcomes require that the patient exhibit certain signs and symptoms, with one set of observations being compared to another using preestablished norms. Signs and symptoms may be detected from laboratory tests or vital signs. In a patient with altered venous circulation, for example, the expected outcome might be, "The patient will be free of circulatory system complications 48 hours postoperatively."

Outcomes must be well formulated to assist the nurse in planning nursing actions. The more specific the outcome, the easier it is to measure the extent to which it is met.

There are four parts of a patient outcome statement: the subject, the terminal behavior, the criterion, and any conditions:

- The *subject* is the patient. The patient is expected to exhibit the behavior.
- The *terminal behavior* is the action or performance required to meet the expected outcome. What action is required for the patient to reach a predetermined health status? For example, for a patient with a below-the-knee amputation, the expected outcome might be, "The patient will walk using a prosthesis and crutches." The action is the patient walking. In the outcome statement, this is the verb, or the action the subject will perform.
- The *criterion* is the standard against which the behavior is measured for acceptable performance. What level of performance are we expecting the patient to achieve? What constitutes "use of a prosthesis"? Will the patient be walking with the use of a prosthesis at discharge, 20 days postoperatively, or when? The criterion should always contain a designated time or date for achieving the behavior.

- The *conditions* are the circumstances or phenomena under which the patient will achieve the expected outcome. Not every outcome has a condition. The condition for the outcome stated above could be, "Patient will walk with a prosthesis assisted by crutches at discharge." The crutches and prosthesis are the conditions under which the patient will walk.

Table 6.1 provides examples of the subjects, terminal behaviors, criteria, and conditions of four different patient outcomes.

Outcomes should be stated as concisely as possible and should be congruent with assessment data, nursing diagnoses, and current knowledge and practice. They should be realistic, usable, measurable, behavioral, achievable, and include a time element.

- Outcomes are *realistic*. Outcome statements should be practical and reasonable. They should not exceed what is possible for that particular patient. An outcome statement that is realistic for a patient having a lumbar laminectomy might be, "The patient will be ambulating 48 hours postoperatively."
- Outcomes are *usable*. Outcome statements should serve the purpose for which they are developed. They should be consistent with the patient's problem and based on the nursing diagnosis. If the nursing diagnosis is "Potential bleeding due to slow clotting time," an outcome statement might be, "The patient will not have excessive bleeding due to surgical procedure."
- Outcomes are *measurable*. Outcome statements must be able to be quantified to determine the extent to which the outcome is met. For example, if the desired outcome for a patient with a fractured femur is, "The patient will arrive safely in the operating room with the leg in alignment and free of pain," this can be measured by the patient's statement that he or she has no pain or by the nurse's observation that the patient does

TABLE 6.1. The Four Parts of a Patient Outcome

Subject (Who)	Terminal Behavior (Action verb)	Criteria (When, where)	Condition (Extent met)
Patient	Will explain what it means to have a colostomy	Prior to administration of medication	Has knowledge
Patient	Will be free of infection	48 hours postoperatively	No infection
Patient	Will have minimal pain	24 hours postoperatively	Minimal pain
Patient	Will ambulate	Up and down hall 1 day postoperatively	With help of walker

not exhibit signs of pain. It may also be measured by the nurse's observation that the traction is on and the patient's leg is in alignment.

- Outcomes are *behavioral*. The patient should be able to verbalize, demonstrate, or exhibit signs or symptoms that can be used in measuring the end result. For example, the outcome statement, "The patient states his knowledge and understanding of the surgical procedure and has signed the informed consent form" defines specific behavioral objectives that are to be met.
- Outcomes are *achievable*. The outcome statement must be able to be carried through and accomplished to achieve the desired result. For example, is the statement "The patient is free of infection 72 hours after a laparoscopic-assisted abdominal hysterectomy" a realistic outcome? Can it be achieved?
- Outcomes have a *time element*. Outcomes should have a time frame that can be used to measure the extent to which the outcome has been attained. For example, if the outcome is "The patient will walk with crutches," the time element might be 72 to 96 hours postoperatively, depending on the patient.

Perioperative nurses must have the ability to predict the outcomes of nursing actions, based on experience with different types of surgical procedures and observations of other patients' postoperative progress. They must have current knowledge of disease processes, types of surgery, and new technology. In addition, perioperative nurses must keep up with the current literature and gain experience in completing patient profiles from medical records.

EVALUATING OUTCOME STATEMENTS

AORN's *Standards of Perioperative Clinical Practice* (2) defines criteria to be used by perioperative nurses when establishing patient outcomes. After devising patient outcome statements, the nurse should evaluate those statements using the following questions:

- Is the outcome derived from a nursing diagnosis? If the diagnosis is that the patient is having considerable pain, the nurse would expect the outcome to be directly related to the patient's pain.
- Is the outcome stated so that it can be observed? Will the nurse be able to observe the patient's response to nursing intervention and determine if

the outcome is met? If the outcome is "The patient will have minimal pain 24 hours postoperatively," the nurse should be alert for signs and symptoms of pain.

- Is the outcome formulated with guidance from the patient, the family, significant others, and other healthcare personnel? Without the cooperation of all these persons, there is no assurance that the outcome is realistic or attainable. The amount of the patient's involvement depends on the illness and type of surgery. When planning care, the nurse has a responsibility to involve the patient and family in identifying important information and organizing, analyzing, and interpreting that information (3).
- Is the outcome congruent with the patient's present and potential physical capabilities and behavioral patterns? This question is answered by reviewing baseline observations made on admission, as well as the nursing diagnoses. The nurse also learns about the patient's potential through the patient's own assessment, the family's impressions, and opinions of other healthcare professionals who have worked with the patient.
- Is the outcome attainable through available human and material resources? Judgment is important in deciding which patient problems are pertinent to the upcoming surgery. In which problems can the nurse realistically intervene? Which problems are appropriate to the nurse's specialty? The services provided by the institution dictate the types of personnel and equipment available. Policies of the operating room are also a factor.
- Can the outcome be achieved within an identifiable period of time? To measure achievement of expected outcomes, the nurse must establish a deadline or a time frame for achievement. An example might be "The patient will be free of wound infection 72 hours postoperatively." The outcome has a clear time period. If the patient shows any evidence of wound infection in this time, such as redness, swelling, or drainage at the incision site, the nurse knows that this goal has not been met. If the wound is clean and dry with no evidence of redness or swelling at 72 hours postoperatively, the nurse could safely say the outcome has been achieved.
- Are the outcomes assigned appropriate priorities? Once identified, outcomes should be ranked in order of importance. The patient, family, nurse, and other members of the healthcare team all participate in assigning priorities. The

nurse must determine what care is required immediately, what care can wait for a time, and what actions may be needed for long-term followup.

AORN's *Patient Outcomes: Standards of Perioperative Care* (1) provides the following six definitive outcomes for measuring patients' responses to surgical intervention:

- The patient demonstrates knowledge of the physiological and psychological responses to surgical intervention.
- The patient is free from infection.
- The patient's skin integrity is maintained.
- The patient is free from injury related to positioning, extraneous objects, or chemical, physical, and electrical hazards.
- The patient's fluid and electrolyte balance is maintained.

- The patient participates in the rehabilitation process.

These six broad outcomes represent potential problem areas for all patients undergoing surgery. It must be noted that even these must be individualized depending on the nursing diagnosis. For example, although not all patients will develop an infection, all have the potential for infection. Thus, "The patient is free from infection" remains an appropriate outcome for all surgical patients. Criteria to measure outcome achievement may differ depending on the site of infection, but can be developed around signs and symptoms.

Developing precise outcomes is a skill worth cultivating. Not only do exact outcomes enable the nurse to plan systematically for individualized care, they contribute to making nursing more scientific. Based on the scientific method, the nursing process is a way of planning care logically instead of instinc-

---

INTRAOPERATIVE PATIENT CARE PLAN
Mr. Ralph Fischer

Nursing Diagnosis	Outcome	Plan	Implementation	Evaluation
PREOPERATIVE				
Knowledge deficit; lack of specific information regarding phenomena that might affect level of functioning	Patient will verbalize understanding of his perioperative care prior to administration of preoperative medications.			
Communication impaired; verbal, resulting from tracheostomy, wired jaw, and possible impaired anatomical structure (tongue)	Patient will be able to communicate postoperatively.			
INTRAOPERATIVE				
Potential for neuromuscular damage due to required positioning and length of surgical procedure.	Patient will be free from neuromuscular complications 24 hours postoperatively.			
POSTOPERATIVE				
Respiration; alteration in, due to tracheostomy	Patient will have patent alternative airway until tracheostomy is closed.			
Increased risk for postoperative (respiratory) complications due to history of bronchitis, history of smoking, exposure to environmental irritants	Patient will be free of respiratory complications 48 hours postop. 1. Infection 2. Atelectasis 3. Aspiration			

FIGURE 6.1.   Intraoperative plan of care showing preoperative, intraoperative, and postoperative nursing diagnoses and outcomes for Mr. Fischer.

tively or haphazardly. Patient outcomes are key in this process, because they distill what the nurse knows about the patient into concise statements that point out what future action the nurse believes will be successful.

Case Example

Outcomes must be realistic, usable, measurable, behavioral, achievable, and include a time element. To illustrate further how these elements are incorporated into outcomes, let us refer again to Mr. Fischer. Mr. Fischer is scheduled for a possible left hemiglossectomy, left mandibulectomy, and neck dissection. Postoperatively he is to have a tracheostomy, nasogastric tube, and wired jaw.

The preoperative assessment indicates that Mr. Fischer's surgery will create a communication problem. That is, the anatomical resection, jaw wiring, and tracheostomy will impair his ability to talk. Therefore, one expected outcome for Mr. Fischer might be "Patient will be able to communicate postoperatively with his physicians, nurses, and family members."

Because Mr. Fischer does not understand everything that will happen to him during the perioperative period, explanations are necessary to assist him in coping with his fear of the unknown. Therefore, another expected outcome related to communication might be "Patient will verbalize understanding of his perioperative care prior to administration of preoperative medications." Both outcome statements based on Mr. Fischer's communication problem meet the criteria described for developing an outcome statement.

Intraoperatively, Mr. Fischer has the potential for neu-romuscular damage because he is elderly, the procedure will be lengthy, and he has some evidence of edema in his extremities. The expected outcome in this regard is "Patient will be free from neuromuscular complications 24 hours postoperatively." This outcome also meets the criteria for developing outcome statements.

During the postoperative period, Mr. Fischer encounters a respiratory problem due to alteration of his airway by the presence of a tracheostomy and the mandibular fixation. In this instance, the expected outcome is simply "Patient will have patent alternative airway until tracheostomy is closed." A potential respiratory problem is his increased risk for postoperative complications because of his history of bronchitis, smoking, and exposure to environmental irritants. The related patient outcome is "Patient will be free of respiratory complications 48 hours postop, including infection, atelectasis, and aspiration." The intraoperative plan of care (Figure 6.1) lists the expected preoperative, intraoperative, and postoperative outcomes for Mr. Fischer.

REFERENCES

1. Association of Operating Room Nurses. "Standards of Perioperative Care." *AORN Standards and Recommended Practices for Perioperative Nursing—1992.* pp. II:7–1 to II:7–2. Denver: AORN, 1992.

2. Association of Operating Room Nurses. "Standards of Perioperative Clinical Practice." *AORN Standards and Recommended Practices for Perioperative Nursing—1992.* pp. II:4–1 to II:4–4. Denver: AORN, 1992.

3. Marriner, A. *The Nursing Process: A Scientific Approach to Nursing Care* 3rd ed. St. Louis, MO: C.V. Mosby, 1983.

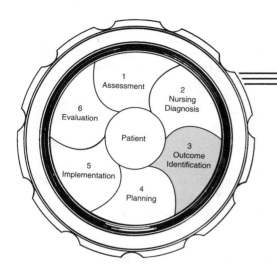

7

The Patient's Understanding of the Surgical Experience

Outcome: Knowledge of the physiological and psychological responses to surgery.

One of the outcomes identified by perioperative nursing is that the patient have a basic understanding of the planned surgical intervention. This outcome is based on the patient's legal right to know. In the 1970s the American Hospital Association published "A Patient's Bill of Rights" and the American Nurses' Association published "The Code for Nurses," providing nurses with written guidance concerning their obligation to confirm that the patient has given informed consent to surgery and is informed about the surgical experience. For several years, patients' rights were a supplemental set of information in the *Accreditation Manual for Hospitals* of the Joint Commission on Accreditation of Healthcare Organizations (JCAHO). Standards were addressed individually in several chapters of the manual. In 1992, an entire chapter was devoted to patients' rights (1).

In addition, the legal doctrine of informed consent requires that the patient understand the risks, benefits, and alternatives of the procedure, in order to be able to make an informed decision about whether or not to proceed with the surgery. Patients who do not receive and understand information about the procedure's risks/benefits and alternatives may sue the surgeon for malpractice. These suits will be successful if patients can demonstrate that they would not have consented if they had understood a risk, benefit, or alternative.

The first of AORN's *Patient Outcome Standards for Perioperative Care* states, "The patient demonstrates knowledge of the physiological and psychological responses to surgical intervention" (2). This statement reflects the commitment of the perioperative nurse to the patient's understanding of surgery. Further, the accompanying interpretive statement refers to the patient's right to information concerning the upcoming procedure and its potential physical and psychological effects. Also discussed is the patient's right to confidentiality, privacy, and maintenance of personal dignity. The criteria identified in the standard are general and address confirmation of consent for the surgery, ability to describe the sequence of events during the perioperative period, and ability to express feelings about the surgery, with realistic expectations regarding outcomes. This outcome is measured by specific criteria, which state that the patient, family, and significant others can:

1. Cite the reason(s) for each of the preoperative instructions provided and exercises explained or practiced
2. State the time surgery is scheduled
3. State the unit to which the patient will return after surgery (e.g., intensive care, same unit, postanesthesia care unit)
4. List anticipated monitoring and therapeutic devices or materials likely to be used postoperatively (e.g., intravenous catheters, transfusion, pain control devices)
5. State the location of family and significant others during the intraoperative and immediate recovery periods

6. Describe in general terms the surgical procedures and subsequent treatment plan (medical and nursing)
7. Describe anticipated steps in postoperative activity resumption
8. Verbalize expectations about pain relief and the measures likely to be taken to alleviate pain
9. Express feelings (anger, fear, anxiety, etc.) regarding surgical intervention and its expected outcomes

These criteria address outcomes directly related to patient teaching that is provided by nurses to assist the patient in participating in his or her care, lowering anxiety, involving the family, and other nursing actions. These patient teaching outcomes must be distinguished from the legal responsibility of the surgeon to provide information regarding the medical risks, benefits, and alternatives of a medical procedure under the informed consent doctrine.

INFORMED CONSENT

The nurse may have a legal responsibility as an employee of the healthcare facility where a surgical procedure is performed to assure that informed consent has been obtained. This responsibility is different from the surgeon's responsibility to obtain the consent. The nurse meets this obligation by following the policies of the individual facility. In facilities that use preprinted consent forms and require that the patient's signature be witnessed by a nurse, the nurse's role as witness is limited to an attestation that this patient signed this form. Figure 7.1 is a sample of such a consent form. The nurse who witnesses the patient's signature on a consent form does not attest to the adequacy or understanding of the information the patient received.

The nurse's legally recognized role in the informed consent process is a narrow one; ethically and professionally, however, the nurse's role is much broader in scope. As an advocate for the patient, the nurse must maintain a delicate balance between respect for the physician–patient relationship and advocacy for a patient with a knowledge deficit. If the nurse assesses a knowledge deficit related to the risks associated with the planned surgical procedure, the probability of success, or any alternatives, the nurse should treat this assessment just like the assessment of any other untoward medical condition. The nurse should first inform the surgeon and request direction; if the nurse feels the surgeon's response is insufficient to address the patient's need,

the nurse should follow the chain of command to bring the situation to the attention of someone with the necessary authority to intervene.

A valid informed consent must cover three specific points:

• The nature of the proposed treatment and the reasons for it
• Risks, complications, expected benefits, or effects of such treatment
• Alternatives to the procedure and their risks and benefits

Although it is the physician's responsibility to inform the patient of the nature, risks, benefits, or alternatives of a surgical procedure, the nurse may have to assess the patient's level of understanding and readiness to sign the consent form. In the preoperative interview, the nurse might ask the patient, "What do you understand about your operation?" If the patient does not have an adequate understanding of the procedure, the nurse may request that the physician talk again with the patient.

Perioperative nurses often question the length of time a consent is valid. Many hospitals specify the number of days consents are valid. Generally speaking, "a signed consent is valid as long as the patient consents to the procedure described. If the procedure changes or the patient withdraws [his or] her permission, then there is no longer consent for the procedure." (3)

The perioperative nurse should check the hospital protocol to remain within the parameters of the specific institution. When dealing with consents, nurses must understand their legal responsibilities. In the event of a lawsuit, it is important that the nurse know and follow hospital policies and procedures.

A good rule of thumb to follow is that if any substance or instrument is introduced into the patient's body space or cavity, a consent is required. The mere act of touching requires consent; without consent, touching may be considered battery. The nurse must know which diagnostic or surgical procedures require consent. Examples of procedures for which consents may be required include bone marrow aspiration, cardiac catheterization, myelogram, and insertion of hemodynamic monitoring devices.

The patient must sign the consent personally if he or she (1) is of legal age, (2) is under age but has a valid marriage certificate, (3) has been designated an emancipated minor (in certain states), or (4) is not presently under legal guardianship. The consent form must be signed by a parent or legal guardian if

Disclosure and Consent
Medical and Surgical Procedures

The Methodist Hospital   Houston, Texas   21-0433   2/88

Name of Patient: _____

TO THE PATIENT: You have the right, as a patient, to be informed about your condition and the recommended surgical, medical, or diagnostic procedure to be used so that you may make the decision whether or not to undergo the procedure after knowing the risks and hazards involved. This disclosure is not meant to scare or alarm you: it is simply an effort to make you better informed so you may give or withhold your consent to the procedure.

1. I (we) voluntarily request Dr. _____ as my physician, and such associates, technical assistants and other health care providers as they may deem necessary, to treat my condition which has been explained to me as: _____

_____

_____

2. I (we) understand that the following surgical, medical, and/or diagnostic procedures are planned for me and I (we) voluntarily consent and authorize these procedures: _____

_____

_____

3. I (we) understand that my physician may discover other or different conditions which require additional or different procedures than those planned. I (we) authorize my physician, and such associates, technical assistants and other health care providers to perform such other procedures which are advisable in their professional judgment.

4. I (we) (do) (do not) consent to the use of blood and blood products as deemed necessary.

5. Any tissues or parts surgically removed may be retained or disposed of by The Methodist Hospital in accordance with its accustomed practice.

6. I (we) understand that no warranty or guarantee has been made to me as to result or cure.

7. Just as there may be risks and hazards in continuing my present condition without treatment, there are also risks and hazards related to the performance of the surgical, medical, and/or diagnostic procedures planned for me. I (we) realize that common to surgical, medical, and/or diagnostic procedures is the potential for infection, blood clots in veins and lungs, hemorrhage, allergic reactions, and even death. I (we) also realize that the following risks and hazards may occur in connection with this particular procedure:

_____

_____

_____

_____

(continued on reverse side)

Patient Identification

FIGURE 7.1.   A sample of a preprinted consent form.

8. I (we) understand that anesthesia involves additional risks and hazards but I (we) request the use of anesthetics for the relief and protection from pain during the planned and additional procedures. I (we) realize the anesthesia may have to be changed possibly without explanation to me (us).

9. I (we) understand that certain complications may result from the use of any anesthetic including respiratory problems, drug reaction, paralysis, brain damage or even death. Other risks and hazards which may result from the use of general anesthetics range from minor discomfort to injury to vocal cords, teeth or eyes. I (we) understand that other risks and hazards resulting from spinal or epidural anesthetics include headache and chronic pain.

10. I (we) have been given an opportunity to ask questions about my condition, alternative forms of anesthesia and treatment, risks of nontreatment, the procedures to be used, and the risks and hazards involved, and I (we) believe that I (we) have sufficient information to give this informed consent.

11. I (we) certify this form has been fully explained to me, that I (we) have read it or have had it read to me, that the blank spaces have been filled in, and that I (we) understand its contents.

Date: _____ Time: _____ A.M.
                                                       P.M.

_____ _____
Patient/Other Legally Responsible Person Sign   Translator or Reader Sign

Witness(s):

_____ _____
Name

_____ _____
Address (Street or P.O. Box)

_____ _____
City, State, Zip Code

· ·

Patient, Do Not Write Below This Line

Identification of Patient Prior to Operation or Procedure

Doctor _____

identified patient as _____

_____
Physician's or Nurse's Signature

                                               ☐ A.M.
Date: _____ Time: _____ ☐ P.M.

FIGURE 7.1. (*continued*)

the patient is a minor or legally considered to be incompetent and is not included in any of the above categories. The nurse must examine the document for the correct date, time, and signatures, which must be in ink (and black ink may be necessary for microfilm copying). The validity of consent forms may have a time limit, such as thirty days.

Other types of consents the nurse may see include emergency consents, sterilization consents, or photograph consents, used as follows:

- In an emergency life-or-death situation in which surgical intervention is required and the patient is unable to sign a consent, the surgeon may legally proceed. Every effort must be made, however, to obtain permission from a responsible family member by telegram, telephone, or, in certain states, court order. In the case of telephone consent, two witnesses must hear the oral consent of the family member or responsible party and must sign the consent form with the name of the responsible party, noting that it is an oral consent by telephone. The surgeon may record, in the doctor's progress notes, the necessity for surgical intervention without obtaining a proper consent. This may release the hospital, operating room nurses, and other personnel from liability.
- Sterilization procedures, including vasectomy, tubal ligation by laparotomy or laparoscopy, and hysterectomy, require a special consent form. The nurse must know who is responsible for signing, that is, both husband and wife or only the individual having the procedure. The nurse should also be aware of any age cutoff for sterility consent. For example, such consent may not be required for a woman over 60 years of age.
- If the surgeon plans to photograph part or all of the surgical procedure, prior permission from the patient is usually required. A special consent form may be available, or the surgeon may add it to the informed operative consent.

For patients admitted to hospitals (but not to ambulatory centers), the Patient Self-Determination Act (42 U.S.C. Sec.1395cc) requires that patients also be informed of their right to formulate advance directives such as living wills and durable powers of attorney for healthcare if these advance directives are recognized by law in the state where the hospital is located. The law only requires that the hospital provide written information about advance directives and the hospital's policies regarding advance directives. However, the nurse must be prepared to answer questions or assist the patient in obtaining appropriate consultation. Therefore, the nurse must be familiar with the laws of the state and the role of the nurse in meeting the needs of the patient regarding advance directives.

ASSESSMENT OF PATIENTS' LEARNING NEEDS

Obvious nursing diagnoses for the preoperative patient are anxiety and knowledge deficit related to the impending surgical intervention. There are many other potential nursing diagnoses, such as ineffective individual coping, anticipatory grieving, altered sexuality patterns, or body image disturbance. These diagnoses may be identified during the assessment phase, depending on the nature and extent of the proposed surgical intervention. They are often arrived at through collaboration among several nurses, since time constraints require that information be communicated from the physician's office, to the hospital admitting area (inpatient or outpatient), and then to perioperative nurses.

Establishing nursing diagnoses and implementing appropriate interventions is a standard of nursing practice that a patient can expect to receive in a hospital accredited by JCAHO. Much of the intervention provided in the preoperative period is designed to help the patient understand the surgical experience. The challenge for the nurse is to rapidly assess the patient's current level of knowledge and his or her receptiveness to learning. Further, an appropriate teaching method must be determined and implemented.

The patient who is admitted the day of surgery or is to return home the same day must receive information in a short amount of time. In today's healthcare environment, where regulations increasingly determine what surgery will be undertaken, when the patient may arrive for preoperative preparation and how long the patient should be hospitalized, more efficient assessment and preoperative teaching methods must be developed. The patient who is admitted the day of surgery has greater learning needs than the patient who will have support from in-hospital nursing staff in answering questions in the perioperative period. Teaching content must be evaluated and expanded for the former patient.

Sufficient information must be provided to permit the patient and/or a support person to care for the patient both pre- and postoperatively. Again, today's healthcare environment is requiring more patients to care for themselves at home. Assessments or interventions previously provided by nurses on surgical units now must be done by patients, their families, or other support persons in the home. These persons must be taught what signs or symptoms they should be alert to and what to do about them should they occur, as well as expected pre- and postoperative activities. Failure to provide adequate teaching to enable patients to safely care for themselves could support a malpractice suit if the patient is injured as a result.

A patient's learning needs can be identified in several ways. If the patient asks questions, comments made during the interview may give clues to his or her understanding, or lack of it. Another way is for the nurse to ask the patient questions. It is important not to make assumptions about what the patient does or does not know. The patient's behavior may imply a lack of knowledge, but this assumption should be validated by questioning. Directed questions such as, "What information did you receive from the doctor's office?" or "Do you have questions about the instructions you received?" establish a baseline. This puts the patient at ease and reinforces the point that it is appropriate for the patient to ask questions about information that has already been given but that needs repeating or clarification.

EFFECTIVE TEACHING METHODS

Hospital and preoperative routines may be explained in many ways. Many hospitals and doctors' offices make videotapes available for patient viewing. Printed materials on hospital and operating room routines are also used widely.

These teaching aids must be supplemented by individualized instruction so that the patient understands the implications of the surgery. Providing information is not the same as teaching. Telling a mother not to give her child anything to eat or drink after midnight or printing it on a list of instructions assures only that information has been given, not that the mother has been taught. Many parents do not consider a glass of water "eating or drinking." Teaching the mother includes an explanation of the need for an empty stomach and the danger of vomiting. The explanation should be tailored to the assessed ability of the mother to understand. Care must be taken, however, not to alarm parents when discussing potential dangers to their children.

Wherever possible, demonstration should be used as an adjunct to teaching. If the perioperative nurse explains deep breathing, coughing, and passive exercises, for example, demonstration and re-

turn demonstration are most effective. Explaining respiratory and circulatory complications should be matter-of-fact, but the nurse should be continually alert to signs of anxiety when discussing complications. A patient who is not coping well with the stress of hospitalization and impending surgery may overreact and enter a crisis phase when such information is discussed. The nurse should be positive, supportive, and reassuring, presenting a decisive, confident image.

Close communication with the patient's physician is another important aspect of effective preoperative teaching. Unusual responses of patients should be reported to the physician immediately so that preoperative anxieties can be handled. It is extremely important for the nurse to realize that patients sometimes demonstrate a stressful reaction when discussing upcoming surgery. The nurse should not feel guilty if all does not run smoothly. It is not abnormal for preoperative patients to demonstrate some anxiety; in fact, a show of anxiety can be therapeutic if it is discussed and handled properly.

Informing the patient of the scheduled time of surgery can be challenging in some institutions. While there are many institutions in which the time of surgery can be predicted with some degree of accuracy, there are just as many in which it cannot be predicted with any certainty. Numerous variables, including the condition of the patient, can have an unforeseen impact on scheduling. It is advisable to discuss an approximate time, explaining that there may be delays and that such delays should not be cause for alarm. Whenever there is the possibility of an alternate plan, it should be explained to the patient. In the unfamiliar hospital setting, patients tend to consider information as absolute. The nurse should be certain that absolute status is not given to something that may be subject to change.

The same holds true when discussing the anticipated unit to which the patient will return, the equipment that will be used postoperatively for monitoring, and drains and other therapeutic devices. Collaboration with other team members is necessary so that accurate preoperative information can be given. Preoperative instruction is useless, and even harmful, if the total plan for the patient is not fully understood. Unit nurses, the surgeon or resident, the operating room supervisor or person who handles scheduling, and other personnel involved in activities that affect the patient can all provide the nurse with information prior to the interview and should be consulted if there are any questions.

A waiting area is usually provided for family or significant others during surgery. When giving this information, the nurse should be informed of the surgeon's routines. Some surgeons, for example, instruct families or friends to wait in the patient's room. Between procedures, the surgeon telephones the room to talk to them and gives them immediate postoperative information. Other surgeons meet families in the waiting area.

A challenging and demanding aspect of preoperative teaching is the delicate discussion of the surgery itself. The nurse must consult the physician before this discussion begins. As mentioned above, discussion of the surgery itself is the surgeon's legal responsibility. Patients sometimes ask very explicit questions of nurses in an effort to test the surgeon, the nurse, or both. If the nurse is to discuss surgical details, this discussion must reinforce the surgeon's prior explanation. In some instances, the surgeon may not wish the operation to be discussed by anyone else. In other cases, the surgeon and nurse mutually agree on what may be discussed. When on doubtful ground, a good rule to remember is to discuss only activities that the nurse is responsible for and that occur while the patient is awake. Whenever there is a discrepancy between the patient's understanding of the upcoming procedure and the actual situation, however, it is imperative that the nurse communicate with other members of the healthcare team, particularly the surgeon.

Perioperative nurses should also be prepared to discuss questions patients might ask regarding their postoperative activity. The opportunity for missing information is great because of the limited time for patients to receive instructions. Patients who will have extensive postoperative care may not be admitted until a few hours prior to surgery. The perioperative nurse shares responsibility for patient support if others are not available to provide it. For example, a patient may ask if the perioperative nurse will come to the intensive care unit to assist with postoperative care. Desire for continuity is indicated in this question. The perioperative nurse must be prepared to support, reassure, empathize with, and inform these patients. Questions that have been forgotten may often be elicited during the preoperative interview.

To determine if the patient understands the usual postoperative course, it is best to begin with broad questions. If the patient does not volunteer information or appears confused, more specific questions can be asked. Consider the following example:

Nurse: Do you have any questions about what happens after surgery?

Patient: No, I don't think so. (This response

may indicate that the patient does not know what to ask.)

Nurse: Do you understand that you will have a tube in your throat after surgery to help your breathing, and that it will be a bit uncomfortable?

Patient: The doctor said a machine would help me breathe for a while. How long will I have it?

Nurse: That will depend on how long it takes for your lungs to resume their normal function. Remember, you won't be able to talk while the tube is in place.

This approach will identify areas that may need reinforcement. Patients may not remember specifics that have already been explained. They only hear what they can cope with, and repetition helps them accept more information as they adapt to the hospital environment. This type of questioning can also be used to determine how much the patient has internalized about therapeutic devices that will be used postoperatively.

Using the word *discomfort* rather than *pain* can help minimize the patient's concern. Patients can be encouraged to discuss concerns and fears about pain, as well as their usual tolerance levels for pain or discomfort. For example, explaining why the patient may have some muscle discomfort can help allay concerns that postoperative discomfort is abnormal. If the patient understands that there is a reason for the discomfort, he or she will be less likely to worry that it indicates a complication. The nurse should discuss ways to relieve discomfort (e.g., by changing positions), as well as the availability of medication for extreme pain. The patient's expectations about pain and its relief can be identified by a question such as, "Do you have any concerns about postoperative discomfort?"

Questions about resuming activities after surgery are frequently spontaneous, requiring less probing. Patients may be eager to talk about the more positive aspects of their recuperation. If the outcome of the surgery is in doubt, however, short-term goals may be all the patient can cope with. The opportunity to express feelings about the surgery and its expected outcome can be provided using broad terms, allowing the patient to set limits on what is discussed.

It is probably unrealistic to expect that all of the patient's questions will be answered, particularly those related to the outcome of an uncertain diagnosis. Nevertheless, the entire staff can assist the patient in managing fears and anxiety by providing as much information as the patient needs or requests. Patients who are not hospitalized must be provided with telephone numbers of resource professionals who can answer any questions that arise after he or she goes home.

FACTORS THAT INFLUENCE EXPECTED PATIENT OUTCOMES

Many factors that can influence the effectiveness of communication between the nurse and the patient occur simultaneously in the perioperative setting. Important internal factors in communicating an understanding of an upcoming surgical procedure include the patient's perception of and attitude toward surgery, emotional state (e.g., anxiety level), and physical and mental readiness for surgery. External conditions such as location and timing of the interview, the involvement of family members or significant others, and the rapport the nurse is able to establish with the patient are also important components in attaining this goal.

Because the preoperative interview is a complex activity, all phases of the nursing process may occur during this period. In fact, the teaching–learning process has many similarities to the nursing process. The first phase of the teaching–learning process is assessment of the learner's abilities, followed by diagnosis of learning needs and setting goals for learning. Principles of learning are used during the planning and implementation phases. Evaluation of the extent to which an identified outcome is attained occurs throughout the perioperative period.

The assessment phase of the preoperative interview is much more subtle than simply observing for physical disorders such a petechiae, bruises, bumps, or limited range of motion. The perioperative nurse must make a nursing diagnosis of the emotional and psychosocial status of the preoperative patient. The teaching plan is initiated with the review of the patient's chart and continues during the interview with the patient and family.

Patient Perceptions and Attitude

The patient enters the hospital with a preconceived idea of what is to happen. This may be based on experience or derived from conversations with others who have had surgery. The nurse assesses the knowledge the patient already possesses and corrects or supplements it with factual information. Questions such as, "What is your understanding of surgery?" or "Do you have any particular concerns about your surgery?" often open up areas for clarification.

Rapport between the perioperative nurse and the patient will do much to change negative attitudes about the surgical experience and will have a positive effect on learning. How the nurse establishes rapport depends on the personality of the patient and the circumstances surrounding the interview.

Emotions

Neutral or slightly positive or negative emotions are generally conducive to learning. Extreme emotion, however, blocks learning. Patients who exhibit high anxiety as the result of shock or fear do not remember information given to them. Often, after the physician has told the patient about the need for surgery, the patient hears nothing else until later, when he or she accepts the situation. Once the patient has been admitted to the hospital or ambulatory surgery, slight anxiety motivates learning about what is likely to happen. For this reason, the time between admitting and surgery is usually a good time for preoperative teaching. In some situations, the stress level remains high, and preoperative teaching may have to be deferred except for minimal information. The patient must have time to accept surgery that is potentially disfiguring or that may result in a serious diagnosis. Nurses must also be aware of their own values and not project discomfort to the patient. How teaching is managed will be determined by how effectively the patient handles the surgical experience.

Patients respond to preoperative stress in the same manner as they cope with other crises or stresses in their lives. If they are unable to cope with stress in a positive way, they may use defense mechanisms temporarily or even as permanent adaptive behavior. For example, it is common to see denial manifested by an inappropriate cheerfulness in a patient who has a serious diagnosis. The patient may ask no questions, joke with the nurse, and try to control the conversation. Rather than confronting the patient's denial, the nurse should offer information in a casual manner, allowing trust to be established, with the patient setting the limitations.

For example, a man who is the director of a large department is admitted for a ptosis procedure under local anesthetic, with sedation and an anesthesiologist in attendance. This man is full of jokes prior to surgery and shows little interest in what will happen. He shrugs off teaching attempts with, "Oh, I know you all will take good care of me." However, after he is sedated, he is quiet and shows signs of marked anxiety. The nurse suggests to the patient that it must feel different to have someone else in charge of everything when he is used to making the decisions. The patient immediately expresses his discomfort at feeling helpless and seems to relax as the nurse instructs him on how to assist in his care for the next few hours. As his anxiety level increases, his defense level shifts from denial to repression and the nurse is able to help him manage. The more information nurses have about their patients, the more they are able to assist in anxiety management. Perhaps the most important factor, however, is the empathy of the nurse.

Patients are sometimes depressed; and sometimes manifest anger and guilt as they emerge from depression. These emotions must be understood and managed before learning can occur. The perioperative nurse who is confronted by a barrage of complaints about the hospital or staff or is told, "You're the fourth person to come in here bothering me," might handle this hostility by saying, "I'm sorry so many of us have interrupted you while you're getting settled. Each of us is involved in your care and we all want to do our best for you. Perhaps I could come back later if you need a little rest."

If the hostility does not have a focus but is simply rude, aggressive behavior, the nurse might ask, "You appear to be angry with me. I'm not sure why." If the patient continues to be hostile, it is best to offer to terminate the interview. Often, however, an open reference to the anger may assist the patient to deal with the reality of the surgery more effectively. In this instance, the patient's learning needs can often be met (Table 7.1).

TABLE 7.1. Facilitating Learning

Response to Anticipation of Surgery	Defense Mechanism	Other Contributing Factors	Nursing Intervention to Facilitate Learning
Anxiety May act jovial and in control. Minimizes or denies symptoms. Misleads the nurse. Uses phrases such as "just a little," "no problem," "no questions." Appears uncomfortable during conversation.	Denial	Patient may not be able to cope with helplessness.	Do not confront the denial. Establish trust. Volunteer some information of a nonthreatening nature and in a matter-of-fact manner. Casually solicit questions. Do not be controlling. Encourage patient through facilitators such as attentive silence, interested posture, etc.
Anger Indicates distrust at questioning. Accusing, suspicious. May complain about physician or other nurses.	Projection	Previous authority figure problems, i.e., angry competitive relationship with parent.	Do not be misled into believing that anger against health team is warranted. Ask about anger.
Frustration Expresses feeling of being thwarted. Anger directed at someone or something.	Projection	May have had bad experience with other hospital personnel, i.e., long wait in admitting department, lab, or x-ray.	Be tactful and firm. Do not side with patient against others on health team. Listen. Let patient vent feelings.
Depression and self-rejection Appears withdrawn, apathetic, silent.	Repression	Physical exhaustion due to illness or strain of admitting procedures. Resignation to feelings of helplessness, despair.	Ask tactful, kind questions about depression. Provide empathic silence. Quietly give major information. Offer availability when the patient feels stronger or feels like talking.
Compulsive behavior Overtalkative, egocentric, hypochrondriacal. Tells symptoms in detail. Asks questions, then apologizes for asking.	Regression	May have unusually dependent personality. May be embarrassed, nervous. May be attempting to be a "good" patient. Clinging, lonely, fear that interviewer will leave. Elderly patients sometimes ramble.	Reassure and support. Be certain patient understands. Ask patient to repeat instructions. Redirect as necessary to accomplish teaching goal.

Physical and Mental Readiness

A patient who is ill and mentally exhausted from coping with the problems associated with hospitalization may not remember or fully understand instructions. The nurse should note this limited readiness for learning and document the need for repeated teaching as the patient's health status improves. Use of the senses to help the patient know what to expect in surgery will help the patient remember. Since hearing remains acute after premedication, even when other senses are dulled, the nurse should warn the patient to expect noises or talking to seem louder. Demonstration, pictures, and descriptions of sights and sounds, for example, assist in preparing the patient for what will happen in the operating room. Describing the hard mattress or the cold room and the availability of warm blankets is useful. If videotapes, pictures, models, or verbal descriptions of what the patient will encounter are used, they should show how the patient will perceive the experience (Fig. 7.2). For example, pictures of the operating room should be taken from the stretcher or bed so that the surroundings are shown as the patient will see them.

Significant Others

Another factor influencing the expected outcome is the patient's support system. The importance of family and friends to the well-being of the patient must be determined. The nurse must identify such a person or persons and consider how to assist them through the surgical experience. The perioperative

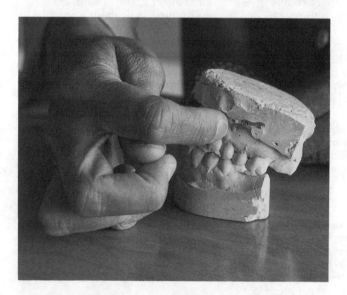

FIGURE 7.2. A model is used to show where the surgery will be and how dentures will be replaced.

nurse demonstrates concern about the comfort of the patient's relatives and friends by providing such information as where they can get coffee and where they should wait during the procedure.

The patient's significant other is the person who provides the major emotional support for the patient (Fig. 7.3). It may be a spouse or relative, but not necessarily. If the patient is alone, the nurse must find out if there is anyone who should be kept informed, or if the staff will be the patient's only support. Professional support may be important for such patients, but the nurse must be careful not to impose, allowing them to maintain their privacy and to depend on their own inner strength if they so desire.

Information obtained during the interview is confidential and should be released only to those immediately involved in the patient's care, unless the patient gives permission otherwise. Particular care should be taken with patients in ambulatory surgery. Messages should not be given to family members or others at the patient's telephone number unless the patient permits it. The patient may choose not to tell others about the surgery. For example, those who have cosmetic or sterilization procedures sometimes do not tell family or friends.

PRINCIPLES OF LEARNING

A review of some principles of learning illustrates ways the nurse can assist patients to achieve identified outcomes.

Patient Participation in the Learning Process

Discussion to determine what information the patient already has and to add or clarify instructions is important. Open-ended questions encourage dialogue and help the nurse assess what the patient anticipates.

Broad questions should be used initially; later, specific questions can be asked to obtain information the patient does not volunteer. Suppose a male patient has been admitted for a thyroidectomy. From reading his chart the nurse knows the patient had a cholecystectomy at another hospital ten years ago. After introducing him- or herself, the nurse might ask, "Have you had surgery before?" The patient might answer, "Yes, I had my gallbladder out several years ago, but I don't remember much about it, except that I was sore for a long time afterward." The nurse could describe some of the hospital routines, referring to the past experience, such as, "Do

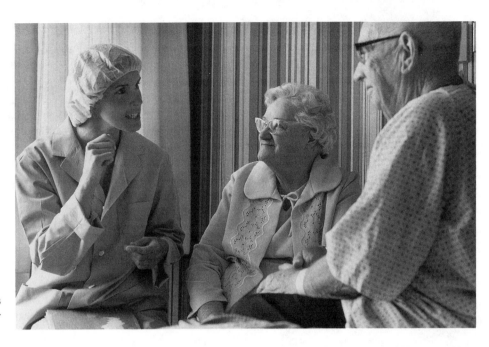

FIGURE 7.3. The patient's wife provides emotional support.

you remember not having had anything to eat or drink after midnight before your previous surgery?" By encouraging participation in this way, the interview is a comfortable dialogue for the patient, not stiff and lecturelike. The patient is contributing to the learning process, not just being bombarded with a lot of information or instructions. What the patient tells the nurse sets the tone for the preoperative teaching. From this information, the nurse can assess what the patient wants to know, what has already been discussed with the physician, and what the patient needs to know.

Repetition and Reinforcement

Repetition and reinforcement are necessary to increase the amount of information the patient retains. A patient who is having surgery under local anesthetic particularly benefits from a preoperative evaluation of the procedure. When instructions are repeated in the operating room, the patient is not dealing with unfamiliar information and finds it easier to comply.

Information discussed with the surgeon must be repeated and reinforced. A patient who is upset at the prospect of having surgery absorbs little information until his or her anxiety level decreases. At that time, questions about the perioperative period arise. Frequently, information or instructions must be repeated several times before a full understanding of events surrounding the operation is reached. The nurse can help patients to remember by asking

them to clarify their understanding of the procedure.

It is important to realize that a patient who denies having been informed about something most probably has forgotten the information. In such cases, nurses tend to assume the patient has not been informed.

Responsibility for preoperative teaching is shared by the surgeon, the anesthesiologist, and the nurses involved in the surgical experience. How effectively patient outcomes are met depends on the professional accountability of these individuals. It is important not only that they communicate with each other, but also that they share respect for each other and for the role each plays in the overall care of the patient. Nurses, in particular, must support each other if continuity of care is to be maintained throughout the preoperative, intraoperative, and postoperative phases of care. Oral communication and written documentation do much to provide this support.

Preoperative teaching is an active process that includes (1) assessment of learning needs and the patient's readiness to learn; (2) teaching, using learning principles; and (3) evaluating the effectiveness of the dialogue by observing the patient's responses.

REFERENCES

1. Joint Commission on Accreditation of Healthcare Organizations. *Accreditation Manual for Hospitals.* JCAHO, Oakbrook Terrace, IL, 1992.

2.   Association of Operating Room Nurses. *Standards of Perioperative Clinical Practice*. Denver: AORN, 1992.

3.   Allen-Bailey, Ann M. "Understanding informed consent." *Today's OR Nurse* 11(12):18, 1989.

SUGGESTED READINGS

American Hospital Association. *A Patient's Bill of Rights*. Chicago: AHA, 1972.

American Nurses' Association. *A Code for Nurses with Interpretative Statements*. Kansas City, MO: ANA, 1979.

Annas, G. J. *The Rights of Hospital Patients*. New York: Avon, 1975.

Coon, D. *Essentials of Psychology Exploration & Application* 5th ed. St. Paul, MN: West Publishing, 1991.

Murphy, E. K. "Informed consent: Part I." *AORN J* 47(April): 1009–1016, 1988.

Murphy, E. K. "Informed consent: Part II." *AORN J* 47(May): 1294–1298, 1988.

Redman, B. K. *The Process of Patient Education* 6th ed. St. Louis, MO: C. V. Mosby, 1988.

Rothrock, J. C. "Perioperative Nursing Records. Part I: Preoperative Psychoeducational Intervention." *AORN J* 49(2 February 1989): 597–614.

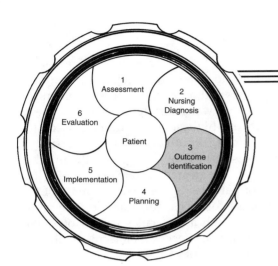

1 Assessment
2 Nursing Diagnosis
3 Outcome Identification
4 Planning
5 Implementation
6 Evaluation
Patient

8

Maintenance of Fluid and Electrolyte Balance

Outcome: Evidence of fluid and electrolyte balance.

Maintaining the water and electrolyte balance of the perioperative patient is a significant responsibility of the perioperative nurse. Under normal circumstances, the body's fluids and electrolytes play a key role in maintaining homeostasis. They transport the necessary oxygen and nourishment to the cells and they remove the waste products of cellular metabolism. They help to regulate the temperature of the body, and they form an integral part of the structure of the body (1).

While the conscious individual is able to regulate the body's fluid and electrolyte requirements by breathing, drinking, eating, and excreting appropriately, the unconscious surgical patient can no longer fulfill these functions alone, and needs the assistance of the perioperative nurse. In fulfilling the AORN standards and practices for perioperative nursing, the nurse will perform an initial preoperative assessment, develop nursing diagnoses and outcome statements, determine a plan of care, implement the plan to monitor and control the fluid and electrolyte status of the patient intraoperatively, and evaluate the effectiveness of the care provided postoperatively (2).

NORMAL FLUID DISTRIBUTION

Most of the weight of human beings is made up of body fluid. This fluid is a solution of water and electrolytes, but the principal ingredient is water. The amount of fluid in the body of the average person is around 57% of his or her weight; in fact, "the total amount of water in an average-sized man weighing approximately 70 kilograms is approximately 40 liters" (1). Approximately 75% of the body weight of infants is composed of water (1). Children also have high proportions of their body weight made up of water. As people age, the amount of water in their body decreases. Women have 10 to 12 percent less body water than men because of their higher fat content (3). In obese individuals the proportion of weight due to water can be as low as 45% (1).

The perioperative nurse can estimate a patient's total body water using the following formula:

Total Body Water (TBW) in liters =

$$\frac{\text{total body weight [lb]}}{4}$$

For a 154 lb (70 kg) man, this works out to be 38.5 liters of water, which is very close to the 40 liters previously mentioned (4). Knowing the approximate amount of body fluid in a patient may provide the perioperative nurse with the basis for a better understanding of fluid replacement during surgical procedures.

In assessing the surgical patient in order to plan care appropriately, the nurse must be aware of the location of the body fluid. There are two main functional fluid compartments in the body: the compartment *within* the cells of the body, or the intracellular compartment; and the compartment *outside* of the cells of the body, or the extracellular compartment.

81

When perioperative nurses assess the hydration status of the patient prior to, during, and after surgery, they usually focus on the patient's blood levels. However, approximately 63% of the fluid in the body (25 liters, assuming 40 liters of total body fluid) is located within the 75 trillion cells of the body, in the intracellular fluid compartment. For this reason, it is also important to assess the adequacy of the intracellular fluid compartment (1).

The extracellular fluid consists of the plasma or intravascular fluid, and the other extracellular fluids such as the interstitial fluid, the fluid in the gastrointestinal tract, and the cerebrospinal fluid (1). Extracellular fluid is approximately 37% of total body water, or approximately 15 liters of the total body fluid in an average 70-kg man (1).

The blood volume of an average individual is commonly considered to be 5000 milliliters. Of this, plasma accounts for approximately 3000 milliliters, and red blood cells for the other approximately 2000 milliliters. Another way of looking at this is that the blood makes up approximately 7.5% of the body weight of adults (5).

Electrolytes in the Body Fluids

The body's fluids contain electrolytes and water. An electrolyte is a substance that will dissociate into ions when it is dissolved in water. These ions carry electric charges. Ions that have a positive charge are known as cations; for example, sodium (Na^+), potassium (K^+), and calcium (Ca^{++}). Ions that have a negative charge are known as anions; for example, chloride (Cl^-) and bicarbonate (HCO_3^-). A balance exists between positive and negative ions in the body fluids.

The constituents of the extracellular fluid (ECF) and intracellular fluid (ICF) compartments are different. Both extracellular fluid compartments (the intravascular compartment and the interstitial compartment) are high in sodium, chloride, and bicarbonate ions. Plasma fluid also contains protein, whereas interstitial fluid does not. The intracellular fluid compartment, in contrast, has large quantities of potassium, phosphates, magnesium, and sulfates, as well as large amounts of protein (1).

The sodium-potassium-ATPase pump maintains the normal electrolyte values in both the intracellular and extracellular compartments. When sodium leaks from the ECF into the cells, for example, it is pumped back into the ECF. If the pump were to fail, the intracellular metabolic processes necessary to maintain life would also fail (3).

Osmosis

The ECF and the ICF are separated by a membrane that is permeable to water, and is selectively permeable to electrolytes and other substances (1). Osmosis is the movement of water through this membrane to the area with the highest concentration of solutes until the concentration of solutes on either side of the membrane is equivalent. The greater the number of these solutes, the greater the rate of osmosis. It is the number of particles rather than the mass of the solute that causes osmosis. For example, one molecule of albumin with a molecular weight of 70,000 has the same osmotic effect as a molecule of glucose with a molecular weight of 180 (1).

The unit of measure used to describe the number of particles is the osmol. *Osmolality* is the term used to express the concentration of a solution in osmols per kilogram of water. *Osmolarity* is the term used to express the concentration of a solution as osmols per liter of solution. In clinical practice, both terms are often used interchangeably (1). Most of the osmolarity of the interstitial fluid is caused by sodium and chloride ions, while most of the intracellular osmolarity is caused by potassium ions (1).

Plasma osmolality ranges from 280 to 295 milliosmols (mOsm) per kilogram (6), while the osmolarity of interstitial and intracellular fluid is slightly less. The greater osmolarity of the plasma is caused by the osmotic effect of the plasma proteins, which tend to hold fluid inside the blood vessels (1). When the perioperative nurse obtains a patient's plasma osmolarity, it is essentially the same as the intracellular and interstitial osmolalities, because all body fluids, except for urine, are in equilibrium (3).

Tonicity refers to the composition of body fluids in solution (4). It is sometimes used interchangeably with osmolality. A solution that has the same osmolality as the cells is said to be isotonic with the cells. A solution that would cause the cells to shrink is said to be hypertonic and a solution that would cause the cells to swell is said to be hypotonic (4).

The Nursing Process Relating to Fluid and Electrolyte Balance

The perioperative nurse following the guidelines spelled out by state nurse practice acts, the competency statements of professional associations (for example, ANA or AORN), and institutional policies will systematically assess the patient throughout each phase of the perioperative experience. Among the preoperative factors that the nurse will consider in relation to the assessment of the patient's fluid and electrolyte status are: (1) any preexisting diseases with their associated treatments/medications, for example, diuretics, aspirin, or nasogastric drainage; (2) the operative procedure and preparations for it, for example, extensive bowel preparations or fluid restrictions; and (3) the age, sex, weight, and general health of the patient. Each of these factors can alter the composition of the patient's fluids and electrolytes. In one study of 100,000 patients, the average perioperative mortality rate was 0.5%, but it increased to 2.1% with obesity, to 7% with ischemic heart disease, and to 15.8% with cardiac failure (7).

After assessing the preoperative condition of the patient, developing nursing diagnoses, and identifying desired outcomes, the perioperative nurse can develop a plan of care that includes measures to enhance patient safety. Wright affirms that unless the surgery is planned to control major hemorrhage or acute pulmonary obstruction, patients should have blood pressure, hematocrit, urine flow, and central venous pressure—all symptoms of fluid and electrolyte imbalance—corrected to within normal limits prior to the surgical procedure (3).

During the intraoperative phase, the nurse will monitor the effect of the type of anesthesia and surgical procedure on the patient's fluid and electrolyte status, the amount of blood loss during the surgery, the loss of fluid from the surgical wound, and the amount of third-space sequestration that may occur. Knowing that derangements in body fluid and electrolytes have widespread physiologic effects, the nurse will measure all the physiologic parameters that are relevant for the particular patient and the specific surgery.

Continuous evaluation throughout the perioperative period is also necessary to ensure that the desired outcomes relating to fluid and electrolyte balance are maintained. Postoperatively, the patient should be free of significant bleeding, have adequate hemodynamic pressures with an effective circulating blood volume, sustain minimal stress-induced postsurgical fluid retention, and should have near normal acid–base and electrolyte readings. The nurse should also ensure that the patient receives adequate metabolic substrates postoperatively, to enable the body to heal the surgical wounds. The nurse must communicate the degree of attainment of desired outcomes to other members of the healthcare team who will be taking over the care of the patient (2).

Some of the specific conditions that the perioperative nurse may encounter relating to the fluid and electrolyte balance of the surgical patient are covered in more detail below, including alterations in fluid volume; decreased and increased levels of sodium, potassium, calcium, magnesium, and phosphorus; and acid–base imbalances.

Fluid Volume Deficit

Fluid volume deficit is the most common fluid and electrolyte derangement that the surgical patient experiences. Fluid volume deficit is an imbalance in isotonic body fluids related to decreased oral intake or abnormal fluid loss (8). Hypovolemia may occur in the perioperative period because of (1) preoperative, intraoperative, or postoperative bleeding; (2) inadequate intake related to previous NPO status or insufficient IV fluid replacement; (3) excessive renal losses, due to hyperglycemia, for example; (4) excessive cutaneous losses from fever and sweating; (5) third-space losses due to bowel obstructions, ascites, peritonitis, or low albumin states; and (6) excessive gastrointestinal (GI) losses resulting from diarrhea, vomiting, GI suctioning, or fistulas (6).

Nursing Assessment: Signs and Symptoms

Patients with fluid volume deficit experience vascular, interstitial, or intracellular dehydration (8). The first step in assessing this dehydration involves a careful history, which should be obtained preoperatively. Findings such as a previous history of diabetes or cardiac disease should alert the nurse to the possibility of intraoperative fluid volume problems. According to the AORN Standards of Practice, the nurse should also assess the philosophical and religious beliefs of the patient regarding possible blood transfusions (2). The preoperative history is an appropriate time for the nurse to meet this standard.

AORN stresses that, in addition to monitoring the patient for loss of body fluids, the nurse should also calculate the effects of excessive fluid losses on the patient (2). In developing a nursing plan of care, the perioperative nurse should be aware that the effects of such losses will depend on how much fluid is lost, and on the rapidity of the loss. A patient who loses a large amount of fluid rapidly will exhibit symptoms of shock, whereas in a slow loss of fluid the intravascular space can help compensate for the loss (9). In surgeries where large losses are anticipated, the nurse will have replacement solutions prepared in advance.

In one study undertaken to validate the indicators of fluid volume deficit related to active isotonic fluid loss, seventeen critical indicators or major defining characteristics were identified (10). Of these critical indicators of dehydration, those that may be assessed clinically by the perioperative nurse include changes in body weight, increased heart rate, thready pulse, decreased pulse volume, decreased venous filling, dry mucous membranes (furrowed, dry tongue and dry lips), and poor skin turgor. Hemodynamic changes include decreased central venous pressure (CVP), decreased blood pressure, postural blood pressure changes, pulmonary capillary wedge pressure values of less than 6 mm Hg, and decreased cardiac output. Laboratory changes include increased urine osmolality and increased hematocrit, while the overall changes in fluid balance show negative intake and output values and decreased urine outputs (10). Other defining characteristics of fluid volume deficit may include thirst, collapsed neck veins in the recumbent patient, an elevated blood urea nitrogen (BUN), and changes in level of consciousness (8).

The nursing diagnosis for this condition is Fluid Volume Deficit. According to Carpenito, "Hypovolemia caused by hemorrhage or NPO states should be considered collaborative problems, not nursing diagnoses." This is because both nursing and medicine act together to treat them. She therefore suggests that they be labeled Potential Complication (PC): Hemorrhage or PC: Hypovolemia (11).

Medical Treatments and Nursing Interventions

Treatment for fluid losses in surgery involves determining what was lost, the effects of the loss on the patient, and the safest replacement solution. The cost-effectiveness of the solution is usually of some consideration in the current cost-conscious healthcare environment.

Crystalloid Fluid Therapy

Functional extracellular fluid is reduced as a result of surgery (12) and needs to be replaced. The fluid lost is isotonic and is usually replaced with isotonic fluids. In choosing among the many available isotonic fluids, the surgeon will usually select one that is as close to the composition of plasma as possible. Crystalloid solutions are mixtures of electrolytes in water; the two that are most frequently used for volume replacement are lactated Ringer's solution and normal saline. Normal saline is composed of 154 mEq/L of sodium and 154 mEq/L of chloride. As Pestana points out, there is nothing "normal" about this solution when we remember that plasma contains approximately 140 mEq/L of sodium and 103 mEq/L of chloride. Sick, elderly patients, patients

with renal impairment, and those undergoing prolonged operative procedures may not be able to deal with the high chloride load contained in normal saline solutions, and may therefore develop intraoperative or perioperative acidosis (9).

Lactated Ringer's is referred to as a "balanced" solution because it resembles plasma more closely than normal saline. It contains 130 mEq/L of sodium, 109 mEq/L of chloride, 4 mEq/L of potassium, 3 mEq/L of calcium, and 28 mEq/L of lactate. The reduced amount of chloride has been replaced by lactate, which is a precursor of bicarbonate (9). Lactated Ringer's is a good choice for surgical patients whose oxygenation status is adequate, because the liver will convert the lactate into bicarbonate. It is not appropriate for patients in lactic acidosis or for patients who have anaerobic metabolism, because they cannot convert the lactate into bicarbonate; instead, it will be converted into lactic acid, causing a deterioration in the patient's condition. There are other balanced solutions (such as acetated Ringer's, which contains acetate instead of lactate as a bicarbonate precursor) that may be more easily converted into bicarbonate in compromised surgery patients (9).

In determining how much solution should be given to the surgical patient, the nurse should remember that, because isotonic crystalloid solutions are similar to extracellular fluid, they become distributed across both compartments of the ECF: the interstitium as well as the intravascular space. When a liter of IV crystalloid solution is infused into the bloodstream, it quickly equilibrates across both extracellular compartments. Of the original 1000 cc, 200 cc remains in the intravascular compartment while 800 cc is in the interstitium (13).

Nursing responsibilities for the care of patients during fluid resuscitation with *large volumes* of crystalloid solutions include:

- Monitoring the patient's intake and output
- Ensuring adequate access with large-bore catheters when large amounts of fluid may be needed
- Using gravity and pressure bags to enhance flow as necessary
- Monitoring electrocardiograms (ECGs), blood pressure, and central venous pressure
- Monitoring the pulmonary artery pressure to evaluate left heart pressures, and/or esophageal ultrasonic Doppler probes to evaluate the cardiac output (if these monitoring devices are in place)
- Monitoring the adequacy of respiration via arterial blood gases, end-tidal capnography, oxygenation saturations, and by auscultating the lung fields for the development of rales
- Monitoring rectal temperatures

Frequent accurate monitoring by nurses and by every member of the perioperative team is particularly important with massive fluid resuscitation. For example, during ruptured aortic aneurysm repair, an average of 15.7 liters of crystalloids and colloids may be infused during the surgery (14). This is three times the blood volume of the average person.

On rare occasions a hypertonic solution will be selected by the surgeon or anesthesiologist. Hypertonic saline solutions, hypertonic Ringer's lactate, and hypertonic sodium lactate have been used experimentally in a few studies for fluid resuscitation during shock states. While improved hemodynamic functions have been reported in comparison to isotonic crystalloids, more research on their use is needed (15).

Infusions of Colloids

Colloid solutions are used as volume expanders, and they act by maintaining colloid osmotic pressure. The advantage of using colloids is that they are more likely to stay within the intravascular space than are crystalloid solutions. Colloids may be natural or synthetic. Albumin and plasma protein fraction (Plasmanate) are natural colloids derived from pooled blood plasma that has been pasteurized with heat to kill the hepatitis B virus. Albumin comes in two strengths: a 5% solution, which is osmotically similar to plasma, and a 25% solution (formerly called salt-poor albumin), which is hyperosmolar and which draws about four times its volume from the interstitium into the circulation. Plasma protein fraction, whose principle ingredient is albumin (83%–90%), comes in a 5% solution (5, 13, 16).

Albumin or plasma protein fraction may be administered to surgical patients in hypovolemic or hemorrhagic shock to expand their intravascular volume; to burn patients; to patients undergoing retroperitoneal surgery/liver resection; to patients with acute nephrosis; and to patients with ascites, peritonitis, or acute liver failure. Nutrition, not albumin, should be ordered for patients with low serum protein values (17).

In administering albumin or Plasmanate, the nurse should monitor the physiological response of the patient to the infusion utilizing the parameters described above, realizing that patients with cardiac disease may be more at risk for circulatory overload. The perioperative nurse should also monitor patients for hives, chills, and rash—signs of an allergic reaction. Because plasma protein fractions and albumin do not contain clotting factors, the perioperative nurse must also watch patients who are receiving large infusions of these products for signs of bleeding.

Synthetic colloids include dextran and hetastarch. Dextrans are glucose polymers that come in two strengths: low molecular weight dextran 40, which is supplied in a 10% solution; and high molecular weight dextran 70, which is supplied in a 6% solution. The use of dextrans for volume replacement in shock is somewhat controversial, because dextrans can cause unwanted reactions. Close monitoring of patients receiving dextrans is essential. Prior to infusing the solution, the nurse should ask the patient about hypersensitivity to dextran as it may also cause anaphylaxis in some individuals. Dextran 1 (Promit) may be given prior to the infusion of dextrans to prevent this. Because dextrans interfere with platelet adhesiveness, they should be administered with caution to patients with coagulation disorders, and the nurse should monitor all patients who receive dextrans for bleeding tendencies. As dextrans also interfere with the typing and cross-matching of blood, the perioperative nurse should ensure that blood is typed and cross-matched before administering dextrans (16).

Hetastarch (Hespan) is a synthetic starch in a 6% solution with an osmolarity of 310 mOsm/L (5). It is used for intravascular volume replacement in hypovolemic and hemorrhagic shock. As with dextrans, the perioperative nurse should monitor patients receiving hetastarch for signs of fluid overload or anaphylactic reactions, and should follow the patients' laboratory values for elevated prothrombin time (PT), partial thromboplastin time (PTT), and bleeding times.

One study explored the use of hetastarch in the immediate postoperative period in a small group of patients who underwent open heart surgery. This study demonstrated some of the benefits of colloid therapy over crystalloid therapy in the perioperative period. The patients receiving the hetastarch exhibited greater hemodynamic stability, needed 2.4 times less fluid than patients who received crystalloids, and had less fluid retention. The weight gain for the patients receiving crystalloids was eight times greater than for those receiving colloids. The patients who received colloids also had shorter stays in the intensive care unit (18). Other studies have found crystalloid therapy to be better in certain circumstances. Frequently, both are used in the operating room. Regardless of which fluid resuscitation strategy is chosen, the perioperative nurse is responsible for evaluating patient responses to therapy.

Homologous Blood Replacement

Blood component therapy involving homologous (banked) blood includes: (1) red blood cells, which should only be given to patients to increase their oxygen-carrying capacity; (2) platelets, which should be given to patients who are at risk of bleeding secondary to decreased platelet counts; and (3) fresh frozen plasma, which should be given to patients who have clotting deficits (5).

Hemorrhage as a consequence of a surgical procedure is significant if it is large and sudden (9). The slow bleeding that may occur in medical patients over days or weeks usually gives the body time to adapt and allows compensation to occur. An acute loss of 10 percent of the total blood volume (500 ml in the average adult, the amount given by blood donors) is usually well tolerated by most individuals.

Blood loss has been divided into four classes, based on the percentage of total blood volume lost (19):

Class I   Blood loss < 15% of total blood volume
Class II   Blood loss 15–30% of total blood volume
Class III   Blood loss 30–40% of total blood volume
Class IV   Blood loss > 40% of total blood volume

Rapid fluid resuscitation is given to Class I and Class II patients; depending on their response and medical condition, these patients may not need blood transfusion. In fact, patients may lose up to one-third of their blood volume (1600 cc in a 70-kg patient) and be treated without blood transfusion (20).

Patients who have lost more than 30% of their blood volume (Class III patients) have hypovolemic, hemorrhagic shock and need immediate crystalloid and colloid replacement in addition to blood transfusions. Shock is defined as inadequate tissue perfusion, and these patients have insufficient blood volume to perfuse their tissues and to ensure that the metabolic needs of the cells are being met. Hypovolemic shock and hemorrhagic shock are fully reversible if the volume is replaced promptly and appropriately with blood transfusions and fluids (9). If the hemorrhage is not stopped promptly, or if sufficient replacement is not instituted without delay, the cellular injury that is the consequence of inadequate tissue perfusion will persist. The body's compensatory mechanisms will fail, and an irreversible condition will ensue in which the cells of the body are incapable of responding to a belated return of tissue perfusion, leading to inevitable death (21).

Perioperative nurses play a key role in monitoring patients who receive banked blood, as surgical patients receive approximately 60% of all the banked blood used in the United States. One-half of this amount is given to patients who need more than four units of blood (22). One of the most important nursing responsibilities relating to blood replacement therapy is to ensure that the patient receives the correct blood. Because human error is the most common cause of hemolytic reactions to blood transfusions (23), the perioperative nurse must ensure that national and institutional standards for the safe administration of blood products, including protocols for patient and blood identification, are adhered to by all present in the operating room at all times.

Prior to implementing blood transfusion therapy, the perioperative nurse should obtain the patient's vital signs. Vital signs should also be obtained immediately following the administration of blood and throughout the transfusion, as the patient's condition and OR policy dictate. The nurse should monitor the patient closely for signs and symptoms of transfusion reactions throughout the transfusion, especially during the first fifteen minutes of infusion. Symptoms of a transfusion reaction may include hives, chills, elevated temperature, dyspnea, wheezing, tachycardia, and flank pain (20). In the unconscious, anesthetized patient, the incompatible cells may continue to be infused until disseminated intravascular coagulation occurs, and the first signs may be generalized bleeding and a sudden drop in blood pressure (24). If a reaction occurs, the nurse should immediately discontinue the infusion, alert the physician and the blood bank, and treat the patient's symptoms under the direction of the anesthesiologist and/or surgeon.

The nurse must also ensure that blood is administered using the appropriate filter for each component and that blood is not mixed with any solution other than normal saline.

The perioperative nurse, together with the entire OR team, has special responsibilities to patients who sustain massive blood loss and receive massive replacement therapy. It is important to monitor these patients for bleeding, because blood stored for more than 24 hours does not contain viable platelets. Fresh frozen plasma may be given to control bleeding, and platelets should be given if there is evidence of bleeding and if the platelet count is less than 50,000. However, even if large amounts of blood are transfused, platelets should not be given prophylactically (20).

Blood loss and replacement of more than one blood volume (5000 ml) may also cause low serum potassium levels. This is a dilutional hypokalemia secondary to replacement by blood and crystalloids low in potassium, even though there are increased levels of potassium in the plasma of transfused blood (25). Massive transfusions of red blood cells have also caused high serum potassium levels. This is because, when blood is stored, some of the potassium that is contained inside the cells begins to leak out into the plasma. The longer the blood is stored, the higher the concentration of potassium in the serum (26). The administration of large amounts of citrated, banked blood may also cause depressed levels of ionized calcium, Approximately 30–40% of multiple trauma patients and 20% of cardiopulmonary bypass patients who have not received calcium develop hypocalcemia secondary to transfused blood. However, this hypocalcemia is usually transient and mild (27).

Patients who sustain large blood losses during surgical procedures, especially children, are also at risk for developing metabolic acidosis because of intravascular volume depletion (25). The nurse should therefore monitor blood gases and electrolyte profiles and report deviations to the anesthesiologist, so that acidosis and electrolyte imbalances can be corrected promptly.

When large volumes of blood components are given to the patient, the blood should be warmed. Arrhythmias and cardiac arrest have been associated with massive infusions of cold blood. The nurse is responsible for verifying that blood-warming equipment is utilized appropriately.

Nurses play a particular role in maintaining universal precautions in relation to blood transfusion practices in the operating room and in developing institutional guidelines for the safe administration and handling of blood products. All blood products and all body fluids should be assumed to be potentially infectious for blood-born pathogens (20).

The nurse, in collaboration with the physician, may educate the patient and family unit about possible options relating to blood transfusions. Family members frequently ask about directed donations, that is, blood collected specifically for the intended recipient. This blood has not been found to be safer than that from anonymous volunteer donors, because directed donors are less likely to discuss risky behaviors (20). One possible option for concerned family members might be for them to obtain donations from a single committed donor. In a study investigating blood donations by the parents of pediatric cardiac surgery patients, the mean decrease in homologous-donor exposure was found to be 57%. In this study, all the blood required by the child was obtained from one of the parents (28).

Autologous Transfusion with Preoperatively Donated Blood

"Autologous transfusion is the collection and reinfusion of the patient's own blood or blood components" (29). Autologous blood transfusions are becoming common because of the chronic shortage in the nation's blood supply, and also because of the risks inherent in transfused blood. It has been estimated, for example, that 10% of all patients who receive donor blood transfusions will contract hepatitis, with non-A, non-B hepatitis being the most common variety (22).

Patients who are scheduled for elective surgery that is anticipated to involve sufficient blood loss to necessitate transfusion may be candidates for preoperative donation. Orthopedic patients, selected "stable" vascular and cardiac surgery patients, elderly patients, children, and a small number of obstetrical patients (for example, those with placenta previa) have all donated autologous blood successfully (29). The perioperative nurse may also see autologous blood used together with colloids such as hetastarch in "luxury" outpatient surgery such as lipoplasty. In such cases, the goal is to keep the patient's hematocrit and hemoglobin as nearly normal as possible, so that the patient can return home to begin early resumption of routine activities, with near-normal red cell mass and albumin levels (30).

The predonation and use of autologous blood by open heart surgery patients is underused, although it has been shown to decrease homologous transfusion use during surgery by at least 30% (31).

Patients may not donate blood for autologous transfusion without the consent of their own physician and the blood bank physician (32). After the decision to donate blood has been made in consultation with the physician, patients may donate as frequently as every 3 days, but donating once a week is more common. Ideally, donations should begin 4 to 6 weeks prior to surgery, and the physician may prescribe ferrous sulfate or other iron supplements during this period. Patients should not donate within 72 hours of surgery. The hemoglobin of patients who wish to donate their blood prior to surgery must be at least 11 g/dL, and their hematocrits must be greater than 33%. Bacteremia is a contraindication for autologous transfusion (29).

Nursing actions related to autologous blood transfusions include collaborating with the physician in identifying suitable candidates for predonation and educating patients about the risks and benefits of the procedure. Vasovagal symptoms are the most common reaction to blood donation, occurring in 2% to 5% of patients (29). The nurse must also inform patients about the actions, dosage, and side effects of oral iron supplementation. In implementing autologous transfusions, the nurse must adhere to the same careful administration standards used for homologous blood.

Perioperative Blood Salvage

"Perioperative blood salvage is the collection and reinfusion of blood lost during and immediately after surgery"(29). The salvage of the patient's blood can take place intraoperatively or postoperatively. Intraoperative blood salvage takes place in the operating room. The primary benefits to the patient are that it is immediately available and that it reduces the risks of disease transmission associated with homologous blood transfusions.

Intraoperative blood salvage has been used in cardiovascular, vascular, neurologic, plastic, and orthopedic surgeries and in liver transplantation. It has also been used in surgeries for ectopic pregnancy and trauma (33). Jehovah's Witnesses who refuse homologous blood on religious grounds, as well as autologous preoperative blood donation processed by a blood bank, have sometimes agreed to intraoperative salvage of blood utilizing systems that are confined to the operating room (33). One further advantage of the intraoperative blood salvage is that 2,3-diphosphoglycerate (2,3-DPG) levels are higher than in banked, homologous blood, so that oxygen delivery to the tissues is improved when it is used (34).

The classic contraindications for intraoperative blood salvage are (1) systemic infections such as osteomyelitis and (2) malignancies. Blood salvage is also contraindicated in cases when the blood is contaminated during the salvage procedure with the contents of the GI tract or with other sources of bacterial infection. There is some controversy over the absolute contraindications for intraoperative blood salvage; in each case, the risks and benefits must be weighed by the surgeon. For example, some authors believe that patients with bacterial endocarditis are at no greater risk during intraoperative blood salvage than they are during reinfusion of blood from the cardiopulmonary bypass machine (33), while others do not use intraoperative blood salvage in patients with endocarditis (35). Primary cancer surgery is considered an absolute contraindication for intraoperative blood salvage, whereas cancer that has already metastasized is not seen to be a contraindication (33). Lost blood that has been contaminated by microfibrillar collagen topical hemostatic agents such as Avitene or Hemopad cannot be used for reinfusion, because of the potential for embolism (33). Similarly, blood is not normally salvaged in the presence of amniotic fluid or prostatic fluid, because of the potential for an amniotic or prostatic fluid embolism.

Intraoperative blood salvage may be accomplished by (1) a centrifuge system (cell saver system) that collects, filters, washes, and reinfuses the red blood cells; (2) a canister system that collects, filters, and reinfuses the red blood cells but does not wash them (34); or (3) a system that collects the blood during surgery and takes it to a centralized unit (e.g., a blood bank) for processing and washing, and reinfuses it back to the patient within 6 hours (35).

Most intraoperative blood salvaging units use a suction system or a roller pump to aspirate the wasted blood. This blood is then reinfused back to the patient instead of being discarded. Suctioning the blood may cause injury to the red blood cells (RBCs), which may then hemolyze and release free hemoglobin. The advantage of washing the salvaged blood with a cell saver is that it will remove most, but not all, of this free hemoglobin and so reduce the risk of transfusion reactions. Washing also removes some of the surgical field debris that may exist (34).

The complement system may become activated when blood is being suctioned for salvage, and this has the potential to activate an inflammatory response throughout the entire body and to cause intraoperative respiratory dysfunction (36). Washing with a cell saver has been shown to remove the activated complement from the blood salvaged during open heart surgery, even after more than a liter of blood was reinfused (37).

With a cell saver system the lost blood is suctioned out of the patient, and an anticoagulant is added to it to prevent clotting during processing. The salvaged blood is then centrifuged to separate the RBCs from the other blood components. The RBCs are washed with normal saline and are returned to the patient utilizing a transfusion filter (38).

Intraoperative blood salvage systems that wash blood require close monitoring by specially trained individuals who should have no other responsibilities during surgery (29). Healthcare personnel who are currently trained to utilize these systems include perioperative nurses, anesthesiologists, nurse anesthetists, and cardiopulmonary bypass technicians (34).

Nurses play a major role in intraoperative blood salvage. In one institution, the Mayo Clinic in Rochester, Minnesota, blood salvage services are provided by a thirteen-member nursing team under the direction of the blood bank physicians (33). In providing nursing care to the patient who is receiving intraoperatively salvaged blood, the perioperative nurse must monitor the patient's hemoglobin and hematocrit values, because the hematocrits of the salvaged blood can vary from lows of 19% (34) to highs of 68% (35). Most cell saver units deliver a product with high hematocrit values back to the patient, because the operator has control over the final hematocrit, and slower fill flows result in higher hematocrits.

Patients receiving large amounts of washed salvaged blood (during cardiac, vascular, or liver surgeries, e.g.) should also be monitored for bleeding problems. All the plasma proteins, including those involved in coagulation, are removed during the blood processing. Most of the platelets are also removed, and those platelets that do remain are functionally impaired. The perioperative nurse should remember that the product delivered by cell savers consists of red cells suspended in saline (34). In surgeries where large amounts of blood have been lost and reinfused (usually over 40–50% of the plasma volume) dilutional coagulopathies may occur. These patients will need homologous transfusions of fresh frozen plasma and platelets from the blood bank stores, and will then be at risk for contracting hepatitis (34). Recommendations for replacement usually involve transfusing one unit of fresh frozen plasma for every four to six units of blood transfused, and the administration of platelets when the platelet count drops below 50,000.

The anticoagulant citrate phosphate dextrose (CPD) is frequently used with cell saver systems. While its use is not associated with coagulopathies, patients with liver dysfunction should be observed for signs of toxicity. The serum calcium and potassium levels, the acid–base status, and the temperature of patients who receive large amounts of salvaged blood must also be monitored by the circulating nurse.

Patients who have received *unwashed* blood that has been treated with heparin as the anticoagulant agent may develop a high level of systemic anticoagulation and should have serial PTTs evaluated by the perioperative nurse. These patients may also be at risk for impaired renal function secondary to hemolyzed red blood cells, and should have frequent urinary output measurements and blood chemistry levels (29). The perioperative nurse should also monitor all patients during autotransfusion procedures for a possible air embolism, a risk that has been considerably reduced with recent advances in blood salvage equipment (29).

The perioperative nurse must also be alert for the signs and symptoms of transfusion-related infection, such as tachycardia and fever, even though infection is not felt to be a significant risk following intraoperative blood salvage (35).

Autologous blood transfusion systems that do not involve suctioning or washing the blood are sometimes used in cases of chest trauma. In cases of intrapleural bleeding or hemothorax, the shed blood may be collected in a system such as that by Sorenson or Pleuravac, and reinfused to the patient using a 40-micron filter. This blood typically does not need anticoagulants because the intrapleural blood is typically defibrinogenated. If, however, blood is collected from a great vessel that is bleeding rapidly, an anticoagulant may be added to prevent the blood from clotting in the collection chamber (39). These systems are used primarily for salvaging mediastinal blood following open heart surgery.

Closed-wound drainage systems can also be used postoperatively, for example, the Solcotrans orthopedic reinfusion system. It is the responsibility of the perioperative nurse to ensure that all autologous blood, including drainage blood, is collected and readministered within the 6 hours mandated by the American Association of Blood Banks (32).

Acute normovolemic hemodilution is another system of sparing blood during the perioperative period. Blood is withdrawn usually just before or after induction of anesthesia, before the surgery is begun, and is replaced with IV solutions of crystalloids or colloids. This blood may be kept at room temperature for up to 4 hours and then transfused back to the patient at the end of the surgical procedure. If the surgery is expected to last longer, the nurse must ensure that the spared blood is kept in a monitored refrigerator that is adapted for blood products. The advantages of this system are that blood loss occurs at lower hematocrits, the circulating blood during the surgical procedure is less viscous, and fresh whole blood with clotting factors is available to the patient at the end of the procedure (29).

Hemofiltration systems have been used to conserve blood during cardiac surgery. "Hemofiltration has the advantage of removing only the excessive fluids from the blood while completely preserving plasma proteins" (40). Small patients and patients with low preoperative hemoglobin levels may need intraoperative blood secondary to the hemodilution that occurs during cardiopulmonary bypass (41). Hemofiltration devices and the hemoconcentration they produce may reduce this need.

Evaluation of Measures to Correct Fluid Volume Deficits

Surgery-related fluid volume deficit and the potential for fluid volume deficit, particularly in the context of high-risk surgery, necessitates accurate and ongoing preoperative, intraoperative, and postoperative monitoring, including invasive monitoring with pulmonary artery catheters. Monitoring is necessary to ensure that appropriate fluid resuscitation measures utilizing crystalloids, colloids, and blood products are instituted rapidly to correct reversible problems and to prevent them from becoming irreversible (42). The professional perioperative nurse plays a vital role in this process.

In evaluating the fluid balance of the patient following surgery, the nurse must be aware that fluid volume deficits may become fluid volume excesses in the immediate postoperative period. The fluids that were administered during surgery may be retained secondary to hypothermia, anesthetic agents, narcotics, stress, and pain. Levels of antidiuretic hormone (ADH) may increase intraoperatively, because ADH is produced when there is more than a 10% decrease in blood volume or blood pressure (43). As long as the patient's other physiologic parameters are satisfactory, the excess water will be eliminated as homeostasis is restored.

Fluid Volume Excess

Fluid volume excess is not as great a concern to the perioperative nurse as fluid volume deficit. It may, however, be present prior to surgery in patients with a history of cardiac, hepatic, or renal disease or in patients with inadequate lymphatic drainage, such as cancer patients. The fluid resuscitation delivered during surgery can also lead to the development of hypervolemia.

Nursing Assessment: Signs and Symptoms

Edema, weight gain, and taut, shiny skin are the major defining characteristics of fluid volume excess (8). Where massive fluid resuscitation is given, the nurse should also assess the patient for the development of hypervolemia, which will be manifested primarily by the symptoms of pulmonary vascular congestion. Patients with impaired cardiac function may develop the symptoms of congestive heart failure secondary to sudden hypervolemia. These symptoms may include dyspnea, bilateral rales, a cough with frothy sputum, and orthopnea. An increased heart rate, distended neck veins, the development of extra heart sounds (S3/S4), changes in blood pressure, diaphoresis, and anxiety may also occur. The arterial blood gases may also show the presence of hypoxia and metabolic acidosis.

"If nursing can prescribe the definitive treatment to reduce or eliminate (the) factors that contribute to (the) edema," the nursing diagnosis for this condition may be identified as Fluid Volume Excess. However, if acute hypervolemia is also present, this should be considered a collaborative problem requir-

ing medical as well as nursing interventions, and may therefore be identified as Potential Complication (PC): Hypervolemia, or PC: Congestive Heart Failure (11).

Medical Treatments and Nursing Interventions

The medical treatment for acute hypervolemia includes oxygen to improve the patient's hypoxia, diuretics to help eliminate the excess fluids, and a vasodilator to reduce the venous return to the heart. If it is not contraindicated, the patient may be placed in a semi-Fowler's position to enhance oxygenation. The nurse may also place the patient's legs in a dependent position, thereby reducing the blood flow to the heart.

Patients with chronic edema will need patient education relating to water and salt intake, skin care, positioning, and the medications and treatments prescribed for their disease process.

SODIUM AND WATER IMBALANCES

Sodium is the major cation in the extracellular fluid (ECF). It plays a major role in maintaining the osmolality and water balance of the extracellular fluid, which, in turn (because cell membranes are permeable to water), affects the intracellular fluid (ICF) volume (1). Sodium is also found to some extent in all the body fluids, and the sodium in bone and connective tissue is exchangeable and can be combined with the sodium in the ECF. Sodium helps to maintain the acid–base balance of the body, and the sodium-potassium pump plays a vital role in neuromuscular activity.

Normal serum sodium is 135–145 mEq/L, while intracellular sodium is considerably lower, at around 14 mEq/L (1). Sodium is ingested via the gastrointestinal tract, is secreted in sweat and the fluids of the gastrointestinal tract, and is excreted by the kidneys.

Sodium and water balance is regulated by a complex series of control mechanisms. These include the intake (thirst) mechanism, the antidiuretic hormone from the posterior pituitary, the renin–angiotensin-aldosterone system, atrial natriuretic peptide from the heart, and intrarenal mechanisms (44). About 26,000 mEq of sodium is filtered by the kidneys each day, while the daily intake of sodium is only around 150 mEq. The kidneys must therefore excrete only approximately 150 mEq (an amount equal to the daily intake) or severe depletion will exist. In maintaining sodium balance, the kidneys play a vital role in reabsorbing sodium. Ninety-two percent of this sodium is reabsorbed in the proximal tubules of the kidney and in the loop of Henle through intrarenal mechanisms, leaving only 8% being presented to the distal tubules (1). When sodium or water levels are low, sodium is reabsorbed in the distal tubules. The amount of sodium that is reabsorbed in the distal tubules is highly variable and is regulated by the presence of aldosterone (1). Eighty percent of the sodium that is reabsorbed is reabsorbed with chloride (45).

Hypertonicity of the extracellular fluid, which is most frequently caused by excess sodium, stimulates thirst in the awake, alert individual to correct the tonicity problem. In elderly patients and in certain disease states, however, the thirst mechanism may be deranged. Antidiuretic hormone is also released by hypertonic body fluids and low-volume states, causing the distal and collecting tubules to reabsorb water (46).

Hyponatremia

Hyponatremia is defined as a serum sodium concentration of less than 135 mEq/L (47). It is one of the most commonly encountered electrolyte abnormalities in hospitalized patients. Hyponatremia is especially prevalent in older patients; it has been observed in 11.3% of hospitalized geriatric patients and 22.5% of patients in a chronic disease facility (47). It has also been seen in previously healthy children who have been admitted to the hospital for minor illnesses or surgery (48).

Hyponatremia is associated with low serum osmolality, except when it is accompanied by high quantities of substances such as glucose or mannitol. It may coexist with normal, elevated, or decreased amounts of water in the ECF. Some of the common causes of hyponatremia include:

I.   Hypovolemic hyponatremia
   A.   Increased excretion of sodium
      1.   Diarrhea
      2.   Diuretic therapy
   B.   Abnormal loss of sodium
      1.   Nasogastric suctioning
      2.   Fistulas
      3.   Ileostomies
      4.   Vomiting
      5.   Serous drainage (e.g., burns, open wounds)
      6.   Third spacing
      7.   GI obstruction
      8.   Pancreatitis
      9.   Postoperative injury

II.   Isovolemic hyponatremia
   A.   Increased water relative to sodium (IV solutions containing no sodium, such as D5W)
   B.   SIADH—the syndrome of inappropriate antidiuretic secretion, which may occur in patients with lung cancer, meningitis, or brain tumors
   C.   Stress secondary to serious illness or surgery
   D.   Adrenal insufficiency (Addison's Disease—aldosterone deficiency)
   E.   Low-salt diet (especially with diuretic administration)
   F.   Drugs (diuretics, morphine, chlorpropamide, aspirin, oxytocin)
   G.   Excessive tap water enemas in bowel-preparation regimens

III.   Hypervolemic hyponatremia
   A.   Congestive heart failure
   B.   Cirrhosis of the liver
   C.   Renal failures
   D.   Nephrotic syndrome

Nursing Assessment: Signs and Symptoms

Water and salt problems go hand-in-hand. When the nurse assesses the effect of low serum sodium values, he or she must also determine the patient's osmolarity levels and hydration status. Patients who have had extensive GI or renal losses prior to or during surgery may develop hypovolemic hyponatremia. As the body attempts to compensate for this volume loss by secreting ADH and aldosterone, the proportion of sodium in the ECF is decreased. These patients have diminished effective blood volumes, and on physical examination may exhibit dry mucous membranes, poor skin turgor, and significant orthostatic hypotension (47).

Patients with isovolemic hyponatremia have an excess of total body water with a normal or slightly decreased total body sodium (47). This is associated with an increased secretion of ADH. Increased ADH may be produced in response to the stress of the surgical experience. Drugs (such as morphine), certain anesthetic agents, and postoperative pain also cause increased secretion of ADH (43). In examining these patients, the perioperative nurse will observe decreased urinary outputs and weight gain.

Patients with hypervolemic hyponatremia frequently have cardiac or liver failure. They retain water and salt in an attempt to compensate for the pressure changes caused by their underlying pathologies. These patients have an increase in total body sodium, but their low serum osmolarities indicate that the increase in water is greater than the increase in sodium (3). Patients with hypervolemic hyponatremia may present with symptoms primarily related to the excess body fluid. These include bounding pulse rates, edema, weight gain, elevated blood pressure, neck vein distention, and dyspnea with rales (8).

Hyponatremia primarily affects the central nervous system; if it develops gradually it may not result in neurological deficits even at low serum sodium levels (less than 110 mEq/L), whereas a sudden onset may lead to brain damage and death (48). The low sodium concentration in the extracellular fluid causes it to become hypotonic. The hypotonic ECF causes the brain to swell due to the osmosis of water from the ECF to the ICF in the brain cells. The swollen brain cells increase the intracranial pressure (ICP). The increased ICP is manifested by neurological systems such as easy fatigability, headache, confusion, lethargy, and muscular weakness, which may progress to seizures, coma, and even death (47).

The perioperative nurse bases the nursing diagnosis on the symptoms of the individual patient. Hyponatremia is a collaborative problem as it requires both medical and nursing interventions. Appropriate diagnostic statements for low-salt states might include: PC: Hyponatremia related to inappropriate ADH secretion, or PC: Hyponatremia related to fistula drainage. The stem *PC* (Potential Complication) is necessary to distinguish nursing actions from medical diagnosis and treatment (8). Fluid Volume Excess related to congestive heart failure may be an appropriate nursing diagnosis for patients with hypervolemic hyponatremia.

The perioperative nurse, in developing a plan of care, may also select diagnoses that indirectly relate to the fluid/electrolyte disorder, for example: Knowledge Deficit concerning medications, or Anxiety related to surgical procedure.

Medical Treatments and Nursing Interventions

Treatment for hyponatremia will depend on the cause and rapidity of onset of the problem. It is dangerous, for example, to rapidly increase the serum sodium of patients who have chronic asymptomatic hyponatremia. In these patients, the central nervous system's osmoregulatory mechanisms have had time to normalize the brain water content (48).

Patients with hypovolemic hyponatremia should be given isotonic saline to increase their fluid volume as well as their serum sodium level. Surgical patients with contracted ECF fluid losses secondary to vomiting, diarrhea, or excessive sweating may need three or more liters of saline to replace their losses (3). If the condition is detected prior to an elective surgery, and if the patient can tolerate it, a high-sodium diet and increased oral fluids should be given. The underlying cause should also be treated.

Patients with isovolemic hyponatremia have an increase in water due to increased ADH secretion with normal total body sodiums. Water restriction is the treatment of choice for these patients, especially for the postsurgical patient who may have a transient stress-induced increase in ADH secretion. Drugs such as demeclocycline may be given to patients with chronic SIADH secondary to lung cancer or other conditions (49).

Patients with hypervolemic hyponatremia frequently present with edema. Treatment for these patients is directed at the underlying disease. Water and sodium restriction may be ordered, and also diuretics. Salt restriction is appropriate for these patients because their total body sodium levels are high, while their serum sodium is low due to the proportionately greater increase in total body water.

The treatment of acute and chronic hyponatremia is different. Patients presenting with acute onset of symptomatic hyponatremia may be treated with a 3% infusion of saline in addition to fluid restriction (47, 48). The aim of hypertonic saline solutions is to stop the seizures and improve the coma, by bringing the serum sodium to 15 mEq/L below the normal level. It is not intended to correct the hyponatremia. Once the serum sodium is 15 mEq/L below the patient's normal level and the symptoms have improved, a slower method of treatment, usually fluid restriction alone, should be instituted (47). The treatment of hyponatremia is controversial, as hypertonic saline may cause the brain to shrink, particularly when the hyponatremia is not acute in onset and the patient's brain has adapted to the condition. Cheng et al. have treated patients with symptomatic hyponatremia with sodium restriction alone, if their urine osmolalities were between 50 and 100 mOsm/kg (47).

The perioperative nurse must initiate frequent neurological assessments to monitor the patient receiving hypertonic saline. Rapid changes in the water content of the brain with shrinking of brain cells (because of the osmosis of the brain water to the higher solute concentrations in the ECF) can occur if hypertonic saline is infused too rapidly. This may cause neurologic damage. Other side effects include symptoms of sudden volume overload (for example, acute pulmonary edema), especially in patients with preexisting cardiac disease.

The 3% saline should be administered via a regulatory controller. Strict intake and output measurements should be obtained hourly, together with frequent urine specific gravities.

Hypernatremia

Hypernatremia is defined as a serum sodium level of greater than 145 mEq/L. Some of the common etiologies of hypernatremia include:

I. Increased intake of sodium
   A. "Hypertonic tube feedings" or parenteral nutrition
   B. Parenteral administration of hypertonic saline

II. Decreased intake of water
   A. NPO
   B. Impaired thirst mechanism

III. Increased excretion of water
   A. Diabetes insipidus
   B. Water diarrhea
   C. Insensible water loss, for example, in hyperventilation
   D. Sweating
   E. Severe burns
   F. Fever

Nursing Assessment: Signs and Symptoms

As with hyponatremia, hypernatremia is also characterized by neurologic manifestations, such as disorientation, agitation, hallucinations, and lethargy, which may progress to seizures, coma, and death (50). The cause of these signs and symptoms is the shrinkage of brain cells with a resultant decrease in cerebral volume, which may cause tearing of cerebral vessels (50). Other symptoms may include a dry, swollen tongue; sticky mucous membranes; and poor skin turgor. The serum osmolality is greater than 295 mOsm/kg, and the urine specific gravity may be greater than 1.015, provided the water loss is from a nonrenal route (6).

The diagnostic label for this collaborative problem may be identified as: PC: Hypernatremia (8).

Medical Treatments and Nursing Interventions

The interventions for hypernatremia vary and are based on the rapidity of onset of the symptoms, the underlying cause of the imbalance, and the fluid volume status of the patient.

The treatment for patients with normal total body sodium levels, whose hypernatremia is due primarily to an acute loss of body water, is replacement of the lost water. Diabetes insipidus, which may be associated with neurosurgical procedures, is an example of hypernatremia brought on by excessive water loss. It is characterized by polyuria and polydipsia (43). Replacement is usually accomplished with 5% dextrose in water; the aim is replacing the deficits that already exist and matching the ongoing urinary losses. The rapidity of the replacement depends upon the patient's symptoms. If seizures or coma are present, D5W should be administered expeditiously until the symptoms have improved, and the remainder of the replacement should then be given over the next 24 to 48 hours (43). For alert patients plain water, administered orally, is preferred.

Patients who have hypernatremia with an increase in total body sodium (e.g., patients who have received hyperosmolar tube feedings or excessive amounts of medications such as sodium bicarbonate) should also receive prompt treatment. Such patients are administered free water, such as D5W, with concomitant administration of a loop diuretic such as furosemide (Lasix) to assist with the removal of the excess sodium by the kidneys. If the patient cannot tolerate diuretic therapy, peritoneal or hemodialysis may be necessary to remove the excess sodium (43).

In patients whose hypernatremia has developed slowly, and who have a concomitant ECF volume deficit with hypertonicity, fluid should be replaced over several days regardless of the etiology (9).

Nursing responsibilities for patients with hypernatremia are monitoring the response of the patient to fluid/diuretic therapy, including frequent monitoring of neurological signs, observing the patient for symptoms of water intoxication, strict intake and output measurements, and ongoing physical assessment of vital signs and respiratory status.

POTASSIUM IMBALANCES

Potassium is the major intracellular cation, and approximately 98% of the body's stores are located within the cells, where the concentration is around 140 to 150 mEq/L (51). Normal serum potassium, on the other hand, ranges from 3.5 to 5 mEq/L. Potassium is necessary for the contraction of both skeletal muscle and smooth muscle. It is therefore necessary for cardiac contractions and for the movements of the gastrointestinal tract. Potassium plays a role in the transmission of nerve impulses by regulating neuromuscular excitability, and in the formation of muscle protein by transporting glucose into the cells with insulin. It is also involved in the maintenance of acid–base balance and intracellular osmotic pressures (52).

The normal dietary intake of potassium is approximately 100 mEq per day which is absorbed in the small intestines (51) from foods such as oranges, bananas, and prunes.

Potassium regulation is achieved by a complex interaction of homeostatic mechanisms which include mineralocorticoids, acid–base balance, body fluid tonicity, insulin, catecholamines, sodium and potassium intake, and the flow rates within the distal tubules of the kidneys (43). Most of the potassium reaching the kidneys is filtered and reabsorbed, but approximately 10–15% reaches the distal convoluted tubules, where the amount of potassium that is excreted is controlled. The amount of potassium excreted varies from 5 to 100 mEq/L in response to the intake of potassium and other metabolic conditions. If serum potassium is elevated, the adrenal cortex secretes aldosterone, which acts on the distal tubules of the kidney, causing it to excrete more potassium in exchange for sodium (43). If the serum potassium is low, potassium is conserved. Even in the face of low potassium stores, the kidneys continue to excrete a minimum of 50 mEq of potassium a day long after intake has ceased (46).

Hypokalemia

Hypokalemia is defined as a serum potassium of less than 3.5 mEq/L (51). Some of the common causes of hypokalemia include:

I.   Insufficient intake of potassium
   A.   Prolonged nausea or anorexia
   B.   Poor diet (e.g., among elderly patients living alone, patients with alcoholism)
   C.   IV therapy without potassium supplements

II.   Gastrointestinal loss
   A.   Vomiting
   B.   Nasogastric suction
   C.   Diarrhea
   D.   Extensive bowel-preparation regimens
   E.   Fistulas

III.   Renal loss
   A.   Diuretic therapy
   B.   Increased diuresis
   C.   Steroid therapy
   D.   Hyperaldosteronism
   E.   Hypomagnesemia

IV.   Shifting of potassium into the cells from the ECF
   A.   Alkalemia
   B.   Insulin administration
   C.   Beta-adrenergic stimulation
   D.   Anabolic tissue repair

Because potassium is so prevalent in the diet, hypokalemia caused by insufficient intake is not common, although it may occur occasionally in elderly, sick patients or iatrogenically in hospitalized patients. Diarrheal fluid contains 35 to 60 mEq/L of potassium and gastric secretions contain approximately 10 mEq/L, so that diarrhea and vomiting over several days without potassium replacement can cause severe hypokalemia (43). Intraoperative suctioning of very large amounts of body fluids may also cause potassium levels to fall (26). Many surgical patients receive diuretic therapy, which causes increased renal flow and contributes to hypokalemia. Other factors that increase renal flow include hypercalcemia and drugs such as mannitol. Patients with high endogenous levels of steroids or those who receive steroid therapy for inflammatory bowel diseases, asthma, or arthritis lose potassium in the distal tubule of the kidney while conserving sodium (6). Other drugs that also cause hypokalemia include amphotericin B, aminoglycosides, beta-2 agonists, cisplatinum, and penicillins (49).

Catecholamines are released by stress, including many of the stressors that face the surgical patient, such as concerns over impending surgery, traumatic injuries, and pain. The increased levels of these stress hormones, such as epinephrine, cause potassium to move from the serum into the muscles and the liver, which may reduce serum potassium levels. Similarly, alkalemia causes potassium to be shifted into the cells in exchange for hydrogen ions, and also causes potassium to be exchanged for hydrogen ions in the kidneys. This is because the body attempts to correct the acid–base imbalance even if it is at the expense of potassium balance (9). During the anabolic phase of tissue repair, potassium also moves into the cells. For this reason, surgical patients who have had extensive injuries or who have had major surgery may be at risk for developing hypokalemia in the postoperative period (52).

Nursing Assessment: Signs and Symptoms

The signs and symptoms of hypokalemia may be nonspecific and difficult for the perioperative nurse to assess. Hypokalemia affects neuromuscular functioning, causing skeletal muscle weakness of the arms and legs, progressing to the trunk and respiratory muscles. The smooth muscle is also impaired, resulting in gastric distention, paralytic ileus, and urinary retention (51). Neuropsychiatric manifestations, such as drowsiness, memory loss, and confusion, may also occur (43).

The cardiac effects of hypokalemia include spontaneous ectopic beats and dysrhythmias, conduction abnormalities, and altered sensitivity to digitalis. The ECG shows flattened T-waves, the development of a prominent U-wave, and also ST depression (43, 51). If the hypokalemia is prolonged, the ability of the kidneys to concentrate urine may be impaired, causing dilute urine, polyuria, and polydipsia (51).

The perioperative nurse should pay special attention to the potassium levels of elderly patients, so that any imbalance can be corrected prior to surgery. Because hypertension and edematous conditions are more common in older patients, they are more likely to be taking diuretics and to be at risk for hypokalemia (53).

Hypokalemia is a collaborative problem rather than a nursing diagnosis, and the perioperative nurse should identify it with the diagnostic label "PC: Hypokalemia" (8).

Medical Treatments and Nursing Interventions

Before undertaking any treatment, the cause of the hypokalemia must be determined and, if possible, corrected. If the deficit is severe and the patient has cardiovascular or other serious symptoms, then IV replacement will be necessary. Hypokalemia associated with preoperative vomiting, and an inability to swallow following surgery is also an indication for IV potassium.

Replacement guidelines will vary depending on the severity of the depletion and the severity of the symptoms. If the patient's serum potassium deficit is above 2.5 mEq/L, intravenous potassium concentrations of 40 mEq/L of IV fluid with infusion rates of 10 mEq/hour are appropriate (49). Patients with potassium levels of less than 2 mEq/L and ventricular dysrhythmias, such as premature ventricular contractions or ventricular tachycardia, need prompt replacement with potassium concentrations of up to 60 mEq/hour and potassium infusions of up to 40 mEq/hour (49). Higher doses of 80 to 100 mEq infused over one hour via two separate IV lines have occasionally been given to suppress life-threatening dysrhythmias (51), but such aggressive therapy is not widely used. Many patients with hypokalemia are volume-depleted and have coexisting electrolyte imbalances, such as insufficient chloride and magnesium levels, which also need to be corrected.

When preparing potassium for administration, the perioperative nurse must be careful to ensure that the potassium is well mixed in the container of IV solution, to avoid the possibility of the patient receiving a sudden fatal bolus. An infusion-regulating controller or pump is desirable when higher doses are administered. The perioperative nurse should monitor the patient for chemical phlebitis, by observing the infusion site for redness, heat, or swelling, and by asking alert patients about site pain (52).

The perioperative nurse should assess the patient for clinical symptoms of potassium overdose, particularly when higher doses of potassium are administered. Serum potassiums should be obtained every 2 to 4 hours. Hourly urine outputs should be obtained, because high doses of potassium may be potentially dangerous in oliguric patients (6).

If the condition is longstanding, and if time permits, correction should be instituted with foods high in potassium or with oral potassium supplements. Oral supplements include liquids, effervescent tablets, and wax or microencapsulated tablets (49). Potassium-sparing diuretics may enhance patient compliance and may be the more appropriate potassium supplements in certain situations, such as diuretic-induced alkalosis (54). If ambulatory surgery patients, in particular, are to receive potassium supplementation following surgery, the responsibility for providing appropriate patient education rests with the perioperative nurse. Patients should be instructed to take liquid or effervescent potassium preparations mixed in fluids. They should be advised not to crush microencapsulated tablets as these are designed to gradually release potassium so that the GI ulceration associated with high doses of potassium is avoided (49).

Hyperkalemia

Hyperkalemia is defined as a serum potassium of over 5.5 mEq/L (43). Some of the common causes of hyperkalemia include:

I. Increased exogenous intake
   A. IV potassium supplements
   B. Drugs containing potassium
   C. Massive transfusions with stored blood

II. Decreased excretion
   A. Renal failure
   B. Hypovolemia
   C. Hypoaldosteronism

III. Shifting of potassium from the cells into the ECF
   A. Acidosis
   B. Insufficient insulin
   C. Beta-adrenergic blockade
   D. Catabolic tissue breakdown

Elevations in potassium rarely occur because of oral intake in patients with functioning kidneys, but IV administration of potassium can cause hyperkalemia (9), especially if the urine output is low. Oliguria may develop during the course of surgery, and should be monitored by the perioperative nurse, as it may lead to a build-up of potassium. Hypovolemic patients are also at risk for developing hyperkalemia because of the decreased flow of water and sodium to the distal tubule of the kidney (43).

Certain drugs also contain hidden sources of potassium, such as the potassium salts that are present in some antibiotics. Salt substitutes, frequently used by patients with cardiac disease, also contain potassium chloride (49).

Blood contains large amounts of potassium within the red blood cells. As the blood is stored, the cells begin to break down, and the potassium that is contained within the cells leaks out. Patients who need massive amounts of stored blood during the operative procedure may, therefore, develop hyperkalemia. Surgery, crush injuries, and burns also cause damage to the cells of the body. The cells then release potassium from the intravascular compartment to the extracellular compartment, raising serum potassium levels.

Many drugs commonly given to surgical patients induce hyperkalemia, including antiinflammatory agents, beta-blockers, captopril, digitalis, heparin, penicillins, and succinylcholine (49). Patients with Addison's disease, elderly diabetic patients who usually have an associated hypoaldosteronism, and patients who take medications that block or reduce the effect of aldosterone (e.g., potassium-sparing diuretics such as spironolactone) are also at risk for developing hyperkalemia (53).

False elevations in potassium may occur in patients with elevated white blood cells counts or because of hemolyzed blood samples. If hyperkalemia is reported on a laboratory value, and it is not correlated with the history or the patient's symptoms, the nurse may wish to draw another sample to confirm the true value.

Nursing Assessment: Signs and Symptoms
As was the case with low-potassium states, the neuromuscular symptoms of hyperkalemia involve both the skeletal muscles and the smooth muscles. Skeletal muscle symptoms include paresthesias and weakness in the arms and legs, which may spread to the trunk, leading to a generalized paralysis that may involve the diaphragm (51). Smooth muscle symptoms include abdominal distention, colic, and diarrhea.

The cardiac manifestations of hyperkalemia are the most serious because excess potassium acts as a cardiac depressant, and, if untreated, can lead to heart block, ventricular arrhythmias, and asystole. The ECG change occurring in hyperkalemia, when the plasma concentration range is from 5.5 to 6.5 mEq/L, is the development of peaked T-waves. As the concentration increases, the QRS widens, the P-wave becomes flatter, and the PR interval increases. Finally, with concentrations over 8 mEq/L, the P-wave disappears, and the QRS takes on the typical sine-wave pattern of severe hyperkalemia (43). If the potassium levels rise suddenly, and if the hyperkalemia is accompanied by low sodium and calcium levels or acidemia, the effects on the heart may be severe, even when the serum potassium is only 6 to 6.5 mEq/L. If, on the other hand, the level of potassium increases slowly, as in chronic renal failure, the effects on the heart may be minimal even at serum concentrations of 7 to 7.5 mEq/L (51).

The perioperative nurse should monitor elderly patients, in particular, for the development of hyperkalemia because of the sluggish response of their aging kidneys to the potential elevations of potassium caused by surgery (53).

After reviewing the data and assessing the patient, the perioperative nurse should identify this collaborative problem with the diagnostic label "PC: Hyperkalemia" (8).

Medical Treatments and Nursing Interventions
The life-threatening cardiac side effects of hyperkalemia must be treated first. Calcium is the agent of choice to counteract the depressant action of potassium on the heart. A 10% solution of calcium gluconate (10–30 ml) is given intravenously at 0.5 to 1 ml per minute (43). Calcium chloride may also be given, but it is more irritating to the veins and may cause local phlebitis. The effects of calcium last from 30 minutes to an hour, so definitive treatment must be administered following this first therapeutic step. The perioperative nurse should maintain constant ECG monitoring to evaluate the patient's response to the calcium administration. If the calcium is ineffective, a transvenous pacemaker may be necessary to maintain an adequate heart rate.

Sodium bicarbonate can be given to cause the serum potassium to move into the cells and in this way to reduce the level of potassium in the plasma. When sodium bicarbonate is administered, the plasma becomes more alkaline. As the body attempts to correct this alkalinity, hydrogen ions are released from the cells into the plasma in exchange for potassium ions. At the same time, more potassium ions and fewer hydrogen ions are exchanged for sodium in the distal tubule in the kidney (46). One ampule of sodium bicarbonate containing 50 mEq may be administered over 5 to 10 minutes (51). If no effect is seen in 10 to 15 minutes, the dosage may be repeated. The perioperative nurse should infuse sodium bicarbonate in a separate IV line as it may precipitate calcium and inactivate pressor drugs. The patient receiving sodium bicarbonate should also be monitored for signs of fluid overload.

Insulin-glucose infusions also cause potassium uptake by the cells. Ten units of regular insulin in 500 ml of a 10% dextrose solution is usually administered over one hour (43). The onset of action should be in approximately 30 minutes, and the duration of action is about 4 to 6 hours (51).

Measures to increase the excretion of potassium with diuretics, such as furosemide (Lasix), bumetanide (Bumex), or ethacrynic acid (Edecrin), which increase sodium flow to the distal tubules of the kidney, may also be tried (43). Potassium may also be removed from the body with a cation exchange resin such as sodium polystyrene sulfonate (Kayexalate). This treatment is rarely seen in the immediate perioperative period, because its onset of action is about 4 to 6 hours (49). Kayexalate is usually administered with sorbitol to induce an osmotic diarrhea which facilitates the excretion of potassium and prevents the constipation that Kayexalate alone may cause. It may be administered orally or via enema. The oral route is preferred because more of the solution is exposed to a greater area of the gastrointestinal tract where the potassium–sodium exchange takes place. Dosages vary, but 15–25 g of Kayexalate with sorbitol is usually given orally, while 50 g of Kayexalate with 50 g of sorbitol in 200 ml is usually given rectally. If the rectal route is used, the enema must be retained for 30 to 60 minutes. This dose can be repeated every 6 hours, and a potassium level should be obtained following each dose (51).

Hemodialysis is a very effective way to remove potassium from the body. Peritoneal dialysis may also be used, but it is less effective than hemodialysis or Kayexalate (51).

In addition to assessing the patient's response to treatment, the perioperative nurse should observe the patient for other electrolyte imbalances that may occur as excess potassium is excreted. "Familiarity with the functions and use of the monitoring equipment," including ECG interpretation, is essential for the care of surgical patients with elevated potassium states. This is particularly true in postoperative settings and local-anesthesia settings where an anesthesiologist may not be present (55).

CALCIUM BALANCE

Calcium is involved in the contractility of all muscle tissue, including heart muscle. It plays a vital role in the conduction of nerve impulses, in blood coagulation, in the activities of various hormones and enzymes, and in cell permeability, division, and movement (27). Ninety-nine percent of the body's calcium is contained in the bones, teeth, and soft tissues, and only 1% in the extracellular fluid compartment (43). The normal value of serum calcium is 8.5 to 10.5 mg/dl (or 4.5 mEq/L).

Calcium is absorbed by the small intestine via active transport under the influence of vitamin D and parathyroid hormone (56). The daily intake of calcium is highly variable and ranges from 200 to 2500 mg/day (57). Foods high in calcium include milk, cheese, yogurt, and other dairy products; fish, such as sardines and salmon; and certain vegetables, such as collards and turnip greens. Calcium is excreted in the urine and feces. Its excretion is similar to that of sodium and is decreased in hypovolemic patients or when the glomerular filtration rate falls. Calcium excretion is increased in hypervolemic states, with osmotic diuresis, and following loop diuretics (57).

Serum calcium levels, as well as phosphate and magnesium levels, are maintained within narrow parameters by a complex interaction between three hormones: parathyroid hormone (PTH), calcitonin, and 1,25-dihydroxycholecalciferol (1,25-DHCC). These hormones influence calcium metabolism in the bone, GI tract, and kidney via interactive feedback mechanisms (58). In response to low serum calcium levels, PTH, which is secreted by the parathyroid gland, causes calcium to be released from the bone supply into the blood. Calcitonin, which is secreted by the thyroid gland, prevents abnormal increases in blood calcium levels. Vitamin D is first converted to 25-hydroxyvitamin D in the liver and this, in turn, is catalyzed to 1,25-DHCC by the kidney. 1,25-DHCC is necessary for the absorption of calcium (59). Magnesium also plays a role in calcium homeostasis, by regulating the secretion of PTH (27).

Calcium is present in the serum in three forms. About 50% of the serum calcium is ionized, and this is the physiologically active component. Another 40% of the calcium is bound to proteins (mostly albumin), while the remaining 10% is complexed with anions such as phosphate, sulfate, and citrate (27, 60). Many factors can influence the availability of the active ionized calcium. The amount of calcium bound to albumin varies with the pH, osmolality, and free fatty acid concentrations of the serum (27). An increase in pH (alkalosis) increases the binding of calcium with albumin and reduces the active ionized calcium in the plasma. A drop in pH (acidosis) decreases the binding of calcium with albumin and increases the active ionized calcium in the plasma. Similarly, the amount of albumin in the blood will affect the ionized calcium levels in the serum. Patients with cirrhosis or nephrotic syndrome, for example, may have low serum albumin levels with low total calcium levels, yet their ionized calcium levels may be normal. For these reasons, direct measurements of ionized calcium levels should be obtained (27). The normal ionized calcium serum levels are 4.0 to 4.8 mg/dl (2.24–2.46 mEq/L) (57).

Hypocalcemia

Hypocalcemia is defined as a total serum calcium level of less than 8.5 mg/dl (< 4.3 mEq/L) and, more significantly, by ionized calcium levels of less than 4.0 mg/dl (< 2 mEq/L) (43). It has been reported to occur in up to 80% of severely ill hospitalized patients and postsurgical patients (27). Some of the common causes for hypocalcemia include:

I. Deficiency or disturbance in metabolism in vitamin D
   A. Inadequate intake
   B. Malabsorption syndrome
   C. Renal disease
   D. Acute pancreatitis
   E. Sepsis

II. Parathyroid hormone deficiency
   A. Hypomagnesemia/severe hypermagnesemia
   B. Neck surgery
   C. Ineffective parathyroid hormone metabolism

III. Miscellaneous
   A. Hypoalbuminemia (e.g., from cirrhosis, starvation, nephrotic syndrome)
   B. Hyperphosphatemia (e.g., from rhabdomyolysis, tumor lysis syndrome)
   C. Chelation after transfusion with citrated blood
   D. Alkalosis

Vitamin D deficiencies can occur in the surgical patient because of an inadequate diet, or because diarrhea or steatorrhea prevent its absorption. Patients with hepatic or renal failure frequently have hypocalcemia because their diseased liver and kidneys are unable to convert vitamin D to its active form. Patients with sepsis and pancreatitis may also have impaired renal hydroxylation of vitamin D (27).

Hypocalcemia can occur following thyroidectomies or radical neck surgeries because of an interruption in the blood supply to the parathyroid glands (60). Low-magnesium states also influence the secretion of PTH. Drugs such as amphotericin B, aminoglycosides, carbenicillin, cisplatin, digitalis, and diuretics can cause hypomagnesemia and therefore hypocalcemia. In fact, in one study, 38% of patients who had received aminoglycosides developed hypomagnesemia (60). Drugs such as calcitonin, cimetidine (Tagamet), furosemide (Lasix), colchicine, magnesium sulfate, mithramycin, and propylthiouracil (PTU) directly impair the secretion and action of parathyroid hormone (43).

Total serum calcium levels can be normal in conditions that cause calcium to chelate, such as blood transfusions, toxic shock syndrome, or following drugs such as edetate disodium (EDTA) (27). Citrate toxicity is rare but may occur when large volumes of blood are being infused during a short period of time (greater than 30 ml/minute), for example, in liver resections (27). It may also occur in patients who have impaired citrate metabolism (e.g., patients with hepatic and renal disease) or in hypothermic patients (27). Phosphates may be released from injured cells or following cancer chemotherapy. The phosphates may then form chelates with calcium or cause calcium to precipitate, both of which will lower the ionized calcium in the serum (27).

Nursing Assessment: Signs and Symptoms

Hypocalcemia causes side effects primarily in the neuromuscular and cardiovascular systems (27). The neuromuscular manifestations of hypocalcemia are indicative of neuronal irritability (27), and include paresthesias, muscle weakness, muscle cramps, Chvostek's sign, Trousseau's sign, and tetany. Tetany with muscle spasm is not commonly seen clinically (60), but the perioperative nurse may assess the patient for the neuronal irritability that occurs with tetany by tapping over the facial nerve to produce a twitch (Chvostek's sign), or by inflating a blood pressure cuff on the upper arm at 20 mm Hg over the systolic blood pressure for 3 minutes to produce a carpal spasm (Trousseau's sign) (56).

The cardiac manifestations of hypocalcemia include hypotension, because the smooth muscles in the arteries are unable to constrict effectively, and diminished cardiac contractility. Dysrhythmias, including bradycardia and ventricular fibrillation, as well as failure to respond to drugs such as digoxin and dopamine, may also occur (27). ECG signs of hypocalcemia may involve lengthening of the QT interval and ST segment. Hypocalcemia can have serious effects on the respiratory system, including bronchospasm and laryngospasm, which may progress to apnea. Psychiatric manifestations, such as anxiety, depression, irritability, and psychosis, may also be observed by the nurse (60).

Having concluded the assessment of the patient with reduced serum calcium levels, the perioperative nurse should identify the problem with the diagnostic level "PC: Hypocalcemia" (8).

Medical Treatments and Nursing Interventions

Acute hypocalcemia with symptoms is a medical emergency, and replacement must be initiated to prevent further deterioration in the patient's condition. An initial bolus of 100 to 200 mg of calcium gluconate administered intravenously over 10 minutes is frequently ordered (27). This may be followed by a maintenance infusion of 1 to 2 mg/kg/hour (43). Calcium chloride may also be used to treat the hypocalcemia but is more irritating to the veins than is calcium gluconate (56). Intraoperative treatment of hypocalcemia (e.g., that occurring secondary to citrate toxicity following large amounts of transfused blood) may be based on serial ionized calcium levels rather than on the development of symptoms. Stone and Benotti initiate calcium replacement during liver resections, when the calcium drops 50% below normal (61).

The decision to replace mild calcium deficits will depend on many factors. Calcium replacements have been shown to be harmful in ischemic and septic states. Zaloga, for example, does not administer calcium supplements routinely to asymptomatic hypocalcemic patients with these conditions (27).

If the patient has concurrent hypomagnesemia or hypermagnesemia, these imbalances should be corrected before calcium therapy is initiated because the response to calcium alone is frequently poor (27, 57). If the patient has tumor lysis syndrome, or other conditions causing high phosphorus and low calcium levels, the administration of calcium can be

dangerous, as it may precipitate. These patients are best treated by lowering their phosphorus levels (27).

The perioperative nurse's role during the replacement of calcium involves monitoring the patient to evaluate the adequacy of therapy. The nurse should observe the ECG for changes signaling hypercalcemia caused by too-rapid replacement. These changes may include ventribular irritability, bradycardia, or heart block (27, 56). Other possible side effects of calcium replacement are hypertension, nausea and vomiting, skin flushing, and angina (27). The IV site should be checked frequently, because calcium is irritating to the veins. Patients who have been taking digitalis should be observed for signs of digitalis toxicity following calcium administration.

The nurse should assess the response of the patient to the calcium replacement clinically by performing Trousseau's sign and Chvostek's sign; by monitoring the patient's blood pressure, pulse, respirations, airway patency and urinary output; and by following the patient's neurological and mental status. Frequent laboratory reports of serum calcium, magnesium, potassium, phosphorus, creatinine, and urinary calcium excretion should also be monitored (27). Seizure precautions should be initiated in any patient demonstrating tetany.

In nonemergency situations, oral calcium replacement is preferred. Dihydrotachysterol (DHT), an analogue of vitamin D, may also need to be taken by patients with hypoparathyroidism or chronic calcium deficiencies. More rarely, the metabolites of vitamin D, 25-hydroxyvitamin D (calcifediol) or 1,25-DHCC (calcitriol) may be prescribed for patients with hypocalcemia that is difficult to manage (62). In the postanesthesia setting, the perioperative nurse has the responsibility for patient education concerning calcium replacement therapy. The nurse should also identify patients at high risk for osteoporosis (e.g., postmenopausal women) and inform them of strategies to prevent further bone loss.

Hypercalcemia

Hypercalcemia is defined as a total serum calcium of over 10.5 mg/dl (5.4 mEq/L) or an ionized calcium of greater than 5.0 mg/dl (2.6 mEq/L) (43). Some of the most common causes of hypercalcemia include:

I. Malignancy
   A. Bronchogenic carcinoma
   B. Breast cancer
   C. Multiple myeloma

    D.   Lymphoma
    E.   Renal cell carcinoma

II. Hyperparathyroidism

III. Increased intake of calcium or calcium metabolites
    A.   Overdosing with vitamins A/D
    B.   Milk alkali syndrome
    C.   Calcium supplements/antacids

IV. Miscellaneous
    A.   Drugs (thiazides, lithium, estrogens, tamoxifen)
    B.   Immobilization
    C.   Granulomatous diseases
    D.   Posttransplant hypercalcemia

Malignancy and hyperparathyroidism together account for approximately 95% of all the cases of hypercalcemia (63). Primary hyperparathyroidism is usually caused by an adenoma or by hyperplasia of the parathyroid glands and occasionally by malignancy (62), and the increased levels of PTH cause increased serum calcium levels. Secondary hyperparathyroidism, on the other hand, may occur because of vitamin D deficiency, a deficiency in calcium intake, or malabsorption of calcium and is not associated with increased calcium levels (62). Hypercalcemia develops in approximately 10 to 20% of all patients with cancer (64), and is the most common life-threatening metabolic abnormality in cancer patients (65).

Thiazide diuretics cause elevations in calcium levels by decreasing the volume of circulating plasma, thereby increasing the serum albumin levels and by increasing the reabsorption of calcium in the kidneys (62).

Nursing Assessment: Signs and Symptoms

Hypercalcemic symptoms may include mental changes such as weakness, fatigue, or lethargy, which may progress to obtundation and coma (63). Gastrointestinal symptoms include anorexia, nausea, vomiting, constipation, and epigastric pain similar to the pain of peptic ulcers or even pancreatitis (43). Renal symptoms include polyuria and polydipsia because the kidneys are not concentrating urine adequately. Kidney stones formed from the excess calcium that is being excreted may lead to renal failure. Cardiovascular symptoms include hypertension and a shortened QT-interval on the ECG (49).

In performing a baseline assessment the perioperative nurse may also notice severe pruritus, which may be due to calcification under the skin,

and the patient may complain of joint pain caused by deposits of calcium in the joint (62). The nurse should also ask the patient whether digitalis is being taken, as calcium potentiates its effects. An appropriate diagnostic label for this problem may be "PC: Hypercalcemia" (8).

Medical Treatments and Nursing Interventions

As with most other electrolyte imbalances, the sudden onset of large amounts of the calcium in the serum demands immediate attention. Acute, life-threatening hypercalcemic crisis may develop and is manifested by calcium levels that are usually above 13 mg/dl, volume depletion, acute renal failure, and coma. The goals of treatment are to increase the intravascular volume, correct the dehydration, and increase the renal excretion of calcium. This is usually accomplished by infusing normal saline and administering loop diuretics. The aim of the saline is to push the kidneys to excrete calcium, because calcium excretion in the distal tubules of the kidney is linked to sodium excretion. When increased amounts of water and sodium are presented to the distal tubules, along with the calcium, the excretion of calcium is boosted (62). Two to 3 liters of normal saline may need to be given with 40 to 100 mg of furosemide (Lasix) over 3 to 6 hours (43). The Lasix increases the excretion of the excess fluids and prevents the calcium from being reabsorbed in the kidneys.

The nurse must monitor these patients, especially patients with cardiac or renal disease, for signs of fluid overload. Frequent physical assessment of the lung fields, observation of vital signs, intake and output measurement and, if possible, central venous pressure and ECG monitoring, should be initiated. In addition, frequent potassium, magnesium, sodium, and calcium levels should be obtained. The nurse should be alert for the possibility that the patient may develop hypokalemia or hypomagnesemia due to the increased urine output, so that early replacement of these electrolytes can be accomplished.

If fluid and diuretic therapy is not effective, or cannot be tolerated, calcitonin (4 IU/kg) may be administered subcutaneously or intramuscularly every 12 hours. Its onset of action is less than 6 hours, and its principle side effect is nausea. The main problem associated with calcitonin is that rapid tolerance is developed, and it is only effective for a short period of time (49). Prednisone, 60 to 80 mg/day, may be given concurrently with calcitonin (49). Glucocorticoids are most effective with hypercalcemia caused by multiple myeloma, and are thought to prolong the effect of calcitonin (64).

Mithramycin, 15 to 25 mcg/kg, may also be given to treat hypercalcemia, but it is associated with multiple side effects, including bone marrow depression and nephrotoxicity. For this reason it is often reserved for patients with hypercalcemia caused by malignancy (62). Its onset of action is usually within 48 hours; the duration of action is variable and ranges from 3 to 15 days (49).

Prostaglandin inhibitors such as indomethacin have been used with selected groups of patients with tumor-related hypercalcemia but without much success (64). Editronate and gallium nitrate have also been used, concurrently with fluids and diuretics, to treat hypercalcemia caused by cancer. In one study the gallium nitrate was successful in 82% of the patient population, while the editronate was successful in only 43% (65).

In the past, intravenous phosphate infusions were given to reduce calcium levels rapidly by the formation of calcium–phosphate complexes. Intravenous phosphates are rarely administered now because they are associated with widespread toxicity, including the deposition of these complexes in the kidneys, causing acute renal impairment (56). Oral phosphates may be given to selected patients with chronic hypercalcemia, and are thought to reduce calcium absorption in the GI tract. If oral phosphates are prescribed, the nurse should stress the importance of follow-up medical appointments, as regular samples of serum calcium, phosphorus, and creatinine levels are required during phosphate therapy. These studies are ordered to ensure that the calcium levels are dropping appropriately and that renal damage is not developing. Phosphate therapy is discontinued if the phosphate level is greater than 3.8 mg/dl (64).

In acute situations, acute hemodialysis with a low-calcium dialysate can be used to reduce high levels of calcium. A recent study described a patient with very elevated calcium levels who was 36 weeks pregnant. She had been drinking five glasses of milk as well as taking 30 calcium carbonate tablets every day. After receiving 3500 ml of normal saline and three doses of Lasix, which caused an hourly urine output of 250 cc/hour, only a slight decrease of serum calcium was observed. Hemodialysis via a right subclavian catheter was instituted, causing a marked reduction of the serum calcium (66). Hemodialysis can reduce excess calcium eight times more rapidly than forced saline diuresis (66).

The treatment of acute hypercalcemia involves treating the symptoms by removing the excess cal-

cium. The treatment of chronic hypercalcemia involves treating the cause whenever possible, for example, by excision of adenomatous parathyroid tumors. In caring for patients who are at risk for developing hypercalcemia, the perioperative nurse should institute measures to prevent its occurrence whenever possible. The nurse should ensure that the patient is adequately hydrated and has an adequate urinary output during the perioperative period. Following surgery, patients should be mobilized as soon as possible.

Education of the at-risk ambulatory surgery patient should include explanations about the importance of weight bearing in preventing hypercalcemia. Patients with hypercalcemia should also be taught about their medications and, if they are ordered, salt supplements. The nurse should also stress the need for a high fluid intake (3–5 L/day) (62).

MAGNESIUM BALANCE

Magnesium is the fourth most plentiful cation in the body, and almost all of it is located within the intracellular fluid compartment. More than 50% of the total amount of body magnesium is located in bones, and most of the remainder is located in muscles and other soft tissues. Less than 1% is in the extracellular fluid (67). Magnesium is necessary for normal bone structure and is a cofactor in many enzyme reactions, including energy production, protein synthesis, and the operation of the sodium–potassium–ATPase pump (68). It is essential for the transmission of nerve impulses and for normal cardiac function (57).

Plasma magnesium ranges from 1.5 to 2.5 mEq/L (1.8–3.0 mg/dl)(6). Magnesium is absorbed in the GI tract, with greater amounts absorbed when the diet is low in magnesium and less absorbed when the diet is high in magnesium. The hormone 1,25-DHCC enhances the absorption of magnesium (69). Magnesium is found in a wide variety of foods, including green vegetables, grains, nuts, meat, fish, and fruits, so that deficiencies rarely result from an inadequate diet alone (46). The daily intake of magnesium is about 20 to 30 mEq (49).

While the GI tract plays a part in magnesium balance, the kidneys control the excretion of magnesium to maintain optimal levels. The kidneys excrete greater amounts of magnesium when serum levels are elevated. Magnesium excretion resembles calcium and sodium excretion, and is inhibited when sodium is not reabsorbed by the kidneys or when diuretics are given. PTH increases serum magnesium levels, but this effect is usually overridden by the hypercalcemia that also occurs with increased PTH levels (69). Magnesium imbalances occur if the kidneys are impaired.

Hypomagnesemia

Hypomagnesemia is defined as a serum magnesium of less than 1.7 mg/dl (67). It has been observed in 10% of all hospitalized patients and in up to 65% of patients in medical intensive care units (70). Some of the common causes of hypomagnesemia include:

I.   Decreased intake
   A.   Protein–calorie malnutrition
   B.   Malnutrition secondary to alcoholism
   C.   Nutritional solutions with inadequate magnesium

II. Decreased absorption
   A.   Small bowel resection
   B.   Malabsorption syndrome (e.g., celiac sprue, radiation enteritis, cystic fibrosis)

III. Increased loss via GI routes
   A.   Nasogastric suctioning
   B.   Chronic vomiting
   C.   Diarrhea
   D.   Laxatives/purgatives

IV. Increased loss via renal routes
   A.   Hypercalcemia
   B.   Hypervolemia
   C.   Diabetic ketoacidosis
   D.   Hyperparathyroidism
   E.   Renal diseases
   F.   Drugs (e.g., diuretics, aminoglycosides, amphotericin-B, cisplatin, pentamidine)

Hypocalcemia occurs in approximately one-third of patients who develop hypomagnesemia (70), because a lack of magnesium interferes with the ability of parathyroid hormone to regulate calcium (68). Forty-two percent of patients with low magnesium also have low potassium (71). This is because magnesium is necessary for the sodium–potassium–ATPase pump to function, and if insufficient magnesium exists, the potassium escapes from the cells and is excreted in the urine (57).

Nursing Assessment: Signs and Symptoms

The signs and symptoms of low magnesium states may be difficult to identify because of the hypocalce-

mia and hypokalemia that frequently coexist with it (67). Hypomagnesemia produces symptoms associated with increased neuromuscular irritability. These include weakness, tremors, tetany, and seizures. The tetany may be due to the hypocalcemia that accompanies the low serum magnesium. The perioperative nurse should check high-risk patients (such as those with hypokalemia, anorexia, or a history of alcoholism or diabetes) for the early signs of tetany with Chvostek's sign and Trousseau's sign.

Hypomagnesemia may cause cardiac dysrhythmias brought on by an increased susceptibility to digitalis toxicity, including premature ventricular contractions (PVCs), ventricular tachycardia, and ventricular fibrillation. In addition, other dysrhythmias, unrelated to digoxin, have occurred. Clinicians have had problems discovering the cause of these hypomagnesemia-induced dysrhythmias, particularly when the patient also has hypokalemia (68). ECG tracings are similar to those seen in hypokalemia and show a prolonged QT-interval, ST-segment depression, and broad, flat T-waves (67).

The nurse may fail to hear bowel sounds when assessing the hypomagnesemic patient, which may be symptomatic of a paralytic ileus. Also, the patient may give a history of anorexia, nausea, and vomiting, all of which may also be indicative of hypomagnesemia (68). Chemical profiles will show reduced serum potassium and calcium, as well as reduced serum and urinary magnesium. An appropriate diagnostic level for this problem may be "PC: Hypomagnesemia"(8).

Medical Treatments and Nursing Interventions

Intravenous replacement of magnesium will be necessary for severely depleted patients who exhibit symptoms such as seizures or dysrhythmias. Magnesium sulfate is usually given via continuous IV infusion at 1 mEq/kg on the first treatment day, followed by 0.5 mEq/kg for the following 3 to 5 days (49). A loading dose of 2 grams (16.3 mEq) may be infused over several minutes (68). The total replacement should take place over several days. The perioperative nurse should use a pump to administer magnesium in order to ensure precise infusion rates.

During replacement for severe hypomagnesemia, the nurse should monitor the patient by checking the deep tendon reflexes (DTRs) to ensure that the replacement is not too rapid. Changes in the DTRs will occur before most other symptoms of excess magnesium appear (69). A complete absence of DTRs with flaccid paralysis usually occurs when the serum magnesium becomes greater than 7% (67).

ECG monitoring should also be initiated, and the nurse may observe prolonged PR- or QT-intervals if the magnesium replacement is too fast, causing elevated serum levels (69). Frequent vital signs should also be taken; a drop or change in respiratory rate or a drop in blood pressure indicate magnesium overdose (71). This is particularly likely to occur in patients with impaired renal function (68).

The perioperative nurse may need to instruct the patient with chronic hypomagnesemia about long-term replacement therapy. Oral preparations include magnesium hydroxide tablets, magnesium acetate solution, liquid milk of magnesia (68), and magnesium oxide. The problem with these preparations is the diarrhea that they cause. To avoid this problem, timed-release tablets of magnesium chloride are now available, but they are expensive for long-term use (71).

Hypermagnesemia

Hypermagnesemia is defined as a serum magnesium of greater than 3 mg/dl, although symptoms are rarely present until the levels exceed 5 mg/dl (67). It occurs much less frequently than hypomagnesemia, and mainly in patients with renal failure because normal kidneys successfully clear excess magnesium from the body. The second most common cause of hypermagnesemia is nosocomial administration. Overdosage may occur when magnesium is given to eclamptic patients or when it is administered for cardiac arrhythmias or myocardial infarction. When magnesium-containing antacids, laxatives, and enemas are given to patients with impaired renal function, the kidneys may not be able to excrete it effectively, and high levels may develop. Overzealous replacement of magnesium deficiency states may also lead to magnesium excess. Occasionally edemas containing magnesium have caused severe hypermagnesemia, especially in children. Hyperparathyroidism, Addison's disease, or lithium therapy may also cause hypermagnesemia, but these are uncommon causes (69).

Nursing Assessment: Signs and Symptoms

Magnesium is a central nervous system depressant; therefore, one of the first signs of hypermagnesemia is weakness. The neuromuscular weakness progresses to paralysis, including paralysis of the respiratory muscles, as the serum levels climb to levels of 13 mEq/L or greater (69). Drowsiness is also evident initially and, if the situation is untreated, deteriorates into coma. The best way for the perioperative nurse to catch the earliest symptoms of neuromus-

cular blockage caused by hypermagnesemia is by monitoring the deep tendon reflexes.

The effects of hypermagnesemia on the cardiovascular system are related to peripheral vasodilation and include hypotension, intracardiac conduction defects progressing to complete heart block, and cardiac arrest (68). The ECG recording shows prolonged PR- and QT-intervals. Hypocalcemia, hyperkalemia, acidosis, and digitalis therapy will increase the cardiac symptoms related to hypermagnesemia (68). The nurse may also observe nonspecific signs, such as flushing and warmth of the skin (indicating peripheral vasodilation), before the more severe manifestations occur. The diagnostic label for this problem may be "PC: Hypermagnesemia"(8).

Medical Treatments and Nursing Interventions

If the hypermagnesemia is severe, calcium gluconate may be administered intravenously to reverse the heart block and to improve the respiratory depression. Calcium antagonizes the action of magnesium in the cardiac conduction system and the central nervous system (68). Ventilatory support with intubation and mechanical ventilation should be instituted for paralysis of the respiratory muscles. Forced diuresis with sodium chloride infusions and loop diuretics may accelerate the renal clearance of magnesium (69). Hemodialysis can be used to remove excessive amounts of magnesium in severely symptomatic patients.

In mild cases of hypermagnesemia, stopping the intake and allowing the kidneys to excrete the excess magnesium may be sufficient treatment (67). Patient education is important in ambulatory surgery settings, particularly for high-risk patients such as those with renal impairment.

PHOSPHORUS BALANCE

Phosphorus is the primary intracellular anion. More than 85% of the body's phosphorus is stored in bone; the remainder is found in soft tissue and skeletal muscle. Less than 1% of the body's phosphorus is found in the extracellular fluid (72). Phosphorus is a major structural component of bone as well as all the body cells, and forms part of the cell membrane phospholipids (73). It is involved in the metabolic processes of the cells, is a source of high-energy chemical bonds, is involved in the release of oxygen by hemoglobin (as 2,3-diphosphoglycerate), and buffers the urine (43).

Plasma phosphorus is normally between 3.0 and

4.5 mg/dl in adults and between 4.0 and 7.1 mg/dl in children (43). Phosphorus is present in the serum as phosphate ions, mostly $H_2PO_4^-$ and HPO_4^-. The proportion of these two forms of inorganic phosphate is dependent upon the pH of the serum. For this reason, phosphate is usually reported as elemental phosphorus (P) (73).

The average American takes in about 800 to 1500 mg of phosphorus a day, mostly from dairy products, red meat, poultry, and fish (49, 57). Its absorption in the small intestine is facilitated by the hormone 1,25-DHCC. Phosphorus is excreted by the kidneys, and the presence of PTH increases this excretion. The regulation of calcium and phosphorus are interrelated.

Hypophosphatemia

Hypophosphatemia is defined as a serum phosphorus of less than 2.7 mg/dl. Some of the most common causes of hypophosphatemia include:

I. Insufficient intake or absorption
   A. Severe starvation (e.g., among hospitalized or alcoholic patients)
   B. Antacids that bind with phosphorus

II. Increased gastrointestinal loss
   A. Prolonged vomiting or nasogastric suction
   B. Chronic diarrhea

III. Increased renal loss
   A. Hyperparathyroidism
   B. Osmotic diuresis
   C. Renal tubular disorders
   D. Rickets/osteomalacia

IV. Shifts from the extracellular compartment
   A. Acute respiratory alkalosis
   B. Carbohydrate ingestion

V. Drugs
   A. Anabolic steroids
   B. Diuretics
   C. Epinephrine
   D. Glucagon

Hypophosphatemia is rarely caused by insufficient dietary intake. However, when phosphorus intake is poor, some patients have been known to develop hypophosphatemia due to malabsorption of phosphates after only 2 weeks of therapy with phosphate-binding antacids (57). Renal loss of phosphorus is seen quite frequently, and hypomagnesemia and hypokalemia may also be present in these patients (43).

Hospitalized patients who receive large amounts of intravenous glucose in hyperalimentation solutions, especially if they have been NPO for some time, may develop the refeeding syndrome. This occurs because the extracellular (serum) phosphorus is depleted during transport of carbohydrates into the cell and during cellular metabolism of carbohydrates (73). Alkalosis will also cause the phosphorus in the ECF to shift into the cells. Acute respiratory alkalosis causes this shift to a much greater degree than metabolic alkalosis, although the reasons for this are unclear.

Severe hypophosphatemia is most frequently seen in alcoholic patients, especially during the withdrawal phase (73).

Nursing Assessment: Signs and Symptoms

The depletion of ATP due to hypophosphatemia causes profound changes in energy metabolism throughout the body. Because of the depletion of ATP, the red blood cells can no longer maintain the integrity of their membranes, and hemolysis may occur. Phosphate is also necessary for the formation of 2,3-diphosphoglycerate (2,3-DPG). If 2,3-DPG levels are insufficient, generalized tissue hypoxia will occur because the red cells will not release oxygen to the tissues effectively (73). The perioperative nurse will need to assess for tissue hypoxia by monitoring arterial blood gases or oxygen saturation levels.

The neuromuscular symptoms of hypophosphatemia are many, including severe weakness, which may progress to respiratory impairment, seizures, and coma. Decreased cardiac contractility and cardiomyopathy may also occur (43). Chronic hypophosphatemia causes structural skeletal problems. An appropriate diagnostic label for this problem may be "PC: Hypophosphatemia" (8).

Medical Treatments and Nursing Interventions

Replacement therapy via the IV route is necessary only when symptoms are severe and serum phosphate is less than 1 mg/dl. As phosphorus is an intracellular ion, the exact dosage is hard to gauge, but 2.5 to 5 mg/kg may be given every 6 hours (43). The phosphorus should be diluted in D5W or normal saline and should be given slowly over 4 to 6 hours (57). IV replacement should stop when the serum phosphorus reaches 2 mg/dl. Because serum potassium levels are also reduced in alcoholic patients and those with diabetic ketoacidosis, half of the replacement amount may be given as potassium phosphate and half as sodium phosphate (73).

During phosphorus replacement the perioperative nurse should monitor the patient for signs of hypocalcemia. Trousseau's and/or Chvostek's signs may be obtained to observe the earliest manifestations of hypocalcemic tetany. Frequent serum phosphorus levels should be obtained, as well as calcium, magnesium, sodium, and potassium.

Oral replacement with whole cow's milk, tablets, or powders is preferred for mild hypophosphatemia and for chronic hypophosphatemia. In instructing patients about their use, the perioperative nurse should emphasize that tablets such as Uro-KP Neutral or Neutra-Phos tablets should be taken with a full glass of water and that the palatability of dissolved products like Fleet Phospho-soda may be improved if they are chilled (57). Strategies for managing diarrhea, which is a frequent side effect of oral phosphorus replacement, can also be discussed. Patient education should also include the signs and symptoms of excess phosphorus and the necessity for ongoing laboratory testing of serum phosphorus levels.

Hyperphosphatemia

Hyperphosphatemia is defined as a fasting serum phosphorus of more than 4.5 mg/dl (43). Renal failure, excessive oral replacement therapy, hypoparathyroidism and acromegaly cause excess serum phosphorus levels (73). Tissue breakdown occurring during chemotherapy, rhabdomyolysis, malignant hyperthermia, and sepsis will cause the intracellular phosphorus to shift into the ECF and raise the serum phosphorus levels (43).

Nursing Assessment: Signs and Symptoms

Tetany due to the hypocalcemia that accompanies hyperphosphatemia is the most frequent symptom seen in the surgical patient. (Serum calcium and serum phosphorus are inversely related; when one rises, the other falls.) The precipitation of calcium phosphate complexes in soft tissues such as the joints, arteries, skin, lung, cardiac conduction system, cornea, and kidneys may occur in uremic patients with chronically high serum phosphorus levels (6, 49). The perioperative nurse should question patients with severe renal disease about their use of phosphate-containing laxatives, as these patients are prone to hyperphosphatemia. The nurse may also want to check the arterial blood gas results of these patients, as high phosphorus levels worsen the metabolic acidosis seen in uremic patients (73). The diagnostic labels for this problem may include "PC: Hyperphosphatemia" (8).

Medical Treatments and Nursing Interventions

If phosphorus levels are elevated, normal saline infusions and 500 mg of acetazolamide (Diamox) every 6 hours may be administered to facilitate renal clearance in patients with functioning kidneys (43). Patients with chronic elevations may be given phosphate-binding antacids such as aluminum hydroxide. These antacids bind with phosphate to form aluminum phosphate, which can then be excreted via the GI tract (49). The intake of phosphorus should be curtailed, and peritoneal dialysis or hemodialysis may need to be implemented in patients with renal failure (43).

ACID–BASE BALANCE

The regulation of acid–base balance is really the regulation of hydrogen ions in the body (1). As the hydrogen concentration in the body increases, body fluids become more acidic; as the hydrogen ion concentration decreases, they become more alkaline. The regulatory systems of the body strive to maintain the acid–base ratio of the body fluids within very narrow limits: slight changes in the normal acidity or alkalinity of these fluids can cause profound changes in the ability of the body to function (1).

Some of the terms commonly used in acid–base management are listed in Table 8.1. Among the most important of these is *pH*, which is used to describe the concentration of hydrogen ions in the body. Put another way, the pH reflects the acidity or alkalinity of the body fluids. The relationship between pH, base, and acid concentrations is explained by the modified Henderson-Hasselbalch equation:

$$pH = pK + \log HCO_3^-/pCO_2$$
(where pK = 6.1, a constant)

The equation shows that the "arterial pH is determined by the logarithm of the ratio of bicarbonate (HCO_3^-) to carbonate dioxide (pCO_2)" (74). This description may seem impractical to the perioperative nurse; in fact, the term *pH* has been described as "obscure to those who are not mathematically inclined" (75). It can be made simpler if the nurse focuses on one essential fact, namely, that a constant relationship between the amount of bicarbonate and the amount of acid is necessary to maintain the pH of the serum. This relationship consists of a constant ratio of one part carbon dioxide (pCO_2) to 20 parts of bicarbonate (HCO_3^-).

Several mechanisms are designed to maintain the serum pH within the limited range that is neces-

TABLE 8.1.   Commonly Used Terms in Acid–Base Management

Term	Definition
Acid	A H^+ donor. When an acid is in solution, it can dissociate to form H^+ and an anion. (Example: $H_2CO_3 \rightarrow 2H^+ + HCO_3^-$.
Acidemia	A decrease in blood pH below 7.35
Acidosis	A process causing acidemia
Alkali	Used interchangeably with base
Alkalemia	An increase in blood pH above 7.45
Alkalosis	A process causing alkalemia
Base	A H^+ acceptor. When a base is in solution it can combine with and remove H^+. (Example: $HCO_3^- + H^+ \rightarrow H_2CO_3$)
pH	"Negative logarithm of hydrogen ion concentration" (74) pH < 7.35 = acidemia (increased H^+) pH > 7.45 = alkalemia (decreased H^+)
Hydrogen ion (H^+)	The positively charged nucleus of the hydrogen atom. Acids are characterized by their ability to release H^+ ions when in solution.

sary for the body to fulfill its metabolic processes. These are the acid–base buffering systems of the body fluids, the respiratory system, and the kidneys (1). The buffer systems are able to act within seconds to respond to pH imbalances and to correct them (1). They help to maintain the pH of the serum and to counteract excessive alkalinity or acidity by combining with strong acids to turn them into weak acids and by combining with strong bases to turn them into weak bases (1).

The most important of these buffer systems is the bicarbonate–carbonic acid buffer system, which is outlined in the following reaction:

$$H^+ + HCO_3^- \rightleftharpoons H_2CO_3 \rightleftharpoons H_2O + CO_2$$

This reaction shows that the hydrogen ion (H^+) donated by a strong acid can combine with bicarbonate (HCO_3^-) to form carbonic acid (H_2CO_3), which in turn dissociates into water (H_2O) and carbon dioxide (CO_2) in the presence of the enzyme carbonic anhydrase (76). The carbon dioxide is then removed by the lungs. The importance of the bicarbonate buffer system cannot be overemphasized, as it accounts for 75 to 80% of the ECF buffering against excess acids (75).

Other buffering systems include the protein buffer system, which is particularly effective in the intracellular environment, and also the phosphate buffer system (1).

Blood gases are obtained to assess the acid–base and oxygenation status of the patient. Arterial blood gases (ABGs) reflect the ability of the lungs to oxygenate the blood adequately. Venous blood gases may also be obtained, to determine tissue oxygenation and the effectiveness of both the circulatory system and the oxygenation system (45). The perioperative nurse plays a role in obtaining blood gas samples. The condition of the patient will determine how frequently blood gas samples are ordered: in open heart surgery, they may be obtained as frequently as every 30 minutes (41).

Table 8.2 shows the normal blood gas values. The pH of arterial blood is maintained between 7.35 and 7.45, with an average of 7.4 at a body temperature of 37°C (77). The pH of venous blood is slightly lower, approximately 7.36. Intracellular pH is even lower, approximately 7.0 (1). A pH of less than 7.35 is considered to be acidic, and a pH of greater than 7.45 is considered alkaline (1). Small changes in pH represent large changes in hydrogen ion concentration. A fall in the pH of 0.30 units, from 7.40 to 7.10, for example, represents a doubling of the hydrogen ion concentration. A rise in the pH of 0.30 units, from 7.40 to 7.70, for example, represents a 50% reduction in hydrogen ion concentration (76). Humans cannot live for more than a few hours at a pH below 6.8 or above 8.0 (1).

Four main acid–base abnormalities may occur: respiratory acidosis, respiratory alkalosis, metabolic acidosis, and metabolic alkalosis. In looking at an ABG, the perioperative nurse must decide whether any of these exist.

Respiratory Acidosis

As the body performs its metabolic functions to produce energy, food is broken down, and the byproducts of this metabolism are energy, water, carbon dioxide (CO_2) and other larger acids, such as sulfuric

TABLE 8.2.   Normal Blood Gas Values

	Arterial	Venous
pH	7.40 (7.35–7.45)	7.36 (7.31–7.41)
pO_2	80–100 mm Hg	35–40 mm Hg
SO_2	95% or greater	70%–75%
pCO_2	40 (35–45) mm Hg	46 (41–51) mm Hg
HCO_3^-	24 (22–26) mEq/L	24 (22–26) mEq/L
Base excess	−2 to +2 mEq/L	−2 to +2 mEq/L

acid. CO_2 is a volatile acid and becomes a true acid when it combines with water to form H_2CO_3 (carbonic acid) which, in turn, can dissociate into hydrogen ions (H^+) and bicarbonate ions (HCO_3^-). While the kidneys can excrete these hydrogen ions along with the other, larger metabolic acids, the lungs remove almost all the CO_2 from the body under normal circumstances. When CO_2 is formed in the cells, it diffuses into the interstitial fluid and then into the bloodstream. The blood carries CO_2 to the lungs, which actively eliminate it by ventilation (1). It is important to remember that the level of the volatile gas (CO_2) is related to the level of the true acid (H_2CO_3). If the level of CO_2 increases, so too does the level of H_2CO_3 (77).

The rate and depth of alveolar ventilation are under the control of the respiratory centers in the brain stem, most importantly, the medulla oblongata. As the production of CO_2 increases (e.g., with the increased energy needs associated with febrile states) the rate and depth of ventilation increases. The normal production of CO_2 is very large; in an average 70 kg man approximately 20,000 mmol CO_2 are removed daily by the lungs (77). Hypoventilation is said to exist if too much CO_2 is present in the blood. Hyperventilation is said to exist if too much CO_2 is removed from the blood. Either of these conditions upsets the 20:1 ration of bicarbonate ions to hydrogen ions that is necessary for the maintenance of normal pH. The respiratory system is able to act within minutes to compensate for acid–base imbalances by controlling pulmonary ventilation (1).

The pCO_2 (the partial pressure or tension exerted by the dissolved CO_2 in the blood) is the parameter in an ABG that indicates the ventilatory status of the patient (45).

Respiratory acidosis is defined as an acidotic condition with a low pH and an elevated pCO_2 (pH < 7.35 and pCO_2 > 45 mm Hg). It occurs when the pulmonary ventilation is not sufficient to keep up with the rate of CO_2 and H^+ production. Many pathological conditions present in surgical patients can cause respiratory acidosis, including diseases of the lung itself or derangements of other structures involved in ventilation, such as the brain centers that control breathing. Some of the common causes of respiratory acidosis include:

I. Lung disease
   A. Chronic obstructive pulmonary disease
   B. Pneumonia
   C. Asthma

II. Diseases/disorders of the extrapulmonary structures involved in ventilation
   A. Rib fractures
   B. Paralysis of the diaphragm
   C. Kyphosis/scoliosis
   D. Pleural effusion

III. Neuromuscular disorders
   A. Guillain-Barre syndrome
   B. Myasthenia gravis

IV. Hypoventilation on mechanical ventilator

V. Problems of the respiratory center
   A. Oversedation with narcotics, sedatives, illegal drugs

Nursing Assessment: Signs and Symptoms

The major effects of acidosis are seen in the central nervous system (CNS). Acidosis acts as a CNS depressant and may initially present as mental confusion, restlessness, headache, or apprehension, which may then progress to coma. Other symptoms may include dyspnea, pallor, and sweating.

Because of the "nearly universal impairment of pulmonary function in the perioperative period," the nurse must ensure that a complete history, physical, and preoperative risk assessment are performed (7). The perioperative nurse should ask the patient about preexisting pulmonary disease, and should identify other risk factors such as obesity, age, and smoking history (7). While hypoxemia is more likely to develop following surgery, the risk of CO_2 retention and respiratory acidosis is increased in patients with preexisting lung disease (78). Upper abdominal surgery may cause diaphragmatic dysfunction in addition to postoperative pain, and both of these may contribute to postoperative hypoventilation (7).

A preoperative visit by the perioperative nurse will frequently help to prevent respiratory complications after surgery. During the visit, the patient can be taught the importance of postoperative deep breathing and coughing and the use of a pillow to splint the incision. The preoperative patient-education session might also include instructions for using an incentive inspirometer to help in preventing atelectasis. The perioperative nurse should also inform the patient about the availability and type of postoperative analgesia.

Some nursing diagnoses that may appropriate for patients with respiratory acidosis include Ineffective Breathing Pattern, Ineffective Airway Clearance, and Impaired Gas Exchange. The nurse may also give this collaborative problem the diagnostic label "PC: Respiratory acidosis" (8).

Medical Treatments and Nursing Interventions

The primary action of the healthcare team in treating respiratory acidosis is to ensure that the patient's ventilation is adequate. The underlying cause, once it is identified, needs to be addressed. Mechanical ventilation may be necessary for patients who cannot achieve effective CO_2 clearance. Drugs such as aminophylline may be prescribed to open up constricted bronchial passages, and oxygen therapy may be ordered for concomitant hypoxemia.

Intraoperatively, the nurse and the anesthesiologist will monitor the adequacy of the patient's ventilatory and oxygenation status via ongoing physical assessment and appropriate blood gas measurements.

After the surgery is concluded the nurse should observe the patient for signs of ineffective ventilation related to any anesthesia, narcotics, and muscle relaxants that may have been given (79). Laryngospasm can develop following intubation and can lead to respiratory acidosis. Constant monitoring will enable the nurse to immediately treat this postoperative complication should it occur.

Other actions the nurse should initiate to prevent the development or exacerbation of respiratory acidosis following surgery include maintaining a patent airway in the patient, administering appropriate amounts of oxygen, monitoring the rate and depth of respirations, providing stimulation (stir-up regimes), and suctioning the tracheobronchial tree if the patient is unable to clear his or her own secretions (79). Positioning the patient in a semi-Fowler's position and a frequent turning schedule (unless contraindicated) also facilitate effective ventilation.

If the patient's ventilations are inadequate, the nurse may need to ventilate the patient manually, with a positive pressure resuscitation ("ambu") bag. The physician should be notified immediately of the development of respiratory acidosis or other respiratory problems. Patients who have had spinal and epidural anesthesia are at risk for respiratory depression and for developing respiratory acidosis, and should be monitored with apnea and end-tidal carbon dioxide monitors and pulse oximeters for 24 hours (80).

Respiratory Alkalosis

Respiratory alkalosis is defined as a high pH and a low pCO_2 (pH > 7.45 and $pCO_2 < 35$). It is more frequently associated with overbreathing than with intrinsic lung disease (1). Some of the common causes of respiratory alkalosis include:

I.   Pathologies of the lung causing hyperventilation
   A.   Pulmonary embolism

II. Generalized conditions causing hyperventilation due to increased demand
   A.   Pregnancy
   B.   Fever

III. Extrapulmonary pathological conditions causing hyperventilation
   A.   Brain injury
   B.   Gram negative septicemia
   C.   Drugs that stimulate the respiratory system

IV. Hyperventilation secondary to hypoxemia from any cause

V.   Hyperventilation secondary to increased altitude

VI. Hyperventilation on a mechanical ventilator

Nursing Assessment: Signs and Symptoms

Overexcitability of the nervous system is the principal symptom of alkalosis, which may manifest itself initially as dizziness, restlessness, agitation, and tingling of the extremities. Later symptoms may include convulsions and widespread tetany, which can cause death if the respiratory muscles are involved (1).

Nursing diagnoses that may be appropriate for this condition include Impaired Gas Exchange, Ineffective Breathing Pattern, Ineffective Airway Clearance, Anxiety related to impending surgery, or Pain related to the surgical incision. Patient education to address these diagnoses prior to surgery may help to prevent their occurrence postoperatively. The nurse may also elect to label this collaborative problem "PC: Respiratory alkalosis" (8).

Medical Treatments and Nursing Interventions

The patient's acid–base and oxygenation levels should be monitored postoperatively, and the physician should be informed of abnormalities. If respiratory alkalosis occurs in the mechanically ventilated patient, the minute ventilation settings should be reduced. Elevated temperatures and pain, both of which may cause hyperventilation and metabolic alkalosis, should be treated promptly. Concomitant electrolyte imbalances should also be corrected.

When the normal 20:1 ratio of bicarbonate and carbonate acid is disrupted, the kidneys act to return the ratio to within its normal parameters by excreting an acidic or an alkaline urine (1). In acidotic conditions the excess hydrogen ions are excreted while the bicarbonate ions are reabsorbed. The maximum acidity that the renal tubules can tolerate is a pH of 4.5, so that excess hydrogen ions need to be transported in a buffer system to prevent the urine from becoming too acidic. The most important of these renal buffers is the ammonia buffer system. Ammonia (NH_3) is synthesized by the renal tubules and combines with the excess hydrogen (H^+) ions to form the ammonium ion (NH_4^+). The positive ammonium ion then combines with a negative ion and is excreted. As most of the negative ions in the ECF are chloride ions, the ammonium ion (NH_4^+) usually combines with the chloride ion (Cl^-) and is excreted as ammonium chloride. If the hydrogen ions were to combine with the chloride ions directly, the resulting hydrochloric acid would exceed the maximum pH of 4.5 that the tubules can tolerate (1). Excess hydrogen ions can also be transported via the phosphate buffer system.

The kidneys control excess base in the body fluids by excreting bicarbonate ((HCO_3^-). When bicarbonate is excreted, it usually combines with sodium (Na^+) to maintain electroneutrality. The renal system is a very powerful acid–base regulator, but it takes time to act, usually several days.

The HCO_3^- (bicarbonate) is the parameter in an ABG that is used to determine the metabolic status of the patient.

Metabolic Acidosis

Metabolic acidosis is defined as a condition with a low pH and a low HCO_3^- (pH < 7.35 and $HCO_3^- < 22$ mEq/L). It can occur for many reasons, including the inability of the kidneys to excrete the normal amount of acid produced in the body; the excessive production of acid; a loss of bicarbonate; and the ingestion of excess acids (1).

Nursing Assessment: Signs and Symptoms

The causes of metabolic acidosis are usually divided into those characterized by an increased anion gap and those identified by no increase in the anion gap. Metabolic acidosis with no increase in anion gap is characterized by a loss of the measured anion bicarbonate, or a gain in the measured anion chloride. The normal anion gap is approximately 15 mEq/L and is obtained by subtracting the two most plentiful anions in the ECF (chloride and bicarbon-

ate) from the most plentiful cations (sodium and potassium) (9):

$$Anion\ gap = (Na^+ + K^+) - (Cl^- + HCO_3^-)$$
$$Anion\ gap = (140 + 4) - (103 + 27)$$
$$= 14\ mEq/L$$

The anion gap represents the anions that are present in the serum but are not usually measured in routine chemistries. These unmeasured anions include sulfates, phosphates, ketones, lactate, and pyruvate. A large anion gap is often associated with metabolic acidosis and infers excess acid production or inadequate acid removal (81). For example, when there is an increase in lactic acid production due to the anaerobic metabolism that occurs in shock states, the body is required to use up its bicarbonate stores to buffer the acid pH. This causes metabolic acidosis with an anion gap due to the build-up of lactic acid (45).

Some of the common causes of metabolic acidosis include:

I. High anion gap: increase in unspecified anions
   A. Severe renal disease: uremia
   B. Uncontrolled diabetes mellitus: diabetic ketoacidosis
   C. Lactic acidosis secondary to shock and cardiopulmonary arrest
   D. Drugs
      1. Salicylates
      2. Methyl alcohol
      3. Ethylene glycol

II. Normal anion gap: no increase in unspecified anions
   A. Losses via the GI tract
      1. Diarrhea
      2. Vomiting (not including gastric contents)
      3. Pancreatic fistulas
      4. Ureteral diversions
   B. Renal tubular acidosis
   C. Drugs such as acetazolamide (Diamox)

The collaborative problem statement for this condition might read "PC: Metabolic acidosis" (8).

Medical Treatments and Nursing Interventions

A careful preoperative history will assist the nurse to identify patients at risk for developing metabolic acidosis intraoperatively and postoperatively. Patients who have had extensive vomiting or diarrhea preoperatively, or who have diabetes mellitus or renal failure, should be carefully monitored for the early signs of metabolic acidosis. The nurse should also anticipate that renal patients may experience postoperative problems. The stress of surgery may overwhelm the ability of their impaired kidneys to cope. The 180 liters of plasma that is filtered each day by the kidneys contains a total of 4500 mEq of bicarbonate. If even a small percentage of this is lost during the surgical procedure, the body's bicarbonate stores would become rapidly depleted, causing severe metabolic acidosis (82). Older patients should also be observed postoperatively for the development of metabolic acidosis. Aging kidneys are less able to excrete metabolic acids, especially during surgical illnesses associated with infection and tissue breakdown (53).

The physician may order IV fluids containing sodium acetate or lactated Ringer's in these high-risk patients to prevent metabolic acidosis in the perioperative period. Sodium acetate can be converted to bicarbonate more readily than sodium lactate, which is a significant factor for patients with concomitant impaired liver function (9).

Metabolic acidosis with very low pH levels (< 7.1) may impair the ability of the heart and other essential organs to function effectively and requires immediate treatment with sodium bicarbonate to buffer the excess hydrogen ions (3). Doses should be calculated based on ABG values, and, depending upon the severity of the acidosis, from 2 to 5 mEq/kg may be infused over 4 to 8 hours (16). Because of the dangers associated with excess bicarbonate levels, a partial replacement should be given to bring the pH toward the normal range (13).

Sodium bicarbonate buffers the excess hydrogen ions by combining with them to form carbon dioxide and water. The lungs must then eliminate the carbon dioxide. The problem with administering sodium bicarbonate is that it generates a large amount of carbon dioxide (260–280 mm Hg for each 50 mEq), and this can diffuse rapidly into the cells causing a paradoxical *intracellular* acidosis. The bicarbonate, on the other hand, crosses into the cells much more slowly (76). The nurse must ensure that the excess CO_2 is removed from the body. This can be accomplished by manually hyperventilating patients whose anesthesia has not been completely reversed, and by encouraging alert patients to breathe deeply. Frequent blood gases should be obtained during the bicarbonate infusion in order to determine the pH and bicarbonate content of the serum. The nurse should also monitor serum osmolarity and serum sodium, both of which can be elevated in patients receiving sodium bicarbonate. The other electrolytes that may be affected by metabolic acidosis and its treatment, such as potassium, chloride, and calcium, should also be measured.

Other agents that may be of use in treating metabolic acidosis include THAM (tromethamine). Dichloracetate (DCA) may also be used to treat patients with metabolic acidosis caused by excess lactate (76).

Metabolic Alkalosis

Metabolic alkalosis is defined as an alkaline condition with a high pH and a high HCO_3^- (pH > 7.45 and HCO_3^- > 26 mEq/L). Some of the common causes of metabolic alkalosis include:

I. Diuretic therapy (except carbonic anhydrase inhibitors)

II. Loss of chloride ions
   A. Vomiting and nasogastric suction of *gastric* contents containing hydrochloric acid

III. Alkali administration: sodium bicarbonate

IV. Excess aldosterone
   A. Cushing's syndrome
   B. Hyperaldosteronism
   C. Administration of exogenous steroids

V. Rapid correction of chronic hypercapnia

Surgical patients may present with metabolic alkalosis secondary to diuretic administration. Diuretics cause an increased amount of sodium ions to flow into the distal and collecting tubules of the kidneys, which must then be reabsorbed into the bloodstream. Because sodium (Na^+) has a positive charge, it must be exchanged for other ions with a positive charge, usually K^+ or H^+. Loss of H^+ ions upsets the 20:1 hydrogen:bicarbonate ratio and causes alkalosis. Cl^- ions, the most numerous ECF ions, are also lost during diuretic therapy, further compounding the alkalosis. Excess aldosterone also causes reabsorption of sodium with losses of potassium and hydrogen.

The nurse may give this collaborative problem the diagnostic label "PC: Metabolic alkalosis" (8).

Medical Treatments and Nursing Interventions

The goal of treatment in metabolic alkalosis is to restore the pH balance to normal limits. This is usually accomplished by allowing the kidneys to excrete excess bicarbonate and to conserve hydrogen ions. Chloride administration is considered a cornerstone of therapy; in fact, some authors categorize metabolic alkalosis as chloride-responsive or chlorine-resistant (75). Chloride is given as an IV infusion of sodium chloride. In excreting the excess volume, the kidneys are able to reabsorb the sodium together with the chloride to maintain electroneutrality while retaining hydrogen ions to correct the alkalosis (9). Potassium chloride is also administered to correct the hypokalemia that usually accompanies metabolic alkalosis.

If the patient has hyperkalemia sodium chloride can be given alone. If the alkalosis is very severe ammonium chloride may be used. Arginine monohydrochloride, a substance that releases hydrochloric acid during metabolism, may also be tried on rare occasions (3).

As in all other acid–base derangements, nursing care plans are directed at prevention as well as treatment. Because alkalosis is associated with hypocalcemia (recall that calcium binds with albumin in alkalotic conditions), the nurse should also monitor the patient for signs of tetany.

Arterial Blood Gas Interpretation

In evaluating an arterial blood gas, the perioperative nurse should use a systematic approach, which might include the following steps:

1. Look at the pH to determine if the ABG is alkaline (pH > 7.45), acidic (pH < 7.35), or within normal limits.
2. Next, look at the pCO_2 to see whether the problem is a respiratory acid–base disorder. If the pCO_2 is elevated (> 45 mm Hg), respiratory acidosis exists. If the pCO_2 is lowered (< 35 mm Hg), respiratory alkalosis exists.
3. Look at the HCO_3^- to see whether the problem is a metabolic acid–base disorder. If the HCO_3^- is elevated (> 26 mEq/L), metabolic alkalosis exists. If the HCO_3^- is lowered (< 22 mEq/L), metabolic acidosis exists.
4. Look to see if compensation exists. The system that is not primarily affected is the one that compensates. If, for example, the problem is respiratory acidosis, the body will compensate by retaining bicarbonate and the HCO_3^- will be elevated. Full compensation is said to exist when the pH values are within normal limits. The body does not overcompensate, and the pH value remains on the side of the primary acid–base abnormality.
5. Look to see whether a mixed acid–base abnormality exists. During cardiopulmonary arrest,

for example, mixed respiratory and metabolic acidosis may be present.
6. Determine the oxygenation status of the patient by evaluating the pO_2 and the SO_2.

Examples of Surgical Blood Gases

1. This first blood gas example was obtained from a patient in the recovery room following a posterior laminectomy and fusion. He was wearing a 60% cool aerosol face mask.

pH	7.34
pCO_2	50 mm Hg
pO_2	251 mm Hg
BE	0
HCO_3^-	25 mEq/L
Hb	9.5 g
O_2 Sat	98%

The interpretation of this ABG is uncompensated respiratory acidosis (low pH, high pCO_2, and normal HCO_3^-). The pO_2 is excessive. The treatment for this patient is to encourage him to ventilate to blow off the excess CO_2. The postanesthesia nurse could also make sure that his airway is clear and that he is not retaining secretions. When the patient is a little more awake, the percentage of oxygen can be reduced.

2. This blood gas was obtained from a patient in the operating room undergoing removal of a bone flap in the left occipital area.

pH	7.53
pCO_2	36 mm Hg
pO_2	157 mm Hg
BE	+8.3 mEq/L
HCO_3^-	32 mEq/L
Hb	9.5 g
O_2 Sat	96%

This ABG represents uncompensated metabolic alkalosis (high pH, high HCO_3^-, and pCO_2 within normal limits). The high pO_2 indicates the oxygen administered by the anesthesiologist, and the pCO_2, at the low end of normal, indicates that the patient is being well ventilated. The anesthesiologist may try cautiously to correct this alkalosis at the conclusion of the surgery. The percentage of oxygen being delivered to the patient will also be titrated postoperatively to maintain the pO_2 within normal limits.

3. This ABG was obtained from a patient in the

operating room undergoing coronary artery bypass surgery.

pH	7.50
pCO_2	27 mm Hg
pO_2	412 mm Hg
BE	+1 mEq/L
HCO_3^-	25 mEq/L
Hb	8.7 g
O_2 Sat	96%

The interpretation of this ABG is uncompensated respiratory alkalosis (high pH, low pCO_2, and HCO_3^- within normal limits). The very high pO_2 reflects the high oxygen concentrations being delivered to the patient during pump oxygenation. The hypothermic condition of the patient also reduces oxygen consumption by the tissues (39). Following surgery, these conditions will be corrected.

4. This ABG was obtained from a patient in the operating room undergoing a radical cystoprostatectomy, ureterectomy, and ileocolonic pouch.

pH	7.32
pCO_2	42 mm Hg
pO_2	142 mm Hg
BE	-4 mEq/L
HCO_3^-	21 mEq/L
Hb	10.1 g
O_2 Sat	95%

The interpretation of this ABG is uncompensated metabolic acidosis (low pH, low HCO_3^-, base deficit of -4, and pCO_2 within normal limits). The pO_2 is elevated, indicating the oxygen gas mixture that the anesthesiologist is using. The pCO_2 (a high normal) indicates that the patient is not being overventilated. Bicarbonate should not be given to this patient, as the HCO_3^- is one point away from normal. The patient can be ventilated a bit more vigorously to blow off some of the excess CO_2, which will probably correct the acidosis.

5. This ABG was obtained from a patient who was scheduled for an exploratory laparotomy for bowel obstruction. He was receiving 100% oxygen via a nonrebreathing mask.

pH	7.26
pCO_2	70 mm Hg
pO_2	59 mm Hg
BE	+2 mEq/L
HCO_3^-	26 mEq/L
Hb	11.3 g
O_2 Sat	87%

The interpretation of this ABG is uncompensated respiratory acidosis (low pH, high pCO_2, and normal HCO_3^-). This patient is unable to ventilate adequately and needs to be intubated and mechanically ventilated to reduce his pCO_2 and improve his oxygenation.

6. This ABG was obtained from a patient during a cardiopulmonary arrest. He had been scheduled for surgery later in the day to revise an access graft.

pH	7.20
pCO_2	33 mm Hg
pO_2	79 mm Hg
BE	-14 mEq/L
HCO_3^-	14 mEq/L
Hb	10.5 g
O_2 Sat	90%

The interpretation of this blood gas is uncompensated metabolic acidosis (low pH, with a low HCO_3^-, and a base deficit of -14). The patient was receiving 100% oxygen with manual resuscitation with an "ambu" bag, which is not that well reflected in the somewhat low pO_2. The adequacy of the manual ventilations is reflected in the low pCO_2. This patient should be given bicarbonate to raise the HCO_3^- level and correct the metabolic acidosis. The cause of the low oxygenation level also needs to be determined.

In caring for surgical patients with any fluid, electrolyte, and acid–base problem, the perioperative nurse practices both the art and science of nursing. The nurse uses the scientific body of knowledge to provide nursing practice which is "flexible, creative, individualized and socially oriented, compassionate and skillful" (83).

REFERENCES

1. Guyton, A. C. *Textbook of Medical Physiology* 8th ed. Philadelphia: W. B. Saunders, 1991.
2. Association of Operating Room Nurses. *AORN Standards and Recommended Practices for Perioperative Nursing–1992.* Denver: AORN, 1992.
3. Wright, H. K. "Fluid, electrolyte, and metabolic acid–base disorders." J. A. McCredie, ed. *Basic Surgery* 2nd ed., pp. 56–64. New York: Macmillan, 1986.
4. Oh, M. S., and Carrol, H. J. "Regulation of extra- and intracellular fluid composition and content." A. I. Arieff and R. A. DeFronzo, eds. *Fluid, Electrolyte, and Acid–Base Disorders*, pp. 1–38. New York: Churchill Livingstone, 1985.
5. Jones, D. H. "Fluid therapy in the PACU." *Critical Care Nurs Clin N Am* 3(1):109–120, 1991.
6. Metheny, N. M. *Fluid and Electrolyte Balance: Nursing Considerations.* Philadelphia: J. B. Lippincott, 1987.

7. Brown, D. L., and Kirby, R. R. "Preoperative evaluation of high-risk elective surgical patients." J. M. Civetta, R. W. Taylor, and R. R. Kirby, eds. *Critical Care*, pp. 137–144. Philadelphia: J. B. Lippincott, 1988.

8. Carpenito, L. J. *Nursing Diagnosis: Application to Clinical Practice* 4th ed. Philadelphia: J. B. Lippincott, 1992.

9. Pestana, C. *Fluids and Electrolytes in the Surgical Patient* 3rd ed. Baltimore: Williams & Wilkins, 1985.

10. Gershan, J. A., Freeman, C. M., Ross, M. C., Greenlee, K., Smejkal, C., Brukwitzki, G., Schneider, K., Jiricka, M. K., Johnson, D., and Anderson, C. "Fluid volume deficit: Validating the indicators." *Heart and Lung* 19(2):152–156, 1990.

11. Carpenito, L. J. *Handbook of Nursing Diagnosis* 4th ed. Philadelphia: J. B. Lippincott, 1991.

12. Shires, G. T. "Important factors in the maintenance of homeostasis in the surgical patient." *Acta Chirurgica Scandinavica Supplement* 550:29–35, 1988.

13. Sommers, M. "Rapid fluid resuscitation: How to correct dangerous deficits." *Nursing 90* 20(1):52–60, 1990.

14. Fietsam, R., Villalba, M., Glover, J. L., and Clark, K. "Intraabdominal aortic aneurysm repair." *American Surgeon* 55:396–402, 1989.

15. Kirby, R. R. "IV therapy for the 90s: Summary." *Proceedings of the Anesthesiology and Critical Care Update Symposium for Physicians, Nurses, and Respiratory Therapists*, pp. 145–149. Lake Buena Vista, FL, November 1990.

16. Gahart, B. L. *Intravenous Medications* 8th ed. St. Louis, MO: Mosby Year Book, 1992.

17. Gianarkis, D. G., Kucich, J. M., and Liotta, C. A. "Evaluating albumin usage in an urban acute care hospital." *Hospital Pharmacy* 26(5):434–436, 1991.

18. Ley, S. J., Miller, K., Skov, P., and Preisig, P. "Crystalloid versus colloid fluid therapy after cardiac surgery." *Heart and Lung* 19(1):31–40, 1990.

19. McCormac, M. "Managing hemorrhagic shock." *Am J Nursing* 90(8):22–27, 1990.

20. National Blood Resource Education Program, Nursing Education Working Group. *National Blood Resource Education Program's Transfusion Therapy Guidelines for Nurses*. NIH Publication No. 90-2668. Bethesda, MD: National Institutes of Health, 1990.

21. Klein, D. G. "Physiologic responses to traumatic shock." D. G. Klein and N. A. Stotts, eds. *AACN Clinical Issues in Critical Care Nursing* 1(3):505–521, 1990.

22. Lampe, G. H. "Blood loss and blood transfusion." *Acta Chirurgica Scandinavica Supplement* 550:88–94, 1988.

23. Litwack, K. "Practical points for transfusion therapy." *J Post Anesthesia Nursing* 11(4):257–261, 1987.

24. Perkins, H. A. "Blood transfusion." J. B. Wyngaarden and L. H. Smith, eds. *Cecil Textbook of Medicine*, pp. 947– 951. Philadelphia: W. B. Saunders, 1988.

25. Brian, J. E., Deshpande, J. K., and McPherson, R. W. "Management of cerebral hemispherectomy in children." *J Clin Anesthesia* 2(2):91–95, 1990.

26. Felver, L., and Pendarvis, J. H. "Electrolyte imbalances: Intraoperative risk factors." *AORN J* 49(4):992–1005, 1989.

27. Zaloga, G. P. " Endocrine crises: Hypocalcemic crisis." *Critical Care Clin* 7(1):191–200, 1991.

28. Brecher, M. E., Taswell, H. F., Clare, D. E., Swenke, P. K., Pineda, A. A., and Moore, S. B. "Minimal-exposure transfusion and the committed donor." *Transfusion* 30(7):599–604, 1990.

29. National Blood Resource Education Program Expert Panel. "The use of autologous blood: The National Blood Resource Education Program Expert Panel." *JAMA* 263(3):414–417, 1990.

30. Hetter, G. P. "Blood and fluid replacement for lipoplasty procedures." *Clinics in Plastic Surg* 16(2):245–248, 1989.

31. Goodnough, L. T., Johnston, M. F. M., Shah, T., and Chernosky, A. "A two-institution study of transfusion practice in 78 consecutive adult elective open heart procedures." *Am J Clin Pathology* 91(4):468–472, 1989.

32. American Association of Blood Banks Standards Committee. *Standards for Blood Banks and Transfusion Services* 14th ed. Arlington, VA: American Association of Blood Banks, 1991.

33. Williamson, K. R., and Taswell, H. F. "Indications for intraoperative blood salvage." *J Clin Apheresis* 5(2):100–103, 1990.

34. Pineda, A. A., and Valbonesi, M. "Intraoperative blood salvage." *Balliere's Clinical Haematology* 3(2):385–403, 1990.

35. Ezzedine, H., Baele, P., and Robert, A. "Bacteriologic quality of intraoperative autotransfusion." *Surgery* 109:259–264, 1991.

36. Sieunarine, K., Wetherall, J., Lawrence-Brown, M. M. D., Goodman, M. A., Prendergast, F. J., and Hellings, M. "Levels of complement factor C3 and its activated product, C3a, in operatively salvaged blood." *Austr and New Zealand J Surg* 61(4):302–305, 1991.

37. Deleuze, P., Intrator, L., Liou, A., Contremoulins, I., Cachera, J. P., and Loisance, D. Y. "Complement activation and use of a cell saver in cardiopulmonary bypass." *ASAIO Transactions* 36(3):M179–181, 1990.

38. Electromedics. *Electromedics, Inc., AT1000 Autotransfusion System Operator's Manual*. Englewood, CO: Electromedics, 1991.

39. Butler, S. "Current trends in autologous transfusion." *RN* November:44–55, 1989.

40. Boldt, J., Zickmann, B., Fedderson, B., Herod, C., Dapper, F., and Hemplemann, G. "Six different hemofiltration devices for blood conservation in cardiac surgery." *Ann Thoracic Surg* 51(5):747–753, 1991.

41. Bell, P. E., and Diffee, G. T. "Cardiopulmonary bypass: Principles, nursing implications." *AORN J* 53(6):1480–1496, 1991.

42. Eisner, R. F., Montz, F. J., and Berek, J. S. "Cytoreductive surgery for advanced ovarian cancer: Cardiovascular evaluation with pulmonary artery catheters." *Gynecol Oncol* 37(3):311–314, 1990.

43. Layton, A. J., and Kirby, R. R. "Fluids and electrolytes in the critically ill." J. M. Civetta, R. W. Taylor, and R. R. Kirby, eds. *Critical Care*, pp. 451–474. Philadelphia: J. B. Lippincott, 1988.

44. Zaloga, G. P. "Hyperosmolar states." J. M. Civetta, R. W. Taylor, and R. R. Kirby, eds. *Critical Care*, pp. 475–481. Philadelphia: J. B. Lippincott, 1988.

45. Broughton, J. O. *Understanding Blood Gases*. Madison, WI: Airco, 1979.

46. Collins, R. D. *Illustrated Manual of Fluid and Electrolyte Disorders* 2nd ed. Philadelphia: J. B. Lippincott, 1983.

47. Cheng, J., Zikos, D., Peterson, D. R., and Fisher, K. A. " Symptomatic hyponatremia: Pathophysiology and management." *Acute Care* 14–15:270–292, 1989.

48. Sarnaik, A. P., Meert, K., Hackbarth, R., and Fleishmann, L. "Management of hyponatremic seizures in children with hypertonic saline: A safe and effective strategy." *Critical Care Med* 19(6):758–762, 1991.

49. Cuddy, P. G. "Fluid and electrolyte disorders." L. Y. Young and M. A. Koda-Kimble, eds. *Applied Therapeutics: The Clinical Use of Drugs* 4th ed., pp. 635–657. Vancouver, WA: Applied Therapeutics, 1988.

50. El-Dahar, S., Gomez, R. A., Campbell, F. G., and Chevalier, R. L. "Rapid correction of acute salt poisoning by peritoneal dialysis." *Pediatric Nephrology* 8(2):602–604, 1987.

51. Smith, J. D., Bia, M. J., and DeFronzo, R. A. "Clinical disorders of potassium metabolism." A. I. Arieff and R. A. DeFronzo, eds. *Fluid, Electrolyte, and Acid–Base Disorders,* pp. 413–509. New York: Churchill Livingstone, 1985.

52. Schwartz, M. W. "Potassium imbalances." *Am J Nursing* 87(10):1292–1300, 1987.

53. Beck, L. H. "Perioperative renal, fluid, and electrolyte management." *Clinics in Geriatric Med* 6(3):557–569, 1990.

54. Womack, P. L., and Hart, L. L. "Potassium supplements versus potassium-sparing diuretics." *DICP, The Annals of Pharmacotherapy* 24(7/8):710–711, 1990.

55. Watson, D. S., and Kaempf, G. *Monitoring the Patient Receiving Local Anesthesia* 2nd ed. Denver: AORN, 1991.

56. Agus, Z. S., and Goldfarb, S. "Calcium metabolism: Normal and abnormal." A. I. Arieff and R. A. DeFronzo, eds. *Fluid, Electrolyte, and Acid–Base Disorders,* pp. 511–574. New York: Churchill Livingstone, 1985.

57. Henderson, L. M., and Barfield, P. S. "The pharmacist's role in calcium, phosphorus, and magnesium replacement in the adult." *Clinical Trends in Hospital Pharmacy* 5(1):1–10, 1991.

58. Arnaud, C. D. "Minerals and bone homeostasis." J. B. Wyngaarden and L. H. Smith, eds. *Cecil Textbook of Medicine,* pp. 1469–1476. Philadelphia: W. B. Saunders, 1988.

59. Bikle, D. D. "Vitamin D." J. B. Wyngaarden and L. H. Smith, eds. *Cecil Textbook of Medicine,* pp. 1577–1479. Philadelphia: W. B. Saunders, 1988.

60. Zaloga, G. P., and Chernow, B. "Hypocalcemia in critical illness." *JAMA* 256(14):1924–1929, 1986.

61. Stone, M. D., and Benotti, P. N. "Liver resection: Preoperative and postoperative care." *Surg Clin N Am* 69(2):383–392, 1989.

62. Arnaud, C. D. "The parathyroid glands, hypercalcemia, and hypocalcemia." J. B. Wyngaarden and L. H. Smith, eds. *Cecil Textbook of Medicine,* pp. 1486–1505. Philadelphia: W. B. Saunders, 1988.

63. Janz, T. G. "Managing the cancer-related emergency." *Emergency Medicine: Acute Medicine for the Primary Care Physician* 22(6):58–82, 1990.

64. Lang-Kummer, J. M. "Hypercalcemia." S. L. Groenwald, M. H. Frogge, M. Goodman, and C. H. Yarbro, eds. *Cancer Nursing: Principles and Practice* 2nd ed. pp. 520–534. Boston: Jones and Bartlett, 1990.

65. Warrell, R. P., Murphy, W. K., Schulman, P., O'Dwyer, P. J., and Heller, G. "A randomized double-blind study of gallium nitrate compared with editronate for acute control of cancer-related hypercalcemia." *J Clin Oncol* 9(8):1467–1475, 1991.

66. Kleinman, G. E., Rodriguez, H., Good, M. C., and Caudle, M. R. "Hypercalcemic crisis in pregnancy associated with calcium carbonate antacid (milk alkali syndrome): Successful treatment with hemodialysis." *Obstet Gynecol* 78(3):496–499, 1991.

67. Lau, L. "Magnesium metabolism: Normal and abnormal." A. I. Arieff and R. A. DeFronzo, eds. *Fluid, Electrolyte, and Acid–Base Disorders,* pp. 575–624. New York: Churchill Livingstone, 1985.

68. Smith, L. H. "Disorders of magnesium metabolism." J. B. Wyngaarden and L. H. Smith, eds. *Cecil Textbook of Medicine,* pp. 1195–1196. Philadelphia: W. B. Saunders, 1988.

69. Van Hood, J. W. "Endocrine crises: Hypermagnesemia." *Critical Care Clin* 7(1):215–222, 1991.

70. Ryzen, E., Wagers, P. W., Singer, F. R., and Rude, R. K. "Magnesium deficiency in a medical ICU population." *Critical Care Med* 13(1):19–21, 1985.

71. Yarnell, R. P., Craig, M. P. "Fluid, electrolyte, and metabolic acid–base disorders." J. A. McCredie, ed. *Basic Surgery* 2nd ed., pp. 56–64. New York: Macmillan, 1986.

72. Kurokawa, K., Levine, B. S., Lee, D. B. N., and Massry, S. G. "Physiology of phosphorus metabolism and pathophysiology of hypophosphatemia and hyperphosphatemia." A. I. Arieff and R. A. DeFronzo, eds. *Fluids, Electrolyte, and Acid–Base Disorders,* pp. 625–659. New York: Churchill Livingstone, 1985.

73. Smith, L. H. "Phosphorus deficiency and hypophosphatemia." J. B. Wyngaarden and L. H. Smith, eds., *Cecil Textbook of Medicine,* pp. 1193–1194. Philadelphia: W. B. Saunders, 1988.

74. Alspach, J. G. *Core Curriculum for Critical Care Nursing.* Philadelphia: W. B. Saunders, 1991.

75. Boysen, P. G., and Kirby, R. R. "Acid–base problem solving." J. M. Civetta, R. W. Taylor, and R. R. Kirby, eds. *Critical Care,* pp. 335–339. Philadelphia: J. B. Lippincott, 1988.

76. American Heart Association. *Textbook of Advanced Cardiac Life Support* 2nd ed. Dallas: AHA, 1990.

77. Adler, S., Fraley, D. S. "Acid–base regulation: Cellular and whole body." A. I. Arieff and R. A. DeFronzo, eds. *Fluid, Electrolyte, and Acid–Base Disorders,* pp. 221–234. New York: Churchill Livingstone, 1985.

78. McConnell, E. A. "Preventing postop complications: Minimizing respiratory problems." *Nursing 91* 21(11):34–39, 1991.

79. Litwack, K. "Managing postanesthetic emergencies." *Nursing 91* 21(9):49–51, 1991.

80. Kaplan, R. E. "Postanesthetic problems." J. M. Civetta, R. W. Taylor, and R. R. Kirby, eds. *Critical Care,* pp. 157–164. Philadelphia: J. B. Lippincott, 1988.

81. Thelan, L. A., Davie, J. K., and Urden, L. D. *Textbook of Critical Care Nursing: Diagnosis and Management*. St. Louis, MO: C. V. Mosby, 1990.

82. Rothstein, M., Obialo, C., and Hruska, K. A. "Renal tubular acidosis." *Endocrinol and Metabolism Clin N Am* 19(4):869–887, 1990.

83. Rogers, M. E. *An Introduction to the Theoretical Basis of Nursing*. Philadelphia: F. A. Davis, 1970.

SUGGESTED READINGS

York, K. "Arterial blood bases: As easy as ABC." *AORN J* 49(5):1308–1329, 1989.

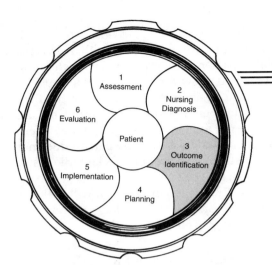

9

The Patient Is Free from Harm

Outcome: Absence of adverse effects related to hazards.

A patient who is undergoing surgery is exposed to a variety of hazards that have a potential for causing harm or injury. The perioperative nurse is obligated to employ safety measures that protect the patient from harm. Safety measures must be employed when the patient is exposed to, or in contact with, electricity, lasers, chemicals, radiation, and internal and external disasters.

One of the six outcome standards for perioperative care defined by the Association of Operating Room Nurses (AORN) is that "the patient is free from injury related to positioning, extraneous objects, or chemical, physical, and electrical hazards" (1). Positioning is discussed in Chapter 20, and the hazards associated with extraneous objects are covered in Chapter 21 (Performing Counts). The following criteria might be used to measure freedom from injury related to chemical, physical, and electrical hazards:

1. The patient will not show evidence of adverse reactions resulting from the use of electrical equipment. The patient will:
   a. be free of burns.
   b. be free of neuromuscular damage.
   c. be free of central nervous system complications.
   d. show no evidence of electrical shock.
2. The patient will be free of harm related to exposure to lasers. The patient will:
   a. be free of burns to the skin.
   b. be free of injury to the eyes.

   c. be free of internal injury related to reflected laser beams.
   d. be free of complications related to inhalation of laser plume.
3. The patient will be free of adverse effects due to exposure to chemical hazards. The patient will:
   a. be free of skin irritation or burns.
   b. be free of respiratory complications.
   c. be free of neurological problems.
4. The patient will show no evidence of excessive exposure to radiation. The patient will:
   a. have no evidence of loss of hair.
   b. have no reduction in white blood cells.
   c. have no evidence of destruction of healthy cells.
   d. show minimal skin irritation, with no ulceration.
5. The patient will be free of harm resulting from an internal or external disaster. The patient will:
   a. not be left unmonitored during warning periods for pending external disasters.
   b. not demonstrate psychological or physical trauma due to internal disasters.
   c. not be unaccompanied during evacuations.

HAZARDS ASSOCIATED WITH ELECTRICITY

As a power source for sophisticated equipment, electricity is an important ally of healthcare providers. Lifesaving devices such as defibrillators, electrocardiographs (ECGs), and dialysis machines depend on electricity. The operating room has many important and complex electrical devices. The most common are electrosurgical units, microscopes, monitors, and lights. Many operating room tables are electrical. Endoscopes are electrically powered, as are lasers, x-ray machines, drills, and video equipment.

Although electrical equipment provides important advantages in surgery, it also introduces potential hazards to patients and personnel. Most hazardous situations in surgical suites are caused by the combination of electrical equipment and combustible materials found there (2). Respect for and basic knowledge of the principles of electricity will do a great deal toward avoiding problems. Basic courses on the theory and application of electricity to patient care should be in the nursing curriculum, because perioperative nurses need a working knowledge of electricity to protect patients properly.

Basic Theory and Principles of Electricity

To understand electricity, it is important to review the following definitions:

Electricity: a form of energy produced by a flow of electrons. Electron movement is caused by creating a higher positive electric charge at one point than at another point on the same conductor. The amount of current flowing is known as *amperage,* or *amps.* The force of the current is known as *volts.* The force (volts) multiplied by the amount of current (amps) equals *watts.*

Conductivity: capacity of a material to transmit electricity.

Resistance: impedance in an electrical circuit to flow of current; measured in *ohms.*

The behavior of electricity can be compared to the functions of the sensory nervous system. The brain acts when it has power (calories) and a stimulus (such as hitting the finger with a hammer). An electrosurgical unit, microscope, or drill also reacts when there is power (electricity) and a stimulus (on-off switch). The power capacity and stimulus produce a reaction.

Think of an electrical device as a brain and the electrical cords as peripheral nerves. Both the cords and the nerves carry messages (currents) to generate an action. The force that drives electrons through a wire conductor is voltage, and the conductors allow

the flow to be continuous. The force that drives a sensation along a nerve is a combination of chemical reactions that also allow the flow to be continuous.

In either case, resistance or blockage of the flow results in improper reactions. If impulses are blocked in the nervous system, say by medication, the arm does not pull back and the person does not say "ouch." If electrical current is blocked, the result is also no action; however, if current is blocked inadvertently, say within a person's body, it will seek the path of least resistance until it reaches ground. This may cause burns or even electrocution.

Common Hazards Related to Electricity

The three most common hazards relative to electricity are fire, burns, and electric shock.

Fire

Many texts say that the fire hazards have been reduced because explosive anesthetic gases are no longer used. But look at the new equipment that has been introduced. Lasers, ultrasonic devices, and video visualization systems all have electrical connections, so fire is still a possibility. High-powered light sources (e.g., 300-watt xenon) are used several times a day per surgical suite. In one case, four alcohol sponges used for skin preparation were placed back into the basin. The basin was set on the lower shelf of the prep table. A nurse pushed the table back against the wall as she rushed to prepare for the procedure. Having finished induction, the anesthesiologist stepped back to plug in the radio. Because the radio was turned on, a spark struck out as connection was made and ignited the alcohol sponges in the basin. The startled anesthesiologist jumped back, upsetting the table. Flames poured across the floor, striking the feet of the circulating nurse, who suffered minor burns on the ankles.

The threat of fire and the control of such a disaster should be on the mind of every hospital employee. Methods of fire prevention should be deeply ingrained in personnel working in patient care areas. The same is true for patients, who should plan an escape route when they are admitted to the hospital, as they would when checking into a high-rise hotel. A fire in an operating room can cost lives, or it can be nothing more than an unpleasant memory if personnel are prepared through adequate planning and rehearsal.

In order for a fire to occur, three elements must be present:

1. A fuel. Potential fuel sources are numerous in the OR. Everything will ultimately burn. Obvi-

ous sources are all types of plastic materials, towels, blankets, and protective attire. The less obvious fuel sources are floor tiles, machines, and human beings.

2. Oxygen. Ambient air contains 29% oxygen and adds to combustion possibilities; however, in the enriched-oxygen atmosphere of the OR, combustion possibilities are increased and can happen rapidly.

3. An ignition source. In the OR, potential ignition sources include electrosurgical unit (ESU) active electrodes, laser free beams or hot fibers, fiberoptic cables, and faulty wiring of any electrical device.

Keeping these three elements apart is the basis for effective fire prevention.

Precautions that can be taken against operating room fires include:

1. Memorize policies and procedures for preventing, fighting, and reporting fires.

2. Know the location of firefighting equipment and fire alarms, and be familiar with the use of fire blankets, water hoses, and fire extinguishers. Never attempt to extinguish an electrical fire with water, because of the added danger of electrocution. Instead, disconnect power sources and use a halon fire extinguisher.

3. Know the guidelines for the prevention of fire hazards in an oxygen-enriched atmosphere.

4. Eliminate the use of explosive gases and liquids.

5. Check all electrical equipment before each use for integrity of function. Are cords intact? Do plugs fit well? Are fixtures securely mounted?

6. Establish and enforce maintenance routines necessary to keep all electrical equipment in perfect operating order.

7. Remove and send for repair any questionable electrical equipment.

8. Plan for sufficient backup equipment to allow for maintenance down-time.

9. Be aware of substances that can be ignited with sparks, such as alcohol and skin-degreasing solutions.

10. Know manufacturers' safety guidelines and usage requirements for all devices used in the operating room, especially high-energy equipment.

11. Practice using firefighting equipment, evacuating, and reporting fires quarterly.

12. Conduct educational programs on fire prevention, firefighting, and evacuating quarterly.

Fires caused by electrical wire or device failures are commonly related to inadequate insulation of cords and cables or to faulty grounding. Insulation protects the user from the electricity traveling through a wire. Insulation material varies but usually consists of rubber or plastic over cotton. Copper wires are usually used as the conductors of the current. In the OR, lightweight cords, heavy-duty cords, and building cables are used. Use of lightweight cords, which typically have two wires, is generally discouraged in the OR, because they are not as sturdy as heavy-duty cords. Three-wire heavy-duty cords are much heavier and have two layers of insulation—one layer for each wire plus a separate outer layer. This type of cord can stand up under heavy use, particularly when there are many users of each cord. The building cable, which brings electricity to the wall outlet, is usually encased in rigid or flexible steel conduit.

All these power cords protect users against contact with "hot" power wires. If the insulation breaks down, electrical current flows between the conducting wires, which generates heat and may start a fire. If a fire starts in the power cord that is attached to a piece of electrical equipment, the electric current can be shut off. If the fire goes to the wall outlet, the steel tubing or conduit prevents it from spreading.

Grounding is another important safety measure associated with the use of electrical equipment. A building's basic grounding system includes two cables, one "hot" and the other "cold." The hot cable carries the electricity from a power company generator to the building. The cold side is connected to an earth ground through large copper rods or pipes driven deep into the ground. One of the best ways to eliminate electrical hazards is to make sure all metal surfaces in an electrical system are grounded. Three-prong safety plugs should be used with all equipment in the OR. One of the three prongs provides a reliable connection to ground, and the plug is constructed so it grips the power cord firmly. The three-prong plug can be opened easily to inspect the connections.

If a fire does start despite all of these precautions, first remove any burning materials from the patient and follow a predetermined evacuation plan to evacuate the patient from the danger zone. Second, shut off anything that is contributing to the fire, including electricity, oxygen, nitrous oxide, or chemicals. Third, activate the disaster plan by reporting the fire and getting help. Fire marshals across the country agree that the best thing for healthcare professionals to do is to get themselves and their patients away from the fire, evacuate the area to safety, and let experienced firefighters eliminate the fire.

Electrical Burns

Tissue burns can obviously be the result of fires; however, burns may occur directly from contact with hot electrical wires, or indirectly from items overheated by electrical wires. High-frequency currents that are dissipated through patient grounding systems, such as those used with electrosurgery or defibrillators, may cause burns. The burn may be due to inadequate contact of the electrode with the patient or faulty wiring in the ground wire while the current is passing through.

The three major kinds of burns associated with electricity are contact, flash, and flame. Contact burns are caused by electrical and thermal coagulation as current enters and leaves the skin. The flash or arc burn results from intense heat generated by electrical current passing through the air from one conductor to another. Arc burns usually produce serious injury to the skin but do not affect internal organs. The defibrillator causes arc burns if the paddles are not placed correctly. Flame burns are the result of an explosion or fire.

Burns are generally classified as first, second, and third degree. First-degree burns damage the epidermis and cause a reddening of the skin area. Second-degree burns damage both epidermis and dermis and result in blistering of the skin. Black charring and tissue desiccation are seen in third-degree burns.

When a patient is burned, three basic principles of treatment should be kept in mind. First, maintain an airway at all times. If the burn is in the head and neck area, there is potential for laryngeal edema and tracheal obstruction. Second, take corrective action to maintain fluid and electrolyte balance. Third, maintain an environment that will prevent infection. With severe burns, there is gross tissue damage and the threat of contamination by bacteria. Usually, if there is necrosis of skin and muscle, debridement can help clean the area, making it easier to thwart potential infection.

Electric Shock

The third common hazard associated with electricity is shock or electrocution. Any direct contact with 110- or 220-volt wiring has the potential for electrocuting patients and employees. This is common household current, which is also used in hospitals. If the voltage is high enough, it can cause damage to the brain and respiratory center, resulting in apnea. In contrast, low-voltage currents frequently affect the heart, causing ventricular fibrillation.

One of the most common complications of electric shock is vascular injury, caused by current following blood vessels. The result may be necrosis, thrombosis, or hemorrhage. Loss of consciousness is another complication due to electrocoagulation of brain tissue. Damage to the respiratory center or paralysis of respiratory muscles leads to cerebral edema, hemorrhage, thrombosis, or apnea. Infections may occur because anaerobic organisms thrive in tissue destroyed by electric current. Cardiac arrhythmias are possible. Eye damage may also be a complication, with blindness occurring due to electrocoagulation of the lens. Precautions can be taken against electrical shock as follows:

1. Establish an uninterrupted power supply to each operating room with a backup emergency power source.
2. Establish and maintain a functional ground detector system that has both audio and visual alarms in each operating room.
3. Know proper grounding devices and secure use-to-grounding panels.
4. Establish policies and procedures for a biomedical engineer to test electrical patient care equipment both when newly installed and at intervals.
5. Do not use equipment that has frayed cords or poor connections.
6. Keep electrical cords off the floor if possible, and never roll equipment over them. Do not use extension cords.
7. Never place liquids on or against electrical equipment.
8. Use laboratory-approved patient grounding systems compatible with the ESU in use.
9. Develop a habit of "nontouch" when electrical equipment is being activated, that is, do not rest against or touch patients, operating room tables, or machinery.
10. Be aware of and stay up to date with records of equipment maintenance, including repairs made.
11. Keep available instructional material on the use of equipment for all personnel.

Electrical Safety Regulations

Basic safety regulations governing hospitals are found in the standards, guidelines, or codes of local, state, and federal agencies as well as voluntary standard-setting groups. The Joint Commission on Accreditation of Healthcare Organizations (JCAHO), the Occupational Safety and Health Administration

(OSHA), and the National Fire Protection Association (NFPA) are some of the most important government and voluntary agencies setting guidelines for patient safety. State and city regulations are promulgated by health boards, licensing bureaus, fire marshals and commissions on health. The U.S. Department of Health and Human Services (DHHS) issues regulations governing all hospitals. Findings of these agencies can influence a hospital's accreditation, certification, or licensure. More important, the hospital's level of compliance can affect the lives and safety of patients and employees.

Being aware of the safety standards published by such agencies is the legal, ethical, and moral responsibility of every employee who provides direct patient care. Electrical safety featuers should be planned and designed from the time of construction of every operating room suite, and safety precautions must be followed routinely every day thereafter. Regulations governing construction of hospitals and operating room suites are set by city, county, and state health departments.

It is impossible to list here all the regulations governing patient safety. The ones governing electricity alone would take many pages. For instance, NFPA has numerous publications dealing with safety in healthcare, each containing many regulations and standards regarding the hazards associated with electricity. DHHS offers a significant number of publications, many of which are relevant to hospital facilities. JCAHO publishes manuals regulating healthcare facilities and the related hazards.

For example, JCAHO requires that accredited healthcare facilities maintain an equipment-management program "designed to assess and control the clinical and physical risks of fixed and portable equipment used for diagnosis, treatment, monitoring, and care of patients and of other fixed and portable electrically powered equipment"(3). All equipment subject to this program must have written equipment-testing procedures and user-training programs designed to manage the clinical and physical risks associated with that equipment. The purpose of this is to provide instructions for use of equipment and eliminate the hazards associated with misuse. Manuals must contain specific information regarding proper operating, safety considerations, and special warnings related to use. It is important to know (1) that these rules exist, (2) how to contact the agencies establishing the regulations, and (3) that the safety measures are to be followed in all patient care areas, including the operating room. Each hospital must have an established method for receiving information from regulatory agencies and communicating safety measures to all concerned. Usually the administrative manager responsible for planning and development is the resource person who has possession of these regulations. The biomedical department and the safety committee are other important resources.

The safe use of electrical appliances is a realistic goal for perioperative nurses and their patients. In order to attain the patient outcome "Absence of adverse effects related to hazards," personnel should know the purpose of the electrical equipment being used and the precautions for preventing accidents.

Electrosurgery Units

The electrosurgery unit (ESU) deserves special attention because it is used in almost every operating room. Although usually used without incident, it can be dangerous. In electrosurgery, a generator delivers high-energy electrical waves into the patient's body through a small, active electrode. The wave of high-frequency electrical energy virtually explodes the tissue cells it contacts, then continues to travel, leaving the body and returning to the generator. Contact with tissue cells causes coagulation, cutting, or fulguration:

- Coagulation eliminates bleeding by thermally sealing the ends of blood vessels as they are dissected (Fig. 9.1).
- Cutting (separation of tissue) is accomplished by high temperatures, which explode the cells contacted by the hot active electrode (Fig. 9.2).
- Fulguration is the destruction of tissue by electrical sparks (Fig. 9.3).

Most ESUs are capable of applying a blended current, which simultaneously provides cutting and coagulation.

Monopolar Electrosurgery

In monopolar electrosurgery, a disposable dispersive electrode (grounding pad) is applied to the surface of the patient's skin, safely carrying the electrical current back to the ESU. The size, shape, and placement of this dispersive electrode are all important to patient safety (Fig. 9.4).

- The pad must be of sufficient *size* to avoid high thermal contact points. Never alter the size of a pad.
- The *shape* must provide for uniform contact with the patient's body. This is critical. If there are gaps between the pad and the patient's skin,

COAGULATION

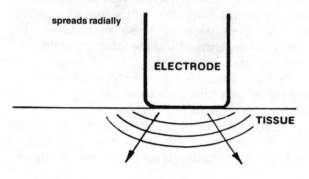

FIGURE 9.1. The coagulation function of electrosurgical units. Coagulation spreads radially. Results are hemostasis and light brown eschar. (Reprinted by permission of Valleylab, Inc., Boulder, Colo.)

CUTTING

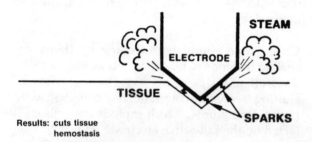

FIGURE 9.2. The cutting function of electrosurgical units. Hot, continuous sparks separate cells, resulting in cut tissue and hemostasis. (Reprinted by permission of Valleylab, Inc., Boulder, Colo.)

electricity may arc across the gap, causing a burn (Fig. 9.5).
- *Placement* of the grounding pad is also crucial. Nothing can be allowed to interfere with the contact surface of the dispersive electrode. The pad is not placed over bony prominences, excess hair is removed, and fluids are not allowed to run or pool near the pad.

The patient's position should be established prior to grounding pad application. Repositioning of a patient during a surgical procedure requires reassessment to be sure that there is secure contact between the patient and the grounding pad.

Poorly applied grounding pads are not the only burn hazard associated with electrosurgical devices.

FULGURATION

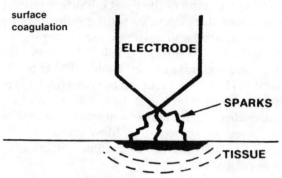

FIGURE 9.3. The fulguration function of electrosurgical units. There is surface coagulation. Hemostasis, deep necrosis, and hard eschar result. (Reprinted by permission of Valleylab, Inc., Boulder, Colo.)

Burns can also occur as electrical current seeks alternative paths out of the body. Electrocardiogram (ECG) electrodes are one of the most common alternative paths. Other locations are points of contact between the patient and metal objects such as intravenous poles and stirrups.

Bipolar Electrosurgery

Bipolar electrosurgery is preferred for certain surgical procedures. The term *bipolar* refers to the means by which the current travels back to the ESU generator. The active and dispersive electrodes are both contained in an instrument that is similar in design to a forcep (Fig. 9.6). Electricity travels along one side of the forcep and returns along the other side when the tips touch or grasp tissue, which completes the flow of current. Because the instrument provides for a complete circuit, a grounding pad is not needed during the use of a bipolar unit.

Routine inservice education for perioperative nurses is the best way to prevent accidents related to electrosurgical devices. Critical topics for the inservice session would be:

- Active electrode safety activities
- Alternative pathways for electricity
- Positioning the patient prior to placing the ground pad
- Placement of the grounding pad as close to the wound site as possible
- Inspection for insulation against any patient–metal contact points

The nurse should always go through a mental checklist to protect patients from the potential prob-

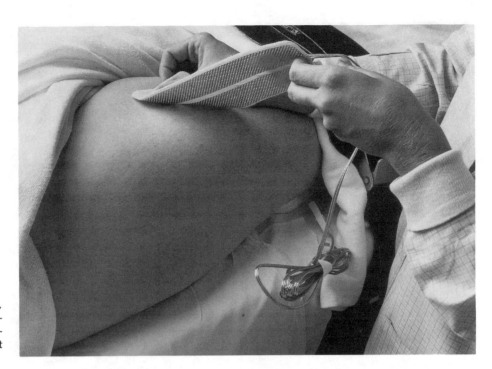

FIGURE 9.4. The size, shape, and placement of the electrosurgical unit grounding pad is important in preventing patient burns.

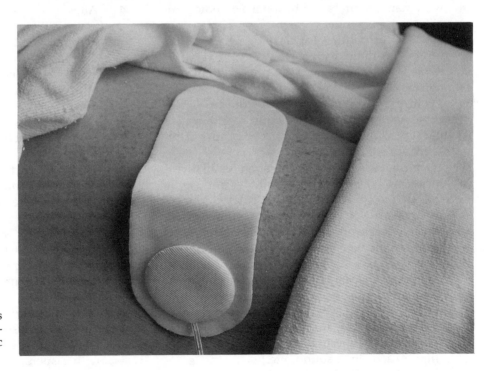

FIGURE 9.5. If there are gaps between the pad and the patient's skin, electricity may arc across the gap, causing a burn.

lems related to ESU electrodes. Electrosurgery is so necessary for performing rapid, precise surgical procedures that its use is worth the risks involved. Risks are minimized when nursing personnel are alert to potential hazards. Continuous prevention includes the following procedures:

1. Choose ESU equipment that is designed to minimize unintentional activation. The cord must be long enough and flexible enough to reach the outlet without stress and without use of an extension cord.

2. Establish a routine maintenance check program

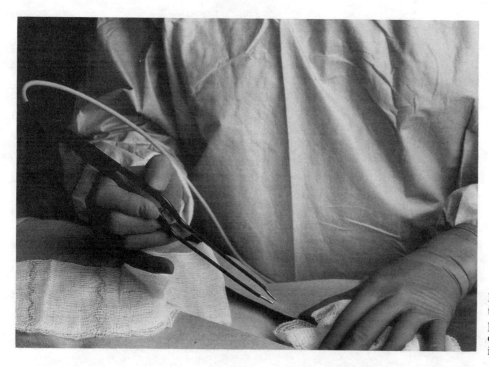

FIGURE 9.6. In bipolar electrosurgery, the active and dispersive electrodes are both contained in an instrument that is similar in design to a forcep.

with manufacturers and hospital biomedical engineering personnel.

3. Establish procedures for cleaning per manufacturers' recommendation.

4. Replace adapters that do not provide tight connections.

5. Avoid placing things on top of the unit. Machine settings can inadvertently be changed if the unit is bumped, and fluid will cause damage if spilled into the unit.

6. Establish a system of shelf rotation for all accessories, such as dispersive electrodes and sterile cords.

7. Assign each ESU an identification number to facilitate documentation of inspections and tracking of problems.

Immediate preoperative precautions against burns should include the following steps.

1. Before each use, inspect all electrical cords, plugs, and connections; test all safety features (lights, activation sound, etc.)

2. Inspect all patient contact areas. Patients must be insulated from contact with metal objects, such as stirrups and head or shoulder braces.

3. Place all electrodes (ECG and electroencephalogram leads, grounding pads, and other conductors of current) after the position of the patient has been determined and established. Repositioning during the intraoperative phase may loosen the dispersive electrode.

4. Allow sufficient time to elapse after skin preparation to permit complete evaporation of any flammable substance, such as alcohol or skin degreasers. Although skin degreasers promote adhesion of electrodes, they can cause burns if not totally removed before electrode application.

5. Be sure gels on grounding pads used to enhance conduction are moist and uniform in quantity.

6. Be sure contact areas between the skin and dispersive electrodes are clean and dry. If necessary, remove excess hair to ensure tight, close adhesion.

7. Place patient grounding devices and ECG monitoring leads away from bony prominences or scar tissue.

8. Place the grounding pad close to the operative site.

9. Place monitoring lead electrodes as far from the operative site as possible.

10. Do not let moisture or liquids come in contact with dispersive electrodes.

During the procedure, power settings should be as low as possible and confirmed orally with the operator prior to activation. Requests for current outputs that are higher than normal may indicate a fault in the electrical circuit. When not in use, but needed ready on the sterile field, place active electrode handpieces in a holster or other clean, dry, nonconductive, highly visible location (Fig. 9.7). Activate

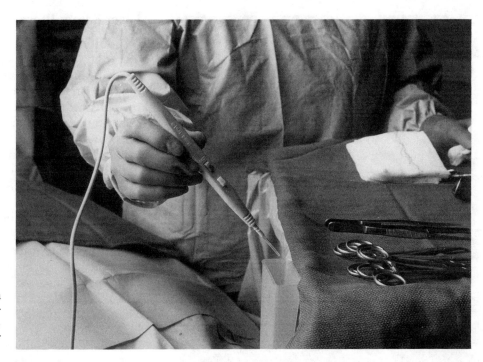

FIGURE 9.7. When not in use, place active electrode handpieces in a holster or other clean, dry, nonconductive, highly visible location.

the ESU only when it is under the direct visual control of the surgeon or assistant. If possible, stop supplemental oxygen at least one minute before and during use of the unit.

HAZARDS ASSOCIATED WITH LASERS

The word *laser* is an acronym for "light amplification by stimulated emission of radiation." It is not an ionizing radiation, as are x-rays. Various-wavelength lasers have been accepted as surgical tools because patients treated with lasers typically experience less bleeding, swelling, and scar tissue formation, as well as shorter hospital stays.

The laser's most important function is precise tissue vaporization, coagulation, or disruption. The high temperatures produced by the carbon dioxide (CO_2) laser, for example, cause the water in the cells to boil and evaporate so fast that the cells explode and vaporize. This action separates the target tissue with minimal thermal damage to surrounding cells. Other thermal lasers have lower energy levels but function in much the same manner.

In addition to the hazards that are associated with any electrical device in the OR, some lasers bring new potential hazards to the intraoperative setting. These additional hazards relate to the high temperatures and thermal action caused by some wavelengths. The amount of electricity (expressed in watts) used by the laser determines, with other factors, the power and density of the laser light beam. The greater the wattage, the more power is converted to light and thus the greater the thermal effect emitted by the laser light. The thermal effect of a laser can be at several hundred degrees Celsius, which will vaporize, cauterize, and sterilize tissue.

Carbon dioxide, argon, neodymium:yttrium-aluminum-garnet (Nd:YAG), and KTP532 are the media most commonly used in medical lasers. Liquid dye and holmium lasers are also available for specific tissue needs. Each of these media has different physical properties. The most important safety issue for all of them is that the beam and its direction must be controlled to prevent undesired tissue damage. The most critical dangers are burns of the eye or skin of patients and personnel.

In establishing their laser safety policies and procedures, individual institutions should be guided by the following:

- "Recommended Practices for Laser Safety in the Practice Setting," offered by AORN (4).
- The American National Standard for the Safe Use of Lasers in Health Care Facilities (ANSI Z136.3–1988), a voluntary guideline established by the American National Standards Institute (5).
- Manufacturing safety regulations set by the Bureau of Radiation Hazards (BRH), part of the federal Food and Drug Administration.

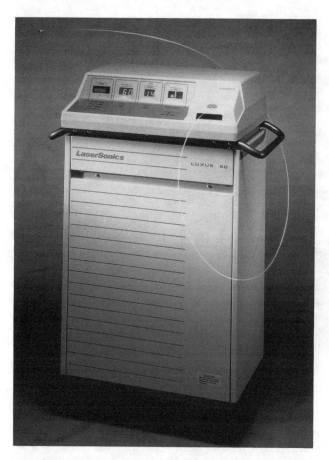

FIGURE 9.8.   Lasers introduce the potential for additional hazards related to high temperature and thermal action. Eye and tissue protection are essential.

Laser Safety Precautions for Personnel

In addition to the normal safety precautions required for any type of electrical equipment, personnel working with lasers need special educational preparation related to each laser to be used. Credentialing committees must establish and evaluate the qualifications required for personnel involved in laser procedures.

In order to prevent injury to personnel working with lasers, a warning sign specific to each laser must be displayed conspicuously at all entrances leading into the room where that laser is in use (Fig. 9.9). All viewing windows should be covered when the laser is in use.

It is critically important that the eyes of patients and personnel be protected from laser beams. Carbon dioxide laser radiation is absorbed in the cornea, causing "welder's flash" or photokeratitis. There is also potential for radiation damage to the lens of the eye, which can be affected by formation of a cataractlike abnormality called *glass-blower's cataract*. Argon and certain other laser wavelengths can also damage the retina. All personnel and awake patients must wear safety glasses, and the optical density of the eyewear chosen must be specific to the wavelength of the laser in use. Protective glasses should be available at the entrance door, next to the laser warning sign, so that anyone coming into the room can put them on before entering.

In addition to eye protection, the skin and other tissues of patients and healthcare workers should be protected from aberrant and reflected laser beams.

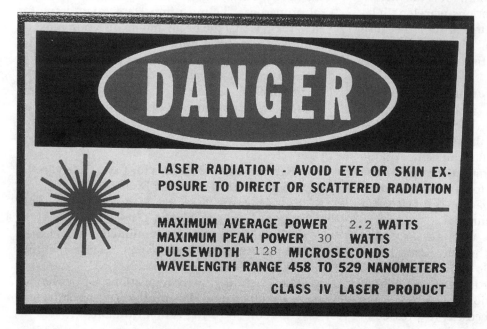

FIGURE 9.9.   A warning sign specific to the laser in use must be displayed conspicuously at all entrances.

Surgical instruments used in laser procedures should have dull, anodized, or matte beaded surfaces to decrease the amount of beam reflection and scatter. In the event of a burn to the fingers or the hand, healthcare personnel should remove surgical gloves immediately and apply water to the burned area.

In order to avoid inadvertent activation of the laser beam, only the physician should have control of the laser foot pedal, and he or she should have only one foot pedal. Assistants should activate all other equipment, such as the bipolar electrosurgery unit. If the physician must use other foot pedals, such as that for the microscope, they should be placed in another location. The laser operating dial should be set on "stand-by," "wait," or "disable" when the laser is set up and on, but not being applied. This prevents inadvertent activation in undesired areas of the surgical field.

Thermal interaction between the laser beam and biological tissue often produces a plume of smoke. Inhalation of this smoke plume has been associated with both biological hazards (i.e., transmission of infectious viruses, bacteria, and cellular material) and chemical hazards (including carcinogens, allergens, or respiratory irritants). In order to avoid hazards associated with laser plume, the following precautions are necessary:

- Use instruments and equipment that help to evacuate smoke. Some speculums and endoscopic instruments have additional evacuation portals to help evacuate laser plume.
- Wear high-filtration masks to deter or delay inhalation of larger carbonaceous particles when lasers are used in procedures that generate a plume of smoke.
- Use a mechanical smoke evacuator system with a high-efficiency filter to remove smoke during plume-generating procedures. Evacuator systems with ultra low-penetration air (ULPA) filters trap particles of even smaller diameter.
- Place the suction hose nozzle as close as possible to the procedure site. (Both the National Institute of Occupational Safety and Health and the Emergency Care Research Institute recommend a distance of 2 inches or less.)
- Change filters on smoke evacuators according to the manufacturer's recommendations; check filters before each procedure. Used filters are considered hazardous waste and should be disposed of accordingly.

If gas cylinders are necessary for the laser's functioning, observe the safety principles outlined in the section on gas cylinders.

Laser Safety Precautions for Patients

Protect the eyes of awake patients with the same protective eyewear used by healthcare personnel. If a patient is receiving a general anesthetic, cover his or her eyes with wet cotton balls, tape, and a wet absorbent towel or eye pads to hold the cotton in place. It is imperative that the cotton stay moist to absorb any reflected beams. Use special protective eye shields for laser treatments close to the eye.

When using thermally intensive lasers, exposed tissue around the operative field should be protected with saline- or water-saturated towels and/or sponges. When using the CO_2 laser in the abdomen, oral cavity, airway, or intracranially, a backdrop should be used behind the tissue being lased to prevent the beam from affecting nontarget tissue. For example, when adhesions are being vaporized intraabdominally, a wet wooden tongue blade, titanium rod, or wet sponge can protect the patient against inadvertent contact of the beam with underlying tissue. For procedures in the perianal area, insert moistened, counted, 4 × 4 radiopaque sponges into the rectum to avoid exploding methane gas. In some anatomical situations, it is not possible to use a backdrop.

Always have a basin of wet solution (such as sterile saline) and a dispensing tool (such as an irrigating syringe) available on the sterile field. Although it is a rare occurrence, drapes, sponges, and towels have been inadvertently ignited by laser beams. Do not use flammable materials near the laser site, such as flammable or combustible anesthetics, prep solutions, drying agents, ointments, or plastics. Use moistened reusable fabrics and/or laser retardant drapes to drape the operative site. Cover non-involved, exposed tissue with wet laparotomy sponges, 4 × 4 radiopaque sponges, or cottonoids, depending on the operative site. Be sure to keep them wet throughout the time the laser is being used. Fill the abdominal or cranial cavities with sterile saline prior to lasing. The solution absorbs the energy of the beam in areas not intended for application.

Prevent patients who have had local anesthesia from moving during laser application. Minimize the potential for movement of a gynecology patient by placing a sheet across her hips and abdomen and tucking it under the mattress. Preoperative teaching and oral reminders during the procedure also help to minimize motion.

Another potential hazard of laser surgery is the possibility of a laryngeal fire. Conventional endotracheal tubes can ignite and support combustion in the presence of the laser's intense heat. All endotracheal tubes used for laser surgery in the aerodigestive tract should be laser-safe. Be sure to read and follow the manufacturer's instructions.

Awake patients should wear high-filtration masks to minimize inhalation of the laser plume.

Laser Safety Programs

Safety is the most critical factor related to the use of any type of laser. Standards published by American National Standards Institute (ANSI) relate specifically to laser safety in manufacturing and use. Regulations developed by the federal government emphasize safety for the manufacturer.

Because the laser beam destroys tissue, it can injure personnel if precautions are not taken. A planned laser safety program can help alleviate concerns. The program should be comprehensive and include the establishment of a laser safety committee. The committee must establish policies related to its composition, purpose, and scope of responsibility, and appointment of new members and specific duties. These duties might include:

- Planning and implementing a full-scope laser service.
- Collaborating with existing planning persons or committees, such as marketing.
- Coordinating the hospital's, office's, or clinic's laser safety needs. This will incorporate any existing safety committees or officers.
- Establishing written policies and procedures and a mechanism for enforcement.
- Developing a laser information resource center.
- Establishing educational programs. Determine how each person operating a laser will become knowledgeable.
- Developing criteria for credentialing with appropriate groups, such as medical–surgical staff.

Committee members should know the goals and objectives of the laser safety program and be willing to work diligently. If planning and implementing decisions take a long time, the goal of an organized, successful laser service may not be realized.

The laser safety committee must interact with individuals responsible for quality assurance within the hospital. Criteria have to be written for evaluating the achievement of desired patient outcomes. A mechanism for reporting laser incidents, for example, when the the laser back-scatters and injures someone's eye, should be developed.

As new technology becomes available for surgical applications, perioperative nurses will be required to expand their knowledge base to incorpo-

rate these sophisticated pieces of equipment safely into treatment modalities.

HAZARDS ASSOCIATED WITH CHEMICALS

In the OR, both personnel and patients are exposed to hazards from liquid chemicals and gases, including sterilizing/disinfecting agents; skin prepping, degreasing, and adhesive agents; environmental cleaning agents; chemotherapy (cytotoxic) agents; and tissue preservatives. These chemicals are all flammable as well as water soluble. The extent to which a chemical is water soluble is useful in determining the type of extinguishing agent that is most effective. For example, alcohol-resistant foam is usually recommended for water-soluble chemicals.

Chemicals have two types of hazards: (1) hazards associated with the inherent properties of the material, and (2) hazards from the toxic products of combustion or decomposition. Personnel in the OR should read and follow all instructions provided on the container label or found on the material safety data sheet (MSDS) provided by the manufacturer. MSDSs must be available to all employees. They identify any hazards, precautions, or special handling necessary; signs and symptoms of toxic exposure; and first aid treatment for exposure.

Chemical hazards are placed in three categories: health hazards, flammability hazards, and reactive hazards. To comply with NFPA standards, health hazards are labeled with blue, flammability hazards with red, and reactive hazards with yellow. Information about hazards related to specific flammable chemicals can be obtained from the NFPA.

Ethylene Oxide

Ethylene oxide (EO) is a colorless gas used to sterilize heat- and moisture-sensitive instruments that cannot be exposed to steam sterilization. It is highly explosive and flammable in the presence of air. It is moderately toxic by inhalation and irritates the eyes and respiratory tract. If it contacts the skin for a prolonged period of time, burns may result. Ethylene oxide has been shown to be a mutagen, which means it can cause changes in the genes of live animal cells. Workers at the American Hospital supply corporation exposed to EO were found to have abnormalities in their chromosomes. The National Institute for Occupational Safety and Health (NIOSH) states that EO should be considered a potential occupational hazard and recommends that workers be monitored for both acute and chronic effects. Upper respiratory irritations and skin rashes are among the short-term acute effects of EO. The gas may have long-term effects on the reproductive, hematological, and neurological systems.

The current OSHA exposure limit for an 8-hour work day is 1 part per million (ppm) ethylene oxide on a time-weighted average. In the air EO can be measured by solid-state sensors, gas chromatographs, infrared spectrophotometry, photoionization detectors, or gas detector tubes. The following precautions are recommended when working with EO:

1. Use of EO should be limited to materials that cannot withstand moist or dry heat sterilization.
2. The biggest risk of EO exposure occurs when items are removed from the sterilizer. Some sterilizers are equipped with factory-installed door exhaust vents. Others should have local exhaust ventilation over the door.
3. Exposure while the sterilizer is being used can be reduced by using local exhaust devices on table-top sterilizers and cycle purges on larger sterilizers.
4. All sterilizers and aerators should be vented directly to the outside atmosphere, an emission control system, or a sanitary floor drain, following the manufacturer's written instructions for venting. The outside exhaust should not be within 25 feet of the air intake for the department or other parts of the hospital.
5. In order to remove residues that can burn workers and patients, EO-sterilized items must be aerated, preferably in an aeration cabinet. Materials that do not absorb EO (metal, glass) do not have to be aerated *unless they were wrapped.* If they were wrapped in muslin, they need at least 30 minutes of aeration. Aeration times depend on the composition, form, and weight of the materials to be sterilized; the sterilization and aeration systems employed; the size, arrangement, and mix of materials being aerated; and the intended application of the items (external or implantable). Items made of polyvinyl chloride (PVC) require the longest aeration times. The Association for the Advancement of Medical Instrumentation (AAMI) recommends the following aeration times for PVC:

At room temperature (70° F)	7 days
120° F in aeration cabinet	12 hours
140° F in aeration cabinet	8 hours

For other materials, the manufacturer's recommendations should be followed. When in doubt about aeration time for a particular item, follow the recommendations for PVC.

6. Regular monitoring of the workplace, especially in and around the sterilizer, is important, including thorough monitoring at least semiannually and system leak checks at least every 2 weeks.
7. Store EO cartridges in a flammable materials cabinet. Do not use outdated cartridges. Mark large canisters with information about flammability, toxicity, and reactivity.

Methyl Methacrylate

Methyl methacrylate is mixed in the operating room for use as a bone cement in artificial-joint replacement. A flammable liquid whose vapor forms explosive mixtures in the air, methyl methacrylate is slightly irritating to the eyes, skin, and respiratory tract. Some patients have experienced hypotension and cardiovascular irregularities. The current OSHA exposure limit is 100 ppm. Exposure levels immediately after methyl methacrylate is mixed can be higher. Local exhaust hoods or other scavenger systems should be used, or mixing should be done in a separate, ventilated area. When stored, methyl methacrylate should be protected from physical damage. Outside storage is preferred. Do not activate electrosurgery pencils or other ignition sources until the chemical reaction has ceased.

Skin Preparation Agents

Iodine and iodophors are two of the best bactericidal solutions used in skin preparation. Drawbacks are that they may stain the skin and they can irritate the skin if the solution is in too high a concentration. These solutions should not be used on instruments because they cause corrosion.

Alcohol is also used in skin preparation. Because it is flammable, precautions must be taken to prevent pooling under the patient. Alcohol should not be the prepping agent of choice when thermal lasers or fiberoptic video equipment are going to be used. Replace any linens that become soaked with alcohol and dispose of alcohol-wet materials in metal containers.

Housekeeping Chemicals

Several chemicals used in housekeeping are potential hazards, especially if used incorrectly. Phenol (carbolic acid) and phenolic derivates are germicides which are colorless or come in white crystals. Phenol is flammable and emits vapors that, when warm, can form explosive mixtures with the air. The phenolics are toxic and can cause severe tissue burns. Systemic absorption of hexachlorophene may lead to convulsions or liver damage. Hexachlorophene, a phenolic compound, was once used for routine hand washing, but it is not recommended for this purpose since it is absorbed through the skin, causing systemic toxicity. Phenolics can also be irritating to the respiratory tract. Personnel should be cautious when handling phenolics. If the solution does come in contact with the skin, water should be used to dilute the phenol and a solution of caustic soda applied to neutralize it.

Chlorine compounds are also used for housekeeping purposes in the operating room. They are highly corrosive to instruments. When using these chemicals, personnel should protect themselves against physical contact because they are irritating to the skin, eyes, and respiratory tract. These compounds should be stored in a well-ventilated, cool, dry area away from combustible materials. The NFPA code for the storage of liquid and solid oxidizing materials provides additional information on these chemicals (6).

Formaldehyde is another hazardous chemical used in the operating room. It produces a colorless gas with a highly irritating odor. Formaldehyde is used in formalin, an aqueous solution of 40% formaldehyde, and as a disinfectant for dialysis equipment. Because of the hazards associated with skin contact, it is a poor choice for other applications. Formaldehyde is potentially carcinogenic and is irritating to the eyes and respiratory tract. Water should be used for spills or to rinse any materials that might come in contact with patients.

Gases

The hazards associated with anesthesia gases in the operating room are discussed in Chapter 17.

Other gases used in the operating room include nitrogen (N_2), which is used for air-powered instruments; CO_2, used for laser equipment; and helium (He), used in the intraaortic balloon pump. These gases are all nonflammable, noncorrosive, and have low toxicity. Carbon dioxide is a colorless gas, liquified at high pressure, and slightly acidic. Nitrogen is a colorless, odorless gas compressed to a high pressure, as is helium.

Carbon dioxide, helium, and, to a lesser degree, nitrogen can act as asphixiants by displacing air and causing suffocation. For this reason, these gases should be stored in well-ventilated areas or kept covered in an outdoor area. When used in the operating room, it is important that ventilation be adequate. The proper exchanges of air per established standard provides adequate ventilation.

Once a common anesthetic agent, ether is now rarely used in the operating room. It has been replaced by nonflammable anesthetic gases, but on occasion, it is used to remove substances on the patient's skin that are difficult to remove with other chemicals. Extremely flammable, ether gas is heavier than air and can travel considerable distances to a source of ignition. Ether should never be stored in the operating room and must be isolated from other combustible material.

The staff should know how to handle and use gas cylinders. If one is knocked over and its neck broken, the cylinder becomes an uncontrollable projectile. Observe the following safety precautions:

- Never turn cylinder valves with oily hands.
- Always secure the cylinder to a solid support with mounting devices or chains.
- Do not drop the cylinder.
- Do not use any cylinder that does not connect easily to the gauge.
- Do not strike the cylinder or cylinder head with a blunt tool if attempting to loosen gauges.
- Close cylinder valves at all times when not in use.
- When a cylinder is empty, close the valve prior to moving it.
- If there is a fire, move gas cylinders away if possible; otherwise, cool them by spraying with water.
- Observe cylinder inspection precautions.

The Compressed Gas Association, a manufacturers' association that establishes standards for safe use of gases, has publications that can be used for teaching purposes. Two groups that also establish standards for chemicals in the operating room are the American Gas Association Laboratories (AGAL) and the NFPA. The AGAL conducts research and laboratory examinations to ascertain if manufacturers are complying with standards related to labeling, handling, and storing gases. The NFPA is the principal organization establishing fire protection standards that may be used as operating standards or legal requirements. Other groups concerned with safe use of hazardous materials are the Institute of Makers of Explosives and the National Safety Council.

HAZARDS ASSOCIATED WITH RADIATION

Diagnostic x-rays, radium implants, and radium-substitute implants are sources of ionizing radiation in the operating room. A less common source is patients who already have radioactive substances in their bodies when they have surgery. Personnel and patients in the operating room are exposed to the same radiation hazards as those in the radiology department. Although the amount of exposure may not be as high, the same education and safety rules should apply in any area where there is a potential hazard due to ionizing radiation.

Radiation is a hazard because it has the ability to modify molecules within body cells. This may cause cell dysfunction, alteration or halt in cell replication, or cell destruction. Cells may be able to recover from radiation damage if exposure is not too high. Effects of radiation are both somatic and genetic. Somatic effects can be observed in patients who are receiving large doses for treatment. Their skin gets very red, they may have a temporary loss of hair, ulcerations may occur, cataracts form in the eyes, and there may be a reduction in white blood cells that predisposes them to infections. Somatic effects vary with the amount of radiation, the age of the person, and what part of the body is exposed. Children are more sensitive than adults, and the unborn fetus is highly sensitive.

Radiation is also associated with reproductive abnormalities such as birth defects and childhood leukemia. Radiation exposure during pregnancy slows the normal growth of the uterus, and children of exposed mothers show reduced growth and increased frequency of mental retardation and leukemia. Radiation exposure is associated with all kinds of cancer and a general shortening of life expectancy.

X-Rays

Sources of x-radiation exposure in the operating room include the portable x-ray machine used to take films in cholangiography and orthopedic manipulations; diagnostic radiology and radiotherapy; fluoroscopy, which directs large doses of intermittent radiation at the patient; and image amplification with television circuitry. Radiation is present from x-rays only while the x-ray tube is energized.

For personnel exposed to radiation, government regulations limit permissible levels to 5 rem per year, for workers over the age of 18 years. (The word *rem* is the acronym formed from *r*oentgen *e*quivalent *m*an.) A dose that exceeds this level is overexposure and requires investigation by a regulatory agency.

The purpose of all protection measures is to reduce the exposure as much as possible and to ensure that the radiation received does not exceed the maximum permissible dose equivalent (MPD). Unnecessary exposure can be avoided in three ways: minimizing the time of exposure, increasing the distance from the source, and placing a shield between the radiation sources and the body.

Radiation exposure is monitored by a film badge clipped to the body. The film badge should be worn for one month, then evaluated. AORN recommends that, if a single monitoring device is used, it should be worn on the same part of the body by all personnel. If two monitoring devices are used, one should be at the neckline outside the apron (to measure head and neck exposure) and one inside the apron (for whole body and gonad exposure) (7).

For pregnant women, the monitoring device should be worn on the waist. If a lead apron is worn, it should be under the lead apron. The pregnant employee is of great concern anywhere in the hospital where there is radiation exposure. The American Society of Radiologic Technologists has adopted guidelines for radiation safety practices for pregnant radiation workers. The recommendations include: (1) during gestation the MPD equivalent to the fetus from occupational exposure should not exceed 0.5 rem; (2) pregnant employees should disclose their pregnancy as soon as they know about it and cooperate with safety practices; (3) the employer should make available to the employee the mandates of the pregnancy disability law, the National Council on Radiation Protection and Measurements (NCRP) guidelines, and the Equal Employment Opportunity Commission (EEOC) guidelines and questions and answers on sex discrimination.

Increasing one's distance from the source is another way of reducing exposure. At 1 foot, personnel receive four times the radiation that is received at 2 feet. Therefore, removal from the radiation source as far as possible will decrease the hazard. Shielding also decreases exposure. Aprons, gloves, shields, and walls that contain or are made of lead reduce radiation exposure by a factor of 10 to 30, depending on the lead equivalent in the material used. Leaded protective devices should not be folded; they should be hung on racks or laid flat on shelves and examined radiographically every 6 months to assure their integrity.

Every hospital radiology department should have a radiation safety program that involves the x-ray department and other departments involved in radiological diagnosis and treatment. Because the operating room has areas where special procedures are done that require personnel and patients to be exposed to radiation hazards, the safety program should include that area.

Regulations for use of ionizing radiation have been established in most states. State departments of health generally have a radiation control division that establishes standards. Regulations for the administration and enforcement of the Radiation Control for Health and Safety Act are also available. Compliance with the regulations is important and should be included in a safety program. The federal Bureau of Radiologic Health is another regulatory body that sets standards for safety.

Compliance with safety regulations is difficult to mandate. A philosophy of safety and caution must be developed that is subscribed to by the entire staff. Potential hazards are real, but at the same time, proper handling and caution greatly decrease any hazard.

Safety for patients having x-rays during surgery includes efficiency in preparing the patient and operating the equipment. Functions related to radiological studies include positioning the patient so that only the area of study is exposed to the film or fluoroscopy, ensuring that the contrast medium selected is effective for the type of study being done, and checking that all equipment is in working order. The patient should be protected by gonadal shielding, when appropriate, for studies of the hips and upper legs.

X-rays to the abdomen and pelvis of pregnant women should be avoided, especially in the first trimester. Leaded shields should be used, when possible, to protect the thyroid during x-ray studies of the upper extremities, trunk, and head. Because any exposure to ionizing radiation carries some risk, all reasonable means should be implemented to reconcile incorrect counts before using x-rays to locate unaccounted-for sponges, needles, and other instruments.

Radiological technologists have a responsibility to protect the patient as much as possible by selecting exposure factors that reduce the need for many x-rays to be taken. The level of exposure is important for viewing purposes, but overexposure simply adds radiation. Focusing the beam on the specific area of study also reduces size of the site exposed to radiation. The technician should always be cognizant of other members of the healthcare team and allow them to leave the room or wear a lead apron or gloves.

Radium and Radium Substitutes

Radium and radium substitutes (iridium-192, cesium-137, and cobalt-60) are used in treatment of cancer. Usually double-sealed in metal tubes, radium remains radioactive indefinitely and is potentially hazardous for thousands of years. When radium or radium substitutes are present in the operating room, the nurse should attempt to stay several arm lengths away from the source. But if it is necessary to be close to the patient, 15 minutes at a half-arm length is no more hazardous than an hour at one arm length. If a radium source is dropped in the operating room, it should be picked up with long forceps and placed in a lead container. To prevent crushing, the source should not be squeezed too hard. An empty emesis basin can be used as a temporary receptacle but should be located several feet from personnel. The sources should not be touched directly. Lead aprons and gloves should not be used. They are not thick enough to offer protection against radium irradiation and usually only increase handling time, which increases exposure. To ensure that no radium is lost in the operating room, linen and trash should be checked with a radiation detector prior to removal.

Radium substitutes are less hazardous because of the principal types of radiation they emit. More radiation is absorbed by the body, but they have less ability to penetrate lead. Distance from the source reduces the hazard. The substitutes only remain radioactive for a few years. The hazards of implantation have been reduced by after-loading techniques. The radioactive sources are not inserted in the operating room, but after the patient is returned to his or her room.

Some treatments consist of permanent implants of short-lived radioactive materials. If these patients require surgery before the material has decayed to a low level, there may be a hazard of irratiation. Precautions are similar to those for patients with radium implants. In addition, radioactive fluids or tissues removed in surgery should be put in strong bottles and handled carefully to avoid breakage. Linens and other waste should be checked for contamination to reduce exposure through distance and shielding.

As with any potential hazard associated with the operating room, personnel and patients can be protected against the dangerous effects of radiation exposure by safe practices. In the healthcare field there may be a tendency to deny the effects because of the common usage of ionizing radiation. All personnel should be educated on safe radiation practices on a continuing basis. Regulations should be reviewed, and updated practices implemented. Personnel safety measures such as monitoring exposure, wearing protective clothing, and following guidelines for the pregnant employee are essential.

HAZARDS ASSOCIATED WITH DISASTERS

Every hospital should have plans for external and internal disasters. For accreditation by JCAHO the plans must be written and rehearsed at least twice a year.

External Disasters

An external disaster is one that originates outside the hospital, such as an airplane crash, train wreck, nuclear accident, or explosion at a chemical plant. Because the hospital has a responsibility to serve the residents in the community, it must be prepared to provide care when an emergency arises. The overall external disaster hospital plan is established according to JCAHO recommendations. The operating room, like other units within the hospital, uses the master plan and individualizes it for the operating room. The plan for the operating room includes the same components as the overall hospital plan. The plan must provide a method of notifying operating room personnel when a disaster occurs. Next, everyone must have an assignment. All personnel may not be assigned to perform surgical procedures; other areas may require additional assistance, so staff could be assigned to those positions. Medical staff is coordinated through the hospital team. Surgeons are assigned to patients needing surgical intervention. The operating room plan includes the availability of supplies, equipment, and instruments, plus their distribution. Procedures for transferring patients to the operating room or surrounding patient care areas are outlined and specific types of personnel capable of monitoring critical patients are specified. The plan includes a physical layout of space available for patients and the types of patients that can be treated in the allocated space.

The hospital has special medical records to be used for disasters. These are available in the operating room for use when needed. When a disaster occurs, it is essential to maintain security. The established plan provides direction as to who should give information to the press or family members calling the hospital.

Internal Disasters

Internal disasters include events that would necessitate moving patients from one unit to another or evacuating them from the hospital. An internal disaster plan should be written and made available to personnel. The plan for an internal disaster must include methods of transferring critical patients to other medical facilities in the immediate vicinity.

Fire is an internal disaster. Hospitals provide personnel with specific instructions as to what they should do in case of fire. Besides continuing education of personnel, regular drills are conducted to evaluate the effectiveness of the plan. Copies of the fire plan are located in an accessible place in the operating room. Personnel are drilled on notification of a fire and how to contain it. They are instructed on use of hospital fire extinguishers, including the types of extinguishers to use on different materials, and the removal of patients. Fire drills are conducted quarterly in an effort to keep staff in a state of readiness.

The purpose of rehearsing the disaster plan twice a year is to maintain readiness of administration, other hospital personnel, and the medical staff. Simulated disasters help all involved to evaluate how they would function in an actual crisis. It is helpful to determine whether equipment used is in proper functioning order and if the physical facility is adequate to treat the victims. The operating room, as well as other units, must evaluate its participation. This includes an assessment of personnel's effectiveness, documentation of problems, and identification of strengths and weaknesses.

Voluntary agencies such as JCAHO and NFPA require hospitals to maintain personnel readiness for disasters. These agencies recommend that employees have formal training on a cyclical basis and that they each sign a form indicating that they have been trained and know their responsibilities related to the plan. The form signed by the employee should be maintained as a part of the employee's personnel file.

ADDITIONAL HAZARDS IN THE OPERATING ROOM

Additional hazards encountered in the operating room include defective or improperly modified instruments, inadequate air exchange, and hazardous waste.

Instrument Safety

Patients have a right to assume that instruments, implants, and equipment are safe and have been tested in accepted ways. Hospital policy should provide for this.

Unauthorized adaptation of equipment and supplies is a difficult hazard to prevent, yet it must be dealt with if patient safety is to be maintained.

AORN recommends that instruments be used only for the specific purpose for which they were designed (8). The practice of some surgeons altering or improvising devices for use in surgery is dangerous. The Bureau of Medical Devices and Diagnostic Products establishes compliance standards that manufacturers must meet. Also, manufacturers will not stand behind their products if they have been changed or applied in an unorthodox manner. The various publications and standards set by the Bureau are available from the Food and Drug Administration and should be accessible in every operating room.

In the old days, doctors brought their own instruments to the hospital and handed them to the nurse. Today, hospitals provide and process instrumentation. There is a legal risk involved with instrumentation no matter who provides it. Hospitals bear the responsibility for making instruments available in sound working order.

Instruments can be damaged from repeated washing, handling, wrapping, and sterilizing. Thus all instruments require routine inspections for damage, wear, and loose parts. Every operating room should have a *standing* policy of equipment and instrument inspection. Responsible hospital personnel should:

1. Set standards related to handling, processing, and use of instruments.
2. Demand quality when purchasing.
3. Demand and support good service from manufacturers.
4. See that all new and repaired instruments are carefully inspected by qualified persons.
5. Reject inadequate instruments at the time of delivery; accept them only when satisfied with precision.
6. Delay marking instruments until they are inspected and accepted.
7. Ascertain what guarantees are promised and insist that they be kept.

The professional nurse employed in a hospital is expected to be alert to potential causes for harm to patients. Nurses are responsible for putting the appropriate administrative and clinical personnel on notice when they recognize a danger to patients.

On November 28, 1991, the Safe Medical Devices Act of 1990 took effect. The Act contains two provisions of special significance to perioperative nurses: user reporting of device problems and implant tracking (9). These provisions require that:

- When a device-user facility becomes aware of information suggesting that a device may have caused or contributed to the death, serious illness, or injury of a patient at the facility, the facility must file a report to the Food and Drug Administration and/or the device's manufacturer within 10 working days.
- Manufacturers must adopt tracking methods for devices when the failure of such devices would be reasonably likely to have serious adverse health consequences, when the device is permanently implantable, or when devices are life-sustaining or life-supporting and are used outside of a device-user facility.

For perioperative nurses, the Act means that incident-reporting systems must be assessed and refined, educational programs developed and conducted, and device-tracking systems enhanced.

Air Exchanges

Inadequate air exchange in the operating room creates a hazard of potential infection. Controlled, filtered air reduces the possibility of contamination and air pollutants. Every operating room should have a controlled, filtered air supply. The number of air exchanges that take place each hour is regulated by JCAHO.

Hazardous Waste

Improper handling of wastes is one of the major causes of employee lost time and accidents in hospitals. Hazardous items include needles, knife blades, and other objects that may cause punctures. The disposal of contaminated drapes, suction canister contents, and other waste that can cause infection should be of concern to the perioperative nurse. Trash compactors, incinerators, and other means of containing and disposing of contaminated materials are required.

LIABILITY FOR PATIENT INJURIES

The obligation of the nurse to use safety measures and to protect the patient from harm are legal obligations as well as professional and ethical ones. Patients who are injured because of a nurse's failure to use reasonable care to protect them from harm can sue him or her for negligence and/or professional malpractice.

The mere filing of a suit does not result in liability. The ability of the patient to successfully sue a nurse for negligence will depend on the ability of the patient and the patient's attorney to introduce sufficient evidence to convince a judge or jury of the following four elements:

1. Duty—What a reasonable and prudent nurse of similar education and experience would have done under similar circumstances.
2. Breach of duty—That the defendant nurse failed to do what a reasonable and prudent nurse of similar education and experience would have done under similar circumstances.
3. Causation—That the defendant nurse's failure to do what a reasonable and prudent nurse would have done was a foreseeable cause of (or failure to prevent) harm to the plaintiff.
4. Damages—how much the patient was in fact injured.

Closer examination of these elements demonstrates how perioperative nurses' focus on safety measures and the expected outcome of keeping patients free from harm combine to result in substantially reduced liability exposure for nurses. If the outcome of absence of adverse effects is realized, the patient cannot become a plaintiff. Unless the patient is injured, there is nothing for which to sue.

In order to examine the first and second elements, the legal system shifts its examination from the patient outcome to the process of a nurse's actions. Even if a patient is injured, a nurse is not liable unless he or she failed to do what a reasonable nurse would have done. Thus, perioperative nurses who are aware of possible adverse effects to patients and who assess, intervene, and implement indicated safety measures are less likely to have their actions judged unreasonable. Without a finding that the defendant nurse's assessments and actions were unreasonable, the nurse cannot be held liable.

Injuries that pose the greatest legal risk to nurses are chemical and electrical burns, neuromuscular damage due to pressure, retained foreign bodies, and those caused by incorrect medications or dosages.

REFERENCES

1. Association of Operating Room Nurses. "Patient outcomes: Standards of perioperative care." *Standards and Recommended Practices for Perioperative Nursing—1992.* Denver: AORN, 1992.
2. Gruendemann, B. J., and Meeker, M. H. *Alexander's Care of the Patient in Surgery* 8th ed. St. Louis, MO: C. V. Mosby, 1987.
3. Joint Commission on Accreditation of Health Care Organizations. *Accreditation Manual for Hospitals Vol. I: Standards.* Oakbrook Terrace, IL: JCAHO, 1992.
4. Association of Operating Room Nurses. "Recommended practices for laser safety in the practice setting." *AORN Standards and Recommended Practices for Perioperative Nursing—1992,* pp. III:10–1 to III:10–5. Denver: AORN, 1992.
5. American National Standards Institute. *American National Standard for the Safe Use of Lasers in Health Care Facilities.* ANSI Z136.3–1988. Toledo, OH: Laser Institute of America, 1988.
6. National Fire Protection Association. *Code for the Storage of Liquid and Solid Oxidizing Materials.* NFPA 43A. Boston: NFPA, 1990.
7. Association of Operating Room Nurses. "Recommended practices for radiological safety in the practice setting." *AORN Standards and Recommended Practices for Perioperative Nursing—1992,* pp. III:16–1 to III:16–7. Denver: AORN, 1992.
8. Association of Operating Room Nurses. "Recommended practices for care of instruments, scopes, and powered surgical instruments." *AORN Standards and Recommended Practices for Perioperative Nursing—1992,* pp. III:9–1 to III:9–9. Denver: AORN, 1992.
9. Koch, Frances A., Solomon, Ronni P., and Nash, Suzanne E. "The Safe Medical Devices Act: What nurses should know about user reporting, implant tracking." *AORN J* 55(2):537–548, 1992.

SUGGESTED READINGS

Association for the Advancement of Medical Instrumentation. *National Standards and Recommended Practices for Sterilization* 2nd ed. Arlington, VA: AAMI, 1988.

Ball, Kay. *Lasers in the OR.* Thorofare, NJ: Slack, 1988.

Buschbaum, W. H., and Goldsmith, B. *Electrical Safety in the Hospital.* Oradell, NJ: Medical Economic, 1975.

Day, J. L., and Lightfoot, D. A. "OR radiation hazards." *AORN J* 20:249, 1974.

Emergency Care Research Institute. "General purpose surgical laser smoke evacuation systems." *Health Devices* 19(1):5–19, 1990.

Harris, F. W. *Desiccation as a Key to Understanding Electrosurgery.* Boulder, CO: ValleyLab, 1978.

InterQual. *Hospital Safety Compliance Guide.* Chicago: InterQual, 1977.

National Fire Protection Association. *Fire Hazard Properties of Flammable Liquids, Gases, Volatile Solids.* NFPA 325M. Boston: NFPA, 1977.

National Fire Protection Association. *Fire Hazards in Oxygen-Enriched Atmospheres.* NFPA 53M. Quincy, MA: NFPA, 1985.

National Fire Protection Association. *Hazardous Chemical Data.* NFPA 4A. Boston: NFPA, 1975.

National Fire Protection Association. *Health Care Facilities.* NFPA 99. Quincy, MA: NFPA, February 5, 1990.

National Fire Protection Association. *Life Safety Code.* NFPA 101. Boston: NFPA, February 2, 1988.

National Fire Protection Association. *Manual of Hazardous Chemical Reaction.* NFPA 491M. Boston: NFPA, 1975.

National Fire Protection Association. *Standard on the Safe Use of Electricity in Patient Care Areas of Hospitals.* NFPA 76B. Quincy, MA: NFPA, 1977.

NDM Corp. *Safer Electrosurgery.* Dayton, OH: NDM, 1981.

Pfister, Judith I., Hicks, Susan H., and Sexton, Linda. "Perioperative nursing care of the patient experiencing laser surgery." *Seminars in Perioperative Nursing* 1(2):96–102, 1992.

Pfister, J., and Kneedler, J. A. *A Guide to Lasers in the OR.* Denver: Education Design, 1983.

Pfister, J. I., Kneedler, J. A., and Purcell, S. K. *The Nursing Spectrum of Lasers.* Denver: Education Design, 1988.

"Radiation protection." *Radiol Technol* 51:525, 1980.

"Radiation protection." *Radiol Technol* 52:321, 1980.

Tuck, C. A., Jr., ed. *NFPA Inspection Manual* 4th ed. Boston: NFPA, 1976.

Union Carbide Corporation. *Specialty Gases: Precautions and Emergency Procedures.* New York: Union Carbide, 1976.

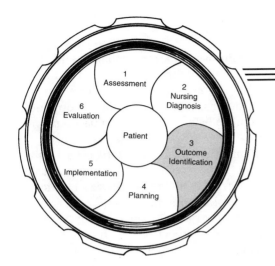

10

Maintenance of Skin Integrity and Wound Management

Outcome: Skin does not show adverse effects from surgery.

A major focus in the perioperative plan of care is the patient's skin. This chapter deals with maintaining the patient's skin integrity, or wholeness. Normal anatomy, preoperative skin preparation, wound care, and the wound repair process are discussed.

The following criteria are indicators that the identified outcome of maintenance of skin integrity is achieved:

1. During the postoperative course, the nurse will observe the patient's surgical incision. The incision will:
   a. Evidence only normal signs of inflammation.
   b. Not exhibit signs of epithelial growth down skin suture tracts.
   c. Have approximated edges.
   d. Not be associated with excessive pain (determined by objective nursing judgment and subjective patient response).
2. Postoperatively, the nurse will observe no burns, pressure ulcers, lacerations, abrasions, contusions, or reddened areas that were not present prior to surgery.
3. Postoperatively, the patient will not exhibit unanticipated sensory impairment.

Certain factors influence how well these criteria are met. The maintenance of skin integrity is influenced by the preoperative condition of the integu-mentary system, preparation of the skin for the surgical procedure, and the patient's wound-healing capacity.

ANATOMY AND PHYSIOLOGY

To plan effective perioperative care, the nurse must have an understanding of the integumentary (skin) system. The skin is the largest "organ" in the body, weighing 6 to 8 pounds and covering approximately 20 square feet in the average adult. As the most visible and accessible body system, the human skin is a sensitive indicator of both physical and emotional status.

The skin is composed of two major layers: the epidermis, or outer layer, and the underlying dermis. Each has specific components and functions, but together with the underlying subcutaneous tissue, they serve to protect and insulate internal body systems.

The skin has the following functions:

1. Protecting the inner body from injury and bacterial invasion
2. Regulating body temperature
3. Preventing body fluid loss
4. Transmitting sensations such as touch, pressure, and pain
5. Providing an interface between the body and the environment

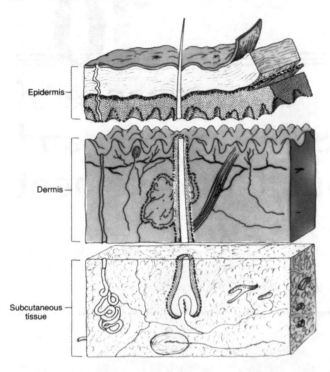

FIGURE 10.1. Layers of the skin: epidermis, dermis, and subcutaneous tissue.

Skin/Soft Tissue Layers

The skin has three principal layers: the epidermis, the dermis, and the subcutaneous tissue (Fig. 10.1).

Epidermis

This thin, avascular layer of skin is composed of five different types of cells. It varies in thickness depending on its location, but averages only 1 mm, or the width of a sharp pencil mark.

The stratum corneum, composed mainly of keratinocytes, is the major chemical and mechanical barrier of the body. Keratin, a protective protein, provides a waterproof cover. Rapidly proliferating epidermal tissue results in dead keratinized cells constantly being replaced by new cells pushing to the top. A new epidermis is formed every 4 to 6 weeks. This normal shedding is a defense mechanism against infection.

Another major type of cell in the epidermis, the melanocytes, release granules of pigment or melanin that provide skin tones.

Langerhans cells are macrophages that ingest potential antigenic compounds and prevent the body from allergic reaction.

The innermost layer of the epidermis, or the basal stratum, is the only layer capable of regenerating by undergoing mitosis to form new cells. Other tissues are repaired by scar formation.

Dermis

The dermis is composed of strong collagen and elastic fibers and provides support and nutrition to the epidermis. This layer contains connective tissue, blood vessels, nerves, and integumentary appendages such as hair follicles, nails, and sebaceous and sweat glands.

Fibroblasts are the most important cells in the dermis. They produce collagen, the protein that gives skin strength. They also synthesize elastic fibers that help the skin stretch.

Other cells include macrophages, which clean up bacterial debris, and leukocytes, which help protect the body during the inflammatory phase of wound healing.

The ground substance of the dermis is a gelatinous matrix containing proteins, enzymes, and immune bodies that cement collagen and elastic fibers.

Subcutaneous Tissue

Sometimes included as a layer of skin, the subcutaneous tissue, or hypodermis, lies under the dermis. It is made up of dense connective and adipose tissue and houses major blood vessels, lymphatics, and nerves. The subcutaneous tissue serves as a shock absorber and heat insulator. Subcutaneous tissue also provides a nutritional "depot" during illness or starvation.

Below the subcutaneous layer is the fibrous fascia, consisting of connective tissue that covers muscle, nerves, and blood vessels. The superficial fascia connects the skin to subjacent parts, facilitating movement. The deep, less elastic fascia forms a sheath or envelope covering for muscles, blood vessels, and nerves.

Vascular and Nerve Supply

A continuous arteriovenous network traverses subcutaneous tissue and extends into the dermis. This network regulates heat and maintains nutrition for skin cells. After an injury, new capillaries quickly form to bring nutrients to the wound-repair area.

Nerves that run through the subcutaneous tissue are divided into sensory and motor nerves. Sensory nerves mediate the sensations of touch, temperature, and pain. Motor nerves control sweat glands, arterioles, and smooth muscle.

Itching and goose flesh are two interesting phenomena involving the integumentary nervous supply. Itching is a mild, painful sensation but differs from frank pain by having a lower impulse frequency that travels along the nerve fiber. Goose flesh is due to traction of the muscle (arrector pili) attached to the hair follicles.

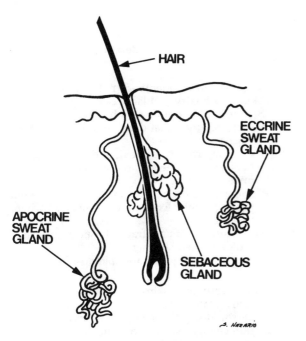

FIGURE 10.2. The two types of skin appendages, cornified and glandular.

Appendages

Skin appendages are of two types, cornified and glandular (Fig. 10.2). These are further separated into more specific groups. Cornified appendages take the form of hair and nails, both of which are keratinized structures. Hair arises from follicles, which are an invagination of the epidermis. An individual's lifelong complement of hair follicles is present at birth. No new follicles will be formed during the lifetime. Hair growth is cyclic, with the anagen (growing) phase or telogen (resting) state being influenced by hormones. This hormonal influence is the most important internal factor in hair growth. A premature resting stage may be caused by stress such as massive illness or childbirth.

With each scalp hair growing approximately 0.35 mm per day, over 100 linear feet of hair are produced daily. Excess male hormone produces baldness; castrated males do not lose their hair.

Nails are also cornified appendages. They are produced by an invagination of the epidermis. Their growth is continuous, although fingernails grow more rapidly than toenails. They protect the tips of fingers and toes, which have a delicate sense of touch.

The other type of skin appendage is glandular. There are two major types of glands—sebaceous and sweat. Sebaceous glands are present everywhere except on the palms of the hands and soles of the feet.

They continuously secrete the products of cell breakdown and produce sebum, a thin lipidal film that covers the skin. Sebum is mildly bacteriostatic and fungistatic. It also retards water evaporation.

Sweat glands are divided into two categories—eccrine and apocrine. Eccrine glands, opening directly onto the skin surface, are controlled by the autonomic nervous system and flood the exterior skin with water for cooling purposes. Eccrine glands are a major factor in maintaining a stable temperature inside the body. Their prime stimulus for function is heat.

Apocrine glands are located in the pubic and axillary areas. The sweat produced in these areas is sterile until it is contaminated by bacteria. It then decomposes, producing body odor. These adrenergic glands are activated by emotional stimulation.

Flora

Healthy skin is host to innumerable bacteria. Normally, these bacteria and the human organisms coexist peacefully. Normal skin bacteria—*Staphylococcus epidermidis* and species of *Corynebacterium* and *Candida*—are especially concentrated in hair follicles and moist areas such as the axillae, groin, and perineum. Their populations remain fairly constant on an individual unless disturbed by such factors as climate changes or antibiotics. Persons with oily, moist skin harbor more bacteria than those with dry skin. Drying is the principal method by which the skin prevents overpopulation of bacteria. The pH of skin normally ranges from 4.5 to 5.5. This is often referred to as the "acid mantle" of the skin, which serves to maintain normal skin flora.

There are two types of bacteria on the skin—resident and transient. Resident bacteria live and multiply on the skin. These bacteria are shed from the body with the movement of old cells and skin secretions from the dermal to the epidermal layer. In this manner they serve as a source of contamination for any break in the skin. Resident bacteria need 6 to 10 minutes of soap and water scrubbing to decrease their population by 50 percent. Bacterial regrowth begins immediately, and in 24 hours 25% will be replaced. Transient bacteria are loosely attached to the skin surface. They are effectively reduced by a 3- to 5-minute scrub.

When planning for maintenance of skin integrity, the perioperative nurse continues the assessment that began with the patient's admission. The primary nurse has assessed the overall health status and specific condition of the patient's skin, considering factors that differ from normal skin and incorporating these into the plan of care (Table 10.1). The

TABLE 10.1. Factors That Influence Preoperative Skin Preparation

Areas of Assessment	Influencing Factors	Considerations
Overall health status		
Age	Pediatric patient	Most pediatric patients are not shaved.
	Geriatric patient	Skin may be dry and lack resiliency.
Nutritional status	Malnourished, obese, hypovolemic	Skin texture and tone may be altered.
Allergy history	Possible sensitivity to soaps and antimicrobial solutions	Select a solution that does not produce a skin reaction.
State of consciousness	Degree of alertness	Positioning may be difficult and require extra personnel for the semiconscious or unconscious patient.
Medical condition	Diabetes (for example)	Diminished circulation to extremities, impaired healing ability. Extra caution exercised when shaving.
Previous surgery	Presence of scars, degree of keloid formation	Scars and keloids are fragile tissue and must be avoided when shaving.
Limitation of motion	Arthritis, contractures, etc.	Attention given to comfortable positioning.
Condition of skin		
Color	Pallor, cyanosis, jaundice, pigmentation changes	These features of skin may not have individual considerations but should all be noted by the
Vascularity	Evidence of bleeding or bruising	person doing the skin preparation. Unusual
Obvious lesions	Allergy reactions, acne, psoriasis	skin changes such as obvious lesions or
Edema	Injury or underlying medical procedures	evidence of bleeding that become evident only after hair has been removed should be reported upon completion of the prep.
Moisture	Dry or sweaty	
Temperature	Warm, hot, cool bilaterally	
Texture	Rough or smooth	
Thickness	Paper thin, fragile, or thick	
Mobility	Decreased due to edema	
Turgor	Decreased due to dehydration	
Examples of surgical procedure/disease		
Carotid artery disease	Plaque in the arteries	Gentle scrub and shave to avoid dislodging plaque.
Breast biopsy	Possible breast carcinoma	Gentle scrub because of possible spread of carcinoma. Axilla and upper arm are shaved.
Fractures	Unstable or open	May be prepped after induction of anesthesia. Attention directed to maintaining alignment of fracture. This requires additional personnel.
Skin lesions	Raised areas on skin surface, i.e., melanomas, basal cell carcinomas, or lesions erupting through skin	Location of lesion noted prior to beginning prep so that the razor does not inadvertently traumatize these areas. Hair on these areas should be closely trimmed with scissors.
Preps after cast removal	Buildup of desquamation skin and scablike patches adhering to skin	The skin will be very sensitive, requiring time to gently soak away adherent patches.

perioperative nurse's responsibility is to continue that assessment and plan intraoperative interventions based on it.

PREOPERATIVE SKIN PREPARATION

Inherent in the goal of maintaining skin integrity is rapid, uncomplicated wound healing. To achieve that goal, a nurse's activities are based on the "minimal interference" concept. Aimed at removing all interference to wound repair, this concept means

preventing contamination and minimizing tissue trauma. Damage to tissues is minimized by gentle handling of wound contents during the surgical procedure. Manipulation of tissues is reduced to the minimum necessary to complete the operation. One of the criteria for maintenance of skin integrity, listed at the beginning of this chapter, is, "Postoperatively there will be no burns, lacerations, abrasions, contusions, or reddened areas that were not present prior to surgery." Presence of any of these increases the body's healing effort for the surgical wound.

Preventing contamination begins prior to the surgical procedure. To prevent contamination, the patient's preoperative hospital stay is as short as possible to avoid unnecessary exposure to bacteria in the environment. The preoperative skin preparation is aimed at making the skin as clean and germ-free as possible.

Surgically Clean Skin

Preparation of the patient's skin begins before admission to the surgical suite. Before surgery, the patient is asked to shower using antimicrobial-containing products. Depending on the procedure, the patient may be asked to repeat the shower the morning of the surgery, paying particular attention to scrubbing the operative site. For example, orthopedic operations requiring implantable devices call for careful skin preparation because of the severe consequences of postoperative infections.

In some situations a preoperative shave is done the night before surgery; however, it is preferable to remove hair in the holding area immediately prior to surgery. Shaving destroys the natural skin defenses and can also create superficial cuts and nicks that encourage bacterial growth. The longer the period between the shave and the surgery, the greater the potential for bacterial growth. Shaving the night before surgery has been associated with increased wound infection. In a study of wounds, Seropian and Reynolds found infection rates of 5.6% when the patient was shaved but 0.6% when there was no shaving or a depilatory was used (1). Cruse and Foord (2) showed that when the hair was neither shaved nor clipped the infection rate was 0.9%; in patients shaved with an electric razor, the infection rate was 1.4%; and shaving with a razor produced a 2.5% infection rate.

Hair should be removed only when necessary. Facial hair of women and children should never be removed. The method that is least damaging to skin is recommended—use of a depilatory if the patient is not allergic to such agents. Hair can also be clipped about 1 cm from the skin with electrical clippers. If hair must be shaved, a wet method should be used, and the razor should be disposable or a terminally sterilized reusable one. Several points should be kept in mind when removing hair:

1. Hair removal should be done as close as possible to the time of surgery to decrease the possibility of wound infection.
2. The patient's privacy should be respected at all times.
3. Skilled personnel should be responsible for hair removal.

Under optimal circumstances all hair is removed with a depilatory, preps are done immediately prior to surgery in a holding area adjacent to the surgical suite, and patient privacy is preserved.

WOUND HEALING

The wound repair process begins the moment an injury occurs and may go on for years. This is true regardless of the type of wound. The injury may occur with a planned incision during a surgical procedure or be the result of some type of skin-tearing trauma.

There are two types of wounds—those with no tissue loss and those with tissue loss (Fig. 10.3). Incised or sutured wounds with no tissue loss heal by primary union, or first intention. The edges of the wound are approximated rapidly with no complications. Contamination is minimized by good aseptic technique and lack of dead space.

Wounds with extensive tissue loss, such as trauma injuries and pressure ulcers, heal by secondary intention. Skin edges cannot be adequately approximated. Granulation tissue must first fill the

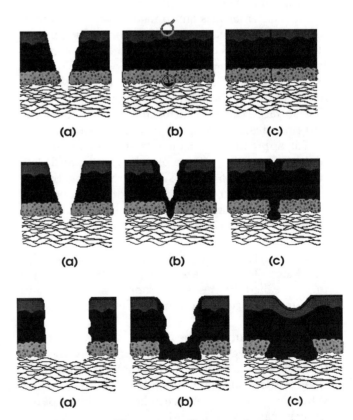

FIGURE 10.3. The top row illustrates healing by primary closure; the middle row healing by delayed primary closure; and the bottom row healing by secondary intention. Least scarring appears in healing by first intention.

area, and then the wound surface can reepithelialize.

Wounds that heal by delayed primary or tertiary intention are those that are left open following wounding, because of significant bacterial contamination. Body cavities such as the peritoneal or pleural cavity are sealed to prevent evisceration but drains are left in situ. The open superficial layers are kept moist with dressings and closed after 4 to 5 days, when the wound develops resistance to infection. Some surgical wounds are healed by this method.

Some body tissues are capable of regeneration. This occurs in "like" cells, such as in an injury involving exclusively epithelial cells. Most injuries involve more than one layer of tissue. Wounds in these tissues heal by scar formation. This is the most common repair process. It involves fibroplasia, contraction, and scarring.

Wounds heal in three phases. These phases overlap and may extend for many years after the injury or incision. The first phase is an inflammatory phase that lasts 1 to 4 days. Also known as the defensive or exudative phase, it begins the moment the surgical incision is made or the moment a traumatic injury occurs. The major activities of the inflammatory phase are hemostasis and phagocytosis. The immediate response is vascular, with vasoconstriction and clot formation to control hemorrhage. Vasoconstriction lasts 5 to 10 minutes and is followed by dilation of the venules. Blood fills the area, and clots form a matrix of fibrin that provides a framework for repair. The surface scab that forms maintains hemostasis and provides protection from contamination.

For approximately 3 days, a substantial amount of fluid containing plasma proteins, water, and electrolytes leaks into the tissues surrounding the injury. As the fluid enters the region, cells become sticky and trap large amounts of interstitial fluid. Therefore the area becomes edematous and warm to the touch.

Leukocytes are the first cells to arrive at the injured area. They squeeze through a vessel wall by a process called *diapedesis*. Macrophages also move to the site and digest and mobilize debris from the injury.

Several hours after the damage, basal cells are activated and begin migration down below the clot that seals the wound. The cells migrate from both sides of the wound and meet within 24 to 48 hours. When both sides meet, cell mitosis begins. Epithelial cells can also migrate down into suture tracts to form so-called stitch abscesses. These are not really abscesses but rather a localized inflammatory reaction.

Fibroblasts begin to multiply 24 to 36 hours after the injury. They move randomly into the wound as the inflammatory process subsides. New capillaries quickly form to provide nutritional substances to newly developing cells. The inflammatory phase is absolutely essential for wound healing.

The second, or fibroblastic, phase, also known as the proliferative or reconstructive phase, begins on approximately the fifth postoperative day and continues to day 20. This phase overlaps the earlier inflammatory stage and likewise overlaps into the later maturing phase of wound repair.

Fibroblasts synthesize collagens, glycoproteins, and mucopolysaccharides. Collagen molecules form into fibers that crisscross into large bundles and give strength to the new connective tissue. Angiogenesis results in new capillaries forming to provide nutrients to the growing, emerging cells. As more collagen is deposited, capillaries begin to disappear. At the end of this phase, collagen synthesis and destruction balance themselves. New connective tissue fibers are associated with the strength of the wound. By the time skin sutures are removed, the wound has approximately 5% of its original skin strength. In one month, the wound has regained 35 to 50% of its original strength.

During the third and final maturation phase, the size and shape of the scar undergo slow, progressive change. The wound gains tensile strength. It will never achieve more than 70 to 80 percent of its preinjury skin strength. The wound reaches this maximum strength in approximately three months. This phase may last a number of months or years. Open wounds decrease in size by contraction, caused by inward movement of fibroblastic cells.

Preoperative Factors That Influence Wound Healing

In the assessment process, the perioperative nurse identifies data pertinent to the patient's total surgical experience. Postoperatively, the incision site and healing process are major concerns. During the preoperative interview, the nurse makes observations and asks questions that relate directly to the patient's ability to respond physiologically to the trauma of the incision.

The nutritional status of the patient is a major factor in wound healing. In response to stress and injury, the basal metabolic rate markedly increases. Protein is essential for collagen formation. In complex wounds, there is increased protein waste. Cortisol levels increase and blood glucose may rise, leading to increased glucose accumulation in cells. This produces an environment conducive to bacterial growth. Vitamin C assists in collagen synthesis and capillary formation. In aged patients and patients who smoke, vitamin C levels are lower. Vitamin A encourages formation of granulation tissue in healing skin incisions. It also seems to have an opposing effect on cortisol during the wound-healing process.

Specific groups of patients have more nutritional problems than the average person. Since the surgical procedure or trauma increases the basal metabolic rate of the body, these patients require careful preoperative nutritional assessment. Frequently, aged patients are in a poor nutritional state and hence exhibit retarded wound healing. Diabetics, obese patients, and those with disease processes requiring irradiation exhibit unique nutritional needs and therefore increased healing time. Electrolytes, enzymes, antibodies, and vitamins are important in wound healing. Known deficiencies should be identified preoperatively and corrected if possible. Surgery may be delayed while patients receive nutritional support. Enteral nutrition is preferred, but some patients may need total parenteral nutrition to overcome nutritional deficits.

The patient's weight may be a factor. Systemic diseases associated with obesity such as cardiovascular disease, hypertension, respiratory disease, and diabetes increase the risk of wound complications. In obese patients, impaired circulation and respiration result in less blood flow and oxygen at the wound area, both of which are important to wound healing. Potential wound complications are infection, incisional hernias, wound dehiscence, and seroma formation. The risk of infection is increased by the longer operating time and trauma to tissue from retraction. Adipose tissue, which is relatively avascular, has little ability to resist infection. Incisional hernias may be caused by increased strain on the incision. Wound dehiscence, often associated with infection, is a common complication. The surgeon may not be able to close the wound so that it will maintain its integrity. In obese patients, there is a greater potential for dead space, which can lead to formation of seromas.

Some disease processes, such as diabetes and cancer, are a concern to the nurse during the preoperative assessment. In the diabetic patient, wound healing is delayed and wound infections are severe and prolonged. Assessment should include the patient's current therapeutic regimen and how well the disease is controlled. Medical history is important, including the age of onset of diabetes. Obesity is also common among diabetics. Patients with cancer may be malnourished and generally debilitated. Their wound-healing ability may also be affected by

therapeutic regimens. If the patient has received radiation, skin in the irradiated area may be fragile and sensitive. The amount of radiation the patient has received, the patient's response to radiation, and his or her overall health should be included in the assessment since they are indicators of postoperative wound healing. Patients with cancer and diabetes may be immunosuppressed, which is also a factor in wound healing. Others who are immunosuppressed include those with congenital, acquired, or age-related deficiencies. Malnourished patients, as well as those with uremic disease, also have impaired immune responses. Immunosuppression may occur as a result of taking agents such as steroids, antiinflammatory agents, and cytoxic drugs.

The data on skin integrity obtained by the nurse are communicated in the plan of care or patient record to other members of the healthcare team so that treatment that might counteract potential complications in wound healing can be instituted preoperatively.

Intraoperative Factors That Influence Wound Healing

The risk of developing a surgical wound infection is largely determined by three factors: the amount and type of microbial contamination of the wound, the condition of the wound at the end of the operation, and host susceptibility (3). Fay (4) describes the etiologic factors in wound sepsis using three categories: environmental, host, and pathogenic. Environmental factors include habits of personnel, surgical technique, air filtration system, OR and hospital environment, effectiveness of sterilization, presence and types of foreign bodies, and failure of drainage systems. Host factors are described as age and general condition of the patient, nature of the illness (systemic disease), effectiveness of host defense mechanisms, anatomic location of injury or surgery, and presence and amount of devitalized tissue. The pathogenic factors include virulence, types, and numbers of contamination organisms.

Wound healing and the potential for infection are affected by intraoperative events. The perioperative nurse is primarily concerned with maintaining environmental asepsis during this period to prevent exogenous contamination of the wound. He or she assures the sterility of the instruments and supplies and is responsible for the skin preparation of the patient. To minimize the potential transfer of contamination from OR personnel to the patient, all members of the team are properly gowned, gloved, and masked. The perioperative nurse observes any breaks in technique and takes corrective action.

The surgeon is responsible for the surgical technique, which influences wound healing. Good surgical technique leads to good wound healing. A sharp, clean incision heals better than one with ragged edges. An electrosurgical knife damages the wound edge and increases the risk of infection. Other factors that affect wound healing are the length of time the wound is open, the handling of tissue, pressure from retractors and other instruments, and hemostasis. Dead space or poor drainage, which permit pooling of fluids, creates a potential for contamination. In some procedures, antibiotics are used prophylactically before and during surgery in wound irrigation.

The type of suture, needle, and stitch used have a bearing on wound healing and susceptibility to infection. Sutures are foreign bodies to which the body reacts. In a study on sutures and wound infection, Sharp and colleagues reported that "synthetic monofilament sutures were far superior to any of the braided sutures, and the synthetic sutures were better than the natural sutures"(5). They recommend that natural sutures not be used for wounds with potential for infection. Sixteen types of suture were tested for their resistance to both gram-positive and gram-negative infections. The diameter of the suture material should be as small as possible. The least amount of suture with the least tension is the best. Staples, now used extensively in surgery, are essentially nonreactive and minimize infection. Because of their B-shape, staples do not crush the skin and nutrients can pass through the staple line to the edge of the incision, reducing necrosis and promoting wound healing. Because the staples are inserted with mechanical devices, tissue handling and operating time are reduced.

The swage or eyeless needle minimizes tissue damage and is more commonly used than eyed needles. The suture is swaged to the needle by mechanical pressure and only a single strand of suture is drawn through the tissue, causing less tissue damage and leakage of fluid. The interrupted stitch is the most widely used and most efficient. Fewer stitches are used, and the skin edges are inverted or everted, promoting wound healing. The fewer the stitches, the less foreign body there is in the wound to cause a reaction.

Postoperative Factors That Influence Wound Healing

Age
As a person ages, wound healing capabilities are diminished. Also, efficiency of the cardiovascular and respiratory systems may be lessened.

Nutrition
Nutritional deficiency can delay healing. Patients with wounds need more calories per day than others, so malnourished patients will have difficulty healing their wounds. In addition, adequate hydration is required. Vitamins A, B, and C are also active in the healing process. Vitamin C is absolutely essential for collagen production. Minerals such as iron, calcium, and zinc are important as well.

Nursing Interventions
Wound healing is also strongly influenced by nursing interventions. During the initial inflammatory phase, observations of the wound, dressing, and surrounding tissue can detect hematoma formation or frank hemorrhage. Drain sites demand the same careful observation as the suture line. Flawless sterile technique must be used when changing dressings to guard against bacterial contamination. Inspection of drainage devices to assure proper function will facilitate correct calculation of the patient's intake and output. The area surrounding pressure dressings must be checked for adequate circulation. Edema of surrounding tissues can lead to increased pain. Elevation of an injured or incised limb above the level of the heart will ease drainage and decrease edema.

Control of circulating fluids is critical for oxygenation of the wounded tissues. Oxygen tension of greater than 15 mm Hg at the wound edges is required for collagen formation. Adequate respiratory movement allows for proper oxygenation of tissues during the healing process. Deep breathing, sighing, yawning, and use of an incentive spirometer increase oxygen exchange as well as stimulate secretory movement from the lungs.

Abdominal stress can seriously affect proper wound healing. Vomiting, the Valsalva maneuver, and deep coughing can produce intraabdominal pressures up to 150 ml water. Contrast this to 29 ml for getting out of bed and 18 ml while walking. Muscles and the wound are stretched, inhibiting the network formation and endothelial and fibroblastic migration necessary for wound healing. Deep coughing may be contraindicated since it can raise intrathoracic pressure to 300 mm Hg. Excessive coughing occasionally causes abdominal wound or muscle disruption.

Although nasogastric (NG) tubes are used to prevent abdominal distention, they can also cause it, since the presence of the NG tube in the throat causes many patients to swallow excessively and take in large amounts of air. Also, channels may form along the tube through which secretions flow and bypass the suction ports. Turning the patients helps collapse these channels and aids maximum, efficient function of the NG tube. A distended bladder also causes muscles to stretch beyond normal capacity and contributes to retarded wound healing.

Pain Control, Rest, and Sleep

Pain can affect wound healing in the postoperative period, leading to vital sign changes. The heart rate increases and blood pressure exhibits instability. Pain medication effectively returns these hemodynamic changes to their normal limits, thus delivering required oxygen to the wound site for healing.

Pain also produces changes in metabolic activity. As metabolism increases, cortisol is produced, which in turn retards wound healing. Patients experiencing pain have a poor appetite and diminished food intake, creating an extra drain on the already compromised nutritional state.

As an adjunct to medication, relaxation can be taught preoperatively to enable the patient to participate in pain control.

Rest and sleep are important factors in wound healing. Since the greatest amount of growth hormone is released during sleep, special times of rest should be included in the care plan. Growth hormone influences protein synthesis, which again influences wound healing by collagen production. Although the relationship is not clearly understood, stress has a negative impact on wound healing. Explanations to the patient and visitors about the importance of rest may be necessary to promote maximum wound repair.

Wound Coverings

Wound coverings protect the wound from trauma and bacterial invasion, assist in exudate removal, and provide a moist environment for reepithelialization. Although wound care used to be aimed at drying the wound and getting a scab to form, it is now known that a moist wound environment is much more conducive to healing. Because they require an adequate blood and nutritional supply to meet energy needs, epidermal cells migrate only over viable tissue. If migrating cells must burrow under and between a scab, resurfacing will be impeded. Exposed wounds are more inflamed and painful, itchier, and have thicker crusts than moist, covered wounds.

The traditional dressing is three layers: a contact layer of nonadherent material; a middle or primary layer, usually gauze, to absorb drainage; and a secondary or outer layer to protect the wound. It is important to have the nonadherent contact layer, because gauze that adheres to the wound will disrupt the reparative process when removed.

Newer options based on moist wound healing research offer some advantages. Semipermeable dressings allow oxygen to communicate with the wound, promoting faster reepithelialization.

Transparent film dressings are adhesive, polyurethane materials that provide a semiocclusive environment, allowing water vapor and gases to pass through, but preventing liquids and bacteria from doing so. They also offer pain reduction. Some have been shown to produce less scarring. Films work best on wounds with light or no exudate. They need to be changed only every 3 to 5 days and offer clear visibility of the incision.

Hydrocolloids are another group of dressings that will maintain a moist wound environment. They are adhesive wafers containing colloids and elastomers that provide an occlusive environment. Hydrocolloids do not require a secondary dressing and will absorb more drainage than the transparent films. They may also be left in place for several days, but the wound is not visible. Some newer formulations are translucent. Pain relief, probably due to protection of nerve endings, is an advantage.

Hydrogels are polymers with high water content. They are moderately absorbent and will provide a cooling, soothing effect to the wound. Since most hydrogels are nonadhesive, a secondary dressing is needed. A transparent film dressing can be used for this purpose.

If a complicated wound is producing a large amount of drainage, a new type of dressing may assist in absorption and healing. Calcium alginates are made from seaweed and form a gel when the calcium ions in the dressing and sodium ions in the wound exchange. Alginates will absorb approximately 20 times their weight. They require secondary dressings as they are nonadherent.

The same wound environment that accelerates healing can also enhance the growth of pathogens. In patients with normal immune status, this will not be problematic. Occlusion is contraindicated in immunocompromised patients or in infected wounds. In other cases, it offers great advantages.

COMPLICATIONS

Even with meticulous nursing and medical care, wounds are subject to complications in the repair process. Keloids, fistulas, adhesions, hematomas, infections, and wound disruptions may complicate healing.

Keloid formation is a hypertrophic scar that results when collagen synthesis exceeds destruction. Fibrous tissue varying in color from white to red extends above the skin surface. This type of scar is treated by injection with corticosteroids or surgical excision. In either case, the keloid tissue tends to recur. It is most common in blacks and dark-skinned Caucasians.

Fistulas may develop during the fibroblastic phase of healing. A tract develops between two epithelium-lined surfaces, allowing unexpected drainage from a particular organ. Patients having surgery of the head and neck, bowel, or genitourinary system are candidates for fistula formation. Some small fistulas may heal spontaneously, but most require surgical intervention.

Wound disruption or dehiscence occurs on approximately the fifth day. Fifty percent of patients with dehiscence exhibit serosanguineous drainage. Total dehiscence leads to evisceration, in which wound contents protrude. If this occurs, the area should be covered with saline dressings and a sterile towel, and the surgeon should be contacted immediately.

Incisional hernias most often occur in patients with abdominal surgery and complicated postoperative courses. Patients exhibit peristalsis under the skin and abdominal protrusion when standing but not while lying down. Incisional hernias can lead to bowel obstruction and must be surgically corrected.

Hematoma formation can occur in the immediate postoperative course, or it may not be evident until days after the surgical procedure. Formation is immediately evidenced by unexpected blood on the dressing and vital sign changes. It may be caused by a vessel not having been ligated or a slipped ligature. These patients are returned to the operating room for surgical correction of the problem.

If a hematoma does not become evident until a wound is in the fibroblastic stage, a small vessel may be slowly leaking blood into the wound space. Evidence of this type of hematoma is generally dehiscence, with discharge of old, dark-red blood. On occasion, the surgeon will tie the vessel and pack the wound, thus allowing for healing by secondary intention.

Adhesion formation is a problem during the final phase of healing. It occurs when two surfaces in the operative area adhere to one another. For example, loops of bowel may bind together, causing pain, dysfunction, and gangrene, necessitating surgical intervention.

REFERENCES

1. Seropian, R., and Reynolds, B. M. "Wound infections after preoperative depilatory versus razor preparation." *Am Surg* 121:251, 271, 1971.
2. Cruse, P., and Foord, R. "The epidemiology of wound infection, a 10-year prospective study of 62,939 wounds. *Surgical Clinics of North America* (February):27–40, 1980.
3. Garner, J. S. "CDC guidelines for the prevention and control of nosocomial infections. Guidelines for prevention of surgical wound infections, 1985." *AMJ of Infection Control* (April):71–80, 1986.
4. Fay, M. F. "Drainage systems, their role in wound healing." *AORN J* 46(September):442–455, 1987.
5. Sharp, W. V., Belden, T. A., King, P. H., and Teague, P. C. "Suture resistance to infection." *Surgery* 91(January):61–63, 1982.

SUGGESTED READINGS

Association of Operating Room Nurses. "Recommended practices, preoperative skin preparation." *AORN J* 48(November):950–968, 1988.
Bernard, L. A. "Wound healing." *AORN J* 35(May):1067, 1982.
Frogge, M. H. "Promoting wound healing in the irradiated patient." *AORN J* 35(May):1088–1093, 1982.
Garibalde, R. A., et al. "The impact of preoperative skin disinfection on preventing intraoperative wound contamination." *Infec Control Hosp Epidemoi* 9(March):109–113, 1988.
Groszek, D. M. "Wound healing in the obese patient." *AORN J* 35(May):132–138, 1982.
Hannigan, L. "Nursing assessment of the integumentary system," *Occup Health Nurs* 26:19, 1978.
Harris, D. R. "Healing of the surgical wound. II. Factors influencing repair and regeneration." *J Am Acad Dermatol* I(September):208–215, 1979.
Keithly, J. K. "Wound healing in malnourished patients." *AORN J* 35(May):1094–1099, 1982.
Kottra, C. J. "Wound healing in the immunosuppressed host." *AORN J* 35(May):1142–1148, 1982.
Masterson, B. J. "Skin preparation." *Clinical Obstetrics and Gynecology* 31(September):736–743, 1988.
Montagna, W., and Parakkal, P. F. *The Structure and Function of Skin* 3rd ed. New York: Academic Press, 1974.
Pillsbury, D. M., and Heaton, C. L. *A Manual of Dermatology* 2nd ed. Philadelphia: W. B. Saunders, 1980.
Rothburn, A. M., Holland, L. A., and Geelhold, G. W. "Preoperative skin decontamination, a study on efficiency and effect." *AORN J* 44(July):62–65, 1986.
Sauer, G. C. *Manual of Skin Diseases* 5th ed. Philadelphia: J. B. Lippincott, 1985.
Schumann, D. "The nature of wound healing." *AORN J* 35(May):1068–1077, 1982.
Westaby, S. *Wound Care*. London: William Heinemann Medical Books, 1985.
Winters, B. "Promoting wound healing in the diabetic patient." *AORN J* 35(May):1083–1087, 1982.
Yordan, E. L., Jr., and Bernhard, L. A. "The surgeon's role in wound healing." *AORN J* 35(May):1078–1082, 1982.

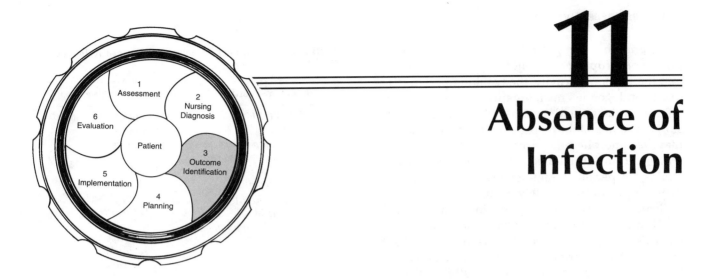

Absence of Infection

Outcome: No evidence of infection related to surgery.

Infection is usually defined as the presence or growth of pathogenic microorganisms (pathogens) on skin or in body tissues or fluids when the presence or growth is accompanied by a clinically adverse effect, either local or systemic. Infection is distinguished from colonization, which is the persistence of microorganisms on skin or in body tissues or fluids but without a clinically adverse effect. Nurses should know the clinical signs and symptoms of infections and should be able to interpret the results of laboratory tests conducted on cultures of skin, body tissues, or fluids to detect the presence of infecting microorganisms.

The perioperative nurse should be conscious of the fact that all patients who undergo operative procedures have the potential to acquire an infection. The desired outcome for all patients is that they will be free from infection postoperatively.

The clinical signs and symptoms of infection differ according to the site of infection. Heat, pain, swelling, and redness occur with most incisional wound, skin, muscle, or joint infections. The heat may occur either locally, at the site of infection, or systemically, as fever; the pain may vary in degree from mild tenderness to severe distress. In addition, the presence of purulent discharge strongly suggests an infection; this discharge can be pus in wound drainage, pyuria (pus in urine), or purulent sputum.

The isolation of one or more microorganisms from a properly collected and processed culture of skin, body fluids, or tissues that appears to be clinically infected usually confirms the presence of an infection and identifies the infecting microorganism(s). Indirect evidence of infection, such as serologic or biochemical results from laboratory tests, and radiologic evidence, such as infiltrates on chest x-rays, can be useful in diagnosing an infection but cannot be used in the absence of clinical or microbiologic data.

SOURCES OF INFECTING MICROORGANISMS

Various microorganisms are capable of causing infections. Those capable of causing infections in healthy persons are commonly referred to as pathogens. Less pathogenic microorganisms, often called opportunistic, are capable of causing disease in persons whose defense mechanisms may be deficient or compromised, including perioperative patients. Commensals, microorganisms that normally inhabit the skin, mucous membranes, and the gastrointestinal tract, are also frequent opportunists in some perioperative patients. Saprophytes, microorganisms abundant in the environment where they are ordinarily of little concern, may cause infections in perioperative patients whose defense mechanisms are deficient or compromised.

Microorganisms capable of causing infections can arise from endogenous or exogenous sources. Endogenous sources of infections are the patient's own microbiologic flora, the normal flora of the skin,

147

nose, pharynx, and gastrointestinal tract. For example, when a ruptured appendix spills bowel contents into the peritoneal cavity, the resulting peritonitis is due to endogenous microorganisms and is therefore referred to as an endogenous infection. On admission to the hospital, the patient's microbiologic flora may become altered, particularly in the pharynx and gastrointestinal tract, by acquiring "hospital strains," especially Gram-negative bacilli. Infections may arise from these newly acquired flora.

Exogenous sources of infection, on the other hand, are those that arise from outside the patient, such as those from infected or colonized patients and hospital personnel, or from inanimate objects in the hospital. For example, epidemics of *Staphylococcus aureus* and Group A *Streptococcus* wound infections usually arise from exogenous microorganisms acquired through person-to-person contact with infected or colonized members of the surgical team. In contrast, the source of *Pseudomonas cepacia* bloodstream infections is usually contaminated intravenous preparations or patient-care objects used intravascularly during the perioperative period.

THE CHAIN OF INFECTION

Microorganisms are ubiquitous. Nevertheless, infection will not occur unless the essential components for infection are present and interaction occurs among them. The essential components are an infectious agent, a susceptible host, and a means of transmission (Fig. 11.1). They are analogous to links in a chain. When they are all present, the chain of infection is complete and infection occurs.

Infectious Agent

The first link in the chain of infection is the infectious agent. Infectious agents can be bacteria, fungi, parasites, or viruses. Bacteria, however, are the most common microorganisms isolated in culture from infections in hospitals. Bacteria are identified in the laboratory by various characteristics, including their staining reactions and their requirement of oxygen for growth. One of the most important and widely

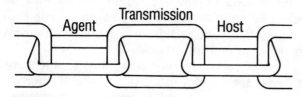

FIGURE 11.1.   Chain of infection.

TABLE 11.1.   Genera of Bacteria Commonly Isolated in Culture from Infections

Gram-Positive	Gram-Negative
AEROBIC	AEROBIC
Cocci	Cocci
Staphylococcus	*Neisseria*
Streptococcus	
Bacilli	Bacilli
Bacillus	*Acinetobacter*
ANAEROBIC	*Campylobacter*
Bacilli	*Citrobacter*
Clostridium	*Enterobacter*
	E. coli
	Klebsiella
	Morganella
	Proteus
	Providencia
	Pseudomonas
	Salmonella
	Serratia
	Shigella
	Yersinia
	ANAEROBIC
	Bacilli
	Bacteroides

used differential staining techniques for bacteria is the Gram stain. This stain rapidly identifies bacteria as Gram-positive or Gram-negative and shows their size and shape when viewed under a microscope.

Bacteria can also be classified according to whether they grow in the presence or absence of oxygen. Aerobic bacteria grow in the presence of oxygen, for example, on the skin, whereas anaerobic bacteria grow in the absence of oxygen, for example, in some deep body organs or tissues. Thus bacteria commonly isolated in culture from infections in the hospital are grouped according to their oxygen requirements, Gram stain, and shape (Table 11.1).

Susceptible Host

The second link in the chain of infection is the susceptible host. Host susceptibility is determined by various factors, such as age, immune status, and type of underlying disease. The extremes of life—infancy and old age—are associated with decreased resistance to infection. Similarly, patients with chronic diseases, such as certain types of cancer and kidney disease, diabetes mellitus, leukemia, or lymphoma, may be more susceptible to infection than other patients. In addition, factors such as nutritional status and lowered local resistance are important contributors to infection in perioperative patients. For example, an incision in the skin interrupts the anatomical barrier to infectious agents, allowing them to penetrate. Moreover, anesthesia interrupts the cough and sneeze reflex and compromises other normal defenses of the respiratory tract, such as the mucous cells and cilia that tend to repel invading infectious agents.

Host susceptibility can also be affected by diagnostic and therapeutic procedures, such as biopsy or surgery, and by treatment with antimicrobial or immunosuppressive agents. Furthermore, the use of invasive devices, such as intravascular catheters and urinary catheters, during the perioperative period also increases host susceptibility to infection.

Means of Transmission

The final link in the chain of infection is transmission of the infectious agent to the susceptible host. Infectious agents are transmitted through one or more of four different means: contact, airborne, common vehicle, and vector-borne transmission.

Contact Transmission
Contact transmission is the most frequent means of transmission of infection in hospitals and can occur by direct, indirect, or droplet contact between the source of the infectious agent and the susceptible host. Direct transmission occurs when person-to-person contact results in the transfer of an agent between the infected or colonized source and a susceptible host. Such transmission can occur from the nurse to the patient and vice versa during routine hands-on perioperative patient care, such as preoperative skin preparation and postoperative dressing changes. Direct contact transmission can also occur by self-inoculation when microorganisms from the patient become the source of the infection.

Indirect contact transmission occurs when the contact between the source and susceptible host involves a contaminated intermediate object, such as some piece of patient-care or surgical equipment that transfers the infectious agent. Droplet contact transmission involves the brief passage of relatively large infectious particles through the air when the infected source and susceptible host are in close proximity, usually within several feet. Such transmission could occur between an infected circulating nurse and the patient during an operative procedure in any setting.

Other Means of Transmission
The remaining three means of transmission of infection—airborne, common-vehicle, and vector-borne—occur less frequently in the perioperative setting than does contact transmission. Airborne

transmission, in contrast to droplet transmission, is relatively infrequent. It involves a true airborne dissemination of infectious agents in droplet nuclei or dust particles that remain suspended in the air for prolonged periods of time and move about as a result of air currents or mechanical movement of air. Common-vehicle transmission occurs when a contaminated inanimate vehicle such as liquid antiseptic, disinfectant, or food is the medium for transmission of the infectious agent from the source to numerous susceptible hosts. Vector-borne transmission occurs when the infectious agent is transmitted through vectors such as mosquitoes, lice, or ticks. Vector-borne transmission rarely occurs in U.S. hospitals.

BREAKING THE CHAIN OF INFECTION

While completing the chain of infection requires that all three essential components be present under the right conditions, breaking the chain requires altering or removing only one of the three components or links. Thus the chain of infection can be broken by (1) destroying the infectious agent, (2) increasing the resistance of the susceptible host, or (3) interrupting transmission of the infectious agent.

Destroying Infectious Agents

Although various cleaning and disinfection procedures reduce the number of microorganisms on objects, the complete destruction or removal of infectious agents on objects in the hospital environment can be accomplished only through sterilization. Infectious agents in waste materials can be destroyed through incineration.

Sterilization
Sterilization is a process designed to completely remove or destroy all forms of microbial life, as compared to disinfection, which kills only some microorganisms. Though it is impossible and unnecessary to attempt to destroy all microorganisms in the perioperative environment, it is particularly important, from an infection-control standpoint, that surgical instruments and certain patient-care items used during the perioperative period be sterile. For example, any object or instrument that enters tissue or the vascular system and any object that blood flows through, such as tubing and catheters, should be sterile.

The most convenient, effective, inexpensive, and

widely used method of sterilization in healthcare settings is steam under pressure, or autoclaving. Steam sterilization is unsuitable, however, for processing certain items with low melting points, such as plastic tubing and catheters, and delicate objects that might be damaged by heat or moisture. In contrast to autoclaving, ethylene oxide gas sterilization is more complex and expensive; it requires special aeration to remove toxic residues of the gas. Its use, therefore, is usually restricted to delicate objects such as lensed instruments and plastics that might be damaged by the heat or moisture of autoclaving.

Chemical germicides can be used for sterilization if the objects are precleaned with a detergent until they are free of organic matter such as blood or mucus. The contact time for sterilization with liquid chemicals varies, depending on their active ingredients and, in most instances, the temperature of the solution. Some liquid chemicals can be used as either disinfectants or sterilants, depending on the duration of contact. The manufacturer's instructions must be carefully followed to achieve the desired result. Moreover, because of their chemical makeup, some of these agents may represent hazards to the user, such as respiratory irritation, dermatitis, chemical burns, or other reactions. Protective equipment such as gloves and eyewear may be required.

Incineration

Infectious agents can also be destroyed by incineration. Some medical wastes, such as pathology and microbiology wastes, may be highly contaminated with infectious agents. Infectious agents in such wastes can usually be destroyed more easily and economically through incineration than through steam sterilization. Even with strict air pollution regulations, incineration of small quantities of infectious wastes is still possible in most communities.

Increasing Host Resistance

Infections cannot occur without a susceptible host, but host resistance is often the most difficult component to alter when attempting to break the chain of infection. Particularly difficult is increasing resistance in patients who undergo an operative procedure. Some host factors that predispose to infection, however, may be altered during the perioperative period if the operation can be delayed until attempts have been made to increase host resistance. For example, the risk of infection in patients with uncontrolled diabetes can be reduced if such patients can have their blood sugar better controlled during the perioperative period. The risk of infection can be reduced in severely malnourished patients if they receive parenteral nutrition perioperatively. The benefits of attempts to increase host resistance must be weighed against the risks associated with the intervention and delay of the operative procedure.

Interrupting Transmission

Since it is difficult to increase host resistance and often impossible and unnecessary to destroy all potentially infectious agents in the surgical environment, attempts at breaking the chain of infection should be directed toward interrupting transmission of microorganisms responsible for infection. Because nurses spend more time with perioperative patients than other healthcare professionals do, it is particularly important that they direct nursing activities toward interrupting transmission of infection.

Handwashing

Handwashing is generally considered to be the single most important method for interrupting transmission of microorganisms and preventing infections. Numerous products, ranging from plain soap to antimicrobial-containing cleansers, are usually available for handwashing in perioperative settings. Soap and detergents suspend easily removable microorganisms on the skin and allow them to be washed off. Antimicrobial-containing products control or kill microorganisms that contaminate the skin and other superficial tissues. Although they do not sterilize the skin, they can reduce the amount of microbial contamination. The degree of reduction depends on the amount and type of contamination on the hands, the type of handwashing product used, the length of exposure to the product, the presence of residual activity of the product, and the technique used.

In the absence of a true emergency, perioperative nurses should wash their hands:

1. Immediately and thoroughly if contaminated with blood and other body fluids containing blood or potentially infective material.
2. Before performing invasive procedures, even if gloves are worn.
3. Before and after touching wounds, whether surgical, traumatic, or associated with an invasive device, even if gloves are worn.
4. Before taking care of particularly susceptible patients.
5. After removal of gloves.
6. After contact with a source that is likely to be

contaminated with virulent microorganisms or hospital pathogens.

7. Between contacts with different patients in high-risk units.

The recommended handwashing technique depends on the purpose of the handwashing. The ideal duration is not known, but washing times of 15 seconds or less have been reported as effective in removing most transient contaminants from the skin. Therefore, for most activities a vigorous, brief (at least 10 seconds) rubbing together of all surfaces of lathered hands, followed by rinsing under a stream of water is recommended. If hands are visibly soiled, more time may be required.

The absolute indications for handwashing with plain soaps and detergents versus antimicrobial-containing products are not known because of the lack of well-controlled studies comparing infection rates when such products are used. For most routine activities, handwashing with plain soap appears to be sufficient, since soap washes off most transient microorganisms.

Preventing Transmission of Blood-Borne Pathogens

In 1985, largely because of the acquired immuno-deficiency syndrome (AIDS) epidemic, infection-control practices in the United States were dramatically altered by the introduction of a new strategy designed to minimize the risk of transmitting the human immunodeficiency virus (HIV), hepatitis B virus (HBV), and other blood-borne pathogens in healthcare settings (1). The new strategy emphasizes that blood is the single most important source of HIV, HBV, and other blood-borne pathogens in the healthcare setting, and that infection-control efforts must focus on preventing exposure to blood and immunization against HBV for healthcare workers (2). The strategy, originally referred to as universal blood and body fluid precautions, is now referred to simply as universal precautions.

The concept of universal precautions emphasizes the need for healthcare workers to consider all patients as potentially infected with HIV, HBV, and other blood-borne pathogens; and to adhere rigorously to infection-control precautions in order to minimize the risk of parenteral, mucous membrane, and nonintact skin exposures to blood and other specified body fluids of all patients. Proper application of these principles will assist in minimizing the risk of transmission of HIV and HBV from patients to healthcare workers, healthcare workers to patients, and patients to patients.

Universal precautions include the following components:

1. Wear glvoes for touching blood and other specified fluids (I.e., amniotic fluid, cerebrospinal fluid, pericardial fluid, peritoneal fluid, pleural fluid, synovial fluid, semen, vaginal secretions, and any other fluid contaminated with blood); for touching mucous membranes and nonintact skin of all patients; for handling items or surfaces soiled with blood and specified body fluids; and for performing vascular access or invasive procedures. Change gloves after contact with each patient, and wash hands immediately after gloves are removed.

2. Wash hands and other skin surfaces immediately and thoroughly if contaminated with blood or other specified body fluids requiring universal precautions.

3. Take care to prevent injuries caused by needles, scalpels, and other sharp instruments or devices during procedures and during handling, cleaning, or disposal after procedures. To prevent needlestick injuries, do not recap, purposely bend, break by hand, remove from disposable syringes, or otherwise manipulate needles by hand. Dispose of used disposable syringes and needles, scalpel blades, and other sharp items in puncture-resistant containers located as close as is practical to the use area. Transport large-bore reusable needles to the reprocessing area in puncture-resistant containers.

4. Wear masks and protective eyewear or face shields to prevent exposure of mucous membranes of the mouth, nose, and eyes during procedures that are likely to generate droplets or splashes of blood or other specified fluids or to generate bone chips.

5. Wear gowns or aprons during procedures that are likely to generate splashes or sprays of blood or other body fluids.

6. Use mouthpieces, resuscitation bags, or other ventilation devices for resuscitation of patients in healthcare settings.

7. Healthcare workers who have exudative lesions or weeping dermatitis should refrain from all direct patient care and from handling patient-care equipment until the condition resolves.

8. Transport linens and articles soiled with blood

or bloody body fluids in bags that prevent leakage.

9. Clean spills of blood and blood-contaminated body fluids with a hospital disinfectant.

10. Use category-specific or disease-specific isolation precautions as necessary if infections other than blood-borne infections are diagnosed or suspected.

Perioperative nurses who participate as members of the operative team should take special care to prevent hand injuries caused by needles, scalpels, and other sharp instruments during surgical procedures. If a glove is torn or a needlestick or other injury occurs, the glove should be removed and a new glove put on as promptly as patient safety permits. The needle or instrument should also be removed from the sterile field.

In addition to universal precautions, other AIDS-related policies and procedures have been establish to prevent transmission of HIV to patients in healthcare settings. These include use of autologous blood transfusions and bone grafts whenever possible, testing all blood and organ donors for HIV antibodies, and following other specified recommendations for preventing transmission of HIV during exposure-prone invasive procedures (3).

NOSOCOMIAL INFECTIONS

Infections in perioperative patients can be classified as either hospital-acquired (nosocomial) or community-acquired infections. Nosocomial infections occur during hospitalization and were neither present nor incubating when the patient was admitted to the hospital. Infections with onset after discharge from the hospital are also considered to be nosocomial if the infecting microorganism is judged to have been acquired during hospitalization. The term *nosocomial* infection, therefore, includes potentially preventable infections from exogenous (external) sources as well as those from endogenous (patient's own) sources.

Nosocomial infections in surgical patients may or may not be related to the surgical procedure. Surgery-related infections involve the surgical wound or surrounding deep organs, tissues, or cavities that are exposed during the operative procedure. Examples of surgery-related nosocomial infections include an incisional wound infection in a patient after laminectomy, a subphrenic abscess in a patient after gastrectomy, or an empyema in a patient after thoracic surgery. Infections that arise in surgical patients but do not involve tissue exposed or manip-

ulated during the operative procedure are not considered surgery-related. For example, purulent thrombophlebitis, postoperative pneumonia, or urinary tract infection in a patient after gastrectomy would not be considered surgery-related.

Surgical patients, more than any other patient group in the hospital, have a high risk of developing nosocomial infections. Many infections in surgical patients are not related to the surgical wound but to instrumentation that invades the urinary and respiratory tracts and intravascular system during the perioperative period. Nevertheless, postoperative wound infections remain a major source of morbidity and an infrequent source of mortality in the surgical patient. Major complications, such as deep sternal wound infections, continue to have a grave impact, increasing the duration of hospitalization five-fold (4). Surgical wound infection following open heart surgery has resulted in a significant loss of reimbursement to the hospital compared with uninfected cases (5).

Definitions of Surgical Wound Infections

In 1988, the Centers for Disease Control (CDC) published a new set of definitions for surveillance of surgical wound infections (6). In these definitions, infections are categorized using both laboratory and clinical criteria. A physician's or surgeon's diagnosis is an acceptable criterion for a surgical wound infection unless there is compelling evidence to the contrary, such as information written on the wrong patient's record or presumptive diagnosis that was not substantiated by subsequent studies. For an infection to be defined as nosocomial, there must be no evidence that the infection was present or incubating at the time of hospital admission. In the CDC definitions, surgical wound infections are classified as either incisional or deep surgical wound infections.

Incisional Wound Infection

An incisional wound infection is defined as an infection that occurs at the incision site within 30 days after surgery, involves skin, subcutaneous tissue, or muscle located above the fascial layer, and any of the following:

1. Purulent drainage from the incision or a drain located above the fascial layer.

2. Organism isolated from culture of fluid from wound closed primarily.

3. Deliberate opening of the wound by the surgeon, unless wound is culture-negative.

4. Surgeon's or attending physician's diagnosis of infection.

Deep Surgical Wound Infection

A deep surgical wound infection is defined as an infection that occurs at the operative site within 30 days after surgery if no implant is left in place, or within one year if an implant is in place. An implant is defined as a nonhuman-derived implantable foreign body (e.g., prosthetic heart valve, nonhuman vascular graft, mechanical heart, or hip prosthesis) that is permanently placed in a patient during surgery. The infection should appear related to surgery, involve tissues or spaces at or beneath the fascial layer, and any of the following:

1. Purulent drainage from a drain placed beneath fascial layer.
2. Spontaneous wound dehiscence or deliberate opening by surgeon when patient has fever greater than 38°C or localized pain or tenderness, unless wound is culture-negative.
3. An abscess or other evidence of infection seen on direct examination, during surgery, or by histopathologic examination.
4. Surgeon's diagnosis of infection.

Classification of Surgical Wounds

One of the most important factors determining the risk of a surgical wound becoming infected is the degree of contamination at the time of surgery. In the mid-1950s, the National Research Council developed a system for classifying wounds based on the degree of contamination of the wound itself and surrounding tissues during the operation (7). This system of stratifying surgical wounds by intrinsic risk of contamination has been adopted for use in various settings. All surgical wounds are divided into four classes: clean, clean-contaminated, contaminated, and dirty or infected.

Class I: Clean Wound

This category includes nontraumatic surgical wounds in which no inflammation is encountered, no break in surgical technique occurs, and no entry is made into the respiratory, alimentary, or genitourinary tract. Examples of clean wounds are thyroidectomy, mastectomy, herniorrhaphy, and laminectomy.

Class II: Clean-Contaminated Wound

This category includes nontraumatic wounds in which only minor breaks in surgical technique occur or in which no significant spillage occur if the gastrointestinal, genitourinary, or respiratory tracts are entered. Examples of clean-contaminated wounds are cholecystectomy, resection of the small or large intestine when no inflammation or infection is present, hysterectomy, oophorectomy, and Caesarian delivery.

Class III: Contaminated Wound

This category includes any fresh traumatic wound from a relatively clean source or one in which there is a major break in surgical technique, gross spillage from the gastrointestinal tract, or entry into the genitourinary or biliary tracts if there is acute nonpurulent inflammation. An example of a contaminated wound is an inflamed but unruptured appendix or gallbladder.

Class IV: Dirty Wound

This category includes wounds in which acute bacterial inflammation or a perforated viscus is encountered, and wounds in which clean tissue is transected to gain access to a collection of pus or abscess. Surgical drainage of an intraabdominal abscess is an example.

Since the classification of a surgical wound can vary depending upon the findings and circumstances during an operation, usually only a member of the operating team can accurately determine the ultimate rating. Ideally, the classification should be made and recorded at the completion of the operation.

Surgical Wound Risk Index

During the last decade, limitations of the traditional wound classification system described above have been recognized and attempts have been made to develop a more meaningful system to predict a surgical patient's risk of developing a surgical wound infection. As a start, a simple risk index was developed during the CDC Study on the Efficacy of Nosocomial Infection Control (SENIC Project)(8). The SENIC surgical wound index consists of counting the number of risk factors present from among the following four factors: (1) an operation that involves the abdomen, (2) an operation lasting longer than 2 hours, (3) an operation classified as either contaminated or dirty-infected, and (4) a patient having three or more diagnoses at discharge. This index has proved to be a better predictor of surgical wound infection risk than the traditional wound classification system.

During the last several years researchers at CDC have modified the SENIC surgical wound index and applied it to data collected on an ongoing basis in the CDC National Nosocomial Infections Surveillance (NNIS) System (9). The NNIS surgical patient risk index consists of scoring each operation by counting the number of risk factors present from among these three:

1. A patient having an American Society of Anesthesiologists (ASA) preoperative assessment score of 3, 4, or 5.
2. An operation classified as either contaminated or dirty-infected.
3. An operation with duration of $> T$ hours, where T depends upon the operative procedure being performed.

In a study recently reported by CDC, rates of surgical wound infections (number of infections per 100 operations) within each category of the traditional wound classification system were compared with surgical wound infection rates using the NNIS surgical patient risk index (9). Within each of the categories of the traditional wound classification system, surgical wound infection rates were 2.1, 3.3, 6.4, and 7.1 respectively. The surgical wound infection rates for the same patients using the NNIS surgical wound index were 1.5, 2.9, 6.8, and 13.0 respectively. The NNIS surgical patient risk index is a better predictor of surgical wound infection risk and provides a better means of comparing surgical wound infection rates among surgeons and institutions, and across time, than the traditional wound classification system.

Microbiology of Surgical Wound Infections

The microorganisms that are isolated from surgical wound infections vary primarily by the site of the surgical procedure. In clean surgical procedures in which no entry is made into the gastrointestinal, gynecologic, or respiratory tracts, *Staphylococcus aureus* from either the patient's own microbiologic flora or exogenous sources is often the cause of infection. In clean-contaminated, contaminated, and dirty surgical procedures, Gram-negative aerobic and anaerobic bacteria that closely resemble the patient's own microbiologic flora at the operative site are the most frequently isolated pathogens (10). The most frequently isolated pathogens from surgical wound infections from the CDC NNIS system for 1986–1989 are: *Staphylococcus aureus*, Enterococci, coagulase-negative Staphylococci, and *Escherichia coli* (11).

Pathogens other than bacteria, for example, fungi and viruses, are rarely reported.

Surveillance of Surgical Wound Infections

Since the beginning of organized infection-control programs, surveillance has been advocated for recognizing nosocomial infection problems and for developing effective prevention measures. Reporting surgical wound infection rates to practicing surgeons has been effective in lowering these rates, as described in numerous studies reported as early as the late 1890s. Therefore, surveillance is promoted by organizations that set standards of care within healthcare facilities, including the American Hospital Association, the Joint Commission on Accreditation of Healthcare Organizations, and the Health Care Financing Administration.

CDC recently introduced two new protocols for surveillance of infections in surgical patients (12). In one protocol, called the detailed option, selected risk factor data are collected on all patients undergoing the operations that are being monitored. That is, hospitals using this protocol select which operative procedures they wish to monitor and collect certain risk factor information on all patients undergoing these procedures. Categories for which risk factor data are collected include: age, sex, date of operation, duration of surgery, wound class, use of general anesthesia, ASA class, whether the operation is an emergency or necessitated by trauma, and the surgeon's name or code. All of the patients undergoing the selected procedures during the same month are observed either for infections at all sites or for surgical wound infections only. Using these data, the infection control nurse can calculate infection rates by each of the risk factors and the NNIS surgical wound index.

In the other protocol, called the limited option, summary data are collected on all patients undergoing operations during the same month. The summary data collected are the number of each type of operative procedures performed, the number of operations in each wound class, and the number of operations performed by each surgeon. As in the detailed option, the hospital can choose to observe the patients for infections at all sites or surgical wound infections only. Infection rates can be calculated for each category for which summary data are collected, for example, surgical wound infection rates by wound class. These rates, however, have limited use since they do not adequately adjust for important risk factors such as intrinsic patient susceptibility to infection.

The Infection Control Nurse

Infection control as a nursing specialty originated in England in 1959, when a nurse was appointed to act as a liaison among all persons concerned with infection control. The concept spread to the United States in the early 1960s, when the infection control nurse (ICN) became the central figure of infection-control programs designed to reduce the ever-present risk of nosocomial infections through consistent surveillance and personnel education. Virtually all U.S. hospitals have established positions for one or more ICNs, and many free-standing surgery centers have established ICN positions on at least a part-time basis.

A wide range of responsibilities and activities are associated with ICNs in U.S. hospitals, including surveillance of nosocomial infections; researching and developing infection control policies; training hospital personnel in infection control; consulting with physicians, nurses, and other personnel or hospital departments; and investigating outbreaks of infection. Through these activities, ICNs work with clinical, administrative, and support service personnel associated with the hospital. Contacts with these persons include informal interaction with nurses about specific patient care or personnel health practices; teaching classes for nurses, physicians, and other members of the hospital staff; and conferences with administrators, department heads, and chiefs of medical services.

The ICN is usually a member of the infection control committee, which is responsible for all policies and procedures related to hospital infection control. The ICN also acts as liaison between the infection control committee and hospital departments (such as the operating room) when policies and procedures are proposed, reviewed, implemented, and evaluated. Moreover, the ICN keeps the director of the operating room informed about the occurrence and outcome of surgical wound infection problems and trends of such infections.

The advent of the AIDS epidemic in the mid-1980s added new responsibilities for most ICNs (13). The additional responsibilities have varied widely, from developing comprehensive and continuing educational programs to inform all hospital personnel about modes of transmission and the corresponding control measures recommended by CDC, to developing programs to monitor and reduce personnel exposures to patients' blood, and interpreting the Occupational Safety and Health Administration (OSHA) regulations for providing a safe work environment (14). AIDS-related infection control issues will continue to play a prominent and ongoing role in ICN activities in the 1990s.

The Infection Control Nurse and the OR Director

The formal relationship between the ICN and the director of the operating room depends in part on the organizational structure of the hospital and the administrative placement of the operating room and infection control departments. Regardless of the organizational structure, however, the ICN and the director of the operating room should discuss and share information about prevention of infections in patients and personnel.

Although the ICN may have limited experience in OR nursing, his or her background and experience with infectious diseases and review of scientific studies can be valuable to the OR director when new policies, procedures, and products are being considered. The ICN is concerned not only about whether the policy, procedure, or product will likely reduce or prevent infections, but whether its infection control benefit outweighs its cost.

The ICN and the OR director bring different knowledge, experience, and perspective to outcome identification for perioperative patients. They should work together closely to ensure that the outcome for perioperative patients is that they will be free from infection postoperatively.

CONTROLLING THE ENVIRONMENT

During the preoperative assessment, the nurse identifies host factors that influence the risk of infection, such as nutritional status, age, and underlying disease. These factors, however, are not usually amenable to change through nursing action during the immediate perioperative period. The primary focus of the nurse in achieving the outcome of freedom from infection for the patient is control of the number and types of microorganisms present during surgery.

Surgery has been described as controlled assault on the human body. Operative intervention breaks down some of the body's primary defenses against infection. Infection can adversely affect the outcome of an operative procedure, and even endanger the life of the patient.

While not all the principles and activities described in this chapter are carried out by nurses, the nurse should understand what is involved in minimizing the microbial population present during surgery. This enables the nurse to coordinate supplies, equipment, and a physical environment that are safe for use in patient care. The nurse must also recognize when conditions or events might make an item or area unacceptable for use in the care of the surgical patient.

Control of microorganisms starts with control of the physical environment of the operative setting. The factors to be considered and the methods of control also apply to other areas where items are prepared for and undergo sterilization. Most infections associated with operative intervention are caused by bacteria, although certain fungi and some viruses are also of concern. Environmental measures are therefore aimed primarily at control of bacterial contamination. The temperature of the operative setting is maintained between 20°C and 24°C (68°F and 75°F), except in situations where the risk of hypothermia to the patient outweighs the benefits of lower temperatures. Such might be the case with infants, because they have immature temperature-regulating mechanisms and physiologic intolerance to cold. Normally, however, patients can tolerate 20°C to 24°C with no difficulty, especially after the surgical drapes are applied. It is thought that most bacteria pathogenic to humans metabolize and reproduce best at temperatures at or near normal body temperature, 37°C (98.6°F). By keeping the room temperature below this level, bacterial growth may be inhibited to some small degree.

A stronger argument for keeping the temperature at these levels is the comfort and thermal regulation of the operative team. When dressed in a scrub suit, cap, mask, and fluid-impervious gown and gloves, operative team members have little body area exposed for heat loss through convection or radiation. If a member of the operative team becomes overheated, the principal cooling method is evaporation of perspiration. This means possible soaking through of clothing and possible dripping of perspiration onto the operative field. This moisture carries bacterial flora and could be a source of infection. Temperatures below 20°C (68°F) may be too cold, even for those dressed in full surgical garb, and involuntary shivering may occur. The attention of the operative team should be on the patient. Variations from the suggested temperature range can produce discomfort and distraction even without provoking the extremes of diaphoresis and shivering.

The relative humidity in the operative setting is maintained at 50 percent ± 10. Bacteria are thought to multiply best in moist environments above 60 percent relative humidity. The 40 to 60 percent range does, however, allow some bacterial growth. The primary reason for the convention of maintaining relative humidity at this level goes back to the time when explosive anesthetics such as ether were in wide use. The potential for static electricity buildup and discharge is greatly lessened if the relative humidity is about 50 percent. Provisions for the control of relative humidity remain a part of most voluntary and regulatory standards for the surgical suite even though explosive anesthetic agents are no longer used. Controlled discharge of large electrostatic charge accumulation sometimes interferes with the operation of electrical monitoring equipment and can cause actual damage to electrical equipment. Also, static shocks that might occur when the operative team member touches the patient could be uncomfortable if the materials in use and the humidity conditions are conducive to static buildup. Therefore, even without explosive anesthetics, there are still reasons to control electrostatic charge buildup through control of humidity.

Air Quality

The ambient air in the operative setting contains microorganisms that could settle into the wound, introducing contamination. Air-handling or ventilation systems of surgical suites being built today are designed to minimize the introduction of contaminants from outside the operating room. The optimal ventilation system delivers air to the room at or near ceiling level from the center of the room. Air exhaust vents are in the periphery of the room, just above floor level. The air currents set up move air down through the surgical field, carrying most airborne particles to floor level and away from the surgical field. In new operating rooms, the rate of air exchange should be at least 20 room volumes per hour. Up to 80 percent of the air may be recirculated, provided the exhausted air is adequately filtered. Recirculation of air conserves energy because minimal heating, cooling, and humidity adjustments are necessary.

The filtration or cleaning of the air is important. In the modern operating room, air-handling systems include a series of filters that remove almost all particulate matter coming from the outside fresh air and that contained in the recirculated air. The air delivered to the operating room is almost sterile. The particle count and thus the bacterial burden, however, rise sharply as the air travels through the operating room because of microbial shedding from the patient and members of the operative team. This shedding increases with activity and cannot be totally eliminated even with modern surgical attire. The 20 air exchanges per hour is sufficient to dilute the bacterial debris from the operative team to a level considered safe for most types of surgery.

Some procedures, however, are thought to require a greater margin of safety because of the potentially catastrophic results of postoperative infections. These include total joint replacements and other procedures in which large amounts of foreign prosthetic material are left in the patient. Procedures on patients who have severely compromised host defense mechanisms, such as severe bone marrow depression, might also fit into this category.

For these patients, some surgeons use laminar airflow systems to create an ultraclean environment where even shedding from the operative team is minimized as a source of airborne contamination. Laminar airflow means unidirectional, nonturbulent airflow. The airflow direction can be either horizontal or vertical, depending on whether the plenum containing the high-energy particulate air (HEPA) filters is on the ceiling or on a wall. In a vertical flow unit, the air enters from the ceiling and exits at floor level. In a horizontal flow unit, the air enters from one side of the room and travels in straight currents across to the opposite wall. What makes this air-handling system different is not the filtration, since most air-handling systems for the operating room have efficient filtration mechanisms, but the speed at which the air travels, which maintains the unidirectional flow. There is a perceptible breeze in rooms using laminar airflow equipment.

Laminar airflow equipment introduces virtually sterile air into the room and blows it across the field at such a rate that particles shed by persons in its path are suspended in the unidirectional currents and not allowed to settle onto the surgical field. It then carries the particulates away from the field to a point where they are captured in a vent or can safely settle out on the floor. In reality, in an occupied operating room, true unidirectional flow is almost impossible to achieve because the air must pass over and around people and objects that break up the laminar flow pattern.

When using laminar airflow equipment, careful planning of the positioning of personnel and equipment is essential. If possible, nothing should obstruct the flow of air from the filter plenum to the wound site. All objects and people should remain downwind or peripheral to this airflow. This is extremely difficult to do, especially in vertical flow units, because the head and shoulders of the surgical team may be over the wound. In these cases, some surgical teams wear special headgear that totally covers the head and face. This may be a plastic face guard similar to those worn by astronauts and a sterile total-hair-cover hood. An exhaust system to remove expired air from the plastic face dome is sometimes used, often more for cooling than for respiratory needs.

There is still a great deal of controversy as to laminar airflow's effectiveness in reducing postoperative infections. Many authorities dispute the claim that it reduces infection by pointing out that the surgeon's speed, proper tissue-handling techniques, appropriate wound drainage, elimination of wound dead space, and the use of prophylactic antibiotics are all significant in keeping the infection low. Laminar airflow equipment is expensive, and many hospitals are reluctant to install it unless its efficacy is clearly demonstrated. If the laminar airflow equipment is misused because of inadequate planning and positioning, the result could be an increase in infection because particles may be driven into the depths of the surgical wound.

Another characteristic of air-handling systems for the surgical suite is the creation of pressure gradients between so-called clean and dirty areas. The actual operating room is considered clean, the adjacent hallway and substerile or scrub areas less clean. The operating room is kept at a slightly (about 10 percent) higher air pressure than the surrounding space so that if a door is opened, air from the less clean space cannot enter the clean space. In surgical suites with a clean core, where only sterile supplies are stored and all personnel wear masks at all times, the clean core has slightly more positive pressure than the operating room. Thus when the door to the clean core is opened, air flows from the "cleaner" core area in to the "clean" operating room.

These pressure gradients are effective only when the doors to the operating room are kept closed except when someone is entering or leaving. Leaving the door open or opening two doors at once disrupts the pressurization and causes turbulent airflow that could increase airborne contamination. In addition, the air-handling system must work harder, thus using more energy and increasing costs.

If air-handling systems are allowed to function as

they were designed to, they deliver high-quality, well-conditioned air. Operating rooms built prior to the 1970s may not have these sophisticated systems in place, and extra care with regard to environmental cleaning, OR apparel, and surgical speed may be appropriate.

Traffic

The greatest sources of bacterial contamination are the persons in the room at the time of surgery, including the patient. This contamination increases with movement and talking.

Every effort should be made to minimize the number of people in the room during an operative procedure. The higher the risk of infection or the greater the consequences of infection for the patient, the more stringent should be the controls on access to the room. This is particularly difficult in teaching hospitals, where residents and students need legitimate access to operative procedures to complete their training. Highly technical or complex procedures that last a long time or require much technical equipment are also of concern. Examples of these are limb replantations and cardiopulmonary bypass procedures.

In these cases, careful planning by nursing personnel can minimize excess movement in and out, as well as within, the operating room. Anticipating supply needs, checking out equipment before the patient arrives, and using an intercom or telephone, if available, can reduce trips in and out of the room. Identifying each person in the room and ascertaining his or her purpose in being present are essential. It may be appropriate to challenge some visitors, using tact and appropriate channels of authority for each institution. The nurse must serve as the patient's advocate in this matter to minimize the risk of infection and to protect the patient's right to privacy.

Traffic flow within the room is governed by the principles of asepsis. Traffic flow within the area in general, outside the actual operative procedure room, is largely dependent on the physical design of the setting. Three components that make up the traffic within any surgical setting are patients, personnel, and supplies and equipment. For each of these, the idea pattern is unidirectional, with entry in one area, travel through the suite, and exit in another area. But few surgical settings are built to permit this ideal traffic pattern, and compromises are usually necessary. These adjustments can be effective and safe in minimizing contamination if they are well thought out and judiciously adhered to. In fact, constructing an ideal surgical setting can be prohibi-

TABLE 11.2. The Three Zones of the Surgical Suite

Zone	Attire	Examples
Unrestricted	People in street attire may enter and mix with those in scrub attire.	Locker rooms, some offices, and the administrative control desk if it is located at the entrance to the surgical suite
Semirestricted	Scrub attire, caps, and shoe covers or clean shoes are required.	Hallways adjacent to the operating rooms, work rooms, and offices located in the interior of the suite
Restricted	Full scrub attire and mask are necessary.	Operating rooms, scrub areas, and the clean core area, if any

tively costly because of the wasted space involved in providing separate corridors and access to them.

For personnel traffic flow, the inpatient or ambulatory surgical suite is usually divided into three zones: the unrestricted or semipublic area, the semirestricted area, and the restricted area (Table 11.2). Personnel can move freely among all three zones if they are appropriately attired. After leaving the suite, however, reentry should be permitted only through the locker room areas, where some or all items of scrub apparel may have to be changed.

Patients usually enter the suite through the public or unrestricted zone and may wait in a holding area where some preoperative assessment and care, such as hair removal, may take place. As patients enter the semirestricted area, their hair is usually covered with a bouffant disposable cap or some other method of containment to minimize particulate shedding during surgery. Patients are in the semirestricted zone only briefly, usually only during transport to the operating room. Patients are not asked to don masks when entering the restricted zone—the operating room. Masks would hinder access to the face and airway and might increase the patients' anxiety, outweighing any small benefit in minimizing bacterial contamination. Masks prevent the spread of respiratory droplets, which usually travel less than 10 feet even with forced exhalation. By keeping the sterile setup well away from the head of the OR bed until after patients are draped, the nurse can minimize the possibility of contamination from their respiratory tract. After surgery, patients usually go to a postanesthesia care unit (PACU) by the same path taken to enter the operating room, through the semirestricted area. If the surgical suite has a clean core, patients are never allowed into this area.

Supply and equipment traffic is probably the most variable in the surgical setting. Separation of clean and dirty items is paramount. Clean and sterile supplies should be taken to the surgical setting on carts that are covered to prevent contamination of the wrappers by dust and respiratory droplets during transport through public corridors and elevators. Corrugated paper boxes and outside shipping containers should be removed before the items enter sterile storage or a patient care area because corrugated boxes generate and collect dust, and the shipping containers are contaminated by handling and transport on common carriers.

At the surgical setting entrance, the dust cover should be removed from the carts and discarded or reprocessed, depending on the material used. Supplies may then be moved to storage locations within the suite or, if a case cart system is in use, directly to the operating room. In a case cart system, all sterile supplies and instruments needed for a surgical procedure are collected and transported on a mobile cart. The cart is usually prepared in the central sterile processing department of the institution and sent to the surgical suite. The cart is taken into the operating room and, if of the appropriate design, may be used as the back table during surgery. At the end of the procedure, all dirty or used items are loaded back onto the cart and the cart is returned to the decontamination area of central sterile processing for item disposal or recycling.

Whether or not a case cart system is used, all soiled items leaving the operative setting must be contained to prevent cross-contamination. These soiled items never enter the clean core if the suite has one. In most instances, soiled items travel approximately the same pathway as clean items, except in reverse. As long as they are contained and are not left next to clean or sterile items for any length of time, this is no problem. Soiled items should not ride on elevators at the same time as patients, food, or clean and sterile supply items, even if enclosed in plastic bags. The turbulent air currents that accompany the rise and descent of the elevators can cause cross-contamination. A separate elevator for soiled material is ideal but seldom realized. If items such as linens and trash are stored in the suite for future pickup and disposal, the storage area should be enclosed and separate from corridors, lounges, and other storage areas.

In addition to traffic patterns, the operative team

must be alert to the need for handwashing. All the separation of clean and dirty breaks down if a nurse goes from the lunch table to opening sterile supplies without washing hands.

Equipment that comes from outside the suite must be damp-dusted with a clean cloth moistened with a germicide safe for use on the equipment. This should be done before the equipment enters the semirestricted zone of the suite. Items that cannot be cleaned adequately, such as compressed gas cylinders with flaking or chipped paint, should be covered with a drape or a cover specifically designed for that purpose before they are moved to the restricted area of the suite.

The use of tacky mats at suite entrances to remove debris from the soles of shoes and cart wheels is discouraged. While the mats collect noticeable amounts of debris, it is questionable whether this debris, already at floor level, represents any real threat of contamination if the surgical suite is properly cleaned each day.

PROCESSES USED IN THE PREPARATION OF SUPPLIES

In addition to control of the environment, the nurse must also be knowledgeable about the preparation and handling of supplies and instruments used during surgical procedures. In the past, these tasks were the sole responsibility of the perioperative nurse. Now, however, these duties are more often assigned to ancillary personnel. Supplies and instruments from the surgical suite are prepared by trained personnel in support areas such as materials management and central sterile processing.

This frees the nurse to spend more time with the patient and in planning patient care. Some nurses see this as a positive move because it allows broader implementation of the perioperative role without increasing staff. Others see this shift of responsibilities as negative, fearing that quality control of sterilization may be lessened. In general, however, quality control in a modern hospital's central processing department meets or exceeds that in the surgical suite. The nurse who cares for patients as well as prepares supplies must divide efforts between the two. Central processing's prime objective is to prepare supplies and equipment for use in patient care.

The division of responsibilities does not relieve the nurse of accountability for determining whether an item is safe for use. That accountability is shared with other healthcare workers but not diminished for the nurse. Therefore, the nurse must still have an understanding of sterilization and disinfection processing as well as storing and handling sterile supplies. In many non-hospital settings nurses may be involved in actual sterilization and disinfection procedures for operative procedures.

The following discussion is theoretical. Techniques and instructions for specific products or equipment are not discussed. If not familiar with an item, a nurse should always consult the operator manual for equipment and the label instructions on cleaning agents or solutions before use.

The preparation of clean and safe supplies is a series of tasks, not a single event. There are three commonly used processes: (1) decontamination; (2) disinfection; and (3) sterilization.

Decontamination

Decontamination literally means "to remove contamination." In health care it has two meanings: (1) to render an object safe for handling by removing infectious material, and (2) to clean an object as the first step leading to sterilization or disinfection. Decontamination assumes that an object has a high but unknown bioburden. Bioburden is the amount and resistance level of microbial contamination on an object at a given time. Blood, feces, sputum, and soil all represent substances that could produce a high bioburden on an object. It is not necessary for gross debris to be visible for the bioburden to be very high. Bacteria are invisible to the naked eye, and millions of them could be present. Decontamination lowers the number of organisms to a level that is assumed to be safe because the body's defense mechanisms can usually cope with small to moderate numbers of microorganisms. Processes for decontamination may use the same type of equipment as that for sterilization, but the goal is different—making the device safe for further handling by personnel who are not wearing any protective attire.

Disinfection

Disinfection is classically defined as the killing of all pathogens by a chemical, usually a liquid. Today, however, we recognize the ability of microorganisms to adapt, transform, and mutate quickly, so that an organism such as *Serratia marcescens*, which was once a nonpathogenic organism cultured in microbiology laboratories for use in demonstrations of bacterial dispersion, is now a highly feared cause of sepsis in hospitals. Therefore, the definition of a pathogen is too variable to rely on in preparing supplies for use in surgery. Spaulding and associates

TABLE 11.3.   Spaulding Classification: Disinfection Levels

Level	Effectiveness
High	Kills all vegetative forms of bacteria, all fungi, and all viruses; highly resistant bacterial spores may survive.
Intermediate	Kills most vegetative bacteria, including the tuberculosis bacillus. Kills most viruses, although an agent that claims to kill the tuberculosis bacillus may not necessarily be an intermediate-level virucide unless that claim is specifically made. Viruses differ in their susceptibility to chemical disinfectants.
Low	Kills most common vegetative pathogens, such as staphylococci and streptococci. May be used as a cleaning agent for inanimate objects.

(15) developed a method of classifying high, intermediate, and low levels of disinfection that has been widely adopted (Table 11.3). Disinfection is an inexact process, and so the definitions of each level are also imprecise. When referring to the preparation of supplies and instrumentation for use in surgery, high-level disinfection is usually meant unless otherwise indicated.

Sterilization

Sterilization is supposed to result in the absolute absence of microbial life on an item. Absolutes, however, are difficult to prove. In this instance, to prove that all life is absent on every object sterilized, each item would have to be cultured thoroughly, rendering it unusable, and the test would still be subject to error.

Therefore, science deals with the probability of an item being sterile. This probability is expressed as a sterility assurance level (SAL), or the chance of a single item being unsterile at the completion of a sterilization process. In general, items that are intended to contact compromised tissue or the vascular system are processed so that they have an SAL of 10^{-6}; that is, there is a 1 in 1,000,000 chance of any single item being unsterile. A lesser SAL of 10^{-3} (1 in 1,000) is allowed for items that will contact only the patient's or caregiver's skin, since the skin itself cannot be sterilized and thus immediately contaminates any topically applied device or drug.

Because sterilization deals with probability, everything that can affect it is relative. Two hemostats, one grossly soiled with blood, the other washed with soap and water, are placed in two identical steam sterilizers. Each sterilizer is run for the same time at the same temperature and steam quality. The time chosen is according to the manufacturer's instructions for sterilization of unwrapped stainless steel instruments. Both items have been through a "sterilization" process, but are both sterile according to the 10^{-6} probability level? No. The clean instrument can be considered sterile. The dirty instrument cannot. Why? Bacteria and other microbes vary, even within the same species, in their resistance to being killed, just as humans vary in their ability to withstand adversity. Studies have shown that, when subjected to heat or a chemical process, not all microorganisms die at once. Ninety percent die in a specific period of time that can be calculated for each species. If exposure is continued for a repetition of that period of time, 90 percent of those surviving the first time will be killed. Successive repetitions of this time will continue to reduce the surviving microbes by 90 percent each time. Thus when starting with 1 million organisms, the first time period will leave 100,000 still alive. The next exposure period will leave 10,000 alive; the next, 1000; the next, 100; the next, 10; the next 1. But 90 percent kill of one organism does not mathematically produce zero—or absolute sterility. It produces 0.1 organisms, or 10^{-1}. Obviously, there is no such thing as 0.1 bacterium, but this is where the sterility assurance level comes in. Just how safe is safe?: A 1 in 1 million chance of a survivor, or 0.0000001 bacterium, is the accepted answer for most items.

If there were 10 million organisms to start with (not a very big clump of bacteria) or if the sterilizing agent had to spend some of the exposure time penetrating organic or inorganic soil to get to the bacteria, as might be true for the dirty hemostat, there would be less than a 10^{-6} assurance level. Indeed, there might be one or two or more whole survivors if the organisms were highly resistant and well shielded.

In hospitals, with many different types of items being sterilized by several different methods, how are sterilizers set to achieve this magic number of 10^{-6}? The sterilizer manufacturers set them. They base the length of time for each cycle on how long it takes to produce a 10^{-6} assurance level for a highly resistant bacterial spore that has been dried to increase its resistance. Most vegetative bacteria and fungi are killed in seconds in a steam sterilization cycle and within minutes with ethylene oxide. Some viruses take longer, and bacterial spores take the longest of all. Bacterial spores are of primary concern to perioperative nurses because several organisms causing postoperative infection, including *Clostridium perfringens*, which causes gas gangrene, are spore formers.

Because of the variability of items being sterilized, there is a certain amount of overkill or safety level built into the sterilization cycle. Manufacturers state in their instructions that items must be clean prior to sterilization, however.

Decontamination, disinfection, and sterilization provide different levels of safety. Choosing the correct processing method for an item that will be used in surgery depends on several factors. Where and how will the item be used? What, if any, are the limitations placed on the processing because of the structure or composition of the item? What are the costs involved, both in materials and time, especially if alternatives are available?

There are some general guidelines. All items that contact blood, body fluids, tissue, or that may indirectly be contaminated by these must be decontaminated prior to further reprocessing. If the item is to be disposed of, this must be done in a manner that does not present danger to those handling the product, the general public health, or the environment. If an item is to contact the vascular system or penetrate the skin, it should be sterile. If the item is to contact mucous membranes or be used in respiratory therapy or anesthesia gas administration, it should be at least high-level disinfected. Items that will be implanted and left in the patient should be packaged appropriately and sterilized. Implants should be held in quarantine until the biological indicator (containing highly resistant, nonpathogenic bacterial spores) that was processed in the same load as the implant has been incubated according to the manufacturer's instructions and shown no evidence of growth, usually for a period of 48 hours.

As with all generalities, there are exceptions to these guidelines in some circumstances. For instance, there is a long-standing controversy over whether laparoscopes and arthroscopes, two types of telescopic apparatuses used to look into body spaces through small incisions, should be sterilized or disinfected. According to the above guidelines, both should be sterilized since they penetrate the skin and contact normally sterile tissue. Yet even the CDC indicates that, while sterilization is recommended for laparoscopes, high-level disinfection is considered adequate. Orthopedic surgeons are divided on the issue of arthroscope disinfection, even though the CDC lists arthroscopes as critical devices that should be sterile prior to patient use. Each institution must be governed by its own policy, based on the opinions of the administration, the surgeons, the infection-control officer, and the institution's liability insurance carrier.

In both cases, the key to safety with high-level disinfection is thorough cleaning prior to disinfection. Without this step, organisms other than a few rare bacterial spores may survive disinfection if they are shielded from the disinfecting agent.

Some materials and types of devices do not tolerate some sterilization or disinfection methods. Polyethylene plastic will not tolerate the heat needed for steam or dry heat sterilization, yet polypropylene can be steam sterilized. Teflon will tolerate radiation sterilization. Electrical appliances may not tolerate immersion in chemicals or the high humidity level in steam. Controls of some flexible fiberoptic endoscopes cannot be immersed in liquids for disinfection.

If an item is to be processed or reprocessed in the healthcare institution, the manufacturer should provide specific written instructions for cleaning, sterilizing, or disinfection. Sales representatives for that manufacturer can provide such instructions.

The cost of various sterilization and disinfection methods varies greatly. In general, steam sterilization is the least expensive and fastest method. Dry heat sterilization is not expensive, but it takes several hours and is suitable for only a few types of products. Ethylene oxide sterilization is relatively expensive and, although sterilization may take only 2 to 4 hours, the aeration process that must accompany it takes an additional 8 to 12 hours at least. Therefore, if an item can be steam sterilized, this is the method of choice.

TASKS IN THE PREPARATION OF SUPPLIES

Decontamination

Items contaminated with blood and body fluids represent a significant risk of infection to anyone handling them without proper personal protective equipment and knowledge of proper work practices. The U.S. Occupational Safety and Health Administration (OSHA) has established regulations to protect workers from blood-borne disease transmission on the job (16). Whether reusable or waste, soiled items should be handled only by persons wearing gloves, a fluid-resistant gown or apron with long sleeves, and, if splashing is possible, a high filtration efficiency face mask and eye protection, such as goggles or a face shield, until such time that the items no longer represent a possible source of infection to

handlers. Items should be contained for transport between the point of use and the point of decontamination and/or disposal so that the inadvertent cross-contamination does not occur, and the container must be marked to indicate that there are biohazardous items within.

For reusable items, adequate cleaning must occur before an item can be processed further. This cleaning can be accomplished by machine, by hand, or a combination of the two. Mechanical cleaning is preferred, since this will minimize handling and therefore minimize the risk of accidental inoculation of workers. Special care must be taken when handling any contaminated device that has sharp edges or parts that could puncture a glove, such as scissors, tissue forceps with teeth, skin hooks, curettes, or gouges. Most mechanical equipment combines cleaning with a process that will kill most or all of the microorganisms present.

Two methods of mechanical decontamination are currently being used: cleaning followed by a steam sterilization process, in machines called washer/sterilizers; and, cleaning followed by a hot water disinfection process, in machines called washer/disinfectors or washer/decontaminators. Both methods are designed to render an item safe to handle by healthy workers with intact skin on their hands and forearms. Some institutions prefer the absolute safety of a washer/sterilization process, but this method has several serious drawbacks. For example, the washing process within the chamber of the washer/sterilizer may not be efficient enough to clean instruments that are grossly soiled or on which the protein soil has dried. Therefore, precleaning is needed. This usually means rinsing the instruments by hand, and possibly using a brief soak in an enzyme-containing detergent to free up the protein soil. These tasks decrease productivity and can add to the risk of infection or injury for employees. If soil is not removed before or during the wash cycle of a washer/sterilizer, it becomes baked on during the sterilization phase, which uses saturated steam at temperatures of 132°C to 141°C (270° to 285°F), and is very difficult to remove. This baked-on soil will be safe to handle for workers, but not acceptable for patient care. Also, washer/sterilizers cost more to purchase than do washer/decontaminators.

With washer/decontaminators, it is possible that small populations of microorganisms may survive the process, but these are not generally sufficient to produce infection in a healthy host, such as most workers in hospitals. Washer/decontaminators do a better job of cleaning grossly soiled instruments, usually without the need for any precleaning by hand. Some units have an enzyme rinse or presoak built in. Once the items are washed, they are subjected to a sustained hot water rinse that varies in duration and temperature, depending upon the model of machine. However, water temperatures are always less than about 90.5°C (195°F). These machines are generally less costly. In today's cost- and risk-conscious healthcare environment, institutions must weigh the options for mechanical decontamination and choose the most appropriate method for their particular needs.

Not all items will tolerate the high temperatures, turbulent conditions, and total immersion involved in mechanical cleaning. For these devices, hand cleaning is the most appropriate. Hand cleaning may also be used as a backup, when mechanical means are not available. Proper protective attire is a must any time items are being hand washed. This should include face mask and eye protection, since splashing can occur. To reduce the risk of splashing and the creation of aerosols, the item being cleaned should be held low in the sink or basin being used. Brushes should be kept under water when in use.

No matter which method of cleaning and decontamination is used, the choice of an appropriate detergent is critical to the process. The detergent must be able to remove the type of soil found on the item, and, at the same time, not damage the item. Protein soil is best removed by detergents that have a pH in the alkaline range (above 7.0). Mineral soils are best removed by acid detergents (below 7.0 pH). In general, it is best to avoid extremes in pH of cleaning solutions, especially when cleaning stainless steel or other hand-held metal surgical instruments. A pH of between 5 and 10 is generally satisfactory, but specific device manufacturer's instructions should be followed. Very acidic or alkaline solutions can damage the inert layer that keeps stainless steel instruments from corroding. Contact with chlorine and other solutions containing chloride ions, such as saline and blood, can also damage stainless steel instruments.

Inspection of all decontaminated devices is essential, both to ensure cleanliness and to assess whether the item still functions as intended. Items that are found to be soiled should be returned to the decontamination area for further cleaning.

An alternative to further hand cleaning for these devices is the ultrasonic cleaner. This machine uses high-frequency sound waves to dislodge debris from the surface of objects. When combined with the appropriate detergent, it is an excellent adjunct to other forms of mechanical or hand washing for diffi-

cult-to-clean objects. Ultrasound has no microbicidal properties but does provide effective removal of fine soil. Instruments must be free of gross soil, as this will interfere with the transmission of the sonic energy. If the ultrasonic cleaner is used prior to exposure to a decontamination process such as a washer/sterilizer or washer/decontaminator, the aerosols created by the action of this machine can present a health risk to any workers in the area not wearing full protective attire (including face mask and eye protection). If used after decontamination, the aerosols will not be hazardous but could contaminate already sterilized items with non-fluid-proof packaging by slightly wetting the wrapper and creating a path for bacterial migration into the package. Therefore, the ultrasonic cleaner should be located in the decontamination area, no matter when it is used in the preparation process. After ultrasonic cleaning instruments should be rinsed to remove debris. Otherwise the material will once again adhere to the instruments. Not all surgical instruments can be placed in the ultrasonic cleaner; some manufacturers of microsurgical instruments advise against it. Instruments that have plated metal and those with telescopic lenses should not be placed in the ultrasonic cleaner.

The care of endoscopes is different from care of other types of surgical instrumentation. These delicate devices, whether rigid or flexible, require special handling. Often they are cleaned and disinfected/sterilized within the surgical suite. As with all other devices, these must be thoroughly cleaned, rinsed, and dried prior to disinfection or sterilization. The manufacturer should be consulted for recommended care, and only individuals trained in these methods should prepare these devices.

Packaging

After decontamination, the second step in sterilization and disinfection is packaging the material, if necessary. Items that are to be disinfected by liquid chemicals do not require packaging. All items undergoing sterilization, however, require some type of packaging, whether they are actually wrapped or are sterilized in an open pan. The packaging selected must be appropriate to the sterilization method and to the conditions of storage and handling that the item will encounter prior to use.

Packaging used for steam sterilization must allow rapid penetration of steam and rapid air removal. For surgical instruments, packaging begins with selection of an appropriately sized tray with holes in the bottom to allow for steam and air movement and drainage of condensate. Next, thought should be given to how the items will be arranged in the tray and how they will be kept in order. Heavy items should be on the bottom or separate from more delicate items. There are many devices on the market to hold, string, clip, or arrange surgical instruments in a specific order, even if the tray is tipped. These can save effort and avoid exasperation on the part of the scrub person asked to set up for the next procedure in 5 minutes or less. Some institutions line the bottom of the instrument tray with a woven fabric towel or other highly absorbent material before beginning to place the instruments. This helps to absorb condensate formed on the instruments during the steam sterilization cycle and speeds drying.

The weight of the instruments should be evenly spread throughout the tray. There is no set limit for the maximum weight of an instrument set. The primary issues in determining how many and what instruments to place in a single tray are (1) the amount of total metal mass (weight) and whether it is evenly spread out or concentrated in a few heavy instruments, and (2) the ease of drainage of condensate formed as steam gives up its energy to the metal to heat the load to sterilizing temperature at the beginning of the cycle and collapses back to water. Sets with too much or too dense metal mass cannot be efficiently dried at the end of the cycle and may come out of the sterilizer still damp or wet, allowing undetected bacterial strike-through and contamination. Small, dense sets may have as many problems as large, heavy sets. In general, sets weighing 17 to 25 pounds are easier to lift and carry.

Pans, basin sets, or other items that can be nested should have a layer of porous material between each layer to facilitate steam penetration. Endoscopes that can be steam sterilized and some microsurgery instruments come in special containers to prevent dislodging or inadvertent crushing should a heavier object be placed on top of them.

Textiles and small items require no tray or pan for steam sterilization. Textiles are folded so that they are ready to use, that is, gowns are folded with the inside out so they can be donned without contamination. Bundles containing several different items are arranged in the order of use, and the warp direction of one item is placed perpendicular to the warp of the next item to facilitate steam penetration and air removal.

Textile bundles must be packaged loosely enough to allow air to leave and steam to easily penetrate all layers yet tight enough to maintain their shape during handling. For cotton and cotton/polyester blends, the maximum density of any textile bundle should not exceed 7.2 pounds per cubic foot, or steam penetration may not occur. Since density is derived by calculating weight divided by width × height × length, textile bundles should not exceed 12 × 12 × 20 inches and weigh no more than 12 pounds. As with instrument sets, small, dense bundles will be as difficult to process as large, oversize bundles.

Many types of woven reusable and nonwoven disposable flat wrappers and peel-open pouches are available today. Whatever the wrap chosen, it should be permeable to the sterilant and resist tearing and puncture. If seals are involved, they should not reseal once opened so that tampering or damage can be detected. The wrapper must be resistant to penetration by airborne bacteria and dust. It should have minimal or no lint, and ideally, if not totally impervious to liquid penetration, the material should discolor or otherwise indicate that it has been inadvertently wet and therefore contaminated, since liquid penetration carries microorganisms with it. The material should be in ready supply, and the cost should be in line with the item's perceived value to the institution.

Rigid sterilization containers have become quite popular. They take the place of wrappers and offer increased physical protection from damage to their contents. Although the initial cost of acquiring such systems may be quite high, the decreased cost per cycle (because no wrapper is used) makes them cost effective in the long run. There are containers made of anodized aluminum, and heat-resistant plastics and stainless steel are also available. The increased weight and steam penetration characteristics may require adjustments in sterilization cycle timing and longer drying times.

Packaging items for ethylene oxide sterilization is not much different than for steam sterilization. The wrapping material must be ethylene oxide compatible and must allow gas penetration and elution. Nylon and aluminum foil are not acceptable. Selection of packaging material involves the same considerations and desirable characteristics discussed under steam sterilization.

For dry heat sterilization, packaging materials should be selected that will not be damaged by high heat—160°C (320°F)—for long periods of time. This usually means metal or glass only. Textiles should be avoided since they will char and burn.

Sterilization

The third step in the preparation of supplies is the actual sterilization or disinfection. Four methods of

TABLE 11.4. Method of Assuring Sterilization and Safe Use of Medical Devices

Classification	Example	Method	Comment
Objects that enter tissue or the vascular system	Surgical instruments and devices, trays, and sets	1. Thoroughly clean objects and wrap or package for sterilization. 2. Follow manufacturer's instructions for use of each sterilizer or use recommended protocol. 3. Monitor time-temperature charts. 4. Use commercial spore preparation to monitor sterilizers. 5. Inspect package for integrity and for exposure of sterility indicator before use. 6. Use before maximum safe storage time has expired if applicable.	Sterilization processes are designed to have a wide margin of safety. If spores are not killed, the sterilizer should be checked for proper use and function; if spore tests remain positive, discontinue use of the sterilizer until properly serviced. Maximum safe storage time of items processed in the hospital varies according to type of package or wrapping material(s) used, the conditions of storage, and amount of handling. Follow manufacturer's instructions for use and storage times.

sterilization are commonly used in hospitals and other healthcare institutions: steam under pressure, ethylene oxide, dry heat, and liquid chemical. A fifth type, widely used in industry for medical devices, is irradiation. Two common methods of disinfection used in hospitals are liquid chemical and pasteurization. Each of these is briefly discussed from the point of view of what the perioperative nurse needs to know.

Steam Sterilization

Saturated steam is placed under pressure so that its temperature in the closed sterilizing chamber will rise. The synergistic action of the moisture and temperature on the microorganism produces death through coagulation of protein. Direct contact with the steam is needed to produce assured sterility. Thus any items with ratchets or with easily removable parts should be processed in the open or disassembled position. While some vegetative bacteria might be killed just through dry heating at the temperatures involved with steam sterilization, others, and certainly bacterial spores, might survive without the synergy of the water and heat at points where metal is tightly approximated to metal, as in a closed hemostat.

There are two basic types of steam sterilizers commonly used. The first of these is the gravity-displacement sterilizer. This type of unit relies on gravity to remove air, which is heavier than steam, from the sterilizer load to allow steam penetration. Saturated steam does not mix with air, and air acts as an insulator to prevent the heating and moisture contact necessary for sterilization. Thus items placed in a gravity-displacement sterilizer must be loaded in such a way as to aid air removal. Textile drape bundles or other bulky, porous packages are placed on end or on their sides. Basin sets and other items that could hold water are placed so that water runs out. Once the cycle begins, the air "runs out" as if it were water. Packs containing metal are not placed above textile packs because condensation at the end of the cycle when the door is opened could drip onto and contaminate the textile packs. If the chamber is overloaded, air will remain trapped in some packages, resulting in sterilization failure.

Once the chamber is loaded, the door is closed and the chamber becomes a pressure vessel. Steam enters the chamber through the upper rear and hits a baffle that disperses it. As steam enters, it displaces the heavier air, which exits through a drain in the bottom front of the chamber near the door. In this drain, there is a temperature sensor reflected in a temperature gauge or recorder at the front of the sterilizer. The pressure inside the chamber is also monitored and may be recorded. As steam continues to enter, all of the air is eventually forced out, if the load is properly arranged. The pressure and the temperature gauges continue to rise. The pressure is necessary to raise the temperature of the steam vapor. At sea level, saturated steam under 15 pounds per square inch pressure according to the gauge (psig), which measures the pressure above the ambient atmospheric pressure, has a temperature of 121°C (250°F).

Commercially available steam sterilizers, by common convention, are set to run at either 121°C or 132°C. At 132°C, the pressure gauge at sea level

TABLE 11.5.   Time and Temperature Relationships for Steam Sterilization

Type of Sterilizer	Temperature	Load	Exposure Time (min)
Gravity-displacement	121°C (250°F)	Wrapped, mixed	15 plus drying time
	132°C (270°F)	Unwrapped, nonporous only	3
		Unwrapped, some porous, or	10
		implants	10 plus drying time
		Wrapped	
Hivac	132°C (170°F)	Unwrapped	4
		Wrapped	4 plus drying time

should read 27 psig. Atmospheric pressure decreases with altitude. To compensate for the lower initial gauge setting, the maximum gauge reading must be increased by 0.5 psig for every 1000 feet of altitude above sea level. Thus a steam sterilizer running at 132°C in Denver (altitude 5280 feet) must have a pressure gauge reading of 29.5 psig to reach the desired temperature.

The second type of steam sterilizer speeds up the evacuation of air by injecting steam and then drawing a partial vacuum in the chamber several times at the beginning of the cycle, which removes the air and heats the load. This type of steam sterilizer, known as a hivac (high prevacuum), is slightly more forgiving of errors in loading some items, but the same rules should be used. In both types, the sterilization cycle has the same elements: the come-up time, during which air is eliminated and steam penetrates the load; the exposure time, which is the period necessary to assure lethality at the 10^{-6} level; and the come-down time, which involves reintroduction of air to the load. If the load contains wrapped articles, drying time is added on before the door can be opened.

Articles can be processed either wrapped or unwrapped in either type of sterilizer at either temperature. Unwrapped articles are most commonly sterilized in either the gravity-displacement type or hivac type at 132°C (270°F). This is referred to as flash, or emergency, sterilization. It is frequently used for unsterile items needed quickly and for instruments that are dropped or otherwise contaminated. These instruments must be cleaned if they are to be sterilized. In the past, prosthetic devices such as orthopedic implants were often flash sterilized. This practice is now strongly discouraged because of the short exposure time. Cycle duration for steam sterilization varies with temperature and with the type of air evacuation used. The come-up time for the hivac is almost instantaneous (Table 11.5).

The advantages of steam sterilization are that it is inexpensive, usually readily available, reliable, free of toxic residue, generally safe to use, and fast. The

disadvantage of steam sterilization is that not all items can tolerate the high moisture, pressure, and temperature necessary.

Steam sterilization is monitored by periodically placing a specially constructed pack containing absorbent reusable towels, or their equivalent, in the bottom front of the sterilizer. This pack also contains dried, live bacterial spores of the *Bacillus stearothermophilus* species in a known concentration. Commercially available spore strips or vials are usually used. This particular species has demonstrated high resistance to destruction by moist heat. The pack is run through an appropriate sterilization cycle for the type of sterilizer and temperature selected. The spore strip or vial is retrieved under aseptic conditions and incubated along with a nonexposed control strip or vial from the same lot number, according to the biological indicator manufacturer's instructions. It should be noted that *B. stearothermophilus* likes high temperatures and should not be incubated in the customary 37°C (98.6°F) clinical incubator. The sterilization cycle is said to be efficacious if there is no growth of *B. stearothermophilus* in the test culture and growth is present in the control. The first, presumptive reading is usually done at 24 to 48 hours incubation; however, 7 to 10 days may be necessary to make sure there is no growth, since some spores may be alive but slow to recover. Biological monitoring is recommended at least once a week for every steam sterilizer and in each load containing implantable devices.

In addition to biological indicators, other process controls are often used with steam sterilizers. These include a recording chart or digital readout recorder that registers maximum temperature and duration for each cycle. That chart is usually on the upper front of the sterilizer and requires frequent changing of the chart paper. Various chemical indicators are also used to monitor temperature, moisture, and time. Not all indicators measure all values and not all are equally accurate. It is important to read the instructions that come with the indicator and be familiar with the color changes or other signs to be expected. With some chemical indicators, it takes a great deal of practice to produce reliable readings. Chemical indicators show that an item has been processed. They do not prove that conditions necessary for sterility were achieved.

Hivac sterilizers are checked daily with a Bowie-Dick-type test for adequate vacuum for air removal. Commercially available sheets have various patterns of heat-sensitive ink on them. One sheet is contained in a specially constructed pack of woven fabric towels placed in the center of an otherwise empty sterilizer. Single-use test packs are also commercially available. The object of the test is to check for uniformity of color change on the test sheet. Lack of uniformity indicates a problem with the vacuum portion of the cycle. The Bowie-Dick-type test does not in any way measure sterility and should not be confused with chemical indicators that monitor one or more of the conditions necessary for sterilization to occur.

Ethylene Oxide (EO) Sterilization

This highly poisonous gas is used under controlled circumstances to produce microbial death. Ethylene oxide sterilizers resemble the pressure vessels used for steam. Sterilization generally occurs at temperatures ranging from room temperature to about 60°C (140°F). Four interrelated factors are necessary to produce sterility using EO: gas concentration, temperature, relative humidity of 30 to 80 percent, and time. Temperature is inversely related to time, so the lower the temperature, the longer the exposure needed. Gas concentration varies with the type of sterilizer used and also has an impact on the exposure time. Adequate relative humidity in the load is vital since desiccated organisms can be highly resistant to EO penetration of the cell wall or cellular membrane. Because of the great variety of sizes and types of EO sterilizers available and the lack of standardization, it is not possible to give time guidelines for the sterilization cycle. Manufacturers' instructions should be followed.

Precautions must be taken when using EO because it is a highly toxic gas that can pollute the working environment. It also leaves residuals in the products sterilized that can be harmful. The current Occupational Safety and Health Agency (OSHA) limit for exposure to EO is 1 part per million (ppm) as an average exposure over an 8-hour period. Long-term inhalation and skin exposure to EO have been implicated as being dangerous to human health.

Operator exposure during EO sterilization can occur at two times. If the gas is not properly vented directly to the outside, exposure may occur when EO is eliminated from the sterilizer chamber. If there is not a continuous, fresh, filtered, air-purge cycle in the unit, exposure may occur when the sterilizer is opened. Hospitals have EO sterilization equipment with dedicated exhaust ventilation systems to reduce worker exposure to a safer level. To minimize exposure when opening an EO sterilizer, it is important to follow the manufacturer's instructions closely. These units differ greatly in determining when the lowest possible concentration in the chamber is reached and in what direction the gas will exit the chamber, which depends on its temperature relative to the ambient temperature in the room. Exposure to EO can also occur when changing gas supply cylinders. Special precautions must be taken to avoid contact with liquid or vaporized EO during this process.

The threshold for detection of the odor of EO is approximately 700 ppm. If an operator smells a strange odor around the EO sterilizer or aerator, the area should be evacuated immediately and the smell reported to appropriate administrative officials. Most hospitals have automatic detection equipment that alerts workers to leaks well below the odor threshold.

Because EO penetrates all porous materials and time is required for it to dissipate, all items sterilized by EO must be aerated before use. The method of choice is to use a filtered, heated forced-air aeration cabinet vented directly to the outside atmosphere. The length of aeration time depends on the nature and composition of the material being sterilized and the type of packaging material used. It is not possible to provide even general time guidelines because of the nature and variety of items that are sterilized. Some material may require in excess of 24 hours of forced-air aeration. The manufacturer of the device being sterilized as well as the manufacturer of the sterilizer and aerator can be consulted for guidance.

If an aeration cabinet is used, the chamber should not be opened until aeration for all items is complete. To do otherwise may expose the person opening the cabinet to unsafe concentrations of EO. If some items require brief aeration and some require longer aeration, ideally they should be separated and sterilized in different loads or aerated in different units. Sorting a load after the sterilization cycle can expose the worker to high levels of EO. If more than one aeration cabinet is available, one alternative is to arrange the load by aeration time, putting each aerator load in a separate metal basket or tray that can be picked up quickly and moved to the appropriate aerator without handling each package.

There may be times when a physician insists on using an instrument or device that is not fully aerated or is in a load that is not fully aerated. This request should not be honored unless everyone involved, with full knowledge and consent, believes that the risk to a patient of not having the device is worth the risk to the worker who must retrieve the device. Hospitals have a responsibility to both patients and personnel to make sure that there is a sufficient supply of such critical devices so that this situation does not arise.

In addition to the EO itself as a toxic residue, two other chemicals can form during the sterilization process. Both are toxic and neither is diminished by aeration. Ethylene glycol forms when EO contacts water. Ethylchlorhydrin forms when EO contacts water and available chloride ions. The key to preventing the formation of both byproducts is to eliminate free-standing water from the load. Thus all items placed in an EO sterilizer should be dried so that no visible water droplets are present before the item is packaged.

Ethylene oxide is an effective sterilant for medical devices. Items must be clean prior to sterilization because dried crystalline debris can effectively block the penetration of EO and allow even vegetative organisms to survive.

The efficacy of the EO sterilization is monitored using live spores of the species *Bacillus subtilis* or *B. globigii*, which have demonstrated resistance to EO. As with steam sterilization, the biological indicator is run in a regular load and then incubated and compared to a nonexposed control. Because of the high degree of possible variability in conditions within the EO sterilizer, each load should be monitored.

Chemical process indicators for EO are available. Some monitor aeration as well.

Dry Heat Sterilization

Dry heat sterilization is seldom used now in hospitals except in the laboratory for glassware. Dry heat at temperatures of 160°C (320°F) produces microbial death by incineration in approximately 2 hours after the item reaches the required temperature. Dry heat sterilization is the method of choice for powders and oils that cannot be sterilized by steam or that retain EO or its byproducts, if these items must be sterilized. Most powders and oils that might be required are commercially available in a sterile state.

Chemical Sterilization

Some chemicals that can produce high-level disinfection are also capable of sterilizing. They are sporicidal if the exposure time is extended. For example, 2% alkaline glutaraldehyde produces sterility in 10 hours. Obviously this requires immersion of the clean, dry device in the chemical for an extended length of time. Few devices will tolerate this repeatedly. Newer technology, using liquids such as peracetic acid or vapors such as hydrogen peroxide, have shortened the exposure time considerably and are more compatible with the delicate devices sterilized in this manner. After sterilization, the sterilant must be removed from the device. For liquids, this means rinsing with sterile water. This rinsing may be accomplished by hand or as part of a mechanical cycle in a machine. The wet item must be moved to the point of use without inadvertent contamination. Items sterilized by hydrogen peroxide in its vapor state undergo a brief detoxification period in which the hydrogen peroxide is broken down to water and oxygen. Chemical sterilization is more expensive than steam sterilization. Furthermore, for most methods of chemical sterilization, there is no means of testing the efficacy of the process without destroying or contaminating the items being sterilized. There are currently no biological indicators for liquid chemical sterilization or disinfection. Chemical indicators that monitor the concentration of active ingredients are available for some solutions. There is a chemical indicator available for hydrogen peroxide vapor.

Radiation Sterilization

Radiation sterilization is used widely in the medical device industry but is not currently used in hospitals in this country. Briefly, it involves the use of gamma ray or electron beam exposure of a product, its package, and usually the shipping container for a specific amount of time so that a carefully calculated dose of radiation is administered. The necessary dose may be determined by government standards and a careful analysis of the known bioburden of the product at the conclusion of manufacture and packaging.

The medical device industry maintains careful control and records of personnel and environment. Protective clothing, special air-handling systems, traffic regulation, and personnel monitoring control bioburden much more effectively than can be done in the diverse environments of healthcare facilities. Thus exact computations of bioburden are possible in industry.

The radiation passes right through the entire product, killing organisms by altering and interfering with metabolism and nucleic acid synthesis. Radiation sterilization leaves no radioactive residue. Not all materials can withstand radiation sterilization because the process may alter chemical structure.

So much is known about the response of certain materials to radiation that some of these substances are used as dosimeters to measure the amount of radiation received by the load. Thus, although biological indicators may be run, the product is released for sale based on the dosimetry readings before biological monitoring can be read.

Radiation sterilization requires special physical facilities and a large degree of technical support. Because of the high cost of initiating such a system, it is not likely to be used by individual healthcare facilities.

Disinfection

Not all items require sterilization prior to use. Some procedures do not require sterile instruments, only disinfected instruments. These procedures usually involve entry through a body orifice, such as the mouth or vagina, that cannot be washed and prepared in the same vigorous manner as intact skin. Thus the operative area remains grossly contaminated with the patient's own organisms. The general principles of asepsis are still applied in these procedures to minimize the introduction of exogenous microorganisms. Because the body's defense mechanisms are less altered than in procedures involving incision through the skin, however, high-level disinfection is considered adequate preparation for smooth, hard-surface devices that can be cleaned readily, such as endoscopes.

Anesthesia and respiratory therapy devices may be a source of cross-contamination if they are reused for several patients. The microorganisms of concern here are vegetative bacteria, fungi, and some viruses, but not bacterial spores. Therefore cleaning followed by high-level disinfection after each patient use should be adequate protection.

Chemical Disinfection
A clean, dry item is immersed in a solution that produces microbial death in a reasonable period of time. The U.S. Environmental Protection Agency (EPA) requires manufacturers who make sterilization or disinfection claims for their products to register with the EPA and submit data in support of these claims. If found acceptable, the product is given a registration number as a sterilant, a disinfectant, or both. This number is to be displayed on the product label. When selecting a chemical disinfectant, look for the EPA registration number and read the label claims carefully to make certain that it is a high-level disinfectant that will kill everything but bacterial spores.

The most commonly used chemical disinfectant is a 2% solution of glutaraldehyde. Halogenated compounds such as sodium hypochlorite (household bleach) are also effective if used in the proper concentration, as are some iodophors. Quaternary ammonium compounds are not acceptable high-level disinfectants and should not be used.

Even though these solutions may disinfect, all chemicals are not safe for all devices. For instance, soaking stainless steel instruments in sodium hypochlorite will damage their surfaces. Therefore manufacturers' recommendations should be followed in selecting chemical disinfectants. Precautions and contraindications on the disinfectant label should be read to determine if the solution is compatible with the type of device to be disinfected.

Chemical disinfection usually takes 20 to 30 minutes of soaking. Much longer periods are required for sterilization. Some people refer to the short exposure period as "cold sterilization," but this is a misuse of the word sterilization.

As with all other processes, disinfection requires that instruments or other devices be clean before immersion. Chemicals require direct contact to kill, and dirt and organic debris can effectively shield microorganisms from the effects of the disinfectant. Devices should also be dry when placed in the disinfectant to avoid further dilution of the chemical by the addition of water.

After the appropriate soaking time has elapsed, the device must be rinsed adequately. Sterile distilled water should be used to avoid reintroducing microorganisms such as those found in tap water. Merely dipping the instrument in a basin of water may not be adequate rinsing, especially if the device has a lumen. Disinfectants are potentially toxic chemicals, and residue may cause injury to the patient's tissues when the device is used. If the device is not going to be used immediately, it should be dried thoroughly prior to storage. Water in the lumen or on the surface can be a suitable environment for bacterial growth over several hours.

Reusable devices should be washed and disinfected immediately after each use to minimize the possibility of environmental contamination. If a device is not to be reused immediately and will be stored for more than a few hours, it should be disinfected again prior to use, if the procedure calls for high-level disinfection. This is because bacterial spores not killed by the chemical could return to the vegetative state and multiply in this interim. Also, it is difficult to package and store an item aseptically after disinfection with any degree of assurance that no contamination occurred during drying and wrapping.

Physical Disinfection
Physical disinfection involves boiling or pasteurization. Boiling is seldom used, because if an item can tolerate that temperature and moisture level, steam sterilization is a better option. Pasteurization is the process of heating the device in water to temperatures at or above 71°C (160°F) and holding the de-

vice there for a period of time, depending on the temperature, usually 15 to 30 minutes. The process is modeled after that used to treat milk and other liquid foods. It kills vegetative bacteria, the tuberculosis bacillus, some viruses, and some fungi. It is not truly high-level disinfection, but more accurately, intermediate-level. The process is suitable for some respiratory therapy devices and anesthesia masks and tubing that does not directly penetrate deep into the airway. Special equipment is used to accomplish pasteurization. Since the process involves nothing but heated water, no rinsing is necessary, but items must be dried before storage in a manner that will not recontaminate them. Forced-air-heated cabinets are available for this purpose.

Handling and Storage

Although disinfected items cannot be stored for any length of time and still be considered free of everything but bacterial spores, wrapped materials that have been sterilized are stored for long periods and still considered sterile. The safe storage of sterile items depends on four factors: whether or not the items was sterile initially; the type of wrapper or barrier used; the amount and type of handling the product receives after sterilization; and the actual conditions of storage. The first factor is obvious but often forgotten. The second factor, the wrapper, deserves discussion. A package wrapper should be resistant to contamination from any condition it may encounter during the handling and storage process. This may include airborne contamination through passive settling of particles. If the package may encounter rough handling, the wrap should resist tearing and the entry of airborne organisms through forced compression and release. If the item may encounter moisture, even as little as the perspiration of workers' hands, the wrapper should be resistant to this.

No one type of wrapper or packaging suits all needs and conditions. The more controlled the handling and storage process, the less concern for the wrapper. Most hospitals, however, do not have well-controlled processes that strictly monitor the number of times an item is subjected to events that might cause contamination. As a general rule, a sterile package should be handled as few times as absolutely necessary between sterilization and use. Everyone handling or transporting the package must be aware of any condition that might lead to contamination. If such a condition is encountered, the package should be regarded as of doubtful sterility and not used.

Storage of sterile items for longer than one or two days should be in closed cabinets to minimize dust accumulation. If open-shelf storage is used, the packaging material should be resistant to dust penetration and capable of having dust accumulation removed before the package is opened. Otherwise, dust from the surface can contaminate the contents during opening.

Wire mesh shelves are preferred to solid shelves to minimize dust accumulation. Shelving should be at least 10 inches from the floor to prevent splashing during floor cleaning. If open shelving is used, the shelves should be at least 2 inches from the wall and allow 18 inches from the tops of items to the ceiling to provide adequate air circulation. Sterile items should be stored separately from clean items and away from soiled or used items.

There are no standard solutions for the problem of shelf life of a particular item. Shelf life is the result of the interrelationship of the four conditions identified earlier. A sterile item can be contaminated at any point after the sterilization chamber is opened. Only planning and awareness by all personnel involved can guarantee delivery of sterile items at the moment needed for patient care. Each institution must set its own guidelines for shelf life, both for products sterilized within the institution and for those purchased sterile, based on the conditions existing in that facility. A package that is sterilized and wrapped in a sealed impervious wrapper will remain sterile forever if the package is not damaged or opened. Shelf life is event-related, not time-related.

The preparation of supplies for use in surgery involves careful attention to cleaning, packaging, sterilizing or disinfecting, and handling and storage. Inadequate care in any process invalidates the whole sequence. The nurse working in the operating room must work with other healthcare personnel involved in these tasks, sharing responsibility and accountability with them for the ultimate delivery of products that are safe for the patient and further the outcome of freedom from infection.

References

1. Centers for Disease Control. "Recommendations for preventing transmission of HIV in healthcare settings." *Morbid Mortal Weekly Rep* 36(suppl 2S):1S–18S, 1987.
2. Centers for Disease Control. "Update: Universal precautions for prevention of transmission of human immunodeficiency virus, hepatitis B virus, and other bloodborne pathogens in healthcare settings." *Morbid Mortal Weekly Rep* 37:377–382, 387–388, 1988.
3. Centers for Disease Control. "Recommendations for preventing transmission of human immunodefi-

ciency virus and hepatitis B virus to patients during exposure-prone invasive procedures." *Morbid Mortal Weekly Rep* 40 (RR-8):1–9, 1991.

4. Taylor, G. J., Mikell,.F. L., Moses, H. W., et al. "Determinants of hospital charges for coronary artery bypass surgery: The economic consequences of postoperative complications." *Am J Cardiol* 65:309–313, 1990.

5. Boyce, J. M., Potter-Bynoe, G., and Dziobek, L. "Hospital reimbursement patterns among patients with surgical wound infections following open heart surgery." *Infect Control Hosp Epidemiol* 11:89–93, 1990.

6. Garner, J. S., Jarvis, W. R., Emori, T. G., Horan, T. C., and Hughes, J. M. "CDC definitions for nosocomial infections, 1988." *Am J Infect Control* 16:128–140, 1988.

7. Howard, J. M., Barker, W. F., Culbertson, W. R., et al. "Postoperative wound infections: The influence of ultraviolet irradiation of the operating room and various other factors." *Ann Surg* 160 (suppl):1–192, 1964.

8. Haley, R. W., Culver, D. H., Morgan, W. M., White, J. W., Emori, T. G., and Hooten, T. M. "Identifying patients at high risk of surgical wound infection: A simple multivariate index of patient susceptibility and wound contamination." *Am J Epidemiol* 121:206–215, 1985.

9. Culver, D. H, Horan, T. C., Gaynes, R. P., et al. "Surgical wound infection rates by wound class, operative procedure, and patient risk index." *Am J Med* 91 (suppl 3B):152–157, 1991.

10. Nichols, R. L. "Surgical wound infection." *Am J Med* 91 (suppl 3B):54–64, 1991.

11. Schaberg, D. R., Culver D. H., and Gaynes, R. P. "Major trends in the microbial etiology of nosocomial infection." *Am J Med* 91 (suppl 3B):72–75, 1991.

12. Emori, T. G., Culver, D. H., Horan, T. C., et al. "National nosocomial infections surveillance system (NNIS): Description of surveillance methodology." *Am J Infect Control* 19:19–35, 1991.

13. Decker, M. D., and Schaffner, W. "Changing trends in infection control and hospital epidemiology." *Infect Dis Clin N Am* 3:671–682, 1989.

14. U.S. Department of Labor, Occupational Safety and Health Administration. "Occupational exposure to bloodborne pathogens: Proposed rule and notice of hearings." *Fed Register* 54:23042–23139, 1989.

15. Favero, M. S. "Chemical disinfection of medical and surgical materials." S. Block, ed. *Disinfection, Sterilization, and Preservation* 3rd ed., pp. 472–477. Philadelphia: Lea and Febiger, 1983.

16. U.S. Department of Labor, Occupational Safety and Health Administration. *Bloodborne Pathogens.* 29 CFR, Part 1910.1030. Washington, D.C.: OSHA, 1991.

SUGGESTED READINGS

American Institute of Architects, Committee on Architecture for Health Care. *Guidelines for Construction and Equipment of Hospital and Medical Facilities.* Washington, D.C.: AIA Press, 1987.

Association for the Advancement of Medical Instrumentation. *AAMI Standards and Recommended Practices. Volume 2: Sterilization.* Arlington, VA: AAMI, 1992.

Association.for the Advancement of Medical Instrumentation. *Good Hospital Practice: Ethylene Oxide Gas—Ventilation Recommendations and Safe Use.* Arlington, VA: AAMI, 1993.

Association for the Advancement of Medical Instrumentation. *Good Hospital Practice: Ethylene Oxide Sterilization and Sterility Assurance.* Arlington, VA: AAMI, 1993.

Association for the Advancement of Medical Instrumentation. *Sterilization and Sterility Assurance in Office-Based, Ambulatory-Care Medical and Dental Facilities.* Arlington, VA: AAMI, 1992.

Block, Seymour S. *Disinfection, Sterilization, and Preservation* 4th ed. Philadelphia: Lea and Febiger, 1991.

Craven, D. E., Steger, K. A., and Barber, T. W. "Preventing nosocomial pneumonia: State of the art and perspectives for the 1990s." *Am J Med* 91 (suppl 3B):44–53, 1991.

Garibaldi, R. A., Cushing, D., and Lerer, T. "Risk factors for postoperative infection." *Am J Med* 91 (suppl 3B):158–163, 1991.

Gross, P. A. "Striving for benchmark infection rates: Progress in control for patient mix." *Am J Med* 91 (suppl 3B):16–20, 1991.

Haley, R. W. "Measuring the costs of nosocomial infections: Methods for estimating economic burden on the hospital." *Am J Med* 91 (suppl 3B):32–38, 1991.

Haley, R. W. "Nosocomial infections in surgical patients: Developing valid measures of intrinsic patient risk." *Am J Med* 91 (suppl 3B):145–151, 1991.

Joint Commission on Accreditation of Health Care Organizations. *Accreditation Manual for Hospitals,* 1993. Chicago, IL: JCAHO, 1992.

Richet, H. M., Chidiac, C., Prat, A., et al. "Analysis of risk factors for surgical wound infections following vascular surgery." *Am J Med* 91 (suppl 3B):170–172, 1991.

Stamm, W. E. "Catheter-associated urinary tract infections: Epidemiology, pathogenesis, and prevention." *Am J Med* 91 (suppl 3B):65–71, 1991.

U.S. Department of Labor, Occupational Safety and Health Administration. *Occupational Exposure to Ethylene Oxide.* 29 CFR 1910.1047. Washington, D.C.: OSHA, 1992.

Wenzel, R. P. and Pfaller, M. A. "Infection control: The premier quality assessment program in United States hospitals." *Am J Med* 91 (Suppl 3B):27–31, 1991.

12

Patient-Centered Surgical Rehabilitation

Outcome: A rehabilitation process based on "partnering" maximizes return to an optimal level of wellness.

The development and implementation of comprehensive programs for the rehabilitation of surgical patients have undergone major changes in recent years. No longer are caregivers independently deciding what patients need or expect as a result of their surgery. No longer are patients and support persons passive participants in the preparation and recovery processes of surgery. This chapter presents a systems model for surgical rehabilitation in which a partnership is formed between the patient, support person, and caregivers. It is a process that enables patients and support persons to participate in decision making before, during, and after surgery—from deciding when and where the surgery will be performed, to setting time frames for discharge. Surgical rehabilitation, as presented in this chapter, is a care delivery system in which patients and support persons have the opportunity, through partnering, to be actively involved and committed to developing and managing surgical rehabilitation activities, which in turn facilitates the patient's return to optimal levels of physical, psychological, and social wellness.

HISTORICAL BACKGROUND

Postoperative rehabilitation, or recovery, is usually seen as the period of time following surgery when the patient is recovering from the effects of surgery and anesthesia. Rehabilitation includes the restoration of the individual to the fullest physical, mental,

social, vocational, and economic states of which he or she is capable. Until the early 1980s, the rehabilitation or postoperative recovery process, like preoperative preparation, was initiated, implemented, and maintained by caregivers (usually nurses) while the patient was in the hospital. This process (care plan) was established by the nurse based on clinical criteria which the nurse believed best met the needs and expectations of physicians and patients. The heavy emphasis on clinical parameters, that is, disease, surgery, and anesthesia, produced a plan of care that was structured to maximize physical outcomes. This traditional approach was narrow in its scope and focus, because it rarely addressed psychosocial needs or solicited information from patients and/or support persons relating to their perceptions of needs, expectations, and/or outcomes of the surgical experience. In addition to limiting planning opportunities, this model had minimal patient and support person involvement in the hospital. It was only when discharge was imminent that the patient and support person became actively involved in surgical rehabilitation.

As a result of this passive, limited involvement with the planning of surgical rehabilitation, nurses and physicians were viewed as owning the process, its implementation, and its outcomes. Patients and their support persons expected physicians and nurses to establish the "dos and don'ts" for them and, likewise, physicians and nurses expected patients and support persons to follow these "dos and don'ts." With professionals in "control," the patient's confidence and willingness to be involved in planning, managing, or evaluating care before, during, or after surgery was limited. While far from ideal, professionally "owned" rehabilitation was not exclusive to surgical patients, but rather was evident in virtually every healthcare delivery service and system.

This professional-control model rapidly became obsolete for surgical patients in the early to mid-1980s, when healthcare services began to shift to outpatient delivery systems. An increase in outpatient/short-stay surgery reduced hospital stays, as day-of-surgery admission and early postoperative discharge became common. The increased volume of procedures and patient acuity, combined with the rising complexity of surgeries performed on an outpatient/short-stay basis, rapidly created a need to re-evaluate established, accepted healthcare methods and practices (1). Patients, support persons, physicians, and nurses voiced concerns about all aspects of the surgical experience, including the rehabilitation/recovery process, and a consensus emerged that change was needed. From identifying postoperative problems and complications to managing postoperative pain, every aspect of the process appeared to require some degree of modification. Key elements under scrutiny included the "exclusive ownership" by professionals of the surgical experience, and limited attention to psychosocial needs and patient/support person involvement in the surgical rehabilitation process.

The 1980s saw the emergence of healthcare delivery systems supporting partnering or "joint venturing" among patients, support persons, physicians, and nurses. In the 1990s this process expanded even further as healthcare consumers demanded to be involved in every aspect of care, from deciding whether or not to have surgery, to learning how to administer intravenous antibiotics at home. Today, patient and support person involvement and participation continues to grow, as does their equal involvement with the professional caregiver in identifying needs, expectations, and desired outcomes involved in surgery. Patients and support persons are actively participating in the development of streamlined, comprehensive surgical rehabilitative delivery systems and processes that can be used with surgical inpatients or outpatients. These new systems begin to address the problems that have emerged as increasing numbers of patients prepare for and recover from surgery outside of the formal hospital system or healthcare facility.

Just as settings for the delivery of surgery have changed, so has the practice of the perioperative nurse. Today's demands and expectations for care require that the perioperative nurse develop professional practices that are compatible with and complementary to current patient needs. According to AORN (2), perioperative nursing begins with a preoperative assessment in the reception area, surgical suite, surgical unit, or home or clinic and continues through the postoperative evaluation, which may take place in the discharge area, surgical suite, postanesthesia area, surgical unit, or home or clinic. Practice settings for perioperative nurses include traditional operating rooms, ambulatory surgery units, physicians' offices, cardiac catheterization laboratories, endoscopy rooms, radiology departments, and other settings where surgery may be performed. Regardless of where perioperative nurses work or the professional services they provide, there is a basic assumption that they will facilitate, educate, support, assist, and lead patients to develop effective programs for recovering from surgery.

SURGICAL REHABILITATION: A SYSTEMS PROCESS

Successful, effective, patient-centered rehabilitation requires an organized, systematic process that enables or "empowers" patients and their support persons to manage recovery in the most beneficial and efficient way. Patient-centered rehabilitation, as a systematic process, provides a foundation on which to establish and maintain systems for easy access to resources; ensures that there is integration of needed services; and promotes collaboration between professional groups, patients and professionals, and patients and support persons. It positions the patient as the central focus for whom care processes are developed, implemented and evaluated. An example of this would be the way preadmission testing services are put together:

- Are preadmission services conveniently located?
- Are appropriate services provided/available during the preadmission process?
- Does the education provided meet patient and support person needs and expectations?
- Are the necessary followup services organized and supplied in a manner that meets the individualized needs of the patients and their support persons?

If not addressed, these seemingly simple elements of an effective rehabilitation process can create real or perceived service gaps. When these service gaps

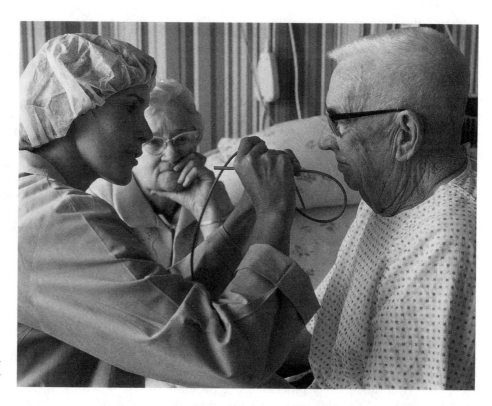

FIGURE 12.1. The nurse explains surgical routines to a patient and his wife before surgery.

occur, patients become paralyzed rather than empowered. They lack the information or resources with which to organize and manage the surgical experience in a way that meets their needs and expectations. This ultimately effects their ability to achieve the desired postoperative outcomes. An organized, all-inclusive system for surgical rehabilitation supports and maintains an environment where partnering and ownership by the patient and support person can thrive. Finally, the systems approach to integrating all elements of surgical rehabilitation provides a foundation that gives the overall program and delivery of service structure and support.

Process Overview

Patient rehabilitation, as an integral part of the surgical experience, needs to be a collaborative, participative process regardless of the scope or intensity of surgery. Patients undergoing open heart surgery, organ transplants, and major reconstructive procedures should be as personally involved in outcome identification, planning, implementation, and evaluation for their surgery and rehabilitation as patients having ambulatory surgery. Both professional caregivers and patients expect support persons to be closely involved in the delivery of care before, during, and after the hospital stay (Fig. 12.1). While this has been the accepted practice for many years for

pediatric patients, increasing numbers of support persons have recently become involved with adult family members undergoing inpatient or outpatient surgery, especially when the surgery involves elderly parents or relatives.

Patient-centered surgical rehabilitation, as a partnership process, requires that the patient, support person, and professional caregivers establish, accept, and commit to mutual recovery goals. These goals can vary considerably, depending upon the condition or intervention from which the patient is recovering. The model presented in this chapter is a trust-based interaction, which assumes that professional caregiver, patient, and support persons actively collaborate and cooperate with each other in all phases of the experience. From identifying desired outcomes at the time surgery is scheduled, to agreeing to appropriate, acceptable time frames for recovery, there is an open environment in which all participants are encouraged to challenge, contribute, and collaborate to reach the mutually identified and established goals and expectations.

This rehabilitation model assumes that the professional and nonprofessional caregivers (nurses, physicians, support persons) and the patient will have individual and joint roles and responsibilities. The overlapping or joint areas include identifying the outcomes that the involved persons anticipate as a result of having surgery performed. Both will need to define the level or status that they are willing to accept as normal functioning or full recovery, but this status generally ought to reflect those physical, psychological, and social parameters that are viewed by society as showing recovery from surgery. Both groups will need to agree to support and participate in activities which promote a return to agreed-upon levels of functioning.

Once outcomes have been agreed upon, participants will need to plan the resources needed to achieve the outcome. Then, there will need to be a clear understanding by all of any and all limitations in accessibility and/or availability of resources as well as the capabilities or limitations in operationalizing them. Nurses and sometimes physicians serve an important role in encouraging and supporting patients and their support persons to take responsibility for (own) the rehabilitative process. Patients and their support persons must accept that their involvement is required if implementation of the plan of care is to lead to optimal recovery. All of the caregivers are equally responsible for establishing and maintaining positive environments where patients can progress in the recovery process. The education of the patient and support person by the nurse or physician about all phases of the surgical experience is an enabling activity that provides them with the information they will need to be active partners in the preparation for surgery and care following discharge (Fig. 12.2). Everyone involved, including the patient, needs to participate in the establishment and maintenance of a collaborative, cooperative, trusting environment. Genuine commitment to attaining mutually agreed-upon outcomes is the responsibility for all of those involved in the process.

Although this partnering rehabilitative process is ideal, it is not always possible. There may be situations where the patient refuses to be involved, is unable to be involved because of physical or psychological deficits, or lacks a support person. Each patient and situation will need to be assessed individually and a plan of care developed that best meets the needs and expectations of the patient. It is important for the nurse to understand and accept that all patients may not be willing to participate in activities that provide them the best opportunity for recovery. Support persons may decide that they do not want to be involved with care, either inside or outside the hospital. In such situations, the nurse must provide a supportive environment where healing and recovery can occur. When patients do not comply with recommended, proven rehabilitative activities, the nurse should pursue the reasons why a patient will not, or cannot, comply, so that prob-

lems in this area can be discovered and perhaps alleviated. It may be appropriate to emphasize to the patient that, by not complying, he or she may be responsible for outcomes that are less than optimal.

THE NURSING PROCESS AND SURGICAL REHABILITATION

Outpatient and short-stay surgeries have been major catalysts in the increased utilization of the nursing process as a framework on which to build a manageable plan of care for surgical patients. Limited contact with patients prior to surgery and shorter stays afterward have increased the need for streamlining methods to quickly assess and educate patients. Organized processes that facilitate positive interactions between patients, professionals, and support persons are critical for successful patient-centered rehabilitation programs.

The nursing process facilitates early initiation of patient assessment and education and joint involvement in planning of care by all involved persons. It provides a foundation on which to assess the patient's needs, capabilities, and resources as they relate to the specific surgical procedure. Rehabilitation/recovery requirements change depending on the type of surgery being performed and the anesthesia being used. For example, the time required before a patient can safely resume a presurgical exercise program will vary considerably with the procedure performed. A patient who undergoes open heart surgery may need more assistance in developing a workable plan to resume his or her preoperative exercise program than a patient who is having a breast biopsy. On the other hand, same-day surgery hernia patients will need different instructions for management of postoperative pain than patients who have had major inpatient surgical procedures. Once the individual patient and procedure-related needs, expectations, and abilities have been determined, the nursing process continues to provide a solid base on which to operate.

Utilization of the nursing process as an operational framework for surgical rehabilitation has the following advantages:

- It ensures that all requirements for individualized, patient-centered surgical rehabilitation plans can be met.
- It ensures that continuity of care will be maintained throughout all phases of the surgical experience, even when the patient requires the intervention or assistance of other healthcare

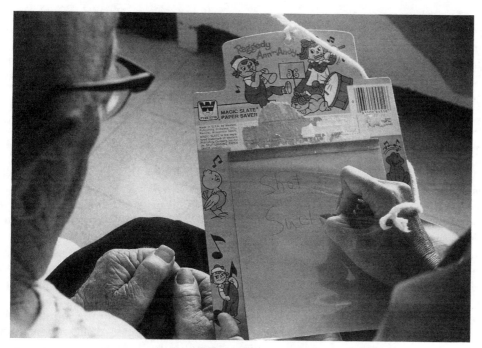

A

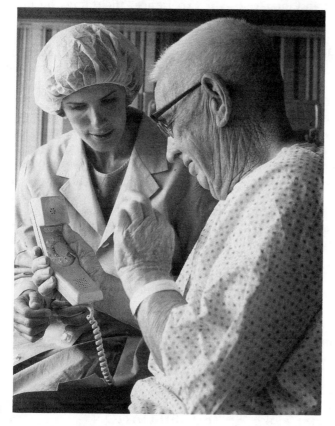

B

FIGURE 12.2. The nurse recognizes the effect that a tracheostomy and wired mandible will have on the patient's ability to communicate postoperatively. A child's magic slate (A) and telephone signals (B) are substituted for oral communication. A patient must be able to initiate or respond to communication if he is to participate in his rehabilitation.

professionals, such as a physical or respiratory therapist, phlebotomist, or EKG technician, before, during, or after surgery.

• It allows for interdisciplinary intervention to be a planned process that is known to the patient and is an accepted part of the total surgical experience.

• It creates and maintains an environment that supports and promotes the involvement of patients and their support persons throughout the surgical experience.

• It helps to identify realistic outcomes.

Responsibility for integrating the nursing process into the care continuum falls to the nurses working directly with patients and their support persons. Often it is the physician's office or preadmission nurse who initiates the surgical rehabilitation process. Regardless of where or when the process begins, the expectations regarding patient preparation for surgery and recovery are the same. It is expected that the professional nurses responsible for the care of the patient will use appropriate strategies and interventions to prepare the patients and their support persons for surgery. Assisting and supporting patients and families to own some, if not all, of the rehabilitative responsibilities is facilitated by utilizing the nursing process.

In organizing effective, comprehensive perioperative care, the involvement and commitment of the patient in the rehabilitative phase is critical for achieving desired outcomes. Patient participation in rehabilitation requires that the patient, family, or significant others:

1. Collaborate with the caregivers (physicians, nurses, and other professionals as appropriate, i.e., physical or respiratory therapists) in setting mutual, realistic postoperative goals by:
   a. identifying the desired outcomes
   b. identifying the individual strengths and weaknesses involved in attaining the desired outcomes
   c. identifying resources needed to attain desired outcomes, and the availability and/or lack of same
2. Collaborate with the caregivers in identifying and defining activities or processes that maximize individual strengths and minimize weaknesses.
3. Recognize major aspects of the surgical experience and how they as individuals are affected by/affect the experience and subsequent rehabilitative process by:

   a. verbalizing physical and psychological changes that occur as a result of the surgical intervention
   b. discussing how they can effectively manage these changes to achieve desired outcomes
   c. organizing and integrating the needed rehabilitative processes into their own activities of daily living
   d. verbalizing an understanding of their responsibilities in the rehabilitative process and activities
   e. expressing their individual concerns or reservations about the surgical experience, desired outcomes, or their involvement in the recovery process
4. Consent and commit to realistic, measurable goals that are consistent with attaining desired outcomes, by setting activity targets that allow/support them in maintaining control by a planned process of increased self-care responsibility throughout all phases of the surgical experience, including the postoperative/rehabilitative period.

The degree to which the desired outcomes of surgery are attained in a timely manner is dependent upon:

1. The level at which the patient, family, and significant others understand, agree, and choose to be involved in and committed to a plan of action to achieve desired outcomes
2. The feasibility and reality of the desired outcomes, given the patient's ability and willingness to be an active participant in the process
3. The ability of the caregivers to guide, direct, adapt, or customize the rehabilitative process (planning and implementation) so that it is consistent with the patient's needs, expectations, capabilities, and/or limitations
4. The timeliness, effectiveness, and appropriateness of discharge planning and followup as it affects and is affected by individual patients, families, and significant others

PATIENT PARTICIPATION IN REHABILITATION

How, when, and where does the patient and his or her support person become involved with setting goals for achieving a return to optimal wellness? This process is a continuum that is initiated when the patient is advised of the need for surgery and agrees to go ahead with the procedure. Regardless of where the process is initiated, it is made up of three basic elements: preparation for surgery, support during surgery, and assistance following surgery.

Rehabilitation begins when the patient decides to have surgery. The process is actualized when the admitting procedure is begun. The admitting procedure can be performed in the physician's office, in an outpatient preadmission testing setting, or in the hospital. The nurse conducts a thorough assessment of the patient's physical, psychological, social, personal, and occupational strengths and weaknesses. This assessment becomes the cornerstone for building a recovery or rehabilitation process that is consistent with the needs, desires, and expectations of the patient, support person, physician, and nurses. Patient participation and involvement during the assessment process initiates the establishment of the partnering process. It provides direction and focus for attaining desired outcomes as the nurse explains the routines involved in the preoperative, intraoperative, and postoperative phases. It is the time when patients and support persons gain the information they will need to actively participate in all phases of the experience, which ultimately facilitates patient, support person, and professional caregiver shared commitment and ownership of all elements of the rehabilitation process.

Patient and support person education is a critical element in an effective program of surgical rehabilitation. Like assessment, education is initiated at the time the patient elects to have surgery. Because patients are spending less time before and after surgery in the hospital, it has become critical to educate patients as early and often as possible. All types of providers, from physicians to home care agencies, have created formal tools that can be used to educate patients and their support persons. The education process is generally initiated in the physician's office, using the following tools:

- Printed brochures that describe the surgical experience from beginning to end
- Videotapes that review the most important aspects of the experience, ranging from preadmission testing to postdischarge exercises
- Individual or group education sessions sponsored by the physician, the hospital, or both
- Audiotapes and patient-focused books that educate patients about the surgical experience and their role and responsibilities

Regardless of the methods used to educate the patient and his or her support person, the desired outcome is to provide information that will empower the patient and the support person to make decisions about how to achieve optimal outcomes through effective management of the overall process.

In order to assess the patient's level of knowledge, educational needs, and expectations, it is essential that preoperative teaching be an organized, systematic process. Utilizing the nursing process within a systems framework ensures that all aspects of surgery, from preparatory information to postdischarge instructions, are reviewed, reinforced, and reemphasized. Again, it is essential that the patient and support person be provided with clear, understandable explanations about procedures and activities they can expect to experience before, during, and after surgery. The success of the partnership model of rehabilitation relies heavily on the patient being informed about all aspects of the upcoming experience. When the patient and support person are informed, it helps them remain in control, thus improving their management of the experience, including the stress that accompanies any surgical encounter.

Another routine part of the preadmission process is to initiate plans for care at home following discharge. The resources available to the patient must be assessed and patients must be provided with information and resources to support the rehabilitation process following discharge. This period can be devastating if the patient and/or support person feels unprepared or unable to effectively manage postdischarge care at home.

On the day of surgery, the perioperative nurse may review the data collected during the preoperative interview, obtain baseline vital signs, review the plan of care with the patient, and reiterate points made in preoperative patient teaching. If feasible, support persons should be permitted to remain with the patient during this time. Allowing support persons to be involved with care and/or remain with the patient has the following positive outcomes:

- It increases comfort and reduces stress for the patient and the support person.
- It reinforces to the patient and support person the willingness of the nurses and physicians to establish and maintain a partnership for care delivery.
- It increases the level of trust and confidence between the patient and professional caregivers.

Intraoperative responsibilities of the perioperative nurse regarding rehabilitation include documenting any unforeseen intraoperative developments that might affect the course of rehabilitation. Postoperatively, the perioperative nurse is responsible for communicating relevant information to nurses in the postanesthesia area. The patient must be provided with physical and psychosocial support until he or she meets criteria for discharge, and discharge instructions must be communicated verbally and in writing.

Example of Patient Participation

The following extended case example demonstrates how nurses are involved with ensuring that rehabilitation is a joint undertaking among patients, support persons, and professionals. It utilizes systems methodology as a foundation for the nursing process, which in turn becomes the basis of surgical rehabilitation activities. As an integrated, organized approach, the nursing process/systems foundation is a simple, easy method for patients and professional caregivers to identify realistic outcomes and then plan and implement appropriate activities to reach maximum recovery potentials.

The case detailed below describes Mr. Forbes, a 68-year-old male patient who was diagnosed with osteoarthritis of the right hip. He had been unable to walk without pain for several years, and his physical activity had been markedly diminished. He entered the hospital for a total hip replacement. The nurses responsible for his care assessed Mr. Forbes's strengths and weaknesses; initiated discharge planning; offered patient education; provided preoperative, intraoperative, and postoperative care; and gave discharge instructions to both the patient and his wife.

Strengths Identified
During the preadmission assessment, the nurse helped Mr. Forbes to identify his strengths. Mr. Forbes described those areas that he felt were an asset to him. He indicated his determination to be able to walk comfortably after surgery. He also indicated to the nurse that, except for his arthritis, he was physically fit. He reported a healthy lifestyle, that is, he did not smoke, participated in a low-impact exercise program, maintained consistent weight over the past 3 years, and had recently undergone a complete physical, the results of which were normal for his age. Mr. Forbes's motivation to regain lost mobility following surgery was supported by the experiences of several of his friends, who had undergone similar operations and were now able to actively participate in normal daily activities.

He was knowledgeable about the need to actively participate in a number of prescribed activities after surgery. He was familiar with the need to exercise regularly, eat a well-balanced diet, and establish a routine for rest and activity. Mr. Forbes's greatest motivation to regain mobility following surgery seemed to be his desire to do as well if not better than his friends had done. He continually emphasized his belief that his surgery would be successful and that he would be out playing golf within 3 months.

Another strength identified by Mr. Forbes and his wife was the support and encouragement that he expected to receive from his family. Mr. Forbes openly discussed his family's support and encouragement for this surgery. According to Mr. Forbes, they had assessed his home environment to identify areas that might require some modification so that potential or real risks to him could be minimized. In addition, they had read all the literature provided to them by the surgeon and were familiar with exercise requirements and other "healthy" living activities that Mr. Forbes would need to adhere to following discharge.

Weaknesses Identified
Mr. Forbes told the nurse that he was concerned about the anesthesia he would be having for surgery. He reported that, in the past, he had experienced several days of severe nausea and vomiting after having general anesthesia. Since the nurse was aware that general anesthesia was the usual choice for a hip replacement, she listed this as a potential weakness to be addressed with Mr. Forbes's surgeon and the anesthesiologist. Mr. Forbes and the nurse decided that it would be appropriate to set up a joint conference with his wife, the surgeon, and the anesthesiologist prior to his admission to the hospital to discuss possible alternatives. It was decided that this should be done within the next week since his surgery was scheduled in 10 days.

Mr. Forbes asked the nurse if she could explain to him about the "living will" he had heard about from several of his friends. The nurse identified this lack of knowledge about patients' rights and responsibilities to be another weakness. She briefly explained the basics of a living will to Mr. Forbes and his wife, provided printed information on the subject, arranged for them to meet with a social worker who could provide them with an in-depth explanation on the subject, and noted on the assessment form that this area needed to be reviewed with them upon his admission to the hospital. The nurse encouraged Mr. and Mrs. Forbes to discuss the living will and medical power of attorney information with their daughter so that their wishes could be known to anyone who might be involved with making decisions about their care in the future.

Discharge Planning
When asked about resources in the home for postdischarge care, Mr. Forbes related that his daughter lived close by

and would drive them wherever they needed to go (e.g., grocery store, church, physician's office). The nurse asked if they were interested in having a visiting nurse stop by and assist them with care following discharge. Mr. and Mrs. Forbes indicated an interest, and the nurse made a note to have the visiting nurse stop by and see them while Mr. Forbes was in the hospital.

Mrs. Forbes indicated that she had already secured a portable toilet with an elevated seat to have downstairs, since their bathroom was located on the second floor. The nurse complimented Mrs. Forbes on her knowledge, since an elevated seat is recommended to decrease potential problems with hip flexion for 8 weeks following surgery. Mrs. Forbes also said that she had moved several throw rugs, since they were a potential hazard if Mr. Forbes needed to use crutches or a walker.

Patient Education

The nurse determined during the assessment that Mr. Forbes had been given a detailed explanation of the procedure using an anatomical model in his physician's office, and printed information and a videotape to review at home. Despite the information provided, Mr. and Mrs. Forbes both indicated that there were some specifics about the immediate postoperative period they did not completely understand. The nurse took this opportunity to identify specific learning needs and expectations as to the extent of information they desired. She learned that they were knowledgeable about many of the general areas (i.e., pain management, deep breathing, coughing and parenteral fluid administration), but had several deficit areas, including postoperative positioning, care of dressing and drains, and recovery room procedures.

In order to eliminate identified knowledge deficits, the nurse described specifics regarding postoperative positioning utilizing the adduction device that Mr. Forbes would use during the first few days after surgery. In addition, she reinforced the need for Mr. Forbes to continue to use a pillow between his knees to maintain adduction following discharge from the hospital. Due to time limitations, the nurse advised Mr. and Mrs. Forbes that they would receive additional instructions and information in the mail on several other techniques that would be involved with bed-to-chair transfers and ambulation. These techniques, she added, would be reviewed on the nursing unit when Mr. Forbes was admitted to the hospital. She noted this information on the plan of care she had developed, which would also be sent to the nursing unit prior to Mr. Forbes's arrival.

The nurse also reviewed specifics related to deep breathing, coughing, and turning that would be carried out by the nurses following surgery. Mr. Forbes was able to successfully demonstrate the ability to deep-breathe and cough appropriately. Mrs. Forbes indicated that she in-

tended to stay with her husband for at least the first 2 days after surgery. She also indicated her interest in being as involved in his care as was feasible. The nurse reviewed with her the 2-hour time schedule that would be used for these activities and encouraged Mrs. Forbes to discuss her interest in participation with the unit nurses at admission time. The nurse also noted on the plan of care that Mrs. Forbes planned to stay overnight on the day of surgery, so that the staff could make the necessary arrangements for a comfortable chair to be placed in Mr. Forbes's room. The nurse reinforced Mr. Forbes's willingness to participate in his recovery and supported his personal involvement in this process. It is essential to identify the expectations of patients and support persons. In the case of Mr. and Mrs. Forbes, their interest and desire to be involved in care activities facilitated collaboration and cooperation in the rehabilitation process.

The nurse working with Mr. and Mrs. Forbes also explained about the suction drain that would be used after surgery. She provided them with a sample of the drain so that they would be familiar with its appearance and operation. The nurse advised Mr. and Mrs. Forbes that its purpose was to drain excess fluid and blood that had collected inside the incision. She told them that the staff would check and record the drainage periodically, and that if there were no problems they could expect the drains to be removed approximately 48 hours after surgery. The nurse reemphasized that the drain and adduction device would be in place when Mr. Forbes awakened from surgery. In keeping with the overall goal of creating an environment where the patient and support person are made aware of all anticipated experiences, situations, and potential procedures, the nurse continued to communicate her commitment to making their experience as consistent as possible with their desire to be knowledgeable about the surgery.

Discussing the drains and splints gave the nurse the opportunity to introduce information regarding the experience and procedures Mr. Forbes could expect to have in the postanesthesia care unit (PACU). She indicated that Mr. Forbes would most likely have an oxygen tube in his nose and that the nursing staff would be checking his blood pressure and pulse frequently. Since Mr. Forbes had had previous problems with postoperative nausea, the nurse told him that the staff would be checking with him frequently as to how he was feeling. Since Mr. Forbes would be responsible for deciding about his pain medication through a patient-controlled analgesia (PCA) pump, the nurse provided a printed information sheet about PCA that was specifically developed for distribution to patients. Mr. and Mrs. Forbes indicated that they were knowledgeable about this system, since Mrs. Forbes had used it when she had had her gall bladder out several months ago. Again, the nurse noted on the plan of care the need to review this process at the time Mr. Forbes was admitted.

As Mr. and Mrs. Forbes gained knowledge about the rehabilitation process and their role and responsibilities, they gained the confidence they would need to actively participate in and contribute to reaching the mutual goal of attaining the highest level of physical, psychological, social, and occupational wellness.

The nurse concluded the preadmission assessment by explaining the activities Mr. and Mrs. Forbes would need to perform at home prior to coming to the hospital. She also provided them with detailed information on when and where to arrive on the day of surgery and what to expect once they arrived. The nurse pointed out the section in their surgical brochure (given to them in the physician's office) that took them step by step through the 2 days preceding admission. She stressed the importance of following the instructions regarding fasting, bathing, and medications. She discussed the rationale for these instructions, that is, the facilitation of safe, controlled conditions for surgery that subsequently enhance recovery to preoperative states of wellness.

Admission to the Hospital

Mr. Forbes arrived at the appointed time and place in preparation for his surgery. He was provided with information on where to go and what he needed to do. All of the instructions were consistent with the information provided during his preadmission visit. After Mr. Forbes had changed his clothes and dressed in a hospital gown, bathrobe, and slippers, the nurse had him and his wife wait in one of the private surgery preparation rooms. The nurse was able to allow Mr. Forbes and his wife several minutes alone so that they could adjust to the new environment and the upcoming surgery. When the nurse returned, she reviewed the data base that had been collected on Mr. Forbes during his preadmission interview. Since there had been no new problems or concerns since that time, the nurse proceeded to take Mr. Forbes's vital signs. She explained the importance of establishing a presurgical information base to measure and compare any changes that might occur during or after surgery. The nurse reviewed the plan of care that had been initiated during the preadmission visit. She asked about their conference regarding anesthesia. They both replied that their meeting had gone very well, and that the anesthesiologist had presented them with several options for anesthetic management. They had all agreed that a general anesthetic would be used, but that the anesthesiologist would modify some of the drugs employed to reduce the potential for postoperative nausea and vomiting.

The nurse utilized this preparatory time to follow up on the transfer techniques that had been covered briefly during the initial interview. Mr. and Mrs. Forbes offered that they had received the promised information in the mail and thoroughly understood the process. They were able to successfully demonstrate two of the transfer techniques without problems. Both Mr. Forbes and his wife communicated to the nurse that they were comfortable with everything that had been done to prepare them for the surgery and felt comfortable proceeding as planned. The nurse asked them if they had talked with the social worker about a living will. Mrs. Forbes provided a copy of the recently executed document, which the nurse placed on the chart.

The nurse then had Mr. Forbes walk to the preoperative holding area, where he was placed on a stretcher. His anesthesiologist inserted the intravenous line that would be used to manage fluid balance during surgery. Mrs. Forbes was allowed to remain with her husband throughout the preparation phase.

Mr. Forbes was then visited by his perioperative nurse. After introducing himself, his nurse reviewed the chart, checked Mr. Forbes's identification band, and verified which hip was to be replaced. The perioperative nurse briefly reviewed the operative process, specifically addressing the procedures that would occur and the expected time in surgery and recovery.

Intraoperative Phase

The perioperative nurse accompanied Mr. Forbes to surgery, where he assisted him to move from the stretcher to the OR bed. He remained close to Mr. Forbes during induction, after which he assumed his role as circulator for the procedure. During the procedure, the perioperative nurse entered relevant information on the nursing assessment portion of the operative record. He noted that the procedure was unusually difficult because of the bony deterioration in the hip joint. Because Mr. Forbes could have a greater than average amount of postoperative discomfort and be slower in regaining his physical strength and mobility as a result of this unexpected problem, this information was incorporated as part of the postoperative plan of care.

Postoperative Phase

Mr. Forbes was accompanied to the PACU by his anesthesiologist and perioperative nurse. They provided the PACU nurse with specifics about the patient's procedure, problems encountered, and special considerations, such as the potential for increased pain as a result of the mechanical difficulties. The PACU nurse assured them that she would communicate this information to the unit nurse when Mr. Forbes was transferred back to the unit. The perioperative nurse then found Mrs. Forbes and provided her with an update on her husband's immediate postoperative status and expected time in PACU. He explained that Mr. Forbes could experience more pain than expected and encouraged her to support him through this difficulty. The perioperative nurse ensured that a continuous care process was carried out after the surgery by communicating relevant information to the nurses in PACU. He also supported the partnering relationship that had been previously established with the patient and his wife by providing Mrs. Forbes with timely updates on her husband's condition.

During the immediate postoperative recovery period, the PACU nurse provided physical and psychosocial support to Mr. Forbes. She encouraged him to cough and deep-breathe, assisted him to turn, assessed vital signs on a regular basis, ensured the integrity of drains and parenteral infusion lines, and administered medication for pain as needed. Mr. Forbes was cooperative throughout his stay in PACU, which the nurse noted on the postoperative nursing flow sheet. The patient's ability and willingness to participate in these activities confirmed that the preoperative education process had been understood.

Mrs. Forbes, after talking with the perioperative nurse, returned to her husband's room. She spoke with his primary nurse, sharing her concerns about Mr. Forbes's determination to "get back to normal" faster than his friends had. The primary nurse thanked Mrs. Forbes for the information and noted it on the plan of care. She reviewed the plan of care, including activity resumption, with Mrs. Forbes and assured her that they would follow this routine to avoid overextending Mr. Forbes.

Mr. Forbes's wife remained with him throughout the night on the day of his surgery. When his primary nurse came to see them on the first postoperative morning, she noted that Mrs. Forbes seemed tired and anxious. She explained the plan of care for the day to both of them. She encouraged Mrs. Forbes to stay and assist her husband for a few hours, but suggested that she then go home and rest for a while. Mr. and Mrs. Forbes indicated that they would discuss this option and get back to the nurse with their answer. They decided that Mrs. Forbes would help her husband with his bath and then leave for a few hours, returning in the late afternoon. Throughout the day, Mr. Forbes's nurse continually kept him updated on any and all activities that were to take place, thus alleviating any unnecessary stress. She encouraged Mrs. Forbes to participate in her husband's care, reinforcing support for her involvement as an active caregiver for her husband. The nurse also communicated appropriately by allowing the couple to discuss when, if at all, they were comfortable with having Mrs. Forbes go home to rest.

The perioperative nurse visited Mr. Forbes on his third postoperative day. He found him out of bed in a lounger chair, visiting with his wife. Mr. Forbes offered that while he was still experiencing a moderate amount of postoperative pain, he had been able to stay comfortable and alert by using the PCA pump. He also noted that he had not had any postoperative nausea or vomiting as with pervious anesthesias. Mr. Forbes told the perioperative nurse that he would be starting physical therapy that afternoon. He explained that his physical therapist had visited the day before and had presented a preliminary plan of exercises

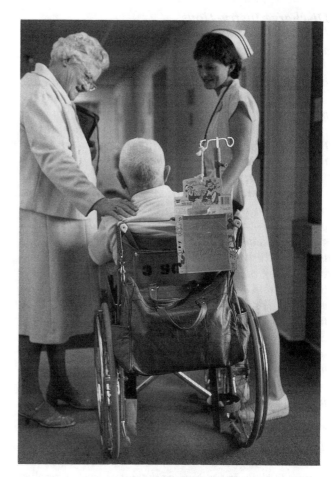

FIGURE 12.3. Going home is a major milestone in rehabilitation. However, many patients continue to need professional nursing service for full recovery at home.

(which helped her to gain the confidence and support of the patient). In creating her action plan, the physical therapist reviewed the patient's record, noting especially Mr. Forbes's determination to "get well fast" and the mechanical difficulties encountered during surgery. (Each of these elements affects the way the therapist develops a plan and presents it to the patient.) After gaining the Forbes's agreement to the overall plan, the therapist reviewed with them those bed exercises that Mr. Forbes could do unassisted. She stressed with Mr. Forbes the importance of proceeding slowly so as not to unnecessarily stress his hip or surrounding tissues.

Mr. Forbes continued to progress satisfactorily, and by the eighth day he was ready for discharge. The visiting nurse stopped by to see the couple, and they agreed that she would come and see them the day after Mr. Forbes was discharged. Mr. Forbes had shown no signs of postoperative infection, his wound was healing well, he was ambulating with minimal assistance, and he had become proficient in doing the active and passive exercises recommended by his physical therapist. His surgeon discharged him on the ninth postoperative day (Fig. 12.3).

Discharge Instructions

Both Mr. and Mrs. Forbes were well informed about the appropriate care that would need to be carried out at home. The nurses observed Mrs. Forbes as she changed the dressing on her husband's incision and assisted him to use the slide-sit maneuver in order to dress himself. The commitment and involvement by the couple throughout the process gave the physicians and nurses the confidence that they were competent to effectively manage the rehabilitative process from this point forward.

The primary nurse provided Mr. and Mrs. Forbes with a brochure and instruction sheet that outlined routine care and covered frequently asked questions. Their primary nurse also told them that she would be calling in a couple of days to check on their progress at home. She urged Mr. Forbes to go slowly with resumption of his previous activities, as he was still in the early stages of healing and unnecessary stress might delay the process. Mr. and Mrs. Forbes asked the primary nurse to extend their thanks to the other staff who had been involved in this experience. They both expressed how pleased they were with all aspects of it, in particular the way they had been allowed and encouraged to participate throughout all phases. They also said that they perceived the education portion of their experience to have been most beneficial.

Conclusion

This patient's experience illustrates that a key element in successful surgical rehabilitation is structuring the process to allow and encourage the fullest level of involvement and participation by the patient and his or her support person. It also demonstrates the need for professionals to educate, educate, educate patients and their support persons. Finally, it emphasizes the need to utilize an organized structure, such as the systems-based nursing process, as a framework on which to operate. Any intervention and subsequent successful recovery relies on the ability of the caregiver to modify the process to meet the unique, individual needs of each person that is directly or indirectly involved with the delivery of service.

This rehabilitation model focuses on a process that is jointly initiated, developed, and maintained by patients and caregivers (nurses, physicians, and support persons) and is not limited to the period of time immediately following surgery. It extends from the time the patient decides to have surgery to the time the patient is deemed fully recovered. It treats the surgical experience as a continuum in which patients move from their normal surroundings to the hospital and back again. It promotes and supports the notion that surgery can and should be a pleasant, smooth, minimally stressful experience in which patients and support persons are included as equal partners and, as such, are allowed to be active participants in the processes of assessment, diagnosis, outcome identification, planning, implementation, and evaluation.

References

1. Llewellyn, J. "Short stay surgery—present practices, future trends." *AORN J* 53(5):1179–1191, 1991.
2. Association of Operating Room Nurses. *AORN Standards and Recommended Practices for Perioperative Nursing—1992.* Denver: AORN, 1992.

Suggested Readings

Caldwell, L. "Surgical outpatient concerns—What every perioperative nurse should know." *AORN J* 53(3):761–767, 1991.

Carmody, S., et al. "Perioperative needs of families: Results of a survey." *AORN J* 54(3):561–567.

Good-Rees, D., and Pieper, B. "Structured versus unstructured teaching." *AORN J* 51(5):1334–1339, 1990.

Kapp, Marshall. "Elder care—Informed, assisted, delegated consent for elderly patients." *AORN J* 52(4):857–862, 1990.

Kneedler, J. A., and Dodge, G. H. *Perioperative Patient Care: The Nursing Perspective.* Boston: Blackwell Scientific Publications, 1983.

Lillcott, N. "Discharge instructions—Advice for knee, shoulder arthroscopy outpatients." *AORN J* 54(5):1015–1028, 1991.

Pool, Madonna. "Opinion—Ambulatory surgery nurses have unique opportunities to provide patient care." *AORN J* 52(4):845–846, 1990.

Wiseman, Susan. "Patient advocacy—The essence of perioperative nursing in ambulatory surgery." *AORN J* 51(3):754–762, 1990.

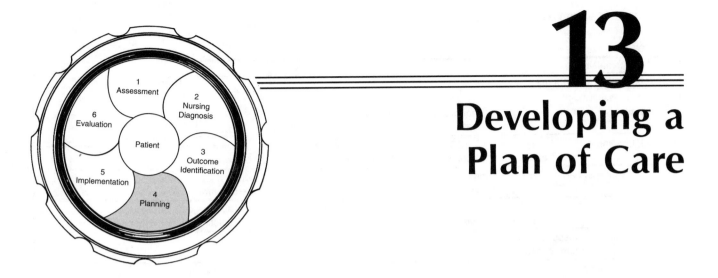

13

Developing a Plan of Care

The plan for nursing care prescribes nursing actions to achieve the expected outcomes.

The perioperative nurse deliberately and actively plans care for the patient having surgery. The planning activity is used to outline solutions to patient problems that can be resolved by nursing intervention. The process requires the nurse to draw upon a solid body of scientific data in order to outline nursing interventions that will result in attainment of the expected patient outcomes. This chapter discusses the purpose of planning, what a plan should entail, methods to communicate a plan to appropriate members of the healthcare team, and the nursing competencies required for planning. An individualized plan is provided as an example.

THE PURPOSE OF PLANNING

A plan of care is an outline of the aim of nursing care and prescribes nursing actions that must be performed to achieve patient outcomes. The plan individualizes care because each patient reacts to care in a different way. Patient-centered care is the objective of every nurse, and this necessitates adapting care to meet the individual needs of patients. If used systematically, the planning process allows for coordination and continuity of care (1).

A plan assures that the necessary information about each patient is available to the staff. Thus, a complete picture of the patient is available at all times. The plan should reflect the acuity level of the patient and validate the amount of nursing care needed. The nurse can then make judgments about

who will be assigned to provide care to the patient. The nurse must be able to review the information and evaluate the effectiveness of care given.

It is important that the plan be flexible so that the information can easily be revised according to the patient's condition. If the plan is not kept up to date, the information becomes meaningless and it can no longer be used to guide care.

The purposes of the plan of care are listed in Table 13.1.

COMPONENTS OF A PLAN OF CARE

A plan of care has traditionally depicted the steps of the nursing process. At one time, it was a requirement of the Joint Commission on Accreditation of Healthcare Organizations (JCAHO) that the plan be in writing on the nursing unit or in each patient's record. Presently, JCAHO requires only that there be evidence in the record that there was a plan of care for the individual patient. This evidence may be

TABLE 13.1.   Purposes of the Plan of Care

- To ensure continuity of care
- To provide a means of individualizing care
- To serve as a method of communicating
- To provide a place to record the care given
- To demonstrate a team approach to care
- To permit the patient's involvement in care planning

1.) Chief complaint:	**Time**

2.) Procedure to be performed: _____

	Time
OR notified	_____
Pt to OPSU	_____
Pt to OR	_____
Pt returned to OPSU	_____
Pt discharged	_____

3.) Pre-op assessment:

a.) Skin: ☐ warm   ☐ cool   ☐ normal color   ☐ jaundice
☐ dry   ☐ moist   ☐ pale   ☐ visible lesions or rash–Site _____

b.) Respiratory: ☐ even   ☐ SOB   ☐ use of accessory muscle   ☐ wheezing
☐ unlabored   ☐ cough   ☐ flaring nostrils   ☐ hoarseness

c.) Cardiovascular: Pulse: ☐ regular   ☐ chest pain   ☐ HX of blood transfusion
☐ irregular   ☐ diaphoritic   ☐ HX of heart surgery

d.) Eyes: sclera   ☐ white   ☐ injected   General: ☐ sunken   ☐ discharge   ☐ tearing
☐ yellow   ☐ red   ☐ puffy   ☐ crusting   ☐ abnormal lesions

e.) Ears: ☐ respond to spoken word
☐ hard of hearing

f.) Neurovascular: ☐ ambulatory   ☐ tremors   ☐ unsteady gait
☐ wheel chair   ☐ paralysis   ☐ use of prosthesis
☐ stretcher   ☐ speech difficulties

Additional comments:_____
_____
_____

4.) Current behavior: calm/relaxed ☐ restless ☐ apprehensive ☐ concerned ☐ child playing ☐ alert ☐ confused ☐ mentally impaired ☐

5.) Patterns of coping/adaptation: communicative ☐ quiet/withdrawn ☐ crying ☐ hostile/angry ☐ normal for age ☐

6.) Discharge Plans:

7.) Preoperative Teaching: a. Patient or significant other oriented to OPS environment and safety limitations ☐

b.) Instructions given regarding surgical procedure, pre & post-operative care ☐

c.) Patient appears to understand instructions given ☐

8.) Outpatient Surgery Nursing Care Plan Implemented   ☐ Yes   ☐ No

NURSING DIAGNOSIS	DESIRED OUTCOMES	NURSING ORDERS			
NURSING DIAGNOSIS	PT GOALS/EXPECTED OUTCOMES AT TIME OF DISCHARGE	M	N/M	N/A	EVALUATION COMMENTS
Alterations in Neuro Function	1. Pre-Op Neuro Status Regained				
Alteration in Cardiac Status	2. Maintain Pre-Op Cardiac Status				
Alteration in Resp. Function	3. Maintain Effective Ventilation				
Nutritional Deficit	4. Maintain Optimal Nutritional Status				
Alteration in Fluid Balance	5. Maintain Body Fluids				
Impaired Physical Mobility	6. Optimum M/S Functioning				
Impairment of Skin Integrity	7. Maintain Skin Integrity				
Alteration in Comfort	8. Minimal Discomfort				
Potential G.I. Alterations	9. No Alterations for G.I. Tract				
Potential for Increased Blood Loss	10. No Increased Blood Loss				
Alteration in Coping	11. Ability to Cope				
Potential for Injury	12. Prevention of Incidents				
Self Care Deficit	13. Resume Activities of Daily Living				

Nurse Signature _____
_____
DATE

MUSKOGEE REGIONAL MEDICAL CENTER
300 Rockefeller Drive
Muskogee, Oklahoma 74401

OUTPATIENT SURGERY — NURSING NOTES

FIGURE 13.1.   Outpatient assessment form.

traced through documentation that reflects the process of care (2). Documenting the plan of care demonstrates accountability to patients and provides evidence of how care is determined based on the desired patient outcome (3).

The nursing process begins with the nursing assessment, or data collection. Figure 13.1 is an example of the types of data collected for outpatients having surgery. The perioperative nurse completes the assessment prior to the patient's surgery.

Based on the nursing assessment, one or more nursing diagnoses is formulated. Figure 13.2 illustrates nursing diagnoses used in an outpatient setting.

Next, the expected outcomes are listed. This enables the perioperative nurse to base nursing actions on the desired results. Figure 13.1 lists thirteen possible expected outcomes and provides space to indicate whether they were met, or not applicable.

This entire process is available on the patient's record and provides a picture of the patient's care during the outpatient procedure.

The factors that should be considered when developing the plan of care include the following:

- The patient's *medical diagnosis*. The plan should reflect that consideration was given to the patient's disease process. This would include nursing actions based on the results of diagnostic tests, the patient's medical history, results of the physical examination, and the type of surgery planned for the patient.
- The patient's *physical condition* and energy resources. The plan outlines nursing activities that will conserve the patient's energy and is realistically based on the patient's physical status. This might include transportation needs and positioning the patient during surgery.
- The *nursing diagnoses* or potential problems of the patient. The plan of care depicts actions that directly relate to identified problems. For example, if a patient lacks knowledge about the surgical experience, the plan should include nursing actions that will result in the patient's being able to verbalize an understanding of the surgery.
- The *involvement of the patient and/or patient's family*. The plan should reflect patient and family input. For example, if the patient is having cataract surgery, the plan needs to include how the patient will get home after surgery and who will be taking the patient home.
- Availability of human and material *resources*. The plan is based on the resources available to carry out the prescribed nursing actions. For instance, a patient having a laparoscopic hernia repair will have to be scheduled when the visual systems are available. Another example is the patient having a hip arthroplasty that requires radiology, or the patient having surgery whose procedure requires additional personnel.
- *Therapeutic effectiveness*. The plan should include nursing actions that have proven to be effective to attain the desired patient outcomes. For instance, if the patient is having a local anesthesia, the nursing actions should include physiological monitoring such as pulse oximetry, blood pressure, and respirations. The desired outcome is that the patient be free of complications due to respiratory or circulatory system failures.
- *Coordination* with the overall medical plan. The plan of care is consistent with the surgeon's treatment regime. Nursing activities planned postoperatively for a patient having a fixation of a right tibial fracture might include elevation of the leg on pillows to reduce or prevent swelling.
- The *psychosocial needs* of the patient. The plan of care addresses the patient's fears and anxiety related to the disease process or the surgical procedure. It also includes nursing actions that provide comfort and well-being. It depicts sensitivity or concern for cultural diversity.

FORMULATION OF NURSING ORDERS

For each expected outcome, one or more nursing actions or nursing orders are written. Nursing actions are measures that the nurse believes must be taken in order for the patient to reach the desired outcome. Orders must be written in a way that is understandable to those putting them into practice. Each nursing order answers all of the following questions:

- What nursing actions should be performed?
- How should nursing actions be carried out?
- When should nursing actions be carried out?
- Where should nursing actions be performed?
- Who should perform the nursing actions?

What Nursing Actions Should Be Performed?

The plan specifies what nursing actions the nurse should perform to achieve the desired outcome. Each activity is usually preceded by an action verb specifying the nature of the action. For example, "Observe and record size and color of ulcerated area on buttock when patient is taken to recovery room," or "Listen to patient's concerns regarding pending surgical procedure."

The plan of care for surgical patients may include nursing orders such as:

- "Explain where patient's family may wait."
- "Identify patient upon admission to OR suite."
- "Verify surgical suite with patient and surgeon, and record."

Nursing orders about human relationships such as, "Give emotional support," might be carried out in various ways by different nurses. Therefore, the action for emotional support should be specific, such as, "Listen to Mr. Jones express his anger." The nurse should also be specific about nursing orders relating to observation of signs and symptoms. The nurse might write on the plan, "Check dressing for bleeding, report amount to head nurse, and chart findings." This same approach could be used for pulse, blood pressure, or other signs that have to be observed closely.

How Should Nursing Actions Be Carried Out?

The nursing order also indicates *how* each action is adapted to the individual patient. Any adaptation or change from the usual procedure should be put in writing. For example, if a patient scheduled for a dilatation and curettage has a hip prosthesis or fused hip that limits her range of motion, the usual lithotomy position will not be appropriate. In this case, the nursing order should state how the patient is to be positioned. The nursing order should also state, "Additional personnel needed to hold extremity during procedure."

When Should Nursing Actions Be Carried Out?

The timing and frequency of the prescribed order must be stated. This simply means the hour, specific time, or frequency of the order. For example, "Mr. Edwards will receive his preoperative medication one hour before the scheduled time for the procedure," or "The nurse will stand by Mr. Edwards during induction." Knowing *when* an action is to occur allows nurses to organize their time and to coordinate the care of a number of patients. An intraoperative example would be counting instruments, needles, and sponges. In abdominal surgery, counts must be made prior to closure of the peritoneum, fascia, and skin. The frequency is three times, and the time is at closure of the specific layers of tissue.

Where Should Nursing Actions Be Performed?

The location of the nursing action must be specified. Does the action occur on the patient care unit, the holding area, the operating room, the recovery area, or the critical care unit? This is important because the order might specify that the patient is to have a shave preparation prior to surgery, and the person assigned must know where this should take place. The order might say, "Shave prep in holding area," "Surgeon will shave head in operating room," or "Shave abdominal area and scrub with antibacterial soap the morning of surgery."

Intravenous fluids may be started in the patient's room or in the holding area. The nursing order might read, "Insert 18-gauge intracath and start 5% dextrose and H_2O in holding area." *When* the activity takes place is important, because if an activity is not timed carefully it can affect the time of surgery, hold up the schedule, create a higher potential for infection, or compromise asepsis.

Who Should Perform the Nursing Actions?

The plan should indicate whether a nurse, licensed practical nurse, technician, or nursing assistant should carry out the nursing order. Prior to assigning personnel to perform nursing activities, the nurse in charge should have a basic understanding of the abilities and educational preparation of the nursing staff.

The need for additional personnel in individual cases is another consideration. For example, elective surgery patients are usually transported by a single transport orderly. For a patient with a fractured femur whose leg must remain in traction during transportation, however, additional assistance will be required. Here, the order might state, "Transport to OR in bed by two orderlies. One orderly maintains leg in alignment with traction." In another situation, a patient in the operating room is showing all the signs of malignant hyperthermia. The nurse in charge carefully selects additional personnel based on their previous experience with carrying out nursing activities necessary for the patient with this condition.

Since nursing orders must be followed consistently and uniformly, the chance of misinterpretation must be minimized. If an order is difficult to understand, the nurses who are putting the plan into action may choose their own nursing actions instead of those prescribed specifically to meet the outcomes for this patient.

Planning the right nursing activity for each patient having surgery is a major part of professional nursing responsibility. Done thoroughly and carefully, it involves logic, experience, and scientific knowledge. Most important, it requires devotion to the principle that each patient is an individual who deserves individualized care planning.

Remember, planning is a continuous process that

is ongoing throughout the perioperative experience. The initial plan is modified or revised on an ongoing basis. When the patient's needs change, the plan of care changes. The plan is simply a guideline that requires periodic revision.

COMMUNICATING THE PLAN OF CARE

The plan of care is an essential mechanism for communicating information to other members of the healthcare team. It may be written in different formats depending on the stage of care and the type of surgery the patient is having.

In an outpatient or ambulatory care setting, the plan will be abbreviated because the patient is there for a short time period. The plan of care for an outpatient usually begins with a telephone call to the patient prior to the day of surgery. Information is obtained in writing and, on the day of surgery, provides valuable data to those providing care. In some situations the patient may come to the ambulatory facility or an area where preadmission information is obtained. Regardless of where they are taken, these data become a part of the patient's plan of care.

The plan is made accessible to those providing the care when the patient arrives for surgery. Additional data, nursing diagnoses, and patient outcomes are added as the patient progresses through the surgical experience.

Preoperative Checklists

Preoperative checklists (Fig. 13.2) are often used to communicate information. Upon arrival in the operating room, the nurse can immediately see what nursing actions or patient responses have been checked off or filled in. When the patient is admitted to the room, the nurse checks off appropriate items such as surgical procedure, verification of patient identity, emotional status upon admission to operating room, position for surgical procedure, known allergies, and presence of prosthetic devices. The operating room checklist is a tool for communicating what care has been given and what is still needed, which is an essential part of any plan.

Perioperative Nursing Record

The perioperative nursing record (Fig. 13.3) is useful for communicating the plan of care during the perioperative period. The notes are used to record nursing activities performed, patient outcomes, and evaluation statements. Data recorded before and during surgery are used by the nurse immediately postoperatively in planning postanesthesia care. The data are also used by others involved in giving patient care. Notes are particularly useful if the charting format follows the nursing process. Other methods the nurse uses to communicate information to those involved in the patient's care include reporting, patient care conferences, and multidisciplinary conferences.

Reporting

Change-of-shift reports take place when one shift of nurses leaves and another comes on. They should always be given at the beginning of the shift, whether morning, afternoon, or evening. Information is shared pertaining to equipment, supplies, types of surgery, and patients. The nurse in charge may conduct the report, but in many situations nurses who have developed a plan of care on specific patients share their plans with the others involved in the care of these same patients. This can be done while the group is convened or on an individual basis.

In some operating rooms, the manager or coordinator for each specialty communicates information about patients to be cared for in each specialty. Other institutions use tape recorders to transmit information from one shift to another. This has proved successful in many situations because it does not require overlapping time at changes in shift. The nurse coming on a shift can listen to the report and then relieve the nurse in the operating room. At the same time, he or she can validate or question any of the information. For example, the following information might be communicated relating to the plan of care for a patient with a fractured femur:

- Maintain fracture limb in alignment.
- Place trochanter roll along right hip.
- Transfer slowly and gently to OR.
- Examine area described as painful for signs of pressure, increased edema, and skin breakdown.
- Maintain traction with free pull.

At the end of a procedure, the perioperative nurse transmits information to other nurses in the operating room, postanesthesia, and patient care units, and to the patient's family. Information is continuously given to carry out, alter, or revise the plan for any patient. The information is provided to vari-

8610-049-87
D1.f136

PRE-OPERATIVE CHECKLIST
Nursing Division

		YES	N/A

I. CONSENTS/DIAGNOSTIC DATA/TEACHING:

Pre-operative teaching completed: Time _5:30 PM_ _10/7/92_ .... ✓

Operative Consent/Special Permits Completed .... ✓

History and Physical/Physician Note on Chart .... ✓

CBC/Hgb. & Hct. results on chart .... ✓

SMAC 7/24 results on chart .... ✓

UA results on chart .... ✓

PTT results on chart .... ✓

PREGNANCY TEST results on chart .... ✓ (N/A)

CHEST X-RAY done .... ✓

EKG copy on chart .... ✓

CARDIOPULMONARY TESTS (Vitalor) on chart .... ✓

BLOOD AVAILABLE FOR SURGERY .... ✓

PHYSICIAN NOTIFIED OF ABNORMAL VALUES/RESULTS .... ✓

INTERM SUMMERY/MEDICATION ON CHART .... ✓ (N/A)

II. PATIENT DATA:

Hearing Aide: ☐ In Place; ☐ Removed .... ✓ (N/A)

Accurate I.D. Band on Unaffected Side .... ✓

Dentures (Partial Plate) ☐ In Place; ☒ Removed .... ✓

Glasses/Contacts, Bobby Pins, Prosthesis removed ... _Rings taped on_. ✓

Make-up removed .... ✓ (N/A)

Disposition of Valuables: _given to family_ .... ✓

PATIENT INSTRUCTED TO STAY IN BED/SIDERAILS UP .... ✓

HT: _5'7½"_ Temp: _98.6_ Pulse: _68_ Resp. _18_ Blood Pressure: _160/90_

WT: _182_ NPO since: _____ Voided at: _7:30 AM_

ALLERGIES: _Ethanol (oral intake) ? Penicillin_

Comments: _____

PRE-OPERATIVE MEDS:

Vistaril 50mg _____ TIME: _7:30 AM_

Robinul 0.2 mg _____ TIME: _7:30 AM_

Ancef Gm I _____ TIME: _7:30 AM_

III. PREPS: ☐ N/A

Scrub/Skin/Shave Prep complete _10/8/92_   _Ann Nichols_   _Toby Parsons_
Date — Signature TPCN — Signature O.R. Personnel

IV. VERIFICATION OF PATIENT IDENTIFICATION WITH O.R. PERSONNEL:

To OR Pre-Operative Holding Area: Time: _7:45 AM_   Date: _10/8/92_

Gwen W. Dodge, RN   _Patricia Crum, RN_
Signature TPCN — Signature O.R. Personnel

V. PRE-OPERATIVE HOLDING:

Arrival Time: _7:55 AM_   Pre-Op Anes. Assessment Verified: _____, MD

COMMENTS/PRE-OP PREPARATION: _____

Signature	Init.	Signature	Init.
Gwen Dodge	_GD_		
Patricia Crum	_PC_		

Date _____   Signature _____

Addressograph

530 126 20   M 79
Fischer, Ralph E.
9. Dodge   10 7 92

FIGURE 13.2. Preoperative checklist. (Courtesy of Porter Memorial Hospital, Denver)

FORM 7211-42-85

PERI·OPERATIVE NURSING RECORD

PERI-OPERATIVE ASSESSMENT

CHECK FOR:
☒ ARMBAND/PT
☒ IDENTIFICATION
☒ LAB
☒ SURGERY VERIFIED

☒ ALLERGY
☒ SURGERY PERMIT

SIDE VERIFIED
☐ R ☒ L ☐ N/A

☐ NPO SINCE 11:00pm 10/7/92 ☒ HISTORY AND PHYSICAL

DISABILITIES
☐ NONE ☒ HEARING ☒ SIGHT
☒ MOBILITY ☒ SPEECH
☐ OTHER _____
_____

SKIN CONDITION
PRE-OP ☒ NORMAL
☐ OTHER _____
POST-OP ☒ NORMAL
☐ OTHER _____
PRE-OPERATIVE STATUS ☒ SEDATED ☐ NON-SEDATED

POSITIONS AND LOCATIONS

FRONT R L Ⓛ BACK R

LOCATION OF DEVICES
SAFETY STRAP = ☒ YES ☐ NO
MONITOR LEADS O ☒ YES ☐ NO
SAFETY STRAP PRIOR TO POSITIONING ☒ YES ☐ NO
K-THERMIA ☐ YES ☒ NO   FULL LENGTH FLOTATION ☐ YES ☒ NO
GROUNDING PAD ☒ PLACED BY: CP   CUT   COAG. 20   CUT   COAG.
☒ YES ☐ NO
TOURNIQUET + ☐ YES ☒ NO   CHECKED BY:
PRESSURE   TOURNIQUET NO.   TIME ON   TIME OFF

POSITION
☒ SUPINE ☐ PRONE
☐ JACKNIFE
☐ LATERAL R L
☐ LITHOTOMY
☐ OTHER

TEMP. PROBE
☐ N/A ☐ AXILLARY R L
☐ SCAPULA R L
☒ ESOPHAGEAL
☐ ANAL
☐ OTHER

PREP., POSITIONING DEVICES, ELECTRICAL EQUIPMENT

PREP SOLUTION
☐ N/A ☒ PROVIDONE/IODINE SCRUB/PAINT
☐ HIBICLENS/HIBITANE ☐ PHISOHEX
☐ ALCOHOL ☐ BABY SHAMPOO
☐ OTHER

POSITIONING DEVICES AND/OR USED
RIGHT ARM Armboard c̄ padding
LEFT ARM at side
HEAD
OTHER Head Rest Egg Crate to heels

ELECTRICAL & IDENT NO.
BIPOLAR # ☐ YES ☒ NO
CAUTERY # 1056 ☒ YES ☐ NO
O.R. TABLE # 6 ☒ YES ☐ NO

AQUATHERMIA # ☐ YES ☒ NO
BLOODWARMER # ☐ YES ☒ NO
FIBRILLATOR # ☐ YES ☒ NO

MEDICATIONS

MEDICATIONS (INCLUDE AMOUNT, TIME, ROUTE, AND PERSON GIVING)
_____
_____
_____

STANDARD OF CARE

☒ GENERIC   ☐ GENERIC PLUS Individualized for patient needs and surgery

EVALUATION OF STANDARD OF CARE

DISPOSITION

DISPOSITION TO
☐ RECOVERY RM. ☐ PATIENT RM.
☐ DOR RECOVERY ☒ ICU/CCU/CSU
☐ OTHER _____

VIA
☐ GUERNEY ☒ PATIENT BED
☐ SURGILIFT
☐ OTHER _____

TRANS WITH
☐ N/A ☒ PORTABLE O₂
☒ EKG MONITOR ☐ IAABP
☒ ARTERIAL MONITOR
☐ EXTERNAL PACEMAKER

NURSE'S SIGNATURE Patricia Crumm
ACCOMPANIED BY Tory Parsons
REPORT GIVEN TO Janice Hotchkiss, RN
REPORT GIVEN BY Patricia Crumm

COMMENTS

ADDRESSOGRAPH

FIGURE 13.3.   Perioperative nursing record. (Courtesy of Porter Memorial Hospital, Denver)

ous members of the team at points throughout the patient's perioperative experience.

Patient Care Conferences

In some facilities, a patient care conference focusing on an individual patient is done in order to provide the best care possible. These conferences may take place before or after surgery.

Conferences prior to the procedure focus on what can be done for the patient. For example, a young teenager is scheduled to have skin grafts. The perioperative nurse who did the preoperative assessment found that the girl had been badly burned as a child and was having a series of procedures to alleviate contractures and improve cosmetic effects. The nurse decided to have a patient care conference and invited the nurse from the adolescent unit to participate. Objectives of the conference for the perioperative personnel were as follows:

- To provide emotional support and comfort during transportation and positioning in the OR
- To gain background information that would assist in planning specifically for the patient's care intraoperatively
- To plan instruments, supplies, and draping
- To prevent infection, since areas of the body were without skin covering

The conference took only about 15 minutes but it was productive. Other OR nurses who had cared for this patient shared what they had done during surgery that was successful. The unit nurse provided information about the patient's likes and dislikes and what would help in relating to her.

This conference was patient-oriented, but others may be disease-oriented. For example, a postsurgery conference was held about a patient who had malignant hyperthermia during surgery. The information shared was invaluable when another patient developed the same condition two weeks later.

Patient care conferences provide an opportunity for group discussion by personnel involved in the patient's care and assist in individualizing the care provided. The staff gains a better understanding of the care they should give. In some instances, policies and procedures are clarified.

The nurse must do advance planning for the conference so that it will run smoothly and everyone will gain information beneficial for nursing care. The time for the conference is arranged with the head nurse or nurse in charge of the operating room. The conference may be conducted at a change of shift, at a specific time when the specialty nurses are available, or during the regularly scheduled time for education or inservice. Short conferences lasting no more than 10 to 15 minutes are preferable.

Care conferences should focus on patients who present nursing care problems that demand immediate, creative solutions. The difficulty may be of a psychocultural nature or an unusual diagnosis, such as myasthenia gravis or Guillain-Barre syndrome, or a patient receiving long-term sternal therapy might be interesting to address. The nurse might discuss how care for the patient having an elective procedure, such as cholecystectomy, compares to that for a patient having an emergency appendectomy. New or revised types of surgical procedures are interesting. A patient having a cochlear implant or laser surgery for cervical intraepithelial neoplasm may provide unusual challenges when planning care.

The nurse should prepare for the conference by conducting a preoperative interview with the patient and gathering data from the nursing unit and the patient record. In some situations, a review of the literature specific to the disease or surgical procedure may be helpful. A literature search can give the nurse added knowledge and provide background for the conference, which will add an educational dimension.

Organizational considerations are important to care conferences. Be sure to start the conference on time. If possible, have the group seated in a circle or at tables in an arrangement conducive to participation. Although members of the group should be encouraged to participate, the nurse should be in control of the discussion. Limit the discussion to the patient and topic being presented, directing the group to recognize patient problems and develop suitable methods for solving them. Because this is a nursing conference, the individualized plan of care should focus primarily on nursing actions. At the end of the conference, review the conference objectives and obtain feedback about how well they were met. The group can suggest what to plan for this patient. After the conference, document the plan and make it available to all participating in the patient's care.

Multidisciplinary Conferences

Multidisciplinary conferences may focus on one patient or a group of patients. A weekly conference might be held for particular types of patients, such as those having open heart surgery. In such a conference, all cases scheduled for open heart surgery that week and all heart surgeries done in the past week would be reviewed; cardiologists, cardiovascular surgeons, and radiologists would attend. Other specialists (e.g., nephrologists, respiratory physicians) might attend when the case involved their services. Nursing representatives from all areas dealing with related preoperative, intraoperative, and postoperative patient care attend. Support personnel, such as the chaplain, are generally also present.

The purpose of presenting a case in a multidisciplinary conference is to increase the quality of care by:

- Sharing information that will allow better nursing care for the patient (e.g., "low pain tolerance," "poor left ventricle," "intraaortic balloon pump will be in place preoperatively," "difficult family members")
- Presenting results of new procedures (e.g., angioplasty) and approving new protocols
- Providing an opportunity for peer exchange to critically evaluate decisions preoperatively and postoperatively

The multidisciplinary conference is becoming an increasingly important method for transmitting patient information to members of the team.

Other multidisciplinary conferences may take place on the patient unit prior to surgery and involve agencies from outside the hospital, such as Reach to Recovery. This group recruits volunteers who have had breast surgery to meet with patients who have been scheduled for a mastectomy. The volunteers also meet with the nurses to provide information that will be important in planning care. Similarly, patients having colostomies should be referred to the wound and continence therapist, who works with patients, nurses, and families preoperatively as well as postoperatively.

The perioperative nurse is a member of the team and attends conferences to share information about the surgical procedure and what will happen to the patient intraoperatively. He or she also learns about the patient and care given on the nursing unit and takes that information into account when planning for the patient during surgery.

Families and patients are involved in some conferences because they are considered members of the team. If they do not understand the illness and what they can and cannot do postoperatively as a result of the surgery, patients will not be able to assist in working toward goal achievement. In confer-

ences where the physician, chaplain, dietitian, nurses, patient, and family attend and the plan of care is discussed, agreed upon, and carried out, patient goals are more likely to be met.

NURSING COMPETENCIES USED IN PLANNING

Specific nursing competencies are required to carry out the planning process. A sound theoretical base is needed, because knowledge must be integrated with motor skills in planning and giving nursing care. Organizational skills are essential to coordinate nursing activities in a sequential, consistent, and systematic manner.

Judgment is a cognitive skill that is essential to the nurse's ability to perceive needs for nursing care and to provide that care. The ability to communicate the plan clearly to the patient, family, significant others, and members of the healthcare team is also important. Finally, nurses must utilize decision-making skills to enable them to make sound decisions when proposing a plan to correct the patient's problems.

Organizational Skills

Organization involves the orderly arrangement of nursing actions. This means nursing actions must be evaluated, ranked, and performed by the appropriate person. Organizational ability is not innate; it is a skill that can be learned. The first prerequisite is knowledge. In developing a plan of care, the nurse must know what problems surgical patients have and how the surgery will affect those problems. This requires the nurse to have an understanding of surgical procedures and what patients experience before, during, and after them. The perioperative nurse should be familiar with the policies and procedures of the facility, job expectations of employees, and surgeon's preferences. The knowledgeable nurse will be able to organize care to foster teamwork and cooperation among all involved.

Six questions that help increase organization skills are: What? Why? When? How? Where? and Who?

- *What* questions provide a list of tasks that must be accomplished. They may be done today, tomorrow, or later in the patient's hospitalization.
- *Why* questions help determine order, as in "What tests will be ordered first?"

- *When* questions help the nurse allocate time. Conflicts can be avoided if a time can be specified. In conducting a preoperative assessment, the nurse must select a time when the patient is not involved in other preparations for surgery.
- *How* questions relate to the institution's policies and procedures.
- *Where* questions ask the location of the patient when an activity is carried out.
- *Who* questions involve personnel, as in "Who is best qualified to perform the task?" Choosing the best-qualified individual involves concern not only for the patient's needs but for those of other nursing personnel.

Nursing Judgment

Making judgments is central to nursing practice. The need to judge sets a profession apart from other occupations. Professionals do not act by rote, nor do they always work under another's direction. They make their own decisions, according to their own knowledge and experience. Nurses use judgment to challenge, question, examine, and validate principles and procedures (4).

Making a nursing judgment to decide on a patient's needs and subsequent care follows a prescribed sequence. It begins with the so-called antecedent phase, when the perioperative nurse decides to become involved in a specific patient's case. The second phase in making a judgment is interactive; the nurse begins to focus on the individuality of the patient and to anticipate potential problems based on what is heard and observed. The final step is the consequent phase, when all possible consequences of the final judgment are evaluated. Table 13.2 provides an example of these phases.

In the example outlined in the table, preventing excessive bleeding is a conscious nursing intervention while the plan of care is being implemented. This entire sequence of events becomes part of the experience the nurse will use when faced with similar situations in the future.

Communication Skills

Communicating is the process by which we understand others and in turn seek to be understood by them. It is a two-way process involving a series of interactions between two or more people. Touching, observing, reading, sharing, emotional stroking, and listening are all methods of communicating. Communication is an art, skill, and science used by the nurse in the role of providing therapy.

The nurse needs communication skills to explain information to the patient, provide instructions, or share data with others. The nurse's knowledge about how people communicate and how nurses can use communication skills enable patient outcomes and nursing activities to be realistic and agreed-upon by the nurse, the patient, and others involved in care. The interaction between nurse and patient many times determines the success or failure of the plan.

For instance, a patient having a mastectomy is seriously concerned about her body image. If she tries to express this concern to a nurse who ignores her need to discuss her concerns and work through her feelings, this creates a communication barrier. The nurse–patient relationship is jeopardized, as is the possibility of planning constructive help for the patient. The patient would be reluctant to express other needs she may have, and meaningful communication ceases.

Effective communication is essential to the nurse–patient relationship. Without it, the plan of care will be unsuccessful. Communication can be verbal, extraverbal, or nonverbal, as follows:

- Verbal communication uses words. The plan, assessment sheet, other written forms, the telephone, and face-to-face discussion communicate verbally.
- Extraverbal communication deals not with what is said but with how it is said. Voice tone, inflection, and speed affect how the receiver translates the message. In written messages, choice of words and punctuation are extraverbal messages.
- Nonverbal communication involves actions and gestures, or body language. We are constantly saying something with our bodies by posture and movements as well as gestures and touching. Understanding nonverbal communication can enhance a nurse's ability to select nursing activities for the patient's plan of care. For example, anxiety may be communicated by certain body actions: wringing the hands, pacing, or fidgeting with buttons. When any of these behaviors is observed, the nurse should plan actions designed to assist the patient with coping.

Decision-Making Skills

During assessment, the nurse collects data and makes a nursing diagnosis. The nursing diagnosis identifies the actual or potential problems a patient may encounter during the planned surgery. The

TABLE 13.2. Antecedent, Interactive, and Consequent Phases of Decision-Making

Antecedent Phase	Example
Nurse makes decision to assess a specific patient and form an opinion regarding care needed prior to and during surgery. In this case, the patient is Carol Jones, admitted for a hysterectomy.	Nurse assesses patient's previous surgical experience by conducting an interview.

Interactive Phase	Example
Nurse anticipates problems as a result of sensory input (e.g., hearing about a patient's problem).	Patient reports bleeding problem during a previous cesarean section.
Nurse seeks more data from patient and other resources.	Nurse discusses past experience and learns patient received eight units whole blood intraoperatively and post-operatively. Nurse reviews current hematology report: hemoglobin 7.9, hematocrit 20, and platelet count 48,000.
Nurse recalls knowledge (concepts) related to hemorrhagic problems.	Nurse reviews current history, finds no mention of previous bleeding problems. Orders previous chart from medical records department and discovers earlier hemorrhagic problem substantiated, plus laboratory records showing clotting times.

Nurse integrates knowledge and facts collected.	*Facts*	*Knowledge*
	Carol Jones's bleeding required blood during previous surgical procedure.	Patient's history indicates potential bleeding for this surgery.
	Slow clotting time recorded in previous history.	Slow clotting times indicate bleeding potential.
	Carol Jones's current hemoglobin is 7.9	Below-normal hemoglobin indicates anemia, possibly due to current bleeding.
	Platelet count is 48,000.	Low platelet count indicates potential for bleeding. Normal platelet count is 200,000 to 350,000 per cu mm.

Nurse analyzes the situation.	Nurse determines Carol Jones has an above-average potential for bleeding.
Prior to concluding what the situation might be, the nurse reflects on all data presented.	All data support previous conclusion.
Nurse affirms judgment and acts accordingly.	Nurse performs the following actions: Informs surgeon and other team members of findings. Verifies availability of additional units of packed cells. Acknowledges and communicates order for additional units. Ensures that intravenous fluid is available with blood administration tubing connected. Increases number of suction bottles on case setup. Adds additional laparotomy sponges on case setup. Documents plan to save blood samples should additional type and cross-match be necessary. Plans for precise measurement of blood loss and irrigation solution.

Consequent Phase	Example
Nurse assesses the outcome or consequences of the final decision and subsequent actions.	The outcome established for Carol Jones was to prevent excessive bleeding and to limit the amount of bleeding. Nursing actions related to this outcome were developed.

nurse studies the identified problems and devises a plan to alleviate or solve the problems and assist the patient to return to the normal activities of daily living.

Ford et al. (5) developed an eight-step model for decision-making. The steps may seem cumbersome but are worth the time involved to follow through on them:

1. Identify, clarify, and order values
2. Formulate behavioral objectives
3. Identify and state the problem
4. Generate and screen options
5. Analyze alternatives for desirability, probability, and personal risk
6. Analyze the problem situation for desirability, probability, and personal risk
7. Make the decision
8. Evaluate the decision

1. Identify, Clarify, and Order Values
The values analyzed may be those of the nurse, the nursing profession, the hospital, or the patient. Values are acquired beliefs or principles that guide individual actions. Together they form personal belief systems that are used in making daily decisions. Every nurse and patient has a value system that is gained through experiences and interactions with other people throughout life.

Nurses acquire additional values through the nursing philosophies and theories they are exposed to during their education. Common values held by most nurses are the worth of life and the preservation of health. If their patients do not hold the same values, it tends to create a conflict for nurses.

Decisions are based on values held by the individuals involved in the decision-making process. It is helpful to identify carefully the values held by those who will be affected by the decision and clarify the impact of those values on the nurse, the institution, the patient, the family, and other members of the healthcare team.

Next, the nurse should rank the values according to his or her own standards. At some point, a choice may have to be made, and values may help the nurse to choose among alternatives.

2. Formulate Behavioral Objectives
The next step is to formulate behavioral objectives. If a nurse's professional value is to provide physical safety to patients going to the operating room, the behavioral objective will be to transport the patient without harm. In other words, objectives are the guidelines for translating values into action. How

the patient will get to the operating room without harm is determined during the decision-making process.

3. Identify and State the Problem
Problem identification is the starting point for the problem-solving process. In identifying the problem, the nurse begins to fulfill the values and objectives. Usually the problem is stated as a question, such as, "How can I transport the patient to the operating room safely?" This question serves as the basis for possible solutions.

4. Generate and Screen Options
The next step is to generate options. The idea is to brainstorm, to produce as many ideas as possible. At this point, options do not necessarily have to be realistic. Options for transporting a patient safely might be to send three nurses and an orderly: one nurse to monitor and maintain respiration, another to keep traction on a fractured limb, and a third to help the orderly in the transport. Another option is to transport the patient in his or her own bed; another is to use a surgical lift. When every option is listed, the desirability of each can be analyzed.

5./6. Analyze Alternatives/Problems for Desirability, Probability, and Personal Risk
Choosing an option goes back to the nurse's values and is determined by what the nurse believes will be best for the patient. Is it possible to use a surgical lift? Perhaps one is not available, or it might not be the best option for this patient. In some cases, more than one option has the potential for solving the problem. Each should be fully explored and analyzed.

Three criteria can be used to determine which alternative is the most applicable to the situation: desirability, probability, and personal risk. Desirability relates to the nurse's value system and involves ranking the alternatives according to personal preference. Probability deals with the chances of the alternative succeeding. Personal risk has three elements: physical, emotional, and social.

Physical risk has to do with the threat to body integrity for nurse or patient. The patient being transferred to the operating room has a potential for physical risk, for example, if traction is not maintained and a fractured extremity is not in alignment. Emotional risk can result from exposing feelings to others, resulting in loss of self-concept. Illness itself may also affect the patient's self-concept. Social risk involves a threat to the individual's role in society, the work environment, or the home situation. In decision-making, the risks are ranked, and the alternative with the lowest probability of resulting in harm is chosen.

7. Make the Decision

The nurse should choose the option or alternative that will best solve the original problem.

8. Evaluate the Decision

Once the decision is made, it should be put into action and then evaluated to determine its effectiveness. If the option selected does not allow the objective to be met, the nurse must reconsider and go through the decision-making process again.

Decision-making is critical in patient care management. Nurses must take responsibility for preparing themselves for complex problems that demand critical thinking. All nurses are involved in making decisions. The skill with which they do so is one factor in determining the extent to which they become autonomous.

Case Example

Even though standards of practice are helpful in determining the plan of care, each patient requires individualized care. The case example used throughout this book illustrates the need for an individualized plan of care.

Mr. Fischer is scheduled for a possible left hemiglossectomy, left mandibulectomy, and neck dissection. The perioperative nurse completed the assessment in the patient's room and collected data pertinent to the procedure. Patient outcomes were determined, and now the plan is being developed.

Communication is one of the most important aspects of Mr. Fischer's plan because he will not be able to talk postoperatively. Part of the plan is to teach Mr. Fischer alternative methods of communicating so that he can let his family and the nurses know how he is doing. The nurse shows him how to use a magic slate that will be kept by his bed. With the slate, Mr. Fischer can write short messages and erase them easily. The nurse also shows him how to use the nurses' call bell.

Because he will have a tracheostomy, the nurse demonstrates hand signals Mr. Fischer can use to communicate, and the patient tries them out. He will use one finger for yes and two fingers for no. The nurse makes a note to have other health team members ask him yes or no questions whenever possible. Since Mrs. Fischer cannot drive, the nurse helps Mr. Fischer plan a way to communicate with her by telephone. He will learn how to tap on the mouthpiece, one tap for yes and two taps for no.

With such complicated surgery, Mr. Fischer does not have a clear idea of all the procedures that will be done.

The nurse explains the activities that will occur during his perioperative experience. Examples are:

1. *Preoperative activities*
   a. *NPO after midnight*
   b. *Preoperative medications*
   c. *Intravenous infusion line*
   d. *Antiseptic scrub*

2. *Intraoperative activities*
   a. *Electrocardiogram*
   b. *Blood pressure monitoring*
   c. *Foley catheter*
   d. *Possible blood transfusions*
   e. *Drains*
   f. *Jaw wiring*
   g. *Tracheostomy*

3. *Postoperative activities*
   a. *Intensive care unit*
   b. *Possible ventilator*
   c. *Frequent suctioning*
   d. *Turning*
   e. *Respiratory therapy*
   f. *Pain medication*
   g. *Dressing changes*

One of the expected outcomes is that Mr. Fischer will be free of neuromuscular complications 24 hours postoperatively. Thus the perioperative plan of care includes such activities as: (1) using positioning devices on the operating room table to prevent pressure over bony prominences (flotation pad, air mattress pad, or egg crate mattress); (2) placing foam pads on heels and elbows, and possibly a foam ring under the buttocks; (3) putting rolled towels under the left shoulder as needed; (4) checking with the anesthesiologist and surgeon regarding padding wanted under the head and neck; (5) checking with the anesthesiologist and surgeon regarding flexion of table or placement of a blanket under the popliteal space to lessen the strain to the lower back; (6) asking the patient about his level of comfort. All the planned actions are based on data collected about Mr. Fischer during the preoperative assessment.

Postoperatively, the plan addresses Mr. Fischer's respiratory problem. He will have a tracheostomy, which will alter his normal airway. To maintain a patent airway, the nurse will check with the surgeon and have available the type and size of tracheostomy tube that will fit the patient. The Postanesthesia Care unit (PACU) will be notified if a ventilator is necessary. Thus the equipment will be available and functioning when the patient arrives in the PACU. For safety during transportation from the operating room to the PACU, an Ambu bag and oxygen tank will

INTRAOPERATIVE PATIENT CARE PLAN
Mr. Ralph Fischer

Nursing Diagnosis	Expected Outcomes	Plan	Implementation	Evaluation
PREOPERATIVE				
Knowledge deficit; lack of specific information regarding phenomena that might affect level of functioning	Patient will verbalize understanding of his perioperative care prior to administration of preoperative medications.	Provide explanations regarding each phase of perioperative period: 1. Preop: NPO, preop meds, IV line, shave, antiseptic scrub, where family can wait, approximate length of surgery, etc. 2. Intraop: EKG, BP, Foley catheter, possible blood transfusions, drains, jaw wiring, trach, etc. 3. Postop: ICU, possible ventilator, frequent suctioning, turning, respiratory therapy, pain meds, dressing change, etc.		
Communication, impaired; verbal, resulting from tracheostomy, wired jaw, and possible impaired anatomical structure (tongue).	Patient will be able to communicate postoperatively.	1. Teach patient to use magic slate and nurses' call bell. 2. Teach patient hand signals (one finger-yes, two fingers-no) 3. Ask patient yes and no questions whenever possible 4. Teach patient to communicate on phone by tapping on mouthpiece		
INTRAOPERATIVE				
Potential for neuromuscular damage due to required positioning and length of surgical procedure.	Patient will be free from neuromuscular complications 24 hours postoperatively.	1. Question patient preop re: any ROM limitations or neurosensory problems 2. Use positional devices on OR table to prevent pressure over bony prominences (i.e., flotation mattress, egg crate, etc.) 3. Place foam pads on heels and elbows and consider foam ring under buttocks 4. Have rolled towel available for affected shoulder (prn) 5. Check with anesthesiologist and/or surgeon re: padding desired head and neck 6. Check with anesthesiologist and/or surgeon re: flexion of table or placement of blanket under popliteal space to lessen strain to lower back 7. After preliminary positioning ask patient about his level of comfort and adjust accordingly 8. Prior to RR transfer check		

FIGURE 13.4. The patient care plan, including preoperative, intraoperative, and postoperative nursing diagnoses, patient outcomes, and plan for Mr. Fischer.

INTRAOPERATIVE PATIENT CARE PLAN
Mr. Ralph Fischer (*continued*)

Nursing Diagnosis	Expected Outcomes	Plan	Implementation	Evaluation
INTRAOPERATIVE				
		bony prominences and buttocks for discoloration, document findings, and communicate abnormal findings to RR		
POSTOPERATIVE				
Respiration, alteration due to tracheostomy	Patient will have patent alternative airway until tracheostomy is closed.	1. Intraop: have ABG kits available 2. Check with surgeon re: type and size of tracheostomy tube 3. Notify recovery room if ventilator necessary 4. Have Ambu bag and oxygen tank ready on patient bed prior to transport 5. If jaw wired, have wire cutters available for recovery room		
Increased risk for postop (respiratory) complications due to history of bronchitis, history of smoking, exposure to environmental irritants	Patient will be free of respiratory complications 48 hours postop 1. Infection 2. Atelectasis 3. Aspiration	1. Preoperatively teach respiratory exercises (coughing, deep breathing, turning); Have patient return demonstrate and state rationale 2. Discuss altered breathing pattern with tracheostomy 3. Explain need for frequent suctioning 4. Due to increased risk of aspiration elevate head of bed per physician's orders and monitor closely for signs of respiratory distress during transport 5. Monitor nasogastric tube for patency and return of gastric secretions		

be ready on the patient's bed prior to transfer. A pair of wire cutters will be with the patient at all times.

Mr. Fischer is susceptible to respiratory complications because of his history of bronchitis, smoking, and previous exposure to environmental irritants. The plan includes preoperative teaching for coughing, deep breathing, and turning. Mr. Fischer demonstrated these activities preoperatively so that the nurse could see that he would be able to do them postoperatively. In addition, the nurse plans to discuss altered breathing patterns due to the tracheostomy and the need for frequent suctioning and coughing (Fig. 13.5). During transportation immediately postoperatively, the head of the bed will be elevated to decrease risk of aspiration or difficult breathing. Figure 13.4 depicts a portion of the plan of care for Mr. Fischer.

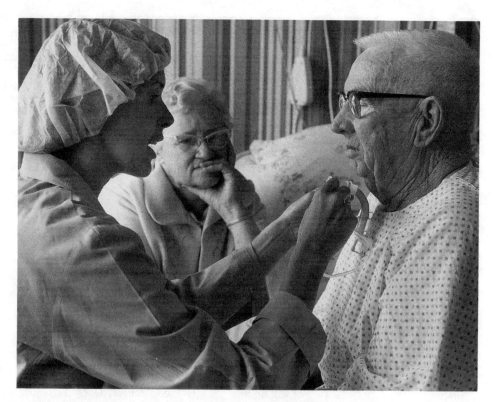

FIGURE 13.5. The plan includes discussing the tracheostomy tube with the patient prior to surgery.

REFERENCES

1. Association of Operating Room Nurses. "Standards of perioperative clinical practice." *AORN Standards and Recommended Practices for Perioperative Nursing—1992*, pp. II:4–1 to II:4–4. Denver: AORN, 1992.
2. Joint Commission on Accreditation of Healthcare Organizations. *Accreditation Manual for Hospitals*. Oakbrook Terrance, IL: JCAHO, 1992.
3. Association of Operating Room Nurses. "Recommended practices for documentation of perioperative nursing care." *AORN Standards and Recommended Practices for Perioperative Nursing—1992*, pp. III:4–1 to III:4–4. Denver: AORN, 1992.
4. Doona, M. E. "The judgment process in nursing." *Image* 8(June):27–29, 1976.
5. Ford, J. G., Trugstad-Durland, L. N., and Nelms, B. C. *Applied Decision-Making for Nurses*. St. Louis, MO: C. V. Mosby, 1979.

SUGGESTED READINGS

Claussen, J. A. "Intraoperative nursing care plan." *AORN J* 44(October):572–574, 1986.

Rothrock, J. C. *Perioperative Nursing Care Planning*. St. Louis, MO: C. V. Mosby, 1990.

Yura, H., and Walsh, M. B. *The Nursing Process: Assessing, Planning, Implementing, Evaluating* 5th ed. Norwalk, CT: Appleton & Lange, 1988.

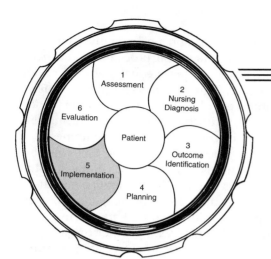

14

Implementing Nursing Interventions

The plan is converted to action.

The fifth component of the nursing process, implementation, begins when the patient's plan of care is put into practice, and ends when all nursing interventions have been carried out and documented. Two important functions are performing nursing actions and documenting the action performed. Interventions should be consistent with the established plan of care and provide continuity for patient care during the perioperative period (1).

What the nurse does with or for the patient is described as a nursing action. Examples of perioperative nursing activities are provided in Table 14.1.

Nursing actions are selected to achieve specific objectives. These actions may be delegated, independent, or interdependent, defined as follows:

- Delegated nursing actions are those that are assigned to another individual to perform. In other words, the perioperative nurse grants permission to technical or ancillary personnel to perform a specific duty, such as picking supplies for a cholecystectomy. This creates an obligation on the part of the other member of the team to perform the duty.
- Independent nursing actions are those provided by the nurse, including assessing, monitoring, and treating the patient based on an identified nursing diagnosis. Explaining to the patient what will happen during the procedure, assess-

ing the patient's level of consciousness, and communicating with the patient's family during the procedure are all examples of independent nursing actions.

- Interdependent actions are those that are shared with other members of the team and relate directly to the treatment plan or medical diagnosis. For example, sponge, needle, and instrument counts are a shared responsibility. The surgeon participates in the actual counting and shares legal responsibility with the nurse. Similarly, nurse and surgeon are both responsible for patient safety in the operating room environment. They jointly monitor apparel, traffic in and out of the operating room, and the containment of contaminants.

Specific activities for each patient are developed in the plan of care prior to the patient's arrival in the operating room. For example, Mrs. Means is scheduled for a breast biopsy and possible subtotal mastectomy. Because Mrs. Means has an arthritic elbow, the nurse notes the need for special padding and extra protection while positioning on the OR bed, includes it in the plan of care, and provides it. As part of the plan, the nurse also uses a soft, gentle voice to explain the procedure to Mrs. Means. This relaxes and comforts the patient. Continuing to carry out the plan, the nurse puts antiembolism stockings on the patient's legs to aid varicosities that create a potential circulatory problem.

201

TABLE 14.1.   Examples of Perioperative
Nursing Activities

Collects Data
  1. Interviews patient, support group
  2. Obtains nursing history
  3. Reviews patient records

Formulates Nursing Diagnoses
  1. Interprets data collected
  2. Sets priorities for data
  3. Identifies patient problem/nursing diagnosis

Identifies Expected Outcomes
  1. Sets mutual expectations with family, support group
  2. Defines measurable criteria for evaluating results
  3. Communicates expected outcomes to appropriate people

Develops a Plan of Care
  1. Identifies nursing actions to achieve desired outcomes
  2. Prioritizes care based on collaboration with the patient and other members of the healthcare team
  3. Communicates plan of care to appropriate people

Implements the Plan of Care
  1. Monitors the physiological and psychological status of the patient
  2. Assigns/delegates appropriate caregivers
  3. Respects the rights and desires of patients, support groups.

Evaluates the Extent to Which Outcomes Are Attained
  1. Determines patients' responses to intervention
  2. Compares patient responses to desired outcomes
  3. Seeks patient's perception and level of satisfaction with care given

---

DETERMINANTS OF NURSING INTERVENTIONS

Several factors determine the types of nursing interventions selected to meet the patients' needs, including the nurse's philosophy and underlying values, the priorities assigned to patient problems, involvement with the family and other members of the healthcare team, the nurse's role perception, policies and procedures, standards of care, available human and material resources, and the nurse's capabilities.

A philosophy of nursing and underlying values are guides in planning care. Actions also are influenced by the importance assigned to the patient's problems and the depth to which they have been explored. The amount of involvement with the family and other members of the team influences activities selected.

The nurse's perception of his or her own role also influences the care planned and implemented. As previously stated, this role encompasses the preop-

erative, intraoperative, and postoperative needs of the patient having a surgical procedure. The perioperative nurse should place equal attention on all segments of care. This includes the patient's need for information regarding the planned surgery prior to the procedure, functional alignment during the procedure, and instructions to follow at home.

Policies and procedures also have a bearing on nursing interventions. For instance, if the institution's policy states that families or significant others are not permitted in the holding area, some nurses follow the policy rigidly, without modifying it to meet individual patients' needs. Other nurses generally follow the policy but in extenuating circumstances realize that the patient's need can only be met by allowing a family member into the area for a short time to provide emotional support or alleviate fear.

Standards of care provide another guide by prescribing nursing orders that have been approved to establish the level of care patients receive. Nurses have a responsibility to individualize standards of care by determining which problems are specific to a certain patient and developing the plan accordingly. In performing an assessment on a patient who is having a cataract removed, for example, the nurse may determine that the patient is apprehensive and hypertensive. The nursing orders in the standard of care for patients having cataract surgery may indicate that the patient should be allowed to verbalize anxieties, express concerns about the impending surgery, and state knowledge regarding the disease process and expected outcomes of surgery. For hypertension, the orders are to notify the anesthesiologist and take and record baseline blood pressure preoperatively. These nursing orders are used in selecting actions appropriate to each patient.

The human resources available also help determine what nursing actions can be used to achieve the desired outcomes. If a patient having palliative surgery for carcinoma of the esophagus is demonstrating a great deal of anger, the nurse may decide that a chaplain or clinical psychiatric specialist should see the patient. If the facility has neither, the nurse could seek out a social worker or an appropriate volunteer.

Nursing actions also depend on the types of equipment and supplies accessible in the facility. If the nurse determines that a patient needs constant cardiac monitoring during transportation to the operating room, the nursing action is to transport the patient with a portable monitor. If this piece of equipment is not available, alternative action should be taken. For example, a nurse skilled in care of the

TABLE 14.2. Knowledge Required by the
Perioperative Nurse

Nursing process
Perioperative standards of practice
Baseline data on the patient having surgery
Cultural differences in patients' responses to surgery
Principles of protective asepsis
Interviewing techniques
Anatomy and physiology
Normal laboratory values
Theories of behavioral psychology

TABLE 14.3. Perioperative Nursing Skills

Identifying the patient on admission to the surgical suite
Performing a physical assessment
Establishing rapport with the patient and family
Coordinating chaplain's visit to meet patient and family needs
Cleansing the patient's skin
Interpreting laboratory data
Interpreting and contributing to data for nursing diagnoses

critically ill could accompany the patient, carefully assessing observable physical signs such as pulse, respiration, and color.

Finally, the nurse's own capabilities determine actions. The nurse's knowledge base, communication skills, interest in others, and concern for the patient all play a role. A nurse who has not performed a procedure or is unfamiliar with it may be unwilling to do it. For instance, a patient is scheduled for a hip fixation, and the orthopedic surgeon requests a specific fracture table. A nurse who has never used this piece of equipment may be reluctant to take on the case unless another person who knows how to use the table is also assigned to the same room.

Remember two important points regarding nursing capabilities. As licensed professionals, nurses are legally accountable for their actions. They should inform their supervisors if asked to perform a procedure for which they are not qualified. At the same time, nurses should take it upon themselves to gain more knowledge and learn new skills.

NURSING CAPABILITIES

A sound educational background in nursing is a prerequisite for the specialty of perioperative nursing. The arts, sciences, and humanities broaden understanding and give the nurse additional resources that influence the type of care patients receive. A perioperative nurse's capabilities are made up of knowledge, skill, and performance.

Knowledge

Knowledge is defined as "an organized body of information, usually of a factual or procedural nature, which, if applied, makes adequate performance of the job possible"(2). Knowledge of perioperative nursing includes a thorough understanding of theories and principles of the science of nursing. It requires that the nurse not only comprehend infor-

mation, but also have the ability to analyze, synthesize, and apply it to a wide variety of situations. Possession of knowledge does not ensure its proper application (2); it simply means that the nurse has the information available to make performing the skill possible. Types of knowledge required by the perioperative nurse are illustrated in Table 14.2.

Skills

Nursing activities also require skills. A skill may be defined as proficient manual, verbal, or mental manipulation of data, things, or persons. Manual skills, involving psychomotor activity, range from very simple tasks to very complex procedures. They include the basic ability to write nurses' notes, as well as the more complicated task of positioning patients on the operating table. Verbal skills are used when interviewing a patient and giving an oral report to a surgeon or supervisor. The perioperative nurse uses mental skills when formulating nursing diagnoses, interpreting laboratory values, analyzing patient problems, and determining a plan of action. Skills required by the perioperative nurse are shown in Table 14.3.

Performance

The third component of a nurse's capabilities is performance, defined as the execution of an action. Possession of knowledge and skill does not necessarily mean that a nursing action will be performed at the expected level or according to established procedures. Attitude plays an important role in performance.

Attitude is hard to define, but its effects are readily visible. The nurse who is warm, caring, friendly, and transmits confidence and cooperation conveys a high level of competence. The nurse's attitude toward a patient can affect the patient's level of tolerance. Combined with knowledge and skill, a caring attitude provides the patient with complete and compassionate support. Thus competent perfor-

TABLE 14.4. Attributes of the Perioperative Nurse

Self-reliance
Sensitivity to human needs
A value system with behavior that is predictable, consistent, and pervasive
Knowledge of one's own strengths and limitations
Tolerance of racial, cultural, and religious differences
Responsibility for one's own behavior

mance entails a variety of intangible qualities. Table 14.4 lists important attributes of perioperative nurses.

SELECTING APPROPRIATE NURSING INTERVENTIONS

Appropriate nursing interventions must be consistent with the plan of care; promote continuity of care; take into account safety, cost, and environmental considerations; protect patients' rights; and be congruent with care provided by others.

Nursing interventions are consistent with the plan of care and are selected to assist the patient toward the desired outcome. For example, the patient who is 6 feet 5 inches tall will need an extension placed on the operating table to maintain body alignment. An obese patient requires armboards and other positioning devices to assure body alignment. Both actions are intended to ensure that the patient is free from harm due to positioning.

Nursing activities provide continuity of care for the patient throughout the perioperative period. Psychological support is an example of a nursing action that demonstrates continuity of care. The patient who demonstrates fear and anxiety about the impending surgery and the operating room requires nursing interventions such as encouraging the patient to express feelings, asking specific questions related to fears, using language appropriate to the patient's level of understanding, and accepting the patient's feelings without being judgmental.

The perioperative nurse collaborates with the unit nurse, other team members, the patient, and his or her family to plan interventions that will prepare the patient for surgery. Assisting the patient to handle anxiety and fear prior to surgery is the initial goal. Intraoperatively, the nurse provides emotional support by reinforcing the patient's adaptive response to fear, giving realistic reassurance, touching, and explaining what is happening (Fig. 14.1). Postoperatively, the patient is told the outcome of surgery, and behaviors that promote recovery are re-

inforced. Psychological support is essential throughout the entire surgical experience because the patient is acutely aware of his or her surroundings and is constantly evaluating the quality of human interaction.

Nursing interventions are selected that demonstrate the nurse's concern for the patient's welfare and also produce the desired effect with a minimum of effort, expense, and waste. Activities that ensure a safe environment might include maintaining asepsis during a procedure; containing and confining soiled sponges, linen, specimens, and instruments; performing equipment checks; and keeping the room temperature and humidity at standard levels.

The judicious use of supplies such as sutures, sponges, needles, and drapes demonstrates the nurse's concern for the patient's expenses. Organization of time and planning of activities will save the patient money in operating room charges. By reducing the time the patient is in the operating room, the nurse reduces the time the patient is exposed to the surgical procedure and therefore may reduce the likelihood of wound infection.

Consideration should be given to use of supplies that impact the environment. Evaluation of products in relation to disposability and the ability to recycle is an important function of the nurse. Segregating infectious and noninfectious waste will decrease costs as well as contribute to resource conservation (3).

The nurse's role includes patient advocacy. As stated in Chapter 7, the patient has rights that must be reflected in nursing actions. Among other things, the patient has a right to information about the upcoming procedure, its potential physical and psychological effects, and any feasible alternatives. Patients also have a right to confidentiality, privacy, and maintenance of personal dignity (4). In addition, the Patient Self-Determination Act requires that patients admitted to hospitals be informed of their right to formulate advanced directives (5).

During transfer from the unit to the surgical suite or operating room table, it is important to preserve the patient's dignity by providing cover, warmth, and comfort. During surgical preparation, the patient should not be exposed more than is necessary. Responding to the patient's questions and explaining procedures are also ways of protecting patients' rights.

The nurse is only one of the several members of the healthcare team who are responsible for the patient's welfare during the surgical experience. Nursing interventions must be congruent with therapies and treatments prescribed by other members of the

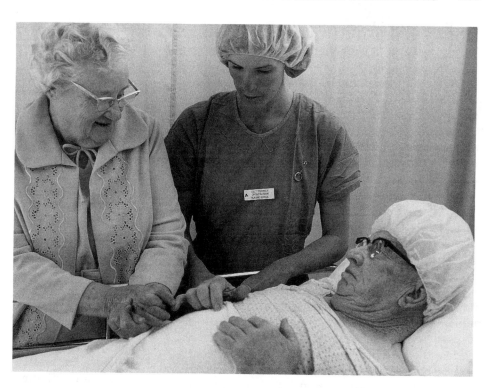

FIGURE 14.1.   The nurse provides emotional support in the holding area.

team. Cooperative effort aids in achieving patient goals. For example, the team must work together when a patient goes into a malignant hyperthermia crisis during the surgical procedure. Nursing actions, such as packing the patient in ice and placing a rectal probe for monitoring temperature, are congruent with therapies employed by the anesthesiologist. Similarly, hemodynamic monitoring prescribed by the physician entails nursing actions such as continuously taking blood pressures and interpreting and communicating data to the physician so that therapeutic measures can be taken.

RESPONSIBILITY FOR DIRECTING PATIENT CARE

The assignment of personnel to perform specific nursing actions takes place in the planning phase and should be incorporated into the patient plan of care. Whatever planned activity is carried out, the registered nurse (RN) is responsible and legally accountable. The nurse has the option of personally performing the nursing activity or assigning it to another individual. When supervising someone else, the nurse must be certain the activity can be carried out competently. The RN also guides activities so the expected outcome will be attained. He or she should ascertain that the best-prepared person is caring for the patient; that the person have appropri-

ate intellectual, interpersonal, and technical skills and the proper educational background. The individual performing the nursing action must be able to make nursing judgments, interpret data, and make decisions about the patient's care.

Once the care has been given, the patient's response is evaluated. This is the responsibility of the nurse assigned to the patient. The patient's response can be evaluated during or after care. Methods for monitoring the effects of nursing activities include observation of nurse performance and patient response, comments from the patient and family, and documentation in the patient record.

Consider the example of the patient having a hernia repair in a free-standing surgery center who is discharged the same day as the surgery. The nurse in this setting still has a responsibility for evaluating and documenting whether the needs of the patient have been met. The nurse does this by communicating with the patient after discharge, either by phone or letter. The information obtained relates to problems such as infection, pain, and mobility.

DOCUMENTING NURSING INTERVENTIONS

Documentation is the recording of individual patient data in the patient record. Both the nursing activity and the patient's response are recorded.

The Purpose of Documentation

The purpose of documentation is to demonstrate that care was given. In the past, recording of preoperative and postoperative patient information by unit nurses was for the most part adequate, but information specific to the patient's surgery was sparse. Greater emphasis is now placed on depicting continuity of care throughout the perioperative period, thus providing a more complete picture of the nursing care given.

Documentation provides a comprehensive review of data about the patient that can be readily retrieved, either concurrently or retrospectively. Therefore it can also be used to measure effectiveness of nursing care in general. Information on patterns and levels of care may be used to improve the overall quality of care, and the information provided may be used for classifying patients for fiscal and administrative accountability. The information also can be used when legal questions arise, to verify and validate the care provided and accurately reflect patient responses. Accurate documentation is a nursing responsibility that demonstrates accountability for nursing actions. Nurses should recognize the importance of their role in assuring the highest level of practice.

Finally, the information documented can be used for research or teaching purposes. In this sense, it becomes part of the body of scientific knowledge for improving the practice of nursing and patient care.

Recording Patient Data

The patient record has several places in which to document nursing care and the patient's response to surgery. One is the preoperative checklist, where the nurse might record preoperative patient teaching, procedures such as insertion of a Foley catheter or nasogastric tube, and identification of the patient upon admission to the surgical suite.

Perioperative records are forms used to record nursing care. They include such data as the placement of electrocardiograph leads and electrosurgical grounding pads; the position of the patient during the procedure; implantable devices; accuracy of sponge, needle, and instrument counts; and other vital information that reflects the nursing care provided.

Relationship to the Plan of Care

When documenting nursing activities, the perioperative nurse uses the plan of care as a guide. The

TABLE 14.5. Examples of Nursing Actions and Expected Outcomes

NURSING ACTIONS	PATIENT OUTCOMES
Patient placed in lithotomy position	Lower extremities maintained in alignment
Both lower extremities simultaneously placed in stirrups	No noticeable dislocation of hips
Both lower extremities padded for protection	No complaints of hip joint pain

information recorded should be consistent with the planned activities. These activities must also lead to expected outcomes since the activities were designed with the patient outcome in mind. For example, if a nursing action is to place the patient in the lithotomy position according to policy and procedure, the expected outcome will be that the patient is free of neuromuscular complications due to positioning. Examples of related nursing actions and outcomes are provided in Table 14.5.

Nursing activities may not be effective in all situations. Accurate documentation reveals a negative response, when the desired result is not attained, as well as a positive one. When this occurs, the nurse reassesses the patient, and the new data are used to formulate a revised plan of action. The entire process is repeated.

Case Example

Mr. Fischer is scheduled for a left hemiglossectomy, left hemimandibulectomy, and left neck dissection. Information pertinent to the operating room schedule has been obtained, nursing diagnoses formulated, outcomes determined, and a plan developed. At this point, perioperative nurses are putting into action the plan of care that was individualized for Mr. Fischer (Fig. 14.2).

One of Mr. Fischer's problems is his lack of knowledge about specific events surrounding the surgical procedure. The perioperative nurse explains to him what will happen. The evening before surgery he will take a shower. In the morning, he should shave as closely as possible because the surgery will involve his face. He should drink no water or fluids from midnight until sometime after surgery. The nurse explains that he will be given medication, a drying agent, in the morning. The drying agent will decrease the secretions in the mouth, which in turn will decrease the potential for aspiration of fluids. He will receive another medication that makes him drowsy. This is to dull his memory of the many activities associated with his transportation, transfer to the operating room table, and preparation for surgery. The nurse tells Mr. Fischer and

INTRAOPERATIVE PATIENT CARE PLAN
Mr. Ralph Fischer

Nursing Diagnosis	Expected Outcome	Plan	Implementation	Evaluation
PREOPERATIVE				
Knowledge deficit; lack of specific information regarding phenomena that might affect level of functioning	Patient will verbalize understanding of his perioperative care prior to administration of preoperative medications	Provide explanations regarding each phase of perioperative period: 1. Preop: NPO, preop meds, IV line, shave, antiseptic scrub, where family can wait, approximate length of surgery, etc. 2. Intraop: EKG, BP, Foley catheter, possible blood transfusions, drains, jaw wiring, trach, etc. 3. Postop: ICU, possible ventilator, frequent suctioning, turning, respiratory therapy, pain meds, dressing change, etc.	• Specific information provided regarding the events surrounding the surgical procedure • Explanations given regarding expectations of the patient and family • Encouraged to express fears and anxieties • Patient explained his understanding of the surgical procedure and anesthesia. • Preoperative instruction regarding postop care: 1-coughing, deep breathing, turning 2-pain 3-drains and tubes 4-IV 5-possible ventilator • Patient demonstrated turning, coughing and deep breathing exercises.	
Communication, impaired; verbal, resulting from tracheostomy, wired jaw, and possible impaired anatomical structure (tongue).	Patient will be able to communicate postoperatively.	1. Teach patient to use magic slate and nurses' call bell. 2. Teach patient hand signals (one finger-yes, two fingers-no) 3. Ask patient yes and no questions whenever possible. 4. Teach patient to communicate on phone by tapping on mouthpiece.	Nurse conducted preoperative assessment • Rapport was established with patient and wife • Patient taught how to use alternative methods of communicating • Patient and wife return demonstrated use of fingers and phone messages.	
INTRAOPERATIVE				
Potential for neuromuscular damage due to required positioning and length of surgical procedure.	Patient will be free from neuromuscular complications 24 hours postoperatively.	1. Question patient preop re: any ROM limitations or neurosensory problems. 2. Use positional devices on OR table to prevent pressure over bony prominences (i.e., flotation order mattress, egg crate, etc.) 3. Place foam pads on heels and elbows and consider foam ring under buttocks	Operating Room: 1. Patient denied ROM limitations preoperatively. 2. Patient placed in supine position with egg crate mattress. 3. Foam pads on both elbows and heels. 4. Rolled towel placed under shoulder. 5. Head and neck slightly extended. 6. O.R. table flexed to	

FIGURE 14.2. Intraoperative patient care plan, including preoperative, intraoperative, and postoperative nursing diagnoses, outcomes, plans, and implementation for Mr. Fischer.

INTRAOPERATIVE PATIENT CARE PLAN
Mr. Ralph Fischer (*continued*)

Nursing Diagnosis	Expected Outcome	Plan	Implementation	Evaluation
INTRAOPERATIVE (*continued*)		4. Have rolled towel available for affected shoulder (prn) 5. Check with anesthesiologist and/or surgeon re: padding desired head and neck 6. Check with anesthesiologist and/or surgeon re: flexion of table or placement of blanket under popliteal space to lessen strain to lower back 7. After preliminary positioning ask patient about his level of comfort and adjust accordingly 8. Prior to RR transfer check bony prominences and buttocks for discoloration, document findings, and communicate abnormal findings to RR	lessen strain on lower back during procedure. 7. Patient states he is comfortable. 8. Physical assessment when transferring to recovery room revealed no evidence of pressure areas or impaired skin integrity.	
POSTOPERATIVE				
Respiration, alteration due to tracheostomy	Patient will have patent alternative airway until tracheostomy is closed.	1. Intraop: have ABG kits available. 2. Check with surgeon re: type and size of tracheostomy tube 3. Notify recovery room if ventilator necessary 4. Have Ambu bag and oxygen tank ready on patient bed prior to transport 5. If jaw wired, have wire cutters available for recovery room.	Operating Room: 1. Blood drawn for ABG and sent to lab. 2. Silastic tracheostomy tube size #7 inserted. 3. Placed on ventilator per ET tube at 50% FIO_2, 1000 tidal volume, rate 12. 4. Ambu bag at bedside. 5. Wire cutters at bedside.	
Increased risk for postop complications due to: 1. History of bronchitis 2. History of smoking 3. Exposure to environmental irritants.	Patient will be free of respiratory complications 48 hours postop. 1. Infection 2. Atelectasis 3. Aspiration	1. Preoperatively teach respiratory exercises (coughing, deep breathing, turning). Have patient return demonstrate and state rationale. 2. Discuss altered breathing pattern with tracheostomy 3. Explain need for frequent suctioning 4. Due to increased risk of	1. Preoperatively the nurse conducted an assessment and taught the patient with return demonstration. 2. Demonstrated altered breathing pattern. 3. Explained need for frequent suctioning. 4. Head of bed elevated immediately postop and until patient returned to nursing unit.	

INTRAOPERATIVE PATIENT CARE PLAN
Mr. Ralph Fischer (*continued*)

Nursing Diagnosis	Expected Outcome	Plan	Implementation	Evaluation
POSTOPERATIVE		aspiration elevate head of bed per physician's orders and monitor closely for signs of respiratory distress during transport. 5. Monitor nasogastric tube for patency and return of gastric secretions.	Postop Unit: 1. Nasogastric tube to gravity drainage with scant amount of light green drainage. 2. Complaining of nausea and NG tube being uncomfortable. 3. Patient vomiting and aspirated secretions into lungs. 4. Physician notified.	

his family when he will be taken to the operating room, where the family can wait, and the approximate time he will return to his room.

The perioperative nurse asks Mr. Fischer if he has any questions and then asks him to explain, in his own words, his understanding of the anesthesia and surgical procedure.

Another important aspect of preparing Mr. Fischer for surgery is the preoperative instruction. The nurse tells Mr. Fischer about coughing, deep breathing, and turning. The nurse then has Mr. Fischer demonstrate these activities in order to evaluate his participation and the potential effectiveness of his actions. The nurse tells him that he will have pain, explaining where it will be and why he will have it. The nurse adds that it is important that he ask for medication before the pain becomes too intense and more difficult to manage. Mr. Fischer will have an intravenous infusion, drains from the operative site, and a nasogastric tube. The nurse explains the reason for these and the part they play in postoperative care.

Because Mr. Fischer is having a temporary tracheostomy, he will be unable to speak and thus will have trouble communicating. The nurse teaches him various methods for postoperative communication. A magic slate is one of the ways Mr. Fischer will communicate his needs. He practices writing the word shot, which means he is having pain. A finger signal is devised by which Mr. Fischer can respond to yes and no questions. One finger means yes; two fingers, no. Because his wife will be calling him

on the phone he will also tap on the mouthpiece. One tap means yes; two taps, no.

The nurse implements the plan of care for patient teaching and has Mr. Fischer and his wife demonstrate the methods selected. The perioperative nurse documents nursing actions on the patient record as well as the operating room care plan.

One of the desired outcomes established for Mr. Fischer is that he will be free of neuromuscular complications 24 hours postoperatively. In the operating room, the nurses place him in a supine position on an egg-crate mattress. Foam pads are put under both elbows and heels (Fig. 14.3), and a rolled towel under the shoulder to extend the head and neck slightly. The operating room bed is flexed to decrease strain on the lower back during the procedure. Mr. Fischer's position is monitored during the procedure, and an evaluation is done by the nurse before he is transferred to the recovery room. There is no evidence of skin impairment or musculoskeletal complications. The nurse documents the activities performed intraoperatively and prepares the postoperative evaluation.

In the postanesthesia care unit (PACU), the perioperative nurse communicates information about Mr. Fischer, his condition, and any needs for special equipment to the recovery room nurse. The PACU nurse then initiates care, placing Mr. Fischer on a ventilator and monitoring physiological and emotional status. When he is discharged from the PACU, the PACU nurse communicates with the family in the waiting room.

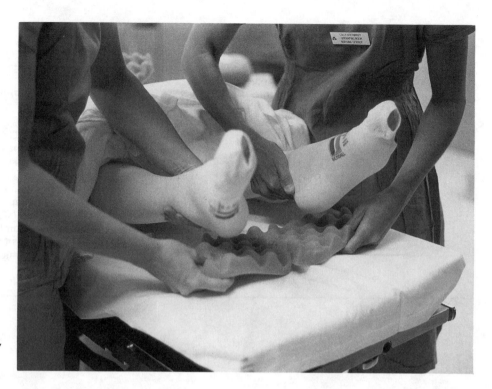

FIGURE 14.3. Intraoperatively, foam pads are placed under both heels.

REFERENCES

1. Association of Operating Room Nurses. "Standards of perioperative clinical practice." *AORN Standards and Recommended Practices for Perioperative Nursing—1992*, pp. II:4–1 to II:4–4. Denver: AORN, 1992.

2. National Certification Board: Perioperative Nursing. *Job Analysis for the Perioperative Nurse and Test Specifications for the CNOR Examination*. Denver: National Certification Board, 1992.

3. National Certification Board: Perioperative Nursing. "A comprehensive waste management program for hospitals." *Hospital Hazards Materials Management* 2(10):1–9, 1989.

4. Joint Commission on Accreditation of Healthcare Organizations. *Accreditation Manual for Hospitals*. Oakbrook Terrace, IL: JCAHO, 1992.

5. "Patient Self-Determination Act," *Omnibus Budget Reconciliation Act of 1990*. PL 101508, Sect. 4206,4751, Nov. 5, 1990. Washington, D.C.: Government Printing Office.

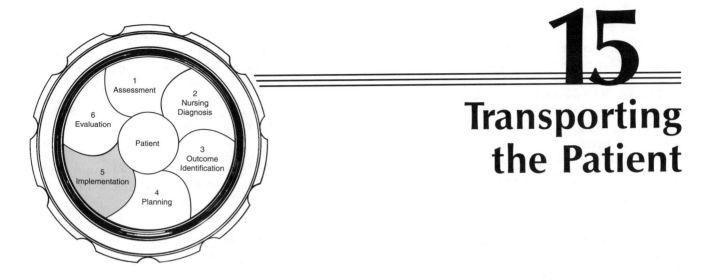

15

Transporting
the Patient

The patient is brought to the operating room safely.

For many patients the preoperative period is a series of frightening and uncomfortable events that can cause extreme anxiety. The trip from the patient's bed to the operating room can be one of these events because the patient is suddenly confronted with the reality of impending surgery.

It is not surprising that patients report feelings of vulnerability, helplessness, and loss of self-esteem during this time. Virtual strangers enter their rooms, remove their possessions, dress them in backless gowns, and strap them to transport vehicles. Then they are whisked off to the operating room, wondering and anticipating.

The process of transporting the patient to the operating room is often viewed by the nursing staff as a nonnursing function and is delegated to ancillary personnel. But the need for nursing care during the transition from the preoperative preparation area to the operating room should not be underestimated. The patient still has physical, psychological, sociocultural, and spiritual needs that must be met. This is a time when the patient requires nursing care.

The purpose of this chapter is to assist the nurse in planning for the perioperative nursing care that should be implemented while the patient is being transported to the operating room. The chapter includes a discussion of the management of transportation, including the role of the transporter, methods that can be used, and specific patient problems that might occur. Finally, the scope of nursing activities that should be accomplished when the patient is transferred to the holding area, to the operating

room bed, to the postanesthesia care unit, and back to the nursing or short-stay unit are all examined.

RESPONSIBILITY FOR TRANSPORTATION

Transporting the patient to the operating room is always a *nursing* responsibility. Ideally, an operating room transporter under the supervision of a nurse transports the patient to the operating room. This provides for continued monitoring by the nurse until the patient is admitted to the operating room and placed under the care of the perioperative nurse. It also provides for continuity of nursing care and communication between nurses.

Even though the transporting task may be delegated, the director of surgery remains responsible and accountable for the welfare of the patient during the transportation period. The director of surgery should ensure that the patient's plan of care provides guidance to the transporters assigned to this task, and that they are thoroughly familiar with the basic transportation protocol. There are times when it is mandatory for a nurse to assist in transporting the patient. In such cases, an agreement between the unit and the operating room will have to be made as to who will accompany the patient.

The Role of the Perioperative Nurse

The perioperative nurse can assure safe transportation by performing a thorough preoperative assessment, planning for transportation in the perioperative plan of care, and communicating the plan to the transporter.

During the preoperative assessment, the nurse should be alert to patient data that can be used in developing diagnoses, outcomes, and nursing actions that pertain to transportation. If the nurse focuses on the following assessment factors, formulating a plan of care will be simpler:

- Age, height, and weight
- Psychological and emotional status
- Sensory status, such as poor eyesight or hearing
- Respiratory status
- Cardiovascular status
- Neuromuscular status
- Presence of medical devices such as catheters, chest tubes, drains, and intravenous infusions

The case of Mrs. Hind illustrates how to abstract pertinent transportation data from the data collected in the preoperative assessment:

Mrs. Hind was admitted to a medium-sized community hospital for a cholecystectomy. The night before surgery a perioperative nurse did a preoperative assessment and collected the following data:

- Age: 43 years; height: 5 feet, 5 inches; weight: 235 pounds.
- Alert and oriented. States she is nervous and dreads going to surgery: "I've never been a patient in a hospital before. Where will my husband wait? He's so worried." Has slight hand tremors, moist palms, and is slightly tearful during the interview.
- Hyperopia and extremely poor eyesight without eyeglasses. Verbalizes concern about not being able to see very well in the postanesthesia care unit (PACU) after surgery.
- States she has a difficult time breathing while lying flat. Labored breathing observed when placed in the dorsal recumbent position.
- History of hypertension controlled by medication. Bilateral varicosities in the lower extremities.
- States she has chronic arthritis in the right shoulder that can cause severe discomfort with weight bearing.

- No medical devices present at the time of assessment. Intravenous infusion will be started in the operating room.

The nurse used these data to develop the plan of care depicted in Table 15.1.

Many patient care problems may occur during transportation. The astute perioperative nurse will be able to identify potential problems and plan appropriate nursing interventions.

EXPECTED OUTCOMES OF TRANSPORTATION

The individual assigned the role of transporter has three fundamental objectives: (1) to transport the patient safely, (2) to assure the completion of planned preoperative actions, and (3) to communicate with the patient and significant others.

Ensuring patient safety during transport is of primary importance. At this time, the patient is vulnerable to environmental hazards. Preoperative medications can cause physiological alterations such as dizziness, weakness, confusion, and sedation, resulting in impaired ability to interpret sensory stimuli. Consequently, the patient becomes more susceptible to accidents.

In order to ensure that preoperative preparations have been completed, the transporter should observe and question the patient about the presence of jewelry, undergarments, and dentures. In addition, the transporter should review the preoperative checklist, ensuring that planned preoperative actions have been completed. The nonnurse transporter is not responsible, however, if the patient arrives in the operating room with unacceptable laboratory test results. The nurse must alert the physician to any abnormal laboratory values before releasing the patient to the transporter.

Communicating with the patient and family members is another important aspect of transportation. So often, the transporter gets caught up in the technical details of the task and ignores the human elements of this patient care activity. Although it can be argued that premedication is more effective if the patient is not unduly stimulated, some form of communication is necessary during transportation. Diligent care during transportation communicates to the patient and significant others, "You're in good hands." Often a sincere touch and a quiet voice say and accomplish more than a whole list of planned therapeutic interventions.

TABLE 15.1. Perioperative Plan of Care Depicting Transportation Problems

Nursing Diagnosis	Expected Outcome	Nursing Intervention
Acute to moderate situational anxiety secondary to impending surgery	During transportation the patient's level of anxiety will not be increased. This will be evidenced by a lack of hand tremors and moist palms.	1. The perioperative nurse responsible for the timing of the preoperative medication will call early enough to ensure that Mrs. Hind receives maximum benefit from the medication. 2. The perioperative nurse dispatching the transporter will give the following instructions: a. The patient is to be moved from the bed to the transport vehicle with minimal stimulation. b. The patient's husband will be encouraged to accompany her to the holding area to provide emotional support. c. During transport, conversation will be kept to a minimum. This will help to provide a quiet environment and enhance the effectiveness of the preoperative medication. 3. The transporter will carry out all instructions and report to the perioperative nurse receiving Mrs. Hind concerning her emotional status during transportation.
Potential for mild respiratory distress and discomfort during transportation to the OR secondary to obesity	The patient will be transported to the OR with no respiratory distress or discomfort. This will be evidenced by the absence of labored breathing. The patient will state that she feels comfortable and is not having difficulty breathing.	The perioperative nurse dispatching the transporter will give the following instructions: 1. After the patient is moved to the transport vehicle, she will be placed in a sitting position of at least 45 degrees. The transporter will accomplish this by elevating the head of the transport vehicle and by placing a pillow behind Mrs. Hind's back. 2. The transporter will ask Mrs. Hind if she is comfortable. If she reports difficulty with breathing, her position will be adjusted as necessary.
Potential for harm during transfer procedures secondary to severe hyperopia	The patient will be transferred from the bed to the transport vehicle and from the transport vehicle to the OR bed without harm.	1. The perioperative nurse dispatching the transporter will give the following instructions: a. The patient will be allowed to wear her eyeglasses to the OR. b. The patient will be assisted from the bed to the transport vehicle by the transporter, who will gently hold Mrs. Hind's arm and guide her during transfer. 2. The circulating nurse will also gently guide Mrs. Hind from the transport vehicle to the OR bed. After she is safely secured to the OR bed, her eyeglasses will be removed. The eyeglasses will accompany Mrs. Hind to the PACU; this will help Mrs. Hind to adapt to the PACU environment and routine after surgery.

As a rule, the transporter should maintain a quiet atmosphere. Family members should be encouraged to accompany the patient to the surgical suite and then be shown to the waiting area. On receiving the patient, the nurse in the preoperative holding area should be told of the whereabouts of the patient's family members. The perioperative nurse should then keep family members informed of the patient's progress, especially if the combined operative and anesthesia time is more than two hours.

METHODS OF TRANSPORTATION

There are a variety of transportation vehicles on the market, and it can be difficult to determine which type to purchase. The decision should be made by the operating room product evaluation committee after a thorough review of the available products. No matter which product is selected, certain design characteristics should be considered essential.

The transport vehicle should be equipped with locking devices on the wheels (Fig. 15.1), restraining

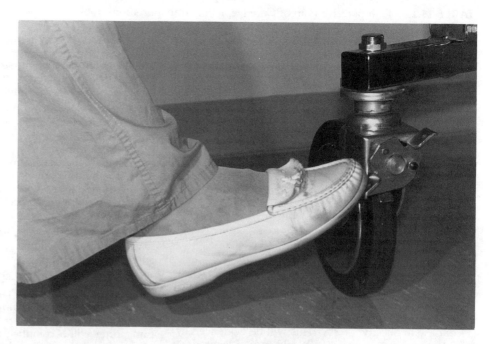

FIGURE 15.1.   The transporter locks the wheel of the transport vehicle.

devices such as safety straps and side rails, rails high enough to prevent a standing child from falling out, intravenous poles or standards with adjustable placement, holding devices for oxygen tanks, positioning capabilities, controls that are easy to operate and within reach of the operator, maneuverability, sufficient size, removable head and foot rails, mattress stabilizing devices, and easily cleaned surfaces (1).

Cribs should be of sufficient size to accommo-

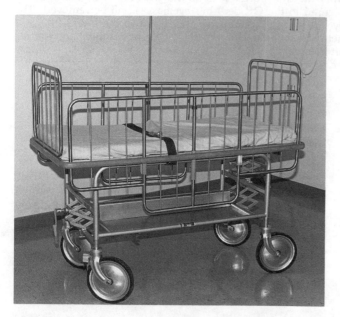

FIGURE 15.2.   A crib with sides partially elevated.

date children up to four years of age, yet small enough to ensure easy handling. Rails with two elevated positions should provide easy access to the patient (Figs. 15.2 and 15.3). The railing at the head of the crib should be removable in case access to the child's head is necessary. Even though it is difficult to restrain a child, safety straps are important and should be available. Like the adult transport vehicle, an intravenous standard with a series of holes for placement is necessary. The crib should have the capability of being put into Trendelenburg's position.

Infant care units are used to transport compromised neonates and infants (Fig. 15.4). These units should provide easy access to the infant, a controlled environment that maintains body temperature, and an oxygen source. The bed portion should have Trendelenburg capability, and there should be a place for securing an intravenous standard.

Another vehicle used for transportation is a surgery lift, which is effective for transporting a comatose patient (Fig. 15.5). The surgery lift facilitates transfer because it fits under the bed and lowers down over the patient, who has been placed on a canvas carrier. The carrier is then attached to the lift with straps. Next, the lift is hydraulically elevated enough for the patient to clear the bed and to be moved to the operating room. This device must be checked periodically, especially the fabric parts, which can deteriorate.

The recovery bed can also be used to transport the patient. It should have the same design characteristics as the transport vehicle except that the bed area should be larger. This is especially important during the postoperative period, when the patient may become hyperactive and begin to toss and turn.

The patient's bed is another possible means of transportation, especially if the patient cannot be moved. Beds that are intended for transportation should be easy to maneuver. The patient coming to the operating room in a bed must be attended by two transporters, one to push and the other to guide the bed. Unfortunately, hospital beds are notorious for having small wheels that have the tendency to become stuck in crevices, especially when disembarking from an elevator. Electrical patient beds should be inspected by the biomedical instrumentation department and certified as safe before being used as transportation vehicles and plugged into operating room electrical outlets.

SAFETY MEASURES

Safety is a top-priority goal of transportation. Measures to ensure patient safety are quite simple, requiring more common sense than advanced cognitive reasoning. Yet accidents still happen, and hospitals continue to be involved in lawsuits because patients have suffered harm during transportation.

Every individual assigned transporter duties should be thoroughly instructed on the equipment to be used and its safety features. Because of the importance of safety, many of these measures are also discussed in the section "Scope of Nursing Activities," below, as tasks that must be accomplished during transportation.

1. All wheels of the transport vehicle must be braked (locked) prior to transferring the patient from a hospital bed to the transport vehicle. If possible, the wheels of the patient's hospital bed should also be locked.
2. Transporters should use their body weight to stabilize the transport vehicle against the bed by leaning against the vehicle during transfer. Likewise, individuals assisting the transporter should use their weight to stabilize the bed next to the vehicle.
3. Safety straps should always be used across the legs and torso to secure the patient.
4. The side rails must be elevated.
5. Intravenous infusion containers should be hung on the standard that has been placed at the side of the transport vehicle, near the middle or at the foot. This will help to protect the patient's head in the event the container becomes dislodged.

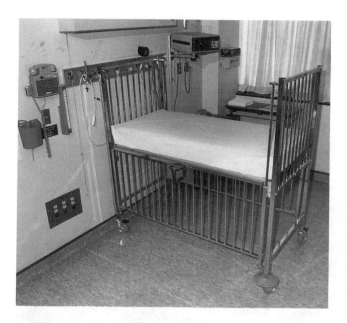

FIGURE 15.3. A crib with the sides down.

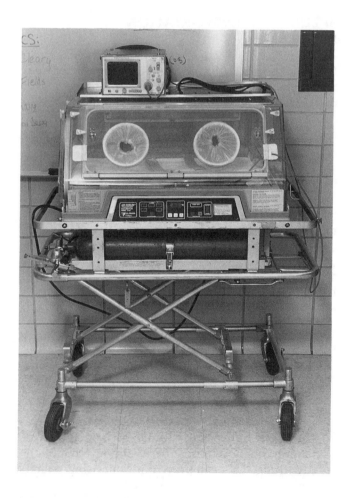

FIGURE 15.4. An infant care unit used in transporting compromised neonates and infants.

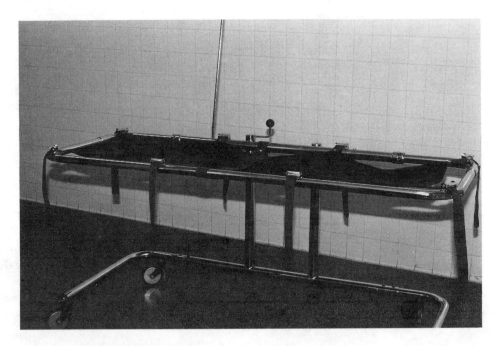

FIGURE 15.5. A surgical lift.

6. The transporter must ensure that the patient's arms remain at the patient's side or folded across the chest. Elbows that protrude from the edge of the transport vehicle can be injured.

7. The transport vehicle should never be used to push through closed doors. This action is hazardous and can result in trauma to the patient's feet. Doors should be held open so the transport vehicle can be pushed through. If there is no second individual present, the transporter should hold the door open by leaning against it and pull the transport vehicle through with both hands.

8. When turning a corner, caution must be exercised to avoid collision.

9. The operating room must ensure that routine preventive maintenance is done on all transportation vehicles. Two areas are of critical concern—the brakes and the side rails. Brakes must stabilize the vehicle, and side rails must lock into position. An unstable side rail can inadvertently release and fall on a patient's arm or hand, causing injury.

If the transporter knows how to operate the equipment, is aware of the possible hazards that can occur, and exercises common sense, transportation should be safe. Note that transporters themselves are also prone to mishaps. Shoes that provide protection should be worn within the surgical environment (2).

SPECIFIC TRANSPORTATION PROBLEMS

It would be ideal if all patients being transported were able to cooperate fully during the process, but this is not always the case. The transporter often encounters a patient who poses special problems and requires extra care. The perioperative nurse should address these problems in the plan of care.

The patient may have an intravenous solution infusing, an indwelling catheter or drainage bag, or a chest tube. The patient may be in respiratory distress, in traction, or pregnant. Pediatric patients also require special considerations.

Patients with Intravenous Infusions

It is the responsibility of the transporter to protect infusion systems during transportation. The following are guidelines for maintaining the integrity of the infusion:

1. Prior to transportation, all connections should be checked to ensure that they are secure and tight.

2. Prior to moving the patient to the transport vehicle, the transporter should ensure that the solution tubing is unobstructed and not caught on anything. This will prevent it from being pulled out.

3. Placing the solution at the right height will en-

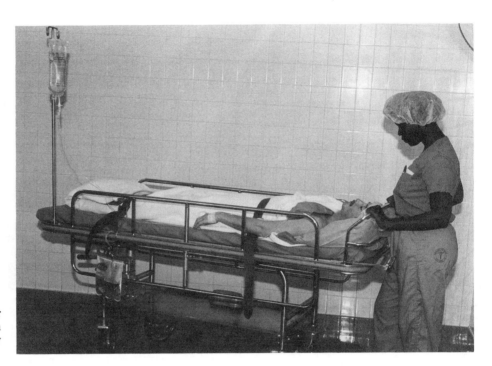

FIGURE 15.6. The proper way to transport a patient with an intravenous line and Foley catheter.

sure that the flow rate remains steady during transportation. If it is too high, the rate will increase; and if it is too low, the rate will decrease. The unit nurse should adjust the height of the solution and check the rate of flow prior to releasing the patient to the transporter.

4. The solution should be hung at the foot or side of the transport vehicle to prevent it from falling on the patient's head if it becomes dislodged during transport (Fig. 15.6).

5. The transporter should check to ensure that the patient is not lying on the tubing and that it is not kinked, since this will impede the flow of the solution.

6. The transporter must not raise the extremity receiving the infusion above the level of the heart. If this occurs, negative pressure will be created into it, causing air to be drawn into it if there are leaks in the infusion system. The result can be an air embolism (3).

7. The transporter must not lower the solution to the level of the patient; this will cause a backflow of venous blood into the tubing.

When the patient arrives in the holding area, the receiving nurse should confirm the patency of the infusion system. At this time, the transporter should report any unusual occurrences during transportation.

Patients with Urinary Catheters and Drainage Bags

Urinary catheters and drainage bags pose problems because personnel often do not know how to handle them. It is the responsibility of the transporter to ensure that patients with catheters have adequate urinary drainage during transportation. The transporter should check to see that the catheter is secured with tape, brought out over the leg, and connected tightly to the drainage bag tubing. Transporters should not place the catheter bag on top of the patient's legs. This is often thought to prevent embarrassment to the patient; however, the drainage bag should not be placed above the level of the bladder because reflux of urine into the tubing can occur and this is a potential source of urinary tract infection (3). All catheters and drainage tubes must be free from kinks, and the drainage bag hung on the side of the transport vehicle during transportation.

Patients with Chest Tubes

Patients with chest tubes should always be transported by a nurse. If the tube becomes disconnected, the physician must be notified immediately. The basic principle is to keep the chest drainage set below the level of the chest and the tubes connected (Fig. 15.7). If the drainage set is elevated above the

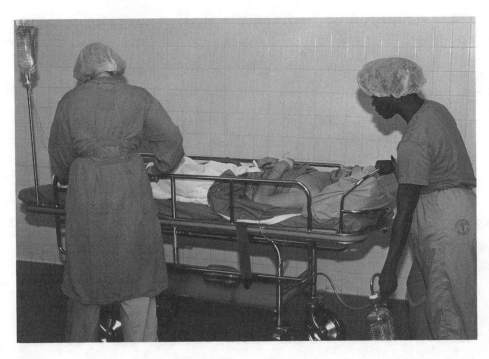

FIGURE 15.7. The proper way of transporting a patient with chest tubes and bottles.

level of the chest, fluid can reflux into the pleural space. If too much fluid enters, the lungs might collapse, leading to a mediastinal shift. If the drainage set is elevated above the level of the chest during transportation, the drainage system can be reestablished by lowering the drainage set. Likewise, if the tubing becomes disconnected, it should be reconnected and personnel should observe the system for proper functioning (3).

There are many nursing implications associated with transporting patients with chest tubes. The presence of a nurse during transportation is justified considering the potential for complications.

Patients in Respiratory Distress

Many patients come to the surgical environment without chest tubes but with some type of respiratory distress. For these patients, it is necessary to facilitate adequate respiratory effort and comfort. Patients with orthopnea can be helped if they are elevated into a sitting position or pillows are placed behind the back. Patients with dyspnea should be placed in the position that is most comfortable, usually the sitting position. If the sitting position does not produce comfort, leaning forward may provide relief by causing the patient to use the accessory muscles (3).

Patients in Traction

Patients who are in traction can be a problem because the traction apparatus makes the bed difficult to maneuver. This is particularly true when the traction apparatus is extensive and cumbersome. A patient may also have to remain in correct body alignment and experience severe pain if traction is compromised and alignment lost. Transporting the patient in traction requires two people, one to maneuver and another to push. A nurse experienced in orthopedics should accompany the patient to ensure that traction is maintained. If it is lost, the nurse can apply manual traction until the mechanical traction is restored. The transporter must know the dimensions of the elevator and doors of the surgical suite because not all patient beds with traction devices fit through these passageways.

Pregnant Patients

Transporting a pregnant patient presents special challenges. Quite often pregnant patients come to the operating room for a cesarean section, which may be an emergency. A pregnant patient should always be accompanied by a nurse, particularly if she is in active labor or seriously ill.

The underlying principle when transporting the pregnant patient is getting her to the operating room as quickly and comfortably as possible. Precautions must be taken to ensure that the intravenous infusion and urinary catheter remain patent. Another important consideration is positioning of the patient on the transport vehicle. The supine position tends to be uncomfortable because of the weight of the pregnant uterus on the internal organs. If the patient is encouraged to lie on her left side, respiration

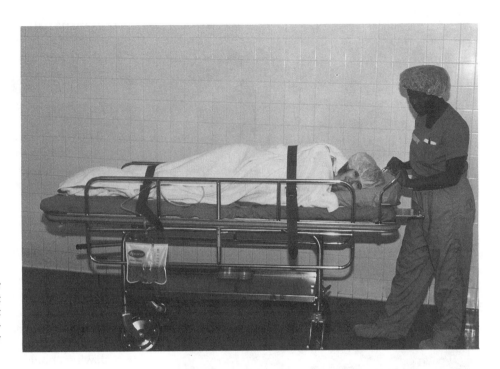

FIGURE 15.8. The proper way of transporting the pregnant patient. She is lying on her left side, which reduces compression on the inferior vena cava by the uterus.

will be easier and compression of the inferior vena cava by the uterus will be minimized (Fig. 15.8).

If the patient has preeclampsia or eclampsia, the transportation period is critical. Since this type of patient is prone to seizures, the nurse and transporter must provide a therapeutic atmosphere that is comfortable and pleasant. The patient should be protected from noise, bright lights, and other noxious or anxiety-producing stimuli. An airway *must* accompany the patient to the operating room. On the patient's arrival, the nurse should check the patient's vital signs, rate of intravenous infusion (especially if there is a magnesium sulfate drip), and the patency of the urinary catheter. Fetal heart tones should also be checked. Suction apparatus and oxygen supply should be readily available in the event of seizure (4).

If a seizure occurs during transportation, the transporter and nurse must take measures to protect the patient from harm. Safety straps should be loose enough to prevent bruising and other trauma, but secure enough to prevent the patient from falling from the narrow transport vehicle. Also, if the transport vehicle has side rails, the patient should be protected from injuring herself on them. After the seizure is over, transportation must be completed as soon as possible and the physician notified immediately.

Pediatric Patients

Pediatric patients have distinct and special needs. Children can be extremely unpredictable and there-

fore are vulnerable to accidents. The correct transportation vehicle should be chosen. When premedication is ordered, it should be given far enough in advance to allow the child to respond emotionally and cause the desired effect. In other words, the child should be allowed to cry and then fall asleep. Once pediatric patients are sedated, caution must be taken not to arouse them. A child who has a special toy or blanket should be permitted to bring it to the operating room. It can provide a great deal of comfort to the patient and will likely facilitate performance of nursing activities.

The operating room supervisor should consider the possibility of alternative methods of transporting the pediatric patient. Nonsedated children may be permitted to walk to the operating room with their parents. Likewise, one of the parents may be allowed to carry an emotionally upset child. A special place set aside in the holding area is convenient, and the parents should be encouraged to stay with the child to offer emotional support. No matter what the arrangement, the pediatric patient must never be left alone. In one instance, a circulating nurse left her six-year-old charge while she went to check an instrument card. When she returned, the boy had disappeared. When finally found, he said, "I was just looking for the bathroom."

SCOPE OF NURSING ACTIVITIES

Specific nursing actions are appropriate at each phase of perioperative transportation, as the patient

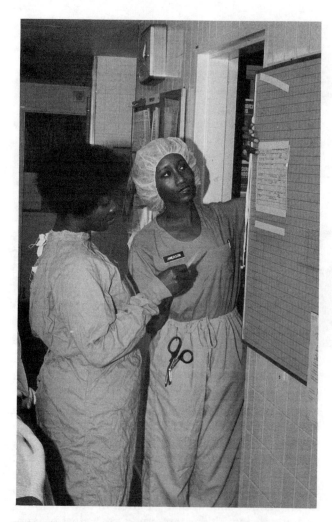

FIGURE 15.9.   The transporter receives her assignment.

is moved from the nursing or short-stay unit to the holding area, to the operating room itself, to the PACU and, finally, back to the preoperative site (5).

Nursing or Short-Stay Unit to Holding Area

Transporting a patient to the holding area can be broken down into steps. These steps are common to all transportation, irrespective of the patient's age or the mode of transport.

1. The transporter should obtain a printed pickup slip from the dispatching nurse or operating room supervisor (Fig. 15.9). The slip should have the patient's full name, age, room number, procedure, and operating room number. This will help to eliminate error when picking up the patient.
2. The transporter should obtain the correct transportation vehicle according to patient need. While most patients come to the operating room on a transport vehicle, there are those who require a different mode of transportation, such as pediatric patients and patients who are extremely obese or too tall to fit on the standard-sized transport vehicle.
3. The transporter should always report to a nurse on arrival on the nursing unit and before approaching the patient. This will help to reduce the potential for error and enable the unit nurse to assist the transporter in moving the patient to the transport vehicle. Furthermore, this will enable the unit nurse to make last-minute additions and adjustments to the patient's record.
4. The transporter should ask the unit nurse or clerk for the patient's record and x-rays (Fig. 15.10). The record and x-ray container must be labeled with the patient's name and identification number. Each facility requires different forms, but the following should always be included:
    a. Informed consent
    b. History and physical examination
    c. Physician progress notes
    d. Laboratory reports, including complete blood count (CBC) and urinalysis
    e. Nursing notes and plan of care
    f. Electrocardiogram (ECG) report, if the patient is over forty years of age
    g. Tissue report
    h. Report of radiographic examination
5. The nurse should review the record and preoperative checklist. The preoperative checklist is a reminder to nursing personnel to complete certain prescribed activities prior to releasing the patient. It is important that the patient receive all ordered preoperative medications prior to being transported. Depending on the type of medication, it may help to decrease pulmonary and oropharyngeal secretions, assist in obliterating vagal reflexes, allay anxiety, reduce blood pressure and pulse, facilitate smoother induction of anesthesia, and/or sedate and relax the patient (6). The transporter can determine if the patient received the prescribed medications by checking with the nurse.
6. The transporter should then ask the nurse the location of the patient. Upon arriving in the patient's room, the transporter should identify him- or herself and the reason for being there; ask the patient's name if the patient is alert and conscious; and make sure that the pa-

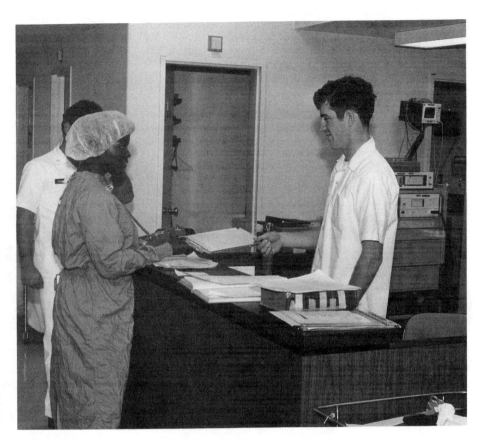

FIGURE 15.10. The transporter is given the patient's record.

tient's record, pickup slip, and identity band match.

7. The transporter should check the patient to ensure that all personal property, clothing, and prostheses have been removed. Patients who use hearing aids should be allowed to wear them to the operating room since this will assist the perioperative nurse during the identification period and help patients understand and follow instructions. Permitting patients with poor eyesight to bring their eyeglasses will help to maintain visual orientation and promote a feeling of security during the transfer process. All clothing should be removed, and the patient should be covered with a hospital gown. This will prevent soiling of the patient's personal clothing and provide perioperative personnel easy access to the patient.

8. The transporter should check and secure all treatment devices, such as urinary drainage bags, chest drainage tubes, and intravenous solution containers. Securing these devices will help prevent breakage and protect the patient from harm. Prior to dispatching the transporter, it should be ascertained whether such treatment devices are being used on the patient. A preoperative assessment is an excellent way of obtaining this information.

9. The nurse and transporter move the patient from the bed to the transport vehicle (Fig. 15.11). This step is crucial, because there is great potential for harm to the patient. To prevent accidental falls, the transport vehicle must be stabilized against the patient's bed, and the wheels of both the bed and transport vehicle must be locked. The patient is then instructed to move from the bed to the transport vehicle. The transporter and nurse lean against both vehicle and bed to provide greater stability. For a patient who cannot easily move from the bed to the transport vehicle, a canvas-covered roller can be used, or a sheet can be placed under the patient to pull him or her onto the transport vehicle. To provide for the patient's modesty, an operating room sheet is placed over the patient prior to transfer. The patient then moves to the transport vehicle while remaining covered with the sheet.

10. Once on the transport vehicle, the nurse should secure the patient. The patient should be covered with enough operating room linens

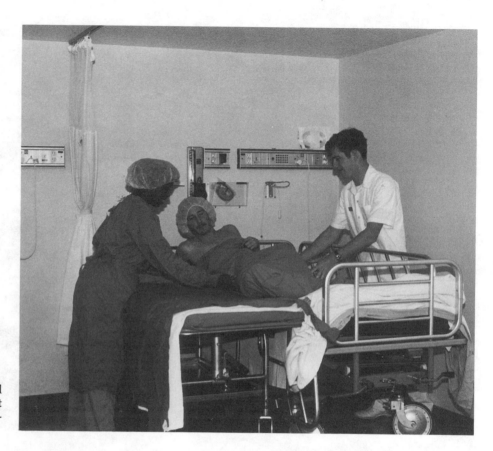

FIGURE 15.11.   The nurse and transporter move the patient from the bed to the transport vehicle.

to ensure comfort. Restraining straps must be placed over the patient and the side rails elevated (Fig. 15.12). A pillow may enhance patient comfort.

11.   The transporter departs from the unit, pushing the patient feet-first. The transporter should avoid swinging the transport vehicle and walking too swiftly, as these actions can cause patient disorientation, nausea, and dizziness. Being near the patient's head gives the transporter immediate access to the airway in case of respiratory distress or vomiting. Caution must be exercised when rounding corners, going through doorways, and entering and leaving elevators. The presence of another individual is especially helpful because he or she can assist in maneuvering the transport vehicle (Fig. 15.13). The transporter should always enter elevators with the patient's head first (Fig. 15.14); this facilitates patient safety. Also, it is very disturbing for the patient to lie with his or her head next to elevator doors that may open and shut a number of times. If feasible, it is desirable to have an elevator dedicated to operating room use during transportation periods. This will help to protect the patient from the curious eyes of other passengers, pro-

vide for a quieter ride, and decrease transportation time because the transporter will not have to wait for an empty elevator.

12.   The transporter releases the patient to the operating room supervisor or other responsible individual. On the patient's arrival in the surgical suite, the transporter should present the chart to the holding area nurse and communicate pertinent patient information (Fig. 15.15).

The Holding Area

In some facilities, the holding area is a separate room in the surgical suite. It is staffed by nurses who care for the patient while the operating room is being prepared. The lighting is usually subdued, and there are facilities for shaving, starting intravenous infusions, inserting catheters, and administering medications. There might even be a rocking chair for frightened children.

This kind of holding area is ideal but unfortunately is not the norm. In many facilities, space is at a premium, and it is not feasible to have an area dedicated for the exclusive purpose of holding patients prior to surgery. Consequently, the patient arrives in the surgical suite and stays in the hallway until the operating room is ready.

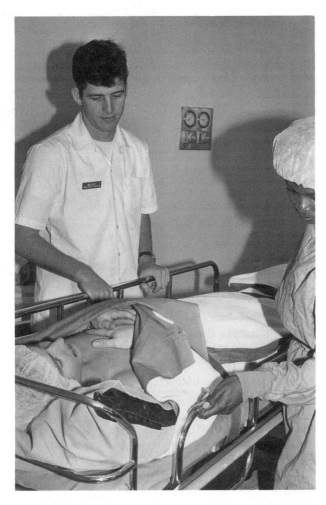

FIGURE 15.12.   The transporter ensures patient safety by elevating the side rails.

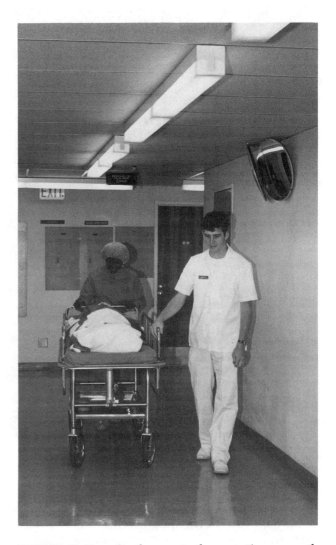

FIGURE 15.13.   On the way to the operating room, the transporter pushes and the nurse guides the transport vehicle.

Whether the patient is in a separate room or a hallway, the following basic nursing activities must be accomplished at this time:

- Verification of the patient's identity, NPO status, allergies, and operative site and procedure
- Review of the operation permit form (informed consent)
- Review of the clinical record, including CBC, urinalysis, electrolytes (if ordered), ECG (if ordered), radiographic report, history and physical examination, nursing notes, and plan of care
- Preoperative assessment or reassessment, initiation of the plan of care, and evaluation of the portion of the plan that pertains to the preoperative period
- Completion of such nursing activities as the shave prep, if the holding area provides privacy for the patient
- Documentation of nursing actions

All of these nursing activities are essential and basic to the perioperative role.

Verification of Patient Information

Some of the activities performed in the holding area are self-explanatory and easy to accomplish, such as identifying the patient and verifying the operative site and procedure.

Because of the serious consequences of aspiration, NPO status cannot be verified too frequently. Some patients say No to the question, "Have you had anything to eat or drink since midnight?" yet still end up vomiting during induction of anesthesia. They may have felt that one cup of coffee could do no harm. A technique for eliciting more accurate information is to ask, "What did you have for breakfast this morning?" Nurses will be surprised by the answers they hear.

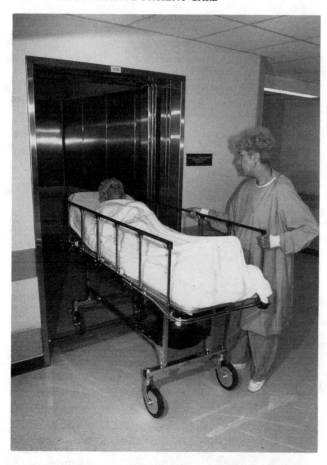

FIGURE 15.14. Always push the patient head-first into the elevator.

Reconfirmation of a patient's allergy status is also important. The nurse should concentrate on allergies and sensitivities to pharmacological agents, detergents, bleaches, tape, and suture products. Again, phrasing the question properly may elicit the most pertinent information. Have you ever had iodine on your body before? Did it cause a rash? What happens when tape is applied to your skin? You say you are allergic to penicillin. What happens if you take it?

Informed Consent

Reviewing the operating permit form is a crucial nursing activity that should be regulated by strict institutional policy. Many arguments have occurred in operating rooms concerning the validity of this form. Unfortunately, a multitude of opinions in books and articles address the issue of informed consent, and it is sometimes difficult to find reliable legal guidance. Each hospital should develop a definitive policy concerning surgical consents. This policy should be a joint effort by the administration, surgical committee, and legal counsel. As a last measure, the board of trustees should review and endorse the policy.

As a general rule, adults eighteen years of age and over who are of sound mind can give informed consent. Those under eighteen should have consent given by a legal guardian. An undecipherable signature scribbled by a confused patient may be worthless and should be approached with suspicion (7). Similarly, consent given by a patient after receiving medication that reduces alertness and comprehension should be questioned (8). Finally, there are instances when it is impossible to obtain a consent, as when the patient is unconscious. When this happens and the situation is life-or-death, the patient may be presumed to have given consent (9).

In reviewing the consent, the nurse should look for the following:

- Clear and concise description of the proposed procedure
- Identification of the surgeon who will perform the procedure
- Signature of the patient, date, and time
- Signature of the individual witnessing the patient's signature
- Any notations of exceptions to the procedure, such as "no photographs to be taken"

Review of Laboratory Reports

Review of laboratory data requires that the nurse, at a minimum, have sufficient knowledge to recognize when those data are not within acceptable norms.

Nursing Process

Ideally, the patient comes to the operating room after the perioperative nurse has initiated a preoperative assessment and prepared a plan of care. The time spent in the holding area can then be used to implement the plan and evaluate its effectiveness. Reassessment should be done to update the plan as needed. There are times, however, when the patient arrives in the operating room without a prior preoperative assessment or plan of care. If this happens, the perioperative nurse should immediately initiate a preoperative assessment and plan of care that at least address the essential patient care needs of the intraoperative period.

Documentation

Documentation is essential throughout the perioperative period. The following example is provided as a guideline for the nurse:

0900 Mrs. Hind arrives in the surgical holding area alert and oriented. According to instructions in the plan of care, she is sitting at a 45-degree angle on the transport vehicle. There are no signs of respiratory distress.

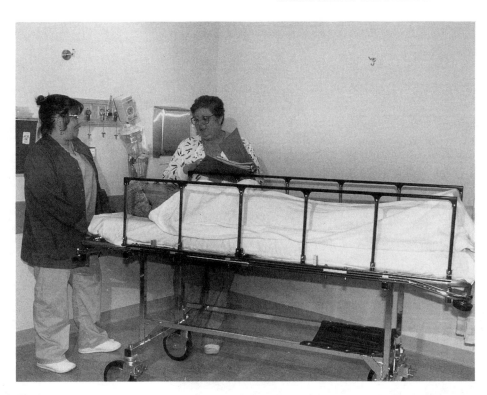

FIGURE 15.15. The transporter gives the holding-area nurse the patient's record and communicates pertinent information.

Identity, operative site, and NPO status are verified. Operative permit is in order. Patient denies allergies or sensitivities to pharmacological agents. Mrs. Hind states, "I feel pretty calm, but I wish I would fall asleep." The patient is given a warm blanket and made comfortable to help induce sedation.

0920 The patient is resting quietly with eyes closed.

It must be mentioned that using the surgical suite hallway as a holding area subjects the patient to a number of unfamiliar and potentially frightening sensory stimuli. Unfortunately, the hallway is not a controlled environment and has a tendency to be busy and noisy. In such situations, the nurse's patient-advocate role takes on new dimensions. It is imperative that the nurse be supportive of the patient and, if necessary, remind other healthcare workers of the patient's presence.

Holding Area to Operating Room

If a formal holding area is available, the patient should be kept there until the operating room is prepared. The trip from the holding area to the operating room should be smooth and relaxed. The circulator should open all supplies and take counts before the patient is transported to the operating room. It is disturbing to a patient to be whisked into the operating room, strapped to the bed, and then

made to watch as the circulator frantically plays catch-up. Once the patient is in the room, he or she must be the center of activity and command the highest priority.

Transport Vehicle to Operating Room Bed

Before the patient is transferred to the operating room bed, the nurse must confirm the patient's identity one more time, and again verify the surgical site. The patient is then transferred to the operating room bed using the same technique employed in transferring from the unit bed to the transport vehicle (Fig. 15.16). Circumstances of transfer are modified according to the age and condition of the patient and the mode of transportation. Once the patient is on the operating bed, the nurse should warn the patient not to move and should place a safety strap across the patient's thighs. In addition, comfort measures are implemented at this point, and the patient is prepared for anesthesia according to the institutional policy. Of all times, this is the time for the presence of the perioperative nurse.

Operating Room Bed to Postanesthesia Care Unit

The time immediately after surgery can be critical for the patient and therefore must be approached with caution by the perioperative nurse. Of primary im-

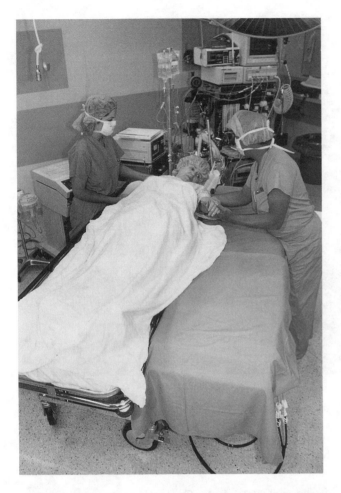

FIGURE 15.16. The patient is transferred to the operating room bed.

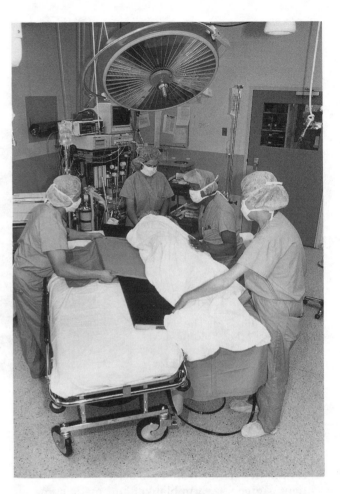

FIGURE 15.17. The patient is transferred from the operating room bed to the transport vehicle.

portance is a smooth transfer from the OR bed to the transport vehicle. If moved too suddenly or roughly, the patient may experience a severe drop in blood pressure. Even though surgery is over, the patient is still in a critical condition and may even experience cardiac or respiratory arrest. The surgical team should be constantly aware of the patient's immediate postoperative vulnerability and alert to possible complications.

The usual method of transportation to the PACU is on a recovery bed. This can be accomplished in a variety of ways. Since the patient's ability to cooperate with transfer is impaired, there should be at least four individuals transferring the patient: one at the head, one at the feet, and one on each side. If the patient is exceptionally tall or heavy, more people may be needed. During the transfer, the anesthesiologist serves as team leader, gives the transfer commands, and maintains the patient's airway while protecting the head.

A lifter sheet that extends from the patient's

shoulders to the buttocks is helpful. The individuals on either side of the patient grasp the lifter sheet securely, while the individual at the foot of the table grasps the patient's feet. The anesthesiologist should reach under the patient's shoulders while cradling the head. He or she then gives the command to move, and the patient is transferred to the recovery bed. All intravenous lines and tubes coming from the patient's body must be unobstructed prior to transfer.

If available, a roller is another device that can be used during transfer (Fig. 15.17). It is particularly helpful when the patient is obese. Its use requires four people: one at the feet, one at the head, and one at each side. One of the drawbacks of a roller, however, is the necessity to log-roll the patient to one side so that it can be placed underneath. If the patient is conscious, this extra movement can be frightening and painful.

If neither a roller nor lifter sheet is available, the patient can still be moved by four people. In this type of transfer, the individuals at the sides reach under the patient and grasp one another's wrists prior to lifting. The anesthesiologist gives the command, and all lift together. If the patient is heavy, extreme caution must be exercised because the individuals at the sides may lack the strength to lift safely.

The surgical lift can also be used to transfer the patient to the PACU. This device is convenient because once the fabric pad is secured to the lift, the patient can be moved smoothly and with a minimum of effort by the surgical team. A drawback of this device, however, is structural stability. If the patient should experience cardiac arrest during transfer, the surgical lift would not provide enough support to conduct cardiopulmonary resuscitation.

The transfer of children to the PACU presents special difficulties. Children are not small adults. Every precaution must be taken to ensure their safety, and this can be a challenge when a patient tries to stand up and look for a parent. The neonate poses the problem of temperature maintenance. It is advisable to transfer neonates in prewarmed incubators.

No matter what the transfer method, the circulating nurse should always accompany the patient to the PACU. This provides for continuity of care and enables the nurse to assist the anesthesiologist in the care of the patient should the need arise. Also, the circulating nurse will be able to report orally to the PACU nurse what transpired during the preoperative and intraoperative phases.

PACU to Nursing or Short-Stay Unit

The patient is released from the PACU after having completely recovered from anesthesia and being cleared by the anesthesiologist. Under normal circumstances, the patient is transported to the nursing unit on the recovery bed. Prior to transport, the postanesthesia nurse should notify the unit nurse that the patient is en route and give a report of the patient's condition. This enables the unit nurse to prepare for the patient's arrival and facilitate an efficient transfer.

Based on a nursing decision, the patient may be transported to the nursing unit by a nurse and/or nursing assistant. In some institutions, a nurse always accompanies the patient to the nursing unit. This promotes continuity of care and provides for skilled nursing care should unexpected complications, such as vomiting or hemorrhage, arise.

The actual transfer of the patient from the recovery bed to the unit bed follows the same procedure used for transfer from the unit bed to the transport vehicle. The only difference is the condition of the patient, who is most likely experiencing pain and may be somewhat stiff. Unless contraindicated, the patient should be encouraged to assist with the transfer. If this is impossible, four people will be needed to move the patient to the bed. The easiest way is to use the bottom sheet of the recovery bed as a lifter. The roller is another option.

The act of transporting the patient from the unit and back again is an important aspect of perioperative care. It takes planning and skill. The patient is vulnerable during this time and may be experiencing any number of problems, from preoperative anxiety to postoperative pain. The presence of the nurse will help alleviate the patient's discomfort as well as provide for continuity of nursing care.

REFERENCES

1. Association of Operating Room Nurses. "Recommended practices for safe care through identification of potential hazards in the surgical environment." *AORN Standards and Recommended Practices for Perioperative Nursing—1992*, pp. III:7–1 to III:7–6. Denver: AORN, 1992.

2. Association of Operating Room Nurses. "Recommended practices for surgical attire." *AORN Standards and Recommended Practices for Perioperative Nursing—1992*, pp. III:3–1 to III:3–5. Denver: AORN, 1992.

3. Luckmann, J., Sorensen, K. C. *Medical-Surgical Nursing* 3rd ed. Philadelphia: W. B. Saunders, 1987.

4. Reeder, S. J., Martin, L., and Koniak, D. *Maternity Nursing: Family, Newborn, and Women's Health Care* 17th ed. Philadelphia: J. B. Lippincott, 1992.

5. Sundberg, Mary. *Fundamentals of Nursing* 2nd ed. Boston: Jones and Bartlett, 1989.

6. Le Maitre, G. D., and Finnegan, J. A. *The Patient in Surgery* 4th ed. Philadelphia: W. B. Saunders, 1980.

7. Regan, W. A. "OR nursing law." *AORN J* 31(June):1225, 1980.

8. Regan, W. A. "OR nursing law." *AORN J* 33(May):1135, 1981.

9. Regan, W. A. "OR nursing law." *AORN J* 32(November):781, 1980.

16

Psychological Support

The nurse assists the patient in coping with anxiety.

Surgery generally has an intense psychological impact on patients. For an adolescent with bone cancer who must have a leg amputated, it can have psychological implications for body image. For an older patient, it may confirm the diagnosis of a terminal illness. For a frightened child in the holding area, it may be the trauma of separation from parents for the first time. On the other hand, surgery may have positive implications. A person may be able to look forward to a better quality of life because of the correction of a physical problem as simple as a hernia that has been causing discomfort or loss of function. Even the illusion of youth may be recaptured through a softening of visible signs of aging. Whatever the reasons for surgery, every patient who comes to the surgical suite has a need for emotional support. This chapter focuses on providing support to the patient throughout the surgical experience.

RECOGNIZING THE NEED FOR SUPPORT PREOPERATIVELY

During assessment, the nurse assesses the patient's mental health status, level of anxiety, and coping methods. In the plan of care, the nurse considers psychological problems and plans nursing actions for them. There are clues that let the nurse know the emotional status of the patient, which may be verbal or nonverbal. Take the example of a forty-two-year-old woman who is having a breast biopsy under local anesthesia. In a brief conversation with her outside the operating room, the nurse discovers she is more concerned about the possibility of finding cancer than the immediate procedure. The nurse touches her hand gently and reminds her that the vast majority of breast lumps are benign. During the procedure, the nurse attempts to sustain the atmosphere of quiet confidence by explaining in a calm and reassuring voice everything that is being done. Common patient responses include fear and anxiety, disorganization, dependency, reduced interpersonal awareness, feelings of loss, and maladaptive behavior (1).

From the time of arrival in the operating room until induction of anesthesia, the patient needs psychological support. Although the contact between nurse and patient may be brief, it should be meaningful to both. The greatest cure for fear is trust. If the nurse is personable and friendly and conveys a caring, supportive attitude, the patient will usually be calmer and less frightened.

Nurses believe that the patient has a right to know, and they often assume that the more a patient knows about the surgery the better. Nurses believe that the greater the patient's knowledge, the lower his or her anxiety will be. This is not true for all patients at all times. Just as they have a right to know, they also have a right *not* to know. Simple explanations are not always effective in reducing anxiety. We must recognize that patients may not be open to hearing the support the nurse is trying to provide. Because the patient plays a vital role in the intervention process, the nurse must be aware of the fact that some patients may not want to know how serious their illness is, their chances of recovery, the likelihood of recurrence, or the expected results of surgery.

In planning for psychological support, the nurse must individualize care as much as in planning for addressing physiological needs. Completing a mental health assessment helps ascertain how much information an individual patient wants and how it will be received. A few patients are calm and confident enough to hear everything that is said, and even ask questions. Many are so anxious that they can absorb little information and may respond better to a general comment and sympathetic touch. It is the nurse's responsibility to determine the best kind of psychological support to offer each patient.

Psychological support is not as easy to prescribe as physiological nursing activities. If a patient's blood pressure drops rapidly, the nurse knows what action to take, but anxiety levels, self-esteem, or coping skills are not as readily measured. Offering the appropriate support depends on the nurse's knowledge of emotional reactions to surgery, sensitivity to others, empathy, and common courtesy. Psychological support is a blend of all these and should be provided throughout the patient's surgery.

The mental health assessment should be done on the unit when the nurse has time to probe the patient's attitudes toward the surgery and assess and reinforce his or her coping mechanisms. If the nurse has an opportunity to see the patient only briefly in the holding area, there will not be enough time to do a complete assessment. The nurse can, however, review the chart for observations about the patient's emotional status by the unit nurse or the perioperative nurse who performed the preoperative assessment on the unit. Even though there is not always a chance to perform a complete assessment, the nurse can reassess the plans for psychological support made during the preoperative interview to see if they are still valid. In a study conducted at Strong Medical Hospital in Rochester, New York, it was found that using audiovisual presentations to supplement verbal explanations was effective in reducing patients' anxiety (2).

Holding area practices vary from institution to institution. In some, the patient is kept in the holding area only until the operating room is ready and then transferred. In others the holding area is where the preoperative medication is given, intravenous infusion started, and other preparation completed. Whatever the procedure, this is an excellent opportunity to provide reassurance and emotional sup-

port. Nurses should explain what they are doing, keep the room quiet, and demonstrate competence.

In some institutions, the patient's family or significant others may remain in the holding area until the patient is transferred to the surgical suite. Having the family there as long as possible may help alleviate fear and apprehension.

If there is any delay in the schedule, the nurse should inform the patient and any family members present. When the patient is transferred to the operating room suite, the staff should create as calm and quiet an atmosphere as possible. Patients who overhear staff conversations may misinterpret them. The nurse should eliminate unnecessary noise and activity around the desk area that could disturb the patient entering or leaving the operating room. Lounge doors should be kept shut to decrease noise in the corridor.

NURSING INTERVENTIONS

The perioperative nurse does not always have a long period of time to intervene and assist the patient and family to work through the immediate stresses that may occur due to the impending surgery. Therefore, the nurse needs to have a good understanding of what can be done in a short period of time. Wheeler (1) outlines short-term interventions that have proven effective. First, the nurse should support the patient's right to dignity by providing for privacy when discussing events related to surgery.

Upon admission to the surgical suite, the patient should be greeted by a nurse who is warm and friendly. The nurse should call the patient by name, and provide introductions to the members of the team while the patient is being transferred to the operating bed. This act of common courtesy may make the environment less alien. The patient may also feel more secure if permitted to witness the nurse checking his or her identity, the procedure to be performed, and the surgical consent form (Fig. 16.1). The surgical patient faces physiological insult that is a personal threat, and the nurse's responsibility is to provide reassurance. The patient should be encouraged to express feelings about having the surgery, and the responses by the nurse should be listening and acceptance.

Another factor in psychological stress is whether the patient sees the surgeon immediately preoperatively. The patient has a need for emotional guidance and rapport with the surgeon. In some cases patients' anxiety and fears escalate to confusion, panic, or despair if they do not see the surgeon. Pa-

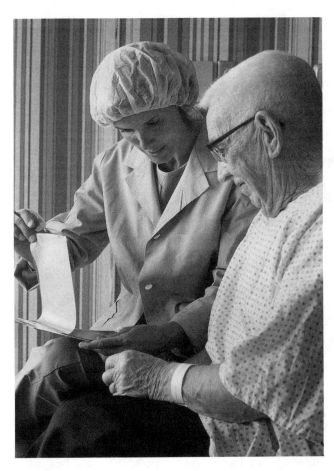

FIGURE 16.1. The perioperative nurse checks the patient's identity, consent form, and validates the surgical procedure to be performed. This gives the patient a feeling of security.

tients want to know the surgeon is there in the operating room because it gives them a feeling of protection. If they do not see the surgeon, they become more threatened. If a physician other than the primary physician does the surgery, it is critical for the patient to know who is to perform the operation and to actually see that person before the anesthetic is given. Constant reassurance and information should be provided to the patient.

As the patient is moved onto the operating bed, the nurse should explain that it is cold and hard. The word *bed* may sound less threatening than the traditional designation *table*. Also, the nurse should explain that because the bed is narrow, a safety strap will be placed over the patient's thighs, and why this is necessary. The nurse should continue to describe what is happening until the anesthesia is given. If the patient is receiving a local anesthetic, the nurse should continue to explain procedures throughout the operative period. These explanations usually focus on stimuli the patient receives and activities that affect the patient directly.

On arrival in the operating room, the patient is usually lying down, which limits range of vision, and the arms and legs are firmly secured (Fig. 16.2). This in itself can be a frightening experience. The patient is secured to a narrow table or bed but may worry about falling off. The nurse can reassure the patient that although the bed is narrow, the safety strap is in place and a nurse will remain by his or her side during induction. The nurse can leave the arm not being used for the intravenous infusion loose at the patient's side. The patient can feel the edges of the table, scratch if necessary, and hold on if this provides additional security. This will relax the patient and provide a sense of safety. The nurse should empathize with the patient, offering a gentle touch or holding the patient's hand.

While the patient is on the operating room bed, prior to being given the anesthetic, the nurses and other members of the team have the responsibility for maintaining an atmosphere that will assist in minimizing fear and anxiety.

Hearing is the last of the senses to leave the patient during induction, and the first to return. Furthermore, there is evidence that patients not only hear comments while they are under anesthesia but remember them. Chance comments of the surgical team may even affect the patient's recovery. Unnecessary noise does not create an atmosphere of trust, calmness, and security. Movements in the room should be kept to a minimum. In last-minute activities, the nurse should attempt to ensure that supplies, instruments, or equipment are not dropped. Counts should be done quietly. Room preparation should be done with a minimum of noise and disturbance. Opening supplies after the patient is on the table may prevent anxiety because the patient will not see the setup during transfer. On the other hand, the nurse may not be able to remain by the patient's side because of the need to prepare for the surgery. In some institutions, the patient is placed on the operating room bed in the corridor, and the patient and bed are transferred to the operating room. The room can be fully prepared and the patient attended the entire time prior to induction. Other hospitals set up the room prior to the patient's arrival and transfer the patient from a stretcher to the operating room bed. No matter which practice is used, the nurse's primary concern is for the patient. It should always be kept in mind that any activity or noise tends to heighten the patient's anxiety.

Overhead operating lights should be kept off until the patient is asleep. If local anesthesia is used,

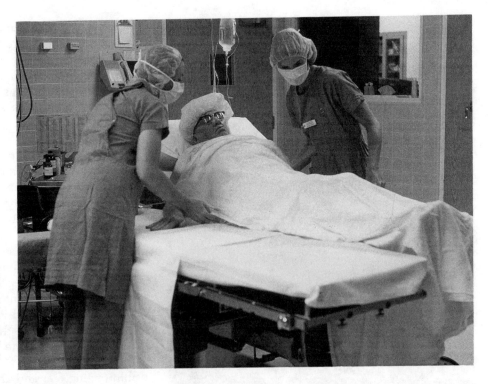

FIGURE 16.2. The patient is experiencing anxiety because of the narrow bed. The perioperative nurse assures him that he will be secure with the safety strap over his thighs and that the nurse will be with him when he goes to sleep.

the lights are turned on after the patient is draped. Lights should be in place and focused on the incision site rather than in the patient's eyes.

While attaching electrodes for cardiac monitoring, blood pressure cuffs, or electrosurgical grounding pads, the nurse should briefly explain the procedure and how it affects the patient. The patient lying on the bed is dependent on the nurse to provide orientation to what is happening. For the patient who is dependent on a hearing aid, physical contact is important. Removal of dentures, eyeglasses, and hearing aids creates a feeling of helplessness; they should be left in place until the last possible moment to decrease the patient's anxiety in this frightening environment (Fig. 16.3).

Conversation at the scrub sink, too, can cause anxiety. A patient who hears that the nurse or surgeon had only four hours of sleep last night wonders if he or she should be involved in the surgery. Laughter and joking give the patient the impression that the surgery is not taken seriously. An older man may believe his hernia repair is risky and that he might not come out of the anesthesia. The woman having open heart surgery is distressed when she hears the nurse asking about the saw blades; she sees herself as a piece of lumber at a construction site. In any case, the tone of the operating room staff should be calm and reassuring.

The nurse should remain close to the patient as anesthesia is administered. Touching the arm, hold-ing the hand, and speaking softly all give the patient a feeling of support and reassurance. Some patients respond to a calm voice saying, "Close your eyes and think of something pleasant," "Have a pleasant fantasy," "Listen to the music and have a beautiful dream." These suggestions help relax the patient and contribute to an uneventful induction. Touch is supportive, but the nurse should realize that reassurance can be communicated through tone of voice, inflection, pauses, facial expressions, and gestures as well.

Once the patient is asleep, the nurse's role as an advocate continues. The patient's modesty and dignity should be preserved. If the patient has expressed concern about the number of people in the room, only essential personnel should be permitted. If people other than the immediate team are to be present, permission should be obtained from the patient and surgeon prior to surgery.

Immediately after surgery, while the patient is emerging from anesthesia, the nurse should again speak to him or her, using the patient's name and staying close during transfer to the stretcher and transport to the postanesthesia care unit.

Special Age Groups

Teenagers
Teenagers undergoing surgery have special needs for psychological support. They experience different

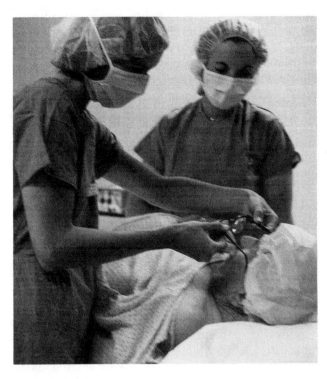

FIGURE 16.3.   The nurse removes the patient's glasses at the last possible minute. This patient's glasses remained with him until induction.

types of problems than adults. Regardless of the kind of surgery, their focus is on body image, disfiguration, and mutilation. They are aware of their appearance and how they look in comparison to peers or current media idols. They are concerned with being whole, with all body parts intact.

Independence is another important concept for them. They are striving to attain their individuality and identity, and when faced with the possibility of surgery they become very ambivalent. They try to be brave but cannot always pull it off. Thus, their behavior is inconsistent. One minute they are demonstrating responsibility and maturity, and the next they are completely the opposite.

Cesarean section can be a traumatic experience, even for adult patients, because many women believe it represents a failure to deliver "normally." The patient may come to cesarean surgery with heightened levels of anxiety due to an exhausting labor and apprehensions about the procedure. For the pregnant teenager, the experience may seem even more overwhelming. Often she has not had the opportunity to attend childbirth education classes. If she is unmarried or the pregnancy is unplanned, she may be facing difficulties beyond the physical rigors of labor and delivery. To a young patient, the threat of disfigurement from the cesarean incision

may be even more disturbing than it is for an adult. Her coping mechanisms may be exhausted, and she may be facing surgery in a state of panic and regression.

Explaining the reasons for the cesarean birth and how long it will last may help reinforce coping skills. The nurse should gently explain what is being done at every step, reassuring the patient and encouraging her to express her feelings. Allowing the father or significant other into the operating room during a cesarean delivery provides support. If no visitors are allowed, the nurse must provide the explanation and reassurance.

Teenagers having abortions are also in need of special emotional support. Due to the circumstances of the pregnancy, they may feel ambivalent and defensive about their decision. They are acutely aware of how they are treated by the staff and sensitive to signs of rejection. The nurse can assist them to cope by showing acceptance, support, and a nonjudgmental attitude.

Children

Children vary in how they cope with the stresses related to surgery. During assessment the nurse should attempt to identify how the child is coping and interpreting the upcoming surgery (3).

The operating room can be especially frightening to a child. For someone under four years of age, separation from parents may be the most traumatic aspect of the procedure. The child may never have faced a threatening experience without a parent. In addition, a child's ability to understand what is happening is limited. Explanations of what will happen during surgery have little meaning. The nurse can best provide support by holding or rocking the child. Letting the child take a special toy or blanket into the operating room may help calm and distract him or her.

Schoolage children have a better understanding of surgery and may benefit from preoperative teaching that includes a tour of the operating room. In some hospitals, nurses take children into the operating room the day before surgery to show them the table, the anesthesia machine, and the mask used to put them to sleep. The next day, when they are admitted for surgery, they are not as frightened and seem better able to cope with separation from their parents.

The child's admission to the operating room may go more smoothly if the room is ready before the patient is brought in. In this way, the child does not have to watch instruments being prepared nor wait for induction. Coordinating the child's arrival from the holding area with that of the surgeon and anesthesiologist also minimizes waiting. When the child arrives, the nurse should be prepared to direct full attention to the patient, call him or her by name, be warm and friendly, and talk quietly.

Before induction, it is a good idea to allow the child to sit up, to be held, or to lie on the operating table without restraints, with the nurse close by. Removing clothing, especially underpants, can be threatening to children. The gown and underpants can be left on until after the child is asleep. A quiet atmosphere is especially important for children because loud talking and clashing instruments may provoke fantasies about what will be done to them.

For induction, the anesthetic may be started and the child then placed on the operating room table and restrained as the stages of anesthesia progress. The nurse should gently hold the child and talk in a soothing voice during induction. Alternatively, the anesthesiologist may talk soothingly while the nurse gently holds the child's hand, then the arms, and finally restrains the patient until the desired anesthesia plane is reached. Then the straps are placed securely to protect the child during the procedure.

Occasionally a parent may be present during induction. This can be reassuring to a frightened child. But each situation must be evaluated individually; such a practice would not be appropriate or desirable in all cases.

Older children may be offered choices of how they are to be induced. They might be asked whether they want to go to sleep with a needle or by breathing through a mask. Whatever choice they make, it should be carried out. Most children can be put to sleep relatively easily with a mask, and the smell of the gas is much more tolerable than it was in the past. Some anesthesiologists use pleasant-smelling extracts such as peppermint or spearmint inside the mask, offering the child a choice of scents. The anesthesiologist encourages the child to breathe deeply and watch the balloon blowing up. This involves the child in the induction process and helps provide a distraction. If the child already has an intravenous infusion line prior to being brought to the operating room, that is the obvious route for administering the anesthetic.

Local Anesthesia

The patient who is awake during surgery has a different perspective from the one having general anesthesia. There is no fear of going to sleep and never waking up again, as with some patients having general anesthesia. However, the patient may be apprehensive about what will happen. The perioperative nurse may have responsibility for monitoring the physiological and psychological status of the patient. In this case the patient's anxiety level should be monitored constantly. For example, the awake patient having a nasal reconstruction may have complete confidence in the surgeon, but the drapes, the heat generated by the drapes and overhead lights, the facial pressure by the surgeon, and the grating and rasping noises all cause anxiety. The nurse can assess how the anxiety is affecting the patient by monitoring vital signs. When anxiety increases, respirations increase, becoming rapid and more shallow. The pulse accelerates, color may change, and perspiring occurs. The nurse must validate that the patient is feeling anxious because other factors such as medication may cause the same symptoms. Muscle cramps, nausea, muscle tenseness, tremor, and facial and body rigidity may indicate a high level of anxiety. Psychological manifestations of anxiety include increased self-awareness, self-consciousness, heightened perception of surroundings, and at times, distraction.

The nurse can intervene by asking an anxious patient how best to help him or her deal with feelings of concern. The nurse may decide to report the patient's anxiety to the surgeon, who may order medication that has a tranquilizing effect. A caring nurse–patient relationship in which the patient feels comfortable will alleviate some of the fear. To provide this type of support, the nurse must:

1. Accept the patient's dependency without feeling threatened by it
2. Give warmth and friendliness without demanding gratitude
3. Adjust to continual and sometimes unexpected change
4. Use empathy to gain insight into patients' needs without overidentifying with their problems

The nurse must be an accepting listener who creates the opportunity for the patient to talk. The nurse's actions must demonstrate a sincere interest in the patient.

During an operation performed under local anesthesia, as during any procedure, the atmosphere in the room is important. The noise level should be kept to a minimum. The traffic in and out of the room should be limited. Conversation must also be limited. The focus is on the patient. The nurse should try to empathize by seeing the surgery through the patient's eyes. Other members of the team, such as the radiologist, pathologist, and con-

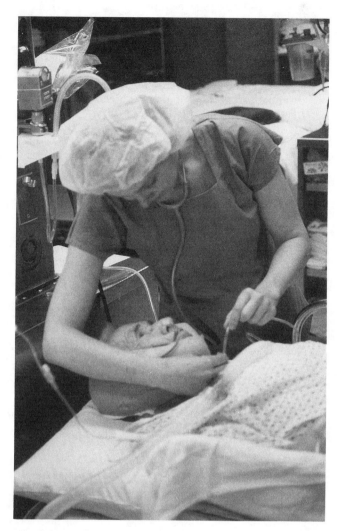

FIGURE 16.4.   The nurse calls the patient by name as he emerges from the anesthesia.

sulting physician, should be alerted to the fact that the patient is awake.

The nurse should assess the patient's comfort. A pillow may ease discomfort from positioning. Drapes should be positioned to provide adequate ventilation around the patient's face.

Some patients want to see what the surgeon is doing, but others do not. The nurse should ask if the patient wants to watch. For example, a nursing educator who was having a mass removed from her right palm asked to have her head propped up so she could see. "One must take advantage of every learning opportunity," she commented. Another patient was curious enough to stare at the operating light, watching his hernia repair in the reflective surface. For the patient who is not inquisitive, though, a screen can be used to separate the operative site from the field of vision.

POSTANESTHESIA CARE

When the patient is transferred to the postanesthesia care unit (PACU), the perioperative nurse should report significant psychological data to the nursing staff. For example, a patient who was resistant and fought during induction may wake up the same way. If the patient went to sleep crying, the same concerns may surface again postoperatively. If a patient requested that dentures be returned immediately on awakening, the PACU staff should be alerted to this. Another patient may be depressed about her mastectomy. In all cases, the PACU nursing staff will need to provide emotional support to all patients as they awaken (Fig. 16.4).

The family is included in psychological support, as in other aspects of the plan of care. While the patient is in surgery, family members or friends are anxiously waiting to hear about their loved one. The nurse who has a sense of commitment to the patient and family will stay in contact with them by going to the waiting room, sending a message, or telephoning. All the nurse has to say is, "The surgery is still in progress," "The surgery is taking a little longer than you were told because we were held up and started later," or "Your husband is now in the postanesthesia care room." If there is a crisis and the family must be told that the surgery was not successful or that a malignancy was found, the nurse may accompany the physician and follow up by having the chaplain present.

Providing psychological support and monitoring the emotional status of patients during the operative period is an important nursing activity. But preoperative preparation of patients has an impact on their behavior during surgery. Patients who have had an opportunity to work through their fears and find coping mechanisms for handling their anxieties are more relaxed when they arrive in the operating room than those who have not. They also recover more quickly and with fewer complications. Psychological support and therapeutic measures are critical to their well-being.

All people deserve to be treated in a warm, caring manner. Remember that every patient coming to the operating room is someone's loved one. To provide the best possible support, the nurse should ask, "How would I want a nurse to care for my loved one?"

REFERENCES

1. Wheeler, Barbara R. "Crisis intervention." *AORN J* 47(5):1242–1248, 1988.
2. Meeker, Bonnie J. "Preoperative teaching: Easing the patient's anxiety." *Today's OR Nurse* 11(8):14–18, 1989.

3. LaMontagne, Lynda L. "Facilitating children's coping." *AORN J* 42(5):718–723, 1985.

Suggested Reading

Aguilera, D. C., and Messick, J. M. *Crisis Intervention: Theory and Methodology* 5th ed. St. Louis, MO: C. V. Mosby, 1986.

Bates, T., and Broome, M. "Preparation of children for hospitalization and surgery: A review of literature." *J of Pediatric Nursing* 1:230–239, 1986.

Bayley, Elizabeth W., and Turcke, Susan A. *A Comprehensive Curriculum for Trauma Nursing.* Boston: Jones and Bartlett, 1992.

Young, C. M. "The postoperative followup phone call: An essential part of the ambulatory surgery nurses' job." *J Postanesthesia Nursing* 5:273–275, 1990.

17

Anesthesia and Perioperative Monitoring

The nurse continually measures the patient's physical status.

This chapter presents an overview of the body's major organ systems, with emphasis on the cardiorespiratory system; summarizes the effects of surgery and anesthesia on these systems; and describes measures for perioperative monitoring.

Professional perioperative nurses must understand the anatomic and physiologic changes patients experience during anesthesia and surgery. As part of the perioperative team, the nurse must be prepared to assist with invasive and noninvasive monitoring, as well as therapeutic intervention. Although a nurse's specific responsibilities for monitoring vary among institutions and according to type of surgical procedure, specific knowledge regarding physiological monitoring, patient responses, and nursing interventions are vital for successful perioperative patient care.

THE CARDIOVASCULAR SYSTEM

Circulatory Anatomy and Physiology

The primary function of the cardiovascular system is the transport of oxygen (O_2), carbon dioxide (CO_2), and nutrients. The heart, enclosed in the pericardium, serves as a pump for the circulatory system. It occupies the lower portion of the mediastinum, between the lungs, anterior to the esophagus and descending thoracic aorta. A septum divides the heart along its long axis into right and left halves, each containing an atrium and a ventricle. Venous blood flows into the right atrium and through the tricuspid (right atrioventricular) valve into the right ventricle by passive flow and the force of atrial contraction. The right ventricle pumps blood through the pulmonic valve into the pulmonary artery. Oxygen and CO_2 exchange occurs in the pulmonary capillaries. Oxygenated blood returns to the left atrium through the pulmonary veins and then flows passively and is pumped through the mitral (left atrioventricular) valve into the left ventricle. Seventy percent of atrial blood flows passively into the left ventricle as the mitral valve opens; the remaining 30% is pumped by the force of atrial contraction. This contraction, termed *atrial kick* is significant in forcing the remaining atrial blood into the ventricle. Left ventricular contraction then pumps the blood through the aortic valve into the aorta and the systemic circulation (1).

The Cardiac Cycle

The cardiac cycle consists of diastole, the period of ventricular relaxation and filling, and systole, the period of ventricular contraction and emptying. The electrocardiogram (ECG) records the electrical activity of the heart, and is described by P-, QRS-, and T-waves. The P-wave represents the electrical impulse (depolarization) generated by the sinoatrial (SA) node located in the right atrium, and initiates atrial contraction. This impulse is conducted to the atrioventricular (AV) node located in the atrioventricular septum, then through the Bundle of His and the Purkinje fibers to cardiac ventricular muscle fibers, causing them to contract. Ventricular contraction initiates systole and is depicted on the ECG by the QRS complex. The QRS complex is followed by the T-wave, which indicates ventricular relaxation (repolarization) and the onset of diastole (1, 2).

Heart Sounds

Characteristic normal heart sounds are vibrations caused by blood flow or valve movement or closure. The first heart sound (S_1) is produced by closure of the tricuspid and mitral valves following atrial contraction. The second heart sound (S_2) is produced by closure of the aortic and pulmonic valves following ventricular contraction. In hearts with poorly functioning ventricles, a third heart sound (S_3) may occur as the ventricles passively fill with atrial blood; and a fourth heart sound (S_4) may be associated with atrial contraction.

Regulation of Cardiac Output and Blood Pressure

Cardiac output is the volume of blood ejected per minute by the left ventricle and is calculated by the following formula:

Cardiac output = stroke volume × heart rate

where stroke volume is the volume of blood ejected by the ventricle with each heart beat.

The amount of blood flowing into the heart from the venous system, called preload, and the force of ventricular contraction, called contractility, are major factors affecting cardiac output. The third major determinant of cardiac output is the vascular resistance to ventricular ejection of blood, or afterload. The heart has an autoregulatory mechanism, termed The Frank-Starling Law of the Heart, that alters the force of ventricular contraction to accommodate fluctuations in venous return. By matching contractility with preload, this mechanism allows all venous blood returning to the heart to be expelled by an adequate ventricular contraction. The force of left ventricular contraction produces a pressure as it propels blood into the aorta, major vessels, and capillaries. Systemic blood pressure is a product of blood flow (cardiac output) and resistance to ventricular ejection of blood (peripheral vascular resistance) (1).

Conditions Affecting Cardiac Function

Conditions that affect cardiac function include aortic valve disease, mitral valve disease, and ischemic heart disease.

Aortic Valve Disease

Aortic valvular stenosis obstructs the egress of blood from the left ventricle. The left ventricle must work harder to overcome this outflow obstruction, resulting in left ventricular hypertrophy. As the lesion progresses, elevated left atrial pressures and pulmonary congestion may develop. Left ventricular hypertrophy and high intracavitary pressures, combined with the pressure gradient across the stenotic valve, may lead to inadequate coronary perfusion. Patients with aortic stenosis do not tolerate rapid heart rates (tachycardia), which decrease cardiac output and coronary blood flow. Symptoms include fatigue, syncope, and angina pectoris.

Aortic valvular insufficiency permits regurgitant blood flow from the aorta to enter the left ventricle during diastole, resulting in left ventricular dilatation and hypertrophy. Patients with aortic insufficiency are particularly sensitive to cardiac rhythm disturbances, especially loss of effective atrial contractions during atrial fibrillation. Symptoms include fatigue, pulmonary congestion, and cerebral and coronary insufficiency.

Mitral Valve Disease

Often associated with rheumatoid disease, mitral valvular stenosis results in a defect that impedes blood flow from the left atrium to the left ventricle during diastole. The stenosis raises left atrial as well as pulmonary artery pressures, leading to atrial dilatation, atrial fibrillation, and pulmonary congestion and edema. Symptoms include dyspnea, orthopnea, and frequent pulmonary infections secondary to pulmonary congestion.

Chronic mitral insufficiency most often results from rheumatic disease, while acute mitral valvular insufficiency results from cardiac ischemia or infarction. Chronic mitral insufficiency results in left atrial enlargement, atrial fibrillation, and ultimately, symptoms of pulmonary congestion. The symptoms of acute mitral insufficiency, occurring in the setting of myocardial ischemia or infarction, usually present as an episode of acute pulmonary edema (severe dyspnea and orthopnea progressing to respiratory failure).

Ischemic Heart Disease

Patients with ischemic heart disease have myocardial O_2 requirements in excess of myocardial O_2 delivery (myocardial blood flow × blood O_2 content).

In this disease condition, coronary blood flow is limited by atherosclerotic plaques, which obstruct the coronary arteries. Ischemia may be precipitated by conditions that decrease myocardial O_2 delivery, such as anemia and tachycardia, or increase myocardial O_2 requirements, such as hypertension. Symptoms of myocardial ischemia include: angina pectoris, fatigue, shortness of breath, and irregular heartbeats (arrhythmias) (3).

THE RESPIRATORY SYSTEM

Respiratory Anatomy and Physiology

Respiration involves the transport of O_2 from the lungs to the body tissues, and CO_2 from the tissues to the lungs for removal. During inspiration (inhalation), air passes through the mouth and nasal passages, trachea, and bronchioles to pulmonary alveoli, where the exchange of oxygen between alveoli and pulmonary capillary blood occurs. From the pulmonary capillary bed, oxygenated blood circulates through the left side of the heart and arterial circulation to the peripheral capillaries. At the tissue level, O_2 release and CO_2 uptake occurs. Carbon dioxide returns to the lungs via the venous circulation, where it is exchanged between pulmonary capillaries and alveoli and removed from the body during expiration (exhalation).

The ventilatory component of respiration requires lung ventilation at a level adequate to eliminate CO_2 from the lungs at the same rate at which it is produced by the tissues. Under normal conditions, this is accomplished through the regulatory functions of the brainstem respiratory center. The respiratory center maintains appropriate arterial carbon dioxide levels ($PaCO_2$) by varying respiratory rate and/or tidal volume to achieve adequate alveolar ventilation (4).

Conditions Affecting Respiratory Function

Chronic obstructive pulmonary disease (COPD) includes respiratory disorders such as chronic bronchitis, emphysema, and asthma, which are characterized by air flow obstruction within pulmonary air passages. Chronic bronchitis is a progressive disorder characterized by bronchial inflammation, increased mucous secretions, and a chronic productive cough. Emphysema, often preceded by or accompanying chronic bronchitis, is characterized by pulmonary alveolar and capillary destruction resulting in hypoxemia from the mismatching of alveolar ventilation with pulmonary capillary perfusion. Asthma can include components of both chronic bronchitis and emphysema, but is usually characterized by increased bronchial smooth-muscle tone and hypersecretion of mucus in response to allergic or environmental stimuli. Expiratory wheezing is a common symptom of an acute exacerbation of asthma or emphysema (5).

In addition to the previously described pathology, patients with COPD, especially those suffering from emphysema, often have a dysfunctional respiratory center and must rely on arterial oxygen levels (PaO_2) sensed by receptors in the aorta and carotid arteries for adjustment and maintenance of an adequate alveolar ventilation. COPD patients who rely on PaO_2 for regulation of breathing are described as breathing on hypoxic drive. If these patients are given excessive oxygen supplementation, their level of alveolar ventilation may actually be reduced as PaO_2 rises past the level required to initiate respiration, resulting in severe CO_2 retention. The capability to assist with ventilation should be readily available whenever patients with COPD receive oxygen supplementation in concentrations greater than those obtained by nasal cannula at oxygen flows of 2 to 3 liters per minute (6).

THE NEUROLOGICAL SYSTEM

The neurological system can be divided anatomically into central and peripheral divisions. Functionally, the nervous system is divided into autonomic and somatic divisions. The somatic division controls skeletal-muscle functions such as movement and phonation. The autonomic division, further subdivided into sympathetic and parasympathetic divisions, is responsible for neurological control of the cardiovascular system (1).

Cognitive, sensory, and motor function can be assessed in the awake patient by evaluating responses to sensation and commands. However, in the anesthetized patient, neurological function must be evaluated by other methods, including the electroencephalogram (EEG) and somatosensory evoked potentials (SSEP) (7).

Conditions Affecting Neurological Function

Vascular conditions that affect neurological function include carotid and cerebral arterial atherosclerosis. These conditions may manifest themselves with symptoms such as transient ischemic attacks (TIAs) and cerebrovascular accidents (CVAs), or strokes (5).

THE RENAL SYSTEM

The kidneys eliminate the end products of metabolism, and regulate body water and its constituents. These functions are accomplished by the formation and excretion of urine. Nephrons, the functional units of the renal system, are composed of glomeruli, tufts of capillaries that filter blood; glomerular or Bowman's capsules, which house the glomerular capillaries and collect the filtrate; and tubules, which concentrate the filtrate through reabsorption of electrolytes and water, producing urine. Urine flows from the kidneys through the ureters to the bladder and urethra for excretion (1). During surgery, urine output is measured by a urethral catheter inserted into the bladder. A urine output of approximately 0.5 ml/kg/hr is generally considered adequate.

Conditions Affecting Renal Function

Patients with acute or chronic renal failure characteristically demonstrate electrolyte and/or fluid volume abnormalities. Renal dialysis, while correcting electrolyte disorders, may result in hypovolemia immediately following dialysis (7).

Agents often administered prior to (and sometimes during) surgery may have a toxic effect on the kidneys. Specifically, iodine contrast media used for coronary, cerebral, or peripheral vascular angiograms and also for cholangiograms may result in acute renal tubular necrosis. Diabetic patients who suffer from preexisting diabetic nephropathy are especially at risk for this complication (3). Intraoperative hypotension and surgical procedures that interfere with renal perfusion (e.g., aortic aneurysm repair) can adversely affect renal function.

THE GASTROINTESTINAL SYSTEM

The digestive tract consists of the mouth, pharynx, esophagus, stomach, small and large intestines, rectum, and anus. It functions to ingest and digest nutrients and eliminate waste products of digestion.

Conditions Affecting Gastrointestinal Function

The body's fluid and electrolyte balance can be altered significantly by nausea, vomiting, and diar-

rhea; bowel obstruction from a variety of etiologies; nasogastric suction; and prolonged "Nil per Os" (NPO) status prior to surgery. Preoperative bowel preparation regimens, designed to make the bowel lumen as clean and free of bacteria as possible, may also produce fluid-volume and electrolyte abnormalities. Responses of the digestive system during surgery and the extent and duration of postoperative paralytic ileus depend on preexisting pathology, the type of procedure performed, and the type of anesthetic administered (7).

THE ENDOCRINE SYSTEM

The endocrine system is, in part, composed of the following glands: the islets of Langerhans in the pancreas, thyroid, parathyroid, adrenal, and pituitary glands. These glands secrete hormones that regulate many aspects of body function. Pancreatic islet cells secrete insulin, a hormone involved in glucose metabolism; the thyroid secretes thyroxine, which regulates metabolic rate; the parathyroid secretes parathormone, an important hormone involved in calcium and phosphate metabolism; the adrenal gland secretes catecholamines (adrenal medulla) as well as glucocorticoids and mineralocorticoids (adrenal cortex); and the pituitary gland secretes a variety of hormones, which function to control many of the activities of the other endocrine glands (1).

Conditions Affecting Endocrine Function

Diabetes mellitus is an endocrine disorder involving inadequate insulin production and/or utilization. Diabetic patients may present to the operating room with hyper- or hypoglycemia depending on the adequacy of their insulin or oral hypoglycemic dosing regimen. Hyperglycemic patients may appear lethargic or somnolent, while hypoglycemia may present with similar symptoms or as anxiety, agitation, and/or convulsion. The perioperative team must be vigilant in assessing the diabetic patient's mental status preoperatively and follow blood glucose levels throughout the perioperative period. An intravenous infusion of glucose with continuous or intermittent insulin administration should be maintained from the time a diabetic patient begins fasting until feedings are resumed postoperatively.

Diabetic patients are also more susceptible to postoperative wound and urinary tract infection, and to skin breakdown over pressure points. Additional care must be exercised in the positioning of

TABLE 17.1.   Guidelines for Monitoring Specific Endocrine Responses

Procedure/Pathology	Specific Concerns	Nursing Activities
Parathyroidectomy	Hypercalcemia Hypovolemia secondary to nausea, vomiting, polyuria	Monitor serum calcium Invasive monitoring Monitor intake and output
Pheochromocytoma	Excessive secretion of epinephrine and norepinephrine Severe hypertension Arrhythmias Hypovolemia	Monitor ECG for arrhythmias Invasive monitoring Vasodilator infusions Alpha and beta blockade
Adrenalectomy	Hyperaldosteronism Hypokalemia Hypervolemia Hypertension	Monitor ECG for arrhythmias Invasive monitoring Monitor electrolytes
Thyroidectomy	Tracheal compression and/or deviation Potential difficult intubation Potential recurrent laryngeal nerve damage	Assist anesthetist with intubation Be prepared for emergency tracheotomy upon anesthetic induction and emergence
Hyperthyroidism	"Thyroid storm" resulting in severe circulatory and metabolic derangement	Monitor ECG for arrhythmias Invasive monitoring Symptomatic management of metabolic derangement
Diabetes Mellitus	Hyperglycemia or hypoglycemia Electrolyte disorders Increased susceptibility to wound and urinary tract infections	Monitor blood glucose Insulin therapy Maintain asepsis, pad pressure points
Hypophysectomy (pituitary adenoma resection)	Hyperadrenocorticism or hypoadrenocorticism Acromegaly (difficult airway) Diabetes insipidus	Invasive monitoring Hydrocortisone administration Assist anesthetist with intubation Monitor intake and output, administer synthetic antidiuretic hormone

these patients and maintaining sterile technique. Guidelines for monitoring responses specific to the endocrine system are presented in Table 17.1.

THE INTEGUMENTARY SYSTEM

The skin covers and protects the external surface of the body. Skin is composed of an outer layer of epithelial cells, the epidermis; and an inner layer, or dermis, composed of connective tissue and containing nerve endings and receptors, sweat glands, hair follicles, and blood vessels.

The skin has three primary functions: protection, sensation, and temperature regulation. The skin protects body structures from mechanical injury and prevents loss of fluids and electrolytes. Nerve endings and receptors communicate sensory information regarding environmental exposure to touch, pressure, pain, and temperature. Conservation and elimination of heat are accomplished by cutaneous vasoconstriction or vasodilation, respectively. Elimination of excess body heat is also facilitated by

evaporative heat loss through the production of perspiration.

A significant amount of body heat is lost to the operating room environment during the perioperative period. Anesthetic agents, which impair the body's thermoregulation abilities, further contribute to the problem of heat loss. Thermal blankets; warm prepping solutions, irrigations, and intravenous fluids; heated and humidified anesthetic gases; and moderate operating room temperatures can minimize operative heat loss.

Conditions Affecting Integumentary Function

Burns are classified by the depth of injury and the percentage of total body surface area involved. First-degree burns involve the epidermis only. Second-degree burns involve the epidermis and superficial dermis. Third-degree burns, the most severe, involve epidermis as well as deep layers of the dermis. Depending on the severity and extent of the burn, significant losses of body heat as well as fluids and electrolytes may occur. Treatment includes minimiz-

TABLE 17.2. Physical Status Classification

Class	Physical Description
I	Healthy patient
II	Mild systemic disease without functional limitation
III	Severe systemic disease without functional limitation
IV	Severe, life-threatening systemic disease
V	Moribund patient
E	Emergency surgery

ing thermal losses, fluid and electrolyte therapy, and burn excision in conjunction with skin grafting. To prevent electrocautery burns during surgery, the dispersion plate should be carefully placed over a flat, dry skin surface, avoiding bony prominences.

Skin preparation solutions, in susceptible individuals, can result in hypersensitivity reactions and skin breakdown. Povidone–iodine solutions have been implicated as a cause of skin injury and should be avoided in patients with a history of such reactions.

THE MUSCULOSKELETAL SYSTEM

The musculoskeletal system includes bones, joints, muscles, and connective tissue, and serves to protect and support the vital organs and soft tissues and provide body mobility. Also, bone marrow serves as a manufacturing site for red blood cells, and bone is a storage area for mineral salts such as calcium and phosphate.

Conditions Affecting the Musculoskeletal System

Malignant hyperthermia (MH), a hereditary disorder involving abnormal skeletal muscle responses to exposure to a variety of anesthetic agents, is uncommon but can result in significant morbidity and mortality. Drugs that can trigger an MH episode in susceptible individuals include the volatile anesthetic agents and the muscle relaxant succinylcholine. MH does not necessarily occur with the susceptible patient's first exposure to triggering agents; in fact, some MH patients have received several anesthetics prior to their initial episode.

The onset of an MH crisis is heralded by a cascade of events. Sign and symptoms include tachycardia, arrhythmias, hypotension, hypercarbia, hypoxemia and cyanosis, hyperkalemia, acidosis, and hyperthermia. Treatment includes cessation

of anesthesia and surgery, hyperventilation with 100% O_2, administration of dantrolene sodium, and symptomatic treatment of cardiovascular responses to the MH crisis. If, during the preoperative assessment, a patient relates a family history consistent with MH susceptibility, a muscle biopsy can be performed under local anesthesia (or general anesthesia with non-MH triggering agents), and the halothane-caffeine contracture test performed on the biopsy specimen to establish the diagnosis (8).

ANESTHESIA

Preoperative Medication

Prior to surgery, the anesthetist makes a visit to perform a focused history and physical examination, formulate an anesthesia plan, and obtain informed consent for the anesthetic. A physical status classification is then assigned to the patient by the anesthetist. Table 17.2 describes a classification system for patient physical status.

Appropriate preoperative medication is prescribed by the anesthetist following preoperative evaluation. Preoperative medication is frequently administered to reduce the patient's anxiety prior to general, regional, or local anesthesia. Medication may also be prescribed for other purposes, for example, to enhance gastric emptying and reduce gastric acidity (8, 9).

General Anesthesia

General anesthetic agents, as well as preoperative sedative medication, can depress cardiovascular and respiratory function. Inhalational anesthetic agents directly depress myocardial contractility and reduce sympathetic vascular tone, resulting in a fall in blood pressure. Although most general anesthetic agents reduce myocardial work and oxygen demand, surgical stimulation may initiate powerful sympathetic responses, which can significantly increase heart rate and blood pressure in the anesthetized patient. In patients with ischemic heart disease, the resultant increased myocardial O_2 demand and decreased supply may provoke myocardial ischemia, requiring prompt therapeutic intervention. Specific drugs used during anesthesia are summarized in Table 17.3 (8).

Regional and Local Anesthesia

Local anesthetics are weak bases and, structurally, are composed of an aromatic section connected to an

TABLE 17.3. Drugs Used During Anesthesia

Inhalation Anesthetics: Used for induction and maintenance of anesthesia

Isoflurane (Forane)
Enflurane (Ethrane)
Halothane (Fluothane)
Nitrous oxide
Sevoflurane (investigational)
Desflurane (investigational)

Sedative-Hypnotics: Used for conscious sedation, induction and maintenance of anesthesia

Barbiturates
Thiopental sodium (Pentothal)
Thiamylal (Surital)
Methohexital (Brevital)

Benzodiazepines
Midazolam (Versed)
Diazepam (Valium)
Lorazepam (Ativan)

Others
Etomodate (Amidate)
Ketamine (Ketalar)
Propofol (Diprivan)

Narcotics

Agonists: Used for sedation and analgesia and, in high doses, for general anesthesia

Morphine
Meperidine (Demerol)
Fentanyl (Sublimaze)
Sufentanil (Sufenta)
Alfentanil (Alfenta)

Agonist-Antagonists: Used for analgesia and partial reversal of narcotic-induced respiratory depression

Nalbuphine (Nubain)
Butorphanol (Stadol)
Dezocine (Dalgan)

Antagonist: Used for reversal of narcotic-induced respiratory depression

Naloxone (Narcan)

Nonsteroidal Anti-inflammatory Drugs: Used for analgesia

Ketorolac (Toradol)

Muscle Relaxants: Used for skeletal muscle relaxation

Short-duration
Succinylcholine (Anectine)

Intermediate-duration
Vecuronium (Norcuron)
Atracurium (Tracrium)

Long-duration
Pancuronium (Pavulon)
Pipercuronium (Arduan)
Doxacurium (Nuromax)

Muscle Relaxant Reversal Agents

Edrophonium (Tensilon)
Neostigmine (Prostigmine)

Anticholinergics

Atropine
Glycopyrrolate (Robinul)
Scopolamine

Beta Blockers

Propranolol (Inderal)
Esmolol (Brevibloc)
Labetalol (Trandate)

Calcium Channel Blockers

Verapamil (Isoptin)
Nifedipine (Procardia)

Antiarrhythmic Agents

Lidocaine (Xylocaine)
Procainamide (Pronestyl)
Bretylium (Bretylol)

Inotropes and Vasopressors

Epinephrine (Adrenalin)
Norepinephrine (Levophed)
Isoproterenol (Isuprel)
Dopamine (Intropin)
Dobutamine (Dobutrex)
Ephedrine
Phenylephrine (Neo-Synephrine)

Vasodilators

Sodium nitroprusside (Nipride)
Nitroglycerin (Tridil)

Malignant Hyperthermia Treatment

Dantrolene (Dantrium)

amine group through an ester or amide linkage. Local anesthetics containing an ester linkage (procaine, chloroprocaine, tetracaine, and cocaine) are metabolized by plasma cholinesterase. A breakdown product of ester metabolism is the compound *p*-aminobenzoic acid, which is associated with hypersensitivity reactions in some individuals. Ester local anesthetics may also produce allergic reactions in patients sensitive so sulfonamides or thiazide diuretics. Local anesthetics containing an amide

linkage (lidocaine, bupivicaine, mepivacaine, and etidocaine) are metabolized in the liver. Amide local anesthetics rarely cause allergic reactions; however, they may contain the preservative methylparaben, which may produce an allergic reaction in a patient sensitive to *p*-aminobenzoic acid (10).

Regional or local anesthetic techniques may be preferable in some patients, especially those with impaired cardiorespiratory function. Spinal (also termed subarachnoid or intrathecal) and epidural anesthetics, brachial plexus blocks, and local field blocks do not require endotracheal intubation and do not directly depress cardiac function.

A more stable and pain-free recovery is also possible through the postoperative administration of spinal or epidural narcotics. Indwelling spinal or epidural catheters for infusion of postoperative narcotics and local anesthetic agents may provide a potentially pain-free surgical recovery.

Hypotension secondary to regional sympathetic block and loss of vascular tone is a potential complication of spinal and epidural anesthetic techniques. Adequate preoperative hydration and prompt, symptomatic administration of intravenous fluids and vasopressors can minimize this complication.

Intravascular injection of a local anesthetic during regional anesthesia can result in convulsions and cardiovascular toxicity. The convulsing patient should be ventilated with 100% O_2 and, if the seizures do not terminate, intravenous diazepam or thiopental may be administered. If the patient develops cardiovascular symptoms such as hypotension or arrhythmias, treatment may include placement in the head-down position and administration of intravenous fluids, vasopressors, and antiarrhythmics (11).

Induction of General Anesthesia, Laryngoscopy, and Endotracheal Intubation

Cardiovascular instability can complicate the transition from wakefulness to the anesthetized state, especially in patients with hypertensive, valvular, and ischemic heart disease. Hypotension results from direct myocardial depression and vasodilation. In patients with coronary atherosclerosis, hypotension (especially when associated with tachycardia) may result in myocardial ischemia and infarction. In order to avoid sudden changes in heart rate and blood pressure, anesthesia should be induced by careful titration of anesthetic dose to desired clinical effect.

The stress of laryngoscopy and endotracheal intubation often results in increases in arterial blood pressure and heart rate. Most patients tolerate these transient changes without developing myocardial ischemia. However, patients with ischemic heart disease and hypertension may experience significantly greater levels of hypertension and tachycardia resulting in ischemia. Patients with hypertension and coronary artery disease should maintain their medication regimen until the day of surgery to prevent or minimize the risk of developing myocardial ischemia during surgery.

During laryngoscopy and endotracheal intuba-

tion, the patient's airway and ventilatory status is continuously assessed by the entire perioperative team. Nursing assistance is often required to facilitate smooth intubation. Many patients, especially those requiring emergency surgery, are at risk of pulmonary aspiration of gastric contents and subsequent aspiration pneumonitis. During intubation, the nurse may be asked to apply cricoid pressure with thumb and second or third finger over the cricoid cartilage, to compress the esophagus against a vertebra in order to prevent passive regurgitation of gastric contents. Discontinuation of cricoid pressure should occur only after the endotracheal tube has been successfully inserted into the trachea, the cuff inflated, and tube position confirmed.

When the anesthetist has difficulty visualizing the larynx during laryngoscopy, the nurse may be asked to apply cricoid pressure. In this case, the goal of cricoid manipulation is to facilitate visualization; thus, the cricoid cartilage should be grasped and pushed cephalad, not posteriorly.

Controlled Hypotension

Controlled hypotension may be initiated for specific surgical procedures in which excessive, uncontrollable blood loss is predicted. These procedures include radical head and neck surgery, intracranial aneurysms and vascular tumors, and major orthopedic procedures. The purpose of controlled hypotension is to decrease operative blood loss, thus reducing the need for transfusion and improving visibility of the surgical field. Inhalational anesthetic agents in combination with sodium nitroprusside or other vasodilators may be used to reduce blood pressure to desired levels. In patients with ischemic heart disease, vigilance must be carefully maintained to detect signs of myocardial ischemia (8).

MONITORING CARDIOVASCULAR STATUS

Intraoperative Monitoring

Monitoring the patient's cardiovascular status throughout the perioperative period is the responsibility of the entire surgical team. Continuous and intermittent data may be collected by capnography (measurement of CO_2), clinical laboratory analysis, invasive and noninvasive blood pressure, ECG, arterial blood gas analysis, central venous and pulmonary artery pressure measurement, urinary volume measurement and urinalysis, temperature monitoring, and pulse oximetry. During the conduct of

TABLE 17.4.   Standards for Basic Intraoperative
Monitoring

1. Qualified anesthesia personnel shall be present in
   the room throughout the conduct of all general anesthetics, regional anesthetics, and monitored anesthesia care.
2. During all anesthetics, the patient's oxygenation,
   ventilation, circulation, and temperature shall be continually evaluated.

Oxygenation

Objective: To ensure adequate oxygen concentration
in the inspired gas and the blood during all anesthetics.

Methods: (1) Oxygen analyzer in the patient
              breathing system
         (2) Adequate illumination and exposure
              of the patient to assess color
         (3) Pulse oximetry

Ventilation

Objective: To ensure adequate ventilation of the patient during all anesthetics.

Methods: (1) Evaluation of clinical signs such as
              chest excursion and auscultation of
              breath sounds
         (2) capnography
         (3) mechanical ventilator disconnect
              alarm

Circulation

Objective: To ensure the adequacy of the patient's circulatory function during all anesthetics.

Methods: (1) Continuous electrocardiogram
         (2) Arterial blood pressure and heart
              rate determined and evaluated at
              least every 5 minutes
         (3) Continual palpation of pulse, aus-
              cultation of heart sounds, or moni-
              toring of intraarterial pressure or
              pulse plethysmography

Temperature

Objective: To aid in the maintenance of appropriate
body temperature during all anesthetics. (Continuous temperature monitoring is used when changes in
body temperature are anticipated).

Source: American Society of Anesthesiologists. *ASA Standards,
Guidelines, and Statements.* Park Ridge, IL: ASA, 1991.

general and regional anesthesias and monitored anesthesia care (MAC), qualified anesthesia personnel
must be continuously present in the operating
room. Perioperative nurses assist the anesthetist
during the conduct of general and regional anesthesia and MAC; however, during some procedures
performed under local anesthesia, the nurse may
have the primary responsibility for patient monitoring. Table 17.4 summarizes current guidelines for
basic intraoperative monitoring.

A precordial or esophageal stethoscope may be

used to monitor heart rate, rhythm, and tones by
auscultation. The sphygmomanometer provides indirect measurement of systolic and diastolic blood
pressure. Several noninvasive blood pressure
(NIBP) measurement devices are available for rapid,
intermittent assessment of blood pressure, while
continuous NIBP measurement is available with the
Finapress BP monitor.

The ECG measures the electrical activity of the
heart. Standard ECG leads II and modified V_5 are
usually monitored. The ECG display allows the
anesthetist and the rest of the perioperative team
to assess cardiac electrical activity continuously, especially during critical periods such as anesthesia induction and intubation, surgical incision, and
emergence from anesthesia. Monitoring the ECG allows recognition of arrhythmias, conduction defects, myocardial ischemia and infarction, as well as
the effects of drugs and electrolyte imbalance. Detection and management of cardiac arrhythmias are
described in Table 17.5.

Pulse oximetry provides a continuous and accurate measurement of oxygen saturation (S_pO_2) in
vessels perfusing a pulsating vascular bed, such as a
finger or ear lobe. The pulse oximeter can rapidly
detect hemoglobin–oxygen desaturation, allowing
early therapeutic intervention. However, any event
that reduces vascular pulsation can interfere with
the instrument's ability to determine oxygen saturation. Adequate peripheral pulsation is often lost
with hypothermia, hypotension, infusion of vaso-
constrictor drugs, and severe peripheral vascular
disease.

Capnography, the measurement of inspired and
expired CO_2, provides continuous assessment of the
adequacy of lung ventilation and perfusion. Capnography permits rapid detection of hyper/hypoventi-
lation, ventilator disconnects and/or malfunction,
and depletion of CO_2 absorbent during anesthesia.
Capnogram wave-form patterns can provide early
detection of bronchospasm, anesthesia machine mechanical problems, partial endotracheal tube occlusion, and air embolus, leading to more rapid
therapeutic intervention. By inserting the capno-
graph sampling port tubing into one side of a nasal
oxygen cannula, spontaneously breathing patients
under conscious sedation can, even while under
surgical drapes, be continuously monitored for ap-
neic episodes (12). In addition to capnography, respiratory status is assessed in the ventilated patient
by an expired volume respirometer, located within
the anesthesia breathing circuit.

Noninvasive intraoperative monitoring of elec-
trophysiologic brain and spinal cord activity during
neurosurgical, neurovascular, and orthopedic verte-

TABLE 17.5 Management of Cardiac Arrhythmias

Arrhythmia	Potential Causes	Treatment
Sinus tachycardia	Stress, fever, anemia, hypoxemia, hyperthyroidism, congestive heart failure	Treat underlying disease
Bradycardia	Geriatric patients, athletes, surgical manipulation of the carotid sinus or eye muscles, vagal stimulation, cardiac disease	Anticholinergic agents such as atropine or glycopyrolate isoproterenol, pacemaker
Premature atrial contractions	Caffeine intake, chronic lung disease, cardiac disease	Treat underlying condition
Paroxysmal supraventricular tachycardia	AV node reentry, cardiac disease	Vagal stimulation, cardioversion, verapamil, beta blockers
Atrial flutter/fibrillation	Cardiac disease, preexcitation syndromes, thyrotoxicosis	Cardioversion, digoxin in combination with verapamil or propranolol, procainamide
Complete (third-degree) heart block	Cardiac disease	Pacemaker, isoproterenol
Ventricular ectopy	Cardiac disease, hypoxemia, electrolyte abnormalities	Oxygenation, lidocaine, treat electrolyte abnormalities
Ventricular tachycardia	Cardiac disease/ischemia, hypoxemia, electrolyte abnormalities	Oxygenation, lidocaine, cardioversion, treat electrolyte abnormalities
Ventricular fibrillation	Cardiac disease/ischemia, myocardial infarction, and cardiac arrest	Cardiopulmonary resuscitation, defibrillation, lidocaine, ventilation and oxygenation
Electromechanical dissociation	Mechanical obstruction of the cardiopulmonary circulation	Treat underlying cause, cardiopulmonary resuscitation
Asystole	Cardiac ischemia/infarction, excessive parasympathetic tone	Cardiopulmonary resuscitation, atropine, pacemaker

bral procedures can be achieved by EEG and SSEP. Cerebral responses to altered hemispheric blood flow conditions, as occur with carotid endarterectomy, are detected by EEG. Diminished hemispheric EEG activity following carotid artery cross-clamping suggests the need for a temporary shunting procedure to restore blood flow. SSEP monitoring is most frequently employed to provide early detection of compromised spinal cord blood flow during surgical procedures involving the spinal cord and vertebral column.

Body temperature monitoring is used routinely during the perioperative period. When changes in body temperature are anticipated during a surgical procedure, continuous temperature monitoring should be employed (13).

Invasive Monitoring

Direct, or invasive, measurement of arterial blood pressure is performed by percutaneous or cut-down arterial cannulation. An advantage of direct arterial blood pressure measurement, compared with NIBP, is accurate assessment of beat-to-beat variations in

blood pressure, allowing more rapid therapeutic intervention when abnormalities are detected. Another advantage is that access to the arterial circulation allows convenient sampling of arterial blood for blood gas analysis. Direct arterial cannulation is most frequently performed in the seriously ill; trauma victims; patients undergoing cardiac, thoracic, major vascular, neurosurgical, or major orthopedic procedures; and patients requiring hypotensive anesthesia.

Monitoring of central venous pressure (CVP) assesses venous filling of the right heart as well as right ventricular function. A catheter inserted into the median cubital, external or internal jugular, or subclavian vein is advanced to the junction of the superior vena cava and right atrium. Position is confirmed and pneumothorax, a risk of insertion, is ruled out by chest roentgenogram. Monitoring CVP is especially useful in determining the extent of perioperative blood loss during procedures where blood loss is extensive or difficult to visually evaluate.

Patients with impaired left ventricular function require measurement of pulmonary artery (PA) pressures for thorough assessment of fluid volume and

TABLE 17.6. Troubleshooting Procedures for Intravascular Pressure Monitoring Catheters

Problem	Causes	Solutions
Arrhythmias	Irritation of endocardium by catheter	Avoid excessive catheter manipulation; CVP catheter may require partial withdrawal; check chest roentgenogram
Infection	Break in aseptic technique Excessive movement of catheter at skin	Main asepsis, change sterile dressing Secure catheter to skin
Pulmonary artery perforation or pulmonary infarction	Overinflation or prolonged inflation of PA catheter balloon Migration of PA catheter into smaller branch of pulmonary artery	Do not overinflate PA balloon or permit prolonged inflation (wedging) Monitor PA tracing for distal catheter tip migration into the wedge position; if detected, partially withdraw catheter
Suspected incorrect values: Overdamping	Blood clot, large air bubble, or kink in catheter or high-pressure tubing Excessive pressure tubing length	Remove clot, bubble, or kink Verify sufficient pressure in heparinized flush solution bag Use shorter length of pressure tubing
Underdamping	Microbubbles in high-pressure tubing or transducer	Carefully flush transducer and high-pressure tubing
Inability to zero transducer or frequent need to re-zero	Malfunctioning transducer or cable Cap remaining on transducer stopcock	Replace malfunctioning transducer or cable Remove stopcock cap to zero
Incorrect zero-pressure reference level	Incorrect transducer height in reference to mid-axilla in supine patient	Adjust transducer level with leveling device

cardiovascular status. Pulmonary artery and pulmonary artery occluded pressure (PAOP) are measured by the pulmonary artery or Swan–Ganz catheter. This catheter is inserted through a percutaneous sheath introducer placed in the internal jugular or subclavian vein. The distal tip balloon is inflated with air and, advanced by blood flow, "floated" through the superior vena cava, right atrium, and ventricle, into the "wedge" position in a branch of the pulmonary artery. In this position, PAOP reflects left atrial and left ventricular end-diastolic pressure. When the balloon is deflated, pulmonary artery pressures are continuously measured.

A critical complication of PA catheterization, pulmonary infarction, can be avoided by vigilant care. This complication occurs when a PA catheter migrates farther into a small branch of the pulmonary artery and occludes its blood supply. Migration and continuous wedging of the catheter can be diagnosed by observing changes in the pressure waveform, and corrected by withdrawing the catheter until the characteristic PA wave-form returns.

The perioperative nurse's responsibilities for set-up, insertion, and troubleshooting of arterial, CVP, and PA invasive pressure lines vary among situa-

tions. However, nurses familiar and involved with invasive pressure lines can provide the most complete perioperative nursing care. Troubleshooting procedures for invasive pressure catheters are described in Table 17.6 (13, 14, 15, 16).

Postanesthesia Recovery

Invasive and noninvasive monitoring, as well as perioperative nursing care, continues throughout postanesthesia recovery. Specific postanesthesia care unit (PACU) discharge criteria vary among institutions and according to patient destination, e.g., intensive care unit, hospital ward, or home. The recovering surgical patient's neuromuscular function, level of consciousness, respiration, circulation, and oxygenation should be evaluated by an anesthetist prior to PACU discharge. Guidelines for PACU discharge are described in Table 17.7 (7, 17).

Positioning
Patient positioning is an example of an intraoperative nursing activity that requires continual monitoring throughout the surgical procedure. The nurse must understand that patients under anesthesia

TABLE 17.7.   Postanesthesia Care Unit Discharge Evaluation

Physical Signs	Discharge Guidelines
Activity	Able to move voluntarily or on command Absence of neurologic weakness
Respiration	Able to cough, deep-breathe, and clear secretions
Circulation	Blood pressure and heart rate within 20% of resting preoperative value Resolution of any new dysrhythmia
Consciousness	Fully awake and oriented Responds to verbal commands and follows simple instructions
Color (oxygenation)	Normal color Acceptable oxygen saturation by pulse oximetry

are vulnerable to injury because they cannot tell us which positions are uncomfortable or painful. Merely elevating a leg or turning a patient's body may produce neurological injury or hemodynamic consequences that must be diagnosed and treated. Prior to moving the anesthetized patient, the anesthetist should be made aware of the planned position change in order to prevent disconnection from monitoring devices and breathing apparatus.

Patient positioning may directly affect cardiovascular and respiratory function. Hypotension can occur secondary to reduced venous return to the heart when patients are placed in the head-up position. In the obese patient, hypoventilation, hypoxemia, and atelectasis due to decreased diaphragmatic excursion and lung ventilation may occur in the supine or head-down position. Chest wall compression, which occurs when patients are placed in the prone position, may also reduce ventilation.

Surgical positioning can also be used to enhance cardiovascular and respiratory function in acute hypotension by enhancing venous return with the head-down, or Trendelenburg's position; and assisting spontaneous breathing in patients with obesity or COPD by placing them in the beach-chair position (7).

CONCLUSION

Understanding body systems and how they are affected by surgery provides a scientific basis for implementing perioperative nursing care. Basic knowledge of major organ systems allows the perioperative nurse to conduct a preoperative assessment that focuses on an individual patient's needs. A thorough and efficient perioperative plan of care can then be formulated to meet the identified needs. During the operative procedure, this background allows the nurse to not only carry out the plan systematically but respond quickly and authoritatively to changes in the patient's condition. Throughout postoperative recovery, nursing involvement in patient assessment and therapeutic intervention is essential for the provision of the most comprehensive and effective perioperative care.

REFERENCES

1. Guyton, A. C. *Textbook of Medical Physiology* 8th ed. Philadelphia: W. B. Saunders, 1991.
2. Thys, D. M., and Kaplan, J. A. *The ECG in Anesthesia and Critical Care.* New York: Churchill Livingstone, 1987.
3. Wyngaarden, J. B., and Smith, L. H., Jr. *Cecil Textbook of Medicine* 18th ed. Philadelphia: W. B. Saunders, 1988.
4. West, J. B. *Respiratory Physiology* 4th ed. Baltimore: Williams & Wilkins, 1990.
5. Stoelting, R. K., Dierdorf, S. F., and McCammon, R. L. *Anesthesia and Coexisting Disease* 2nd ed. New York: Churchill Livingstone, 1988.
6. Comroe, J. H. *Physiology of Respiration* 2nd ed. Chicago: Year Book Medical Publishers, 1974.
7. Barash, P. G., Cullen, B. F., and Stoelting, R. K. *Clinical Anesthesia.* Philadelphia: J. B. Lippincott, 1989.
8. Miller, R. D. *Anesthesia* 3rd ed. New York: Churchill Livingstone, 1990.
9. Firestone, L. L., Lebowitz, P. W., and Cook, C. E. *Clinical Anesthesia Procedures of the Massachusetts General Hospital* 3rd ed. Boston: Little, Brown, 1988.
10. Stoelting, R. K. *Pharmacology and Physiology in Anesthetic Practice* 2nd ed. Philadelphia: J. B. Lippincott, 1991.
11. Raj, P. P. *Clinical Practice of Regional Anesthesia.* New York: Churchill Livingstone, 1991.
12. Goldman, J. M. "A simple, easy, and inexpensive method for monitoring $ETCO_2$ through nasal cannulae." *Anesthesiology* 67:606, 1987.
13. Blitt, C. D. *Monitoring in Anesthesia and Critical Care Medicine* 2nd ed. New York: Churchill Livingstone, 1990.
14. Ream, A. K., and Fogdall, R. P. *Acute Cardiovascular Management.* Philadelphia: J. B. Lippincott, 1982.
15. Hensley, F. A., Jr., and Martin, D. E. *The Practice of Cardiac Anesthesia.* Boston: Little, Brown, 1990.
16. Nelson, P. S., and Goldman, J. M. "Laser-assisted transducer alignment." *Anesthesia and Analgesia.* Abstract; p. S218; supplement to 1992 editions.
17. Aldrette, J. A., and Kroulik, D. "A postanesthetic recovery score." *Anesthesia and Analgesia* 49:924, 1970.

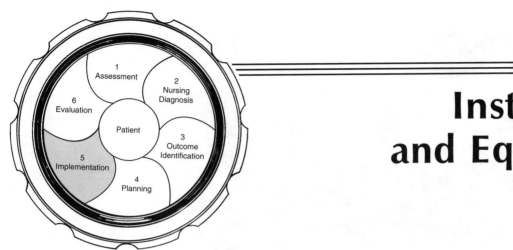

18

Instruments and Equipment

The nurse uses instruments and equipment appropriately.

The function and use of instruments and equipment in the operating room comprise a large segment of the body of knowledge needed by the experienced perioperative nurse. It is essential for students and beginning registered nurse practitioners to learn this information systematically in order to give knowledgeable, safe, professional perioperative nursing care. Knowledge of equipment and instruments gained from other areas of nursing can be applied and used in providing perioperative patient care.

The professional nurse in the operating room functions primarily in the role of circulating nurse, although it is also important to have a complete understanding of the role of the scrub person. Most nurses speak enthusiastically about the role of scrubbing; many state that they prefer this job, although it is a technical one.

In this chapter some of the equipment and instruments commonly used in the care of patients in the operating room are discussed. This discussion is not inclusive by any means. The equipment commonly used in some of the specialty services is also mentioned. How the circulating nurse and scrub person use each type of equipment and instruments is discussed.

EQUIPMENT

The nurse should become familiar with all the equipment in the operating room itself (Fig. 18.1). This can be accomplished by moving it about, cleaning it, and raising and lowering the surgical table and Mayo stand. Once the nurse knows how they are used safely, switches can be turned on and off. Handling the equipment is important since it familiarizes nurses with everything they will be working with during surgery.

Operating Room Table

The operating room table is an expensive, complex piece of equipment used for all surgical procedures (Fig. 18.2). It has been designed specifically to meet the needs of the surgical patient. Several types of tables are available for use in general surgical, orthopedic, urologic, and other procedures.

In order to position the patient safely, it is essential that the circulating nurse be proficient in the manipulation of the operating table. The nurse must be familiar with all parts of the table and its available accessories.

Prior to the patient's arrival in the operating room, the table should be checked for cleanliness and completeness according to the procedure scheduled. Attachments should be readily available as required, including stirrups for patients to be placed in the lithotomy position, or a table extension for patients who are over 6 feet 6 inches tall. Padding for the accessories may be necessary and should be readily available.

As most modern operating room tables are electrically operated, it is necessary to perform an electrical safety check prior to use, including all cords and plugs.

These tables are versatile and can be arranged for

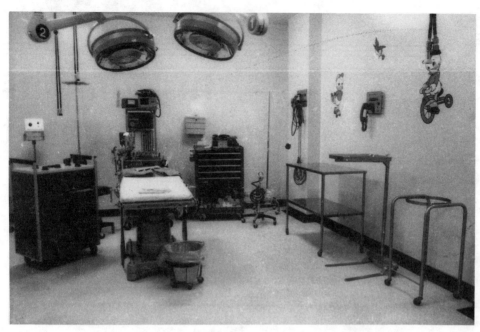

FIGURE 18.1. A basic operating room shows the variety of equipment the nurse uses to care for the patient intraoperatively. The surgical table is the center of activity.

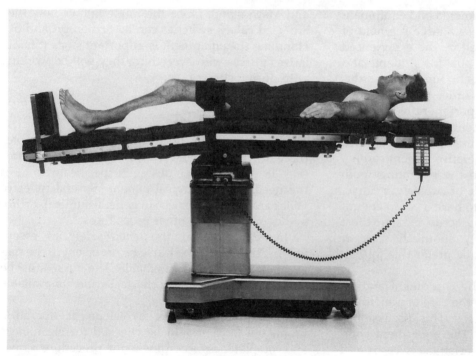

FIGURE 18.2. The basic surgical table in supine position. The tunnel immediately under the padding and supports allows the placement of x-ray cassettes under the patient during surgery for intraoperative x-rays. The push-button control panel for changing the table's position is located on the right side of the table. (Photograph courtesy of AMSCO/American Sterilizer Company, Erie, PA 16512.)

numerous positions, such as Trendelenburg's, lateral (Fig. 18.3), lithotomy (Fig. 18.4), jackknife, a slight left or right tilt, and many others. Knowledge of the control panel is essential to assist with positioning of the patient. The nurse may also be asked to make adjustments to the table and patient position during the intraoperative period.

Many surgical tables have been designed to allow x-rays to be taken during the operative procedure.

The tops of these tables are penetrable by x-rays, and a chamber underneath the table top holds the x-ray film or cassette in a variety of positions.

Many parts of the operating table are removable or have specialized attachments; for example, the head section may be removed to allow the insertion of a headrest for a craniotomy. Again, it is the nurse's responsibility to know all parts of the table, how to remove them, and how to add attachments

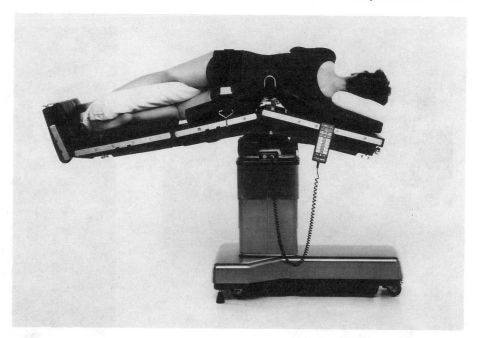

FIGURE 18.3.   Lateral position demonstrates the break in the table at the midpoint. Safety straps and arm rest are in position. (Photograph courtesy of AMSCO/American Sterilizer Company, Erie, PA 16512.)

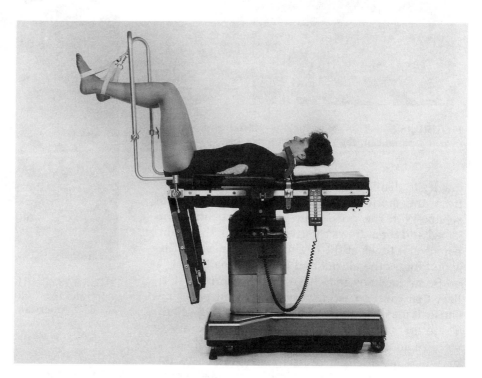

FIGURE 18.4.   Lithotomy position demonstrates the use of the cane stirrup attachments, anesthesia screen at the patient's head, and the folding down of the foot end of the table. (Photograph courtesy of the AMSCO/ American Sterilizer Company, Erie, PA 16512.)

quickly and safely. It is recommended that nurses who are new to the operating room be thoroughly oriented to this equipment and allowed time to practice manipulating the accessories into numerous positions.

It is the responsibility of the circulating nurse to be sure that the table is locked in place prior to moving the patient from the transport vehicle to the table. Once the patient is on the table, the safety strap must be secured in position (Fig. 18.5).

Sterilizers

One of the pieces of equipment used daily by operating room personnel is the sterilizer. It is essential that the perioperative nurse understand the principles of sterilization, including the operation of sterilization equipment.

Most modern operating rooms have either a gravity-displacement or a prevacuum sterilizer. In the gravity displacement sterilizer, the unit relies on

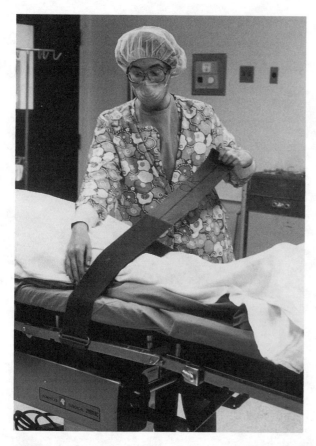

FIGURE 18.5. The safety belt is placed and secured over the patient on the operating room table.

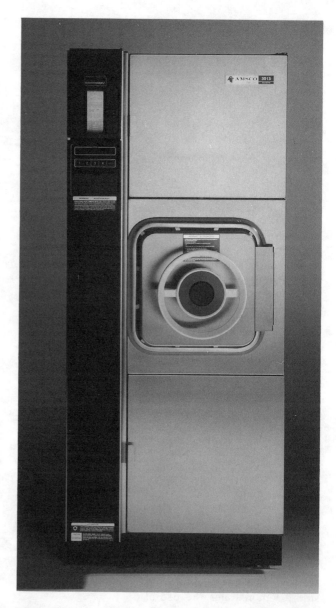

FIGURE 18.6. The AMSCO 3013 computerized emergency sterilizer with flash cycle. (Photograph courtesy of AMSCO/American Sterilizer Company, Erie, PA 16512.)

gravity to displace air, which is heavier than steam, from the sterilizer load to allow penetration of steam. With the prevacuum sterilizer, steam is injected and then draws a partial vacuum in the chamber several times at the beginning of the cycle. This action forces the air out and heats the load.

Some facilities may have a computerized sterilizer that can be used for a variety of purposes because it has different types of cycles (Fig. 18.6). There are situations where it may be necessary to sterilize an instrument that has been contaminated, or when an emergency arises. In this case, unwrapped instruments are placed in a computerized sterilizer or the gravity displacement sterilizer and sterilized for either 3 or 10 minutes. Traditionally, this has been referred to as flash sterilization. Today it is called the unwrapped method and used only when necessary.

In Figure 18.7, the computerized sterilizer illustrated has four cycles: express, prevac, flash, and gravity. These cycles are selected based on the packaging material and the size and type of item(s) being sterilized.

A monitoring system provides permanent daily graphs of temperature during all cycles. These graphs provide a visual record of the chamber temperature. They are kept on file as documentation of proper sterilization. Whenever an item is removed from the sterilizer, the operator must check the graph to be absolutely certain the correct sterilization temperature has been reached. For additional safety, a sterilization indicator must be placed in the tray and checked at the time of removal from the sterilizer.

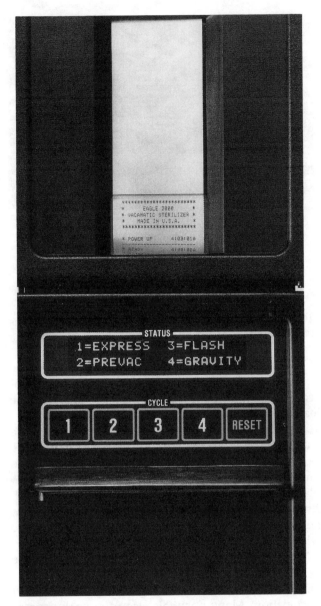

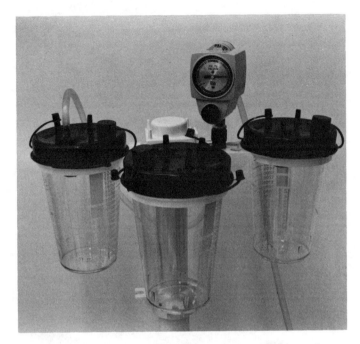

FIGURE 18.8.   A basic double-container floor suction unit used for surgery. This must be checked and in working order prior to the patient's arrival.

FIGURE 18.7.   Closeup of the computerized control panel for the AMSCO 3013 sterilizer. The mechanism for marking the autoclave graph is a part of this panel. (Photograph courtesy of AMSCO/American Sterilizer Company, Erie, PA 16512.)

Suction

Suction equipment is essential for safe patient care in the operating room. This equipment must be checked and in good working order prior to the patient's arrival (Fig. 18.8).

There must be at least two sets of suction apparatus in the room ready for use. The anesthesiologist uses one to assist in maintaining the patient's airway by removing accumulated secretions. This equipment must be available throughout the procedure. In suctioning, the anesthesiologist uses either a Yankauer tonsil tip or a suction catheter. The suction catheter is used while the airway or endotracheal tube is in place. After these are removed at the end of the procedure, the tonsil suction tip is more useful.

In addition to the suction apparatus used by the anesthesiologist, a second or even third setup may be used by the surgeon or assistant at the operative site. Suction is used to remove blood, secretions, and/or irrigating solutions to maintain a clear field where the surgeon is working. Should hemorrhage occur, it is essential to find the point of bleeding quickly so that it can be controlled. Of course the bleeding point has to be seen before it can be clamped.

Once the patient has been draped, the scrub person brings to the operative site the sterile suction tubing with tip. Often the surgeon attaches and arranges these as the scrub person brings up the Mayo stand and the circulating nurse brings in the back table and basins.

The distal end of the suction tubing is passed off the field to the circulating nurse, who attaches the end to the appropriate unit and turns the unit on.

Monitors

It is standard practice to monitor the patient during all operative procedures. In the past, perioperative

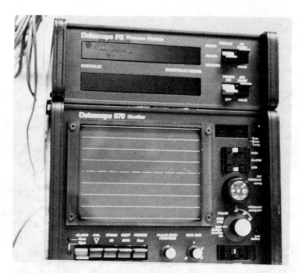

FIGURE 18.9. An example of a basic cardiac monitor used intraoperatively. The type shown also has digital readout of pulse and alarm systems that can be set to specific levels to alert personnel to possible problems.

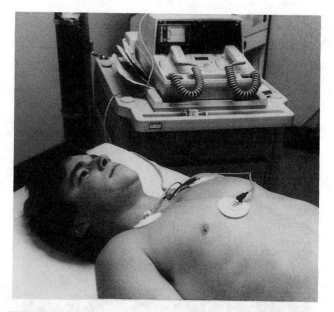

FIGURE 18.10. Correct placement of the electrodes is crucial to obtain accurate patterns.

nurses were not greatly involved in this area. Today, however, expertise in monitoring is essential.

In basic cardiac monitoring, the perioperative nurse may be responsible for anything from applying the leads to actual interpretation. Interpretation skills are becoming more important as operating rooms are used more for outpatient surgery and other procedures for which an anesthesiologist may not be present (Fig. 18.9).

As the experience, knowledge, and skill of perioperative nurses increase, they will become involved in more complex patient care activities. More complex monitoring systems will be employed to follow the patient's status throughout the procedure. The circulating nurse will assist with more complex procedures, such as inserting central venous pressure and Swan-Ganz lines.

The most basic monitoring system is an automatic vital sign monitor, which includes blood pressure and pulse. These monitors can be set at specific time intervals, and some equipment has prior data memories.

The next component in cardiac monitoring is the electrocardiograph (ECG). An ECG records the electrical impulses that instigate atrial and ventricular contractions. Leads are attached to the patient to pick up these impulses and transfer them in the form of a wave-tracing or an oscilloscope screen or readout graph paper.

Two leads are essential to pick up these impulses, with a third applied as a grounding wire (Fig. 18.10). These electrodes are placed on the patient's chest or extremities. The pads used are available pregelled and disposable and snap onto the lead wires. The clarity of the tracing on the oscilloscope depends on the proper placement of these leads.

Basically, there is a relationship between the wave displayed on the scope or paper strip and the cardiac physiology at that moment. It is essential to know the various ECG waves, intervals, and complexes, and what is normal and what is abnormal. Knowledge of the relationship of the P-wave, QR interval, and QRS complex, and the width of the whole pattern is necessary for interpretation.

A course in basic arrhythmias is helpful to the perioperative nurse. Many courses in advanced cardiac life support are offered by the American Heart Association. Many hospitals also offer such courses for their critical care nurses, which include perioperative nurses.

Numerous types of ECG monitors are available, some with only a basic oscilloscope screen and others that include displays of heartbeat and blood pressure. Some ECG monitors, such as the LIFE-PAK6 system (Fig. 18.11), are sold as a total lifesaving system in combination with a defibrillator.

Hypoxia is a critical condition that can occur at any time during a patient's perioperative experience. Pulse oximetry is a new, noninvasive monitoring procedure that continuously measures arterial hemoglobin–oxygen saturation. A simple clothespin-type detector is placed on the patient's finger, toe, or earlobe, and the oxygen saturation level is indicated on a monitor. The oximeter has become part of the

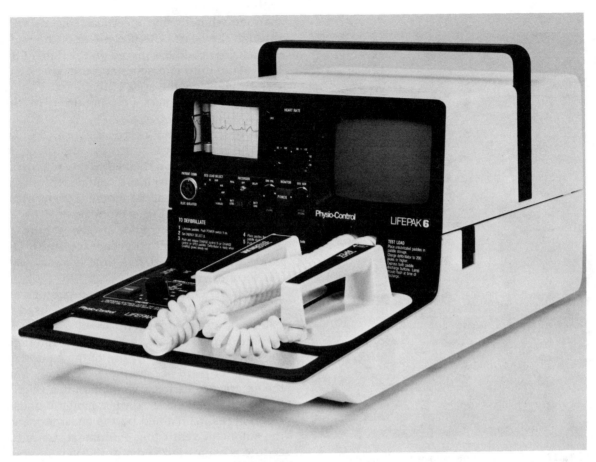

FIGURE 18.11.   The LIFEPAK 6 is a combination defibrillator and cardiac monitor found on many emergency carts. The external paddles are left attached and in full view, ready for use. (Photograph by Bob Peterson, courtesy of Physio-Control Corp., Redmond, WA 98052.)

standard monitoring devices used by anesthesiologists. For patients undergoing local procedures, the nurse monitoring the patient can detect hypoxic episodes quickly and intervene with appropriate therapy.

Emergency Equipment

Any patient, whether under general anesthesia or local block, can react adversely at any time to a medication, the stress of the procedure, or intraoperative hemorrhage. Cardiac or respiratory arrest can occur in any patient at any moment during the intraoperative period. General anesthesia has a certain level of morbidity even for patients in good condition who are undergoing elective surgery. The team must be even more alert to patients who are known beforehand to be poor surgical risks.

For the protection of the patient, it is imperative that the surgical team be intimately familiar with the emergency equipment available in their particular suite. When a crisis occurs, the response must be swift and efficient in order to be lifesaving. Emergency equipment and drugs must be reviewed routinely with the nursing staff so that expertise in their use is maintained. In addition, outdated drugs must be replaced and the functioning of equipment must be tested on a routine schedule.

Where is the equipment located? The nurse should find it on the first day in the operating room and review policy and procedure with respect to its use. Most operating rooms have an emergency crash cart where everything needed for cardiac and respiratory arrest is together in one spot and on wheels, so that it can be moved quickly to the patient's side (Fig. 18.12).

Usually the defibrillator and monitor are plugged in, in order to recharge their batteries, when the cart is in its home spot. These items must be unplugged before attempting to move the cart to the patient's side.

The nurse should know the emergency call signals, where they are located, and how to activate them. These signals may include a call light or

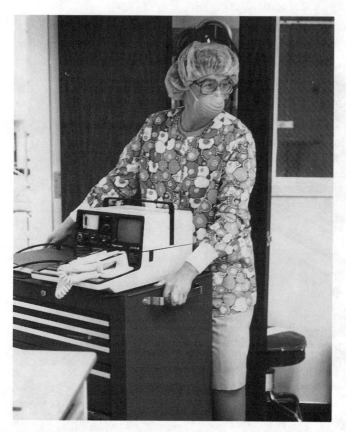

FIGURE 18.12. A typical emergency cart is painted red and has several drawers that contain all the necessary medications, syringes, needles, IV solutions, and tubes. The defibrillator and paddles with monitor sit on top for easy accessibility. This cart must be checked daily for completeness.

buzzer that should remain on until enough people have gathered to care for the patient.

The cardiac monitor is an integral part of the crash cart. Use of the ECG has already been reviewed.

The cardiac defibrillator provides an electrical force that is applied to the patient's chest at the time of cardiac arrest to stimulate the heart muscle to contract. Defibrillation was first used by Bech in 1947. This method has now progressed to external application to stop ventricular fibrillation. To be most effective, defibrillation should be done in the first minute of arrest. With every passing minute the patient has less chance of survival.

The defibrillator is basically a condenser of stored electrical energy that is discharged when needed. Today's equipment can be small, portable, and combined with a cardiac monitor, as in the LIFEPAK6 (Fig. 18.11).

To apply the electrical force, two metal paddles with conductive gel are placed on the patient in a manner whereby the electrical current will pass through the heart. The placement of the paddles is crucial. One paddle is placed on the right of the sternum at the third interspace and the other on the anterior wall below the apex of the heart. The paddles must have skin contact. Pressing firmly on the paddles provides good contact.

In order to avoid electrical shock, the operator must be careful not to touch the electrodes, the patient, or the metal on the bed. Everyone involved in care at this time must avoid contact with the patient and these elements at the moment of electrical stimulation. Also during the moment of defibrillation, the cardiac monitor and oxygen to the patient should be turned off to prevent explosions. The level of electrical current at this time is about 300 watts per second.

After use, the defibrillator and paddles must be cleaned properly. The conductive gel used on the paddles must be removed carefully to prevent formation of metal oxide, which could interfere with the electrical flow in later use of the equipment.

Another piece of equipment generally found on the emergency cart is a ventilation bag (Fig. 18.13). While the patient is under general anesthesia, breathing is maintained by the anesthesiologist using automatic ventilating equipment. Once the procedure is completed and anesthesia is reversed, the patient begins to respond and breathe independently. Some patients may respond slowly and continue to need ventilatory assistance, particularly during transportation from the operating room to the postanesthesia recovery room. Others may purposely be kept heavily sedated in the immediate postoperative phase with continued intubation and attachment to automatic ventilating equipment. Again, the ventilation bag is essential to transport such patients from one place to another. This bag is used in emergency situations throughout the hospital where patients' respirations need to be maintained.

Electrosurgical Equipment

Increasingly complex electrical equipment is being used in modern operating rooms. Orientation should include instruction, demonstration, and return demonstration of all these electrical units. Written instructions available from the manufacturer are most helpful.

Any electrical unit can be hazardous to both patient and staff. For the well-being of all involved in the procedure, safety precautions must be followed meticulously.

All equipment should be checked prior to use to

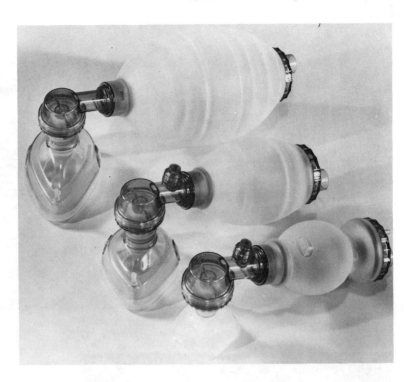

FIGURE 18.13. The Laerdal ventilation reservoir bag and mask can be used to maintain the patient's respirations during an emergency or to transport ventilator-dependent patients. (Photograph courtesy of Laerdal Medical Corp., Armonk, NY 10504.)

ensure that it is in good working order. All cords and plugs should be checked for exposed wires or frays in the insulation. The alarm system for that piece of equipment and the general alarm system within the suite should also be checked. Damaged units or electrical equipment that is not working properly should never be used. Faulty items should be reported, labeled, and removed immediately. A continuing preventive maintenance program for all electrical equipment is mandatory in all hospitals.

Wrapping cords tightly damages their insulation and wiring. Running over the electrical cords with other equipment can damage cords as well. Three-pronged plugs are required for all electrical equipment, with larger explosion-proof plugs being required in the operating room. The nurse has legal responsibility for the proper functioning of any equipment attached to the patient. And safety checks must be completed prior to the entry of the patient into the operating room.

Use of electrical equipment in the operating room should be documented. All electrosurgical equipment must be numbered so that the name, number, and settings used can be entered on the patient's chart.

The prime piece of electrical equipment used for most patients in surgery is the electrocautery unit. It is called by several other names, the most common being Bovie, after Dr. F. Bovie who in the 1920s was one of the prime developers of the present electrocautery system.

The electrocautery unit uses a high-frequency electrical current to cauterize bleeding vessels. By changing the current, this electrical flow can also be used as a cutting edge. The cauterization current is used most frequently.

The controlled electrical current in a Bovie is passed from the main transformer to the patient by a sterile electrode (pencil) attached to the equipment by a wire. The pencil is activated by hand control or foot switch (Fig. 18.14). Electrosurgical pencils can be either disposable or reusable and may be presterilized by either steam or gas.

With the advent of modern technology this equipment is now solid-state. Since the module is more compact than earlier models, it occupies less space and is more mobile.

With monopolar electrocautery, safe completion of the electrical circuit requires that a ground-dispersion plate or pad be in contact with the patient's skin (Fig. 18.15). Any fleshy part of the body is appropriate, but bony areas and/or scar tissue should be avoided. The grounding pad returns or drains the electrical current back to the electrocautery unit. If the current does not return to the electrocautery unit through the grounding pad, burning can occur at any point of contact on the patient. Today's pads are flexible and self-adhering, with impregnated electrolyte gel on a foam pad. A used pad should never be reapplied.

With bipolar electrocautery (Fig. 18.16) the output of current is isolated between the tips of the cautery forceps, allowing safe use of the coagulation current in close proximity to vital structures. Be-

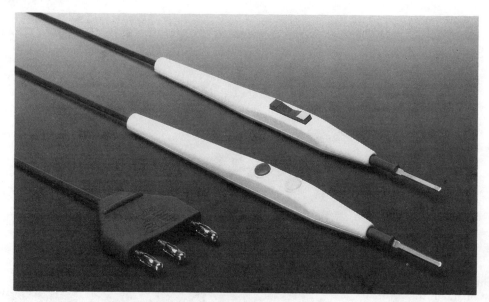

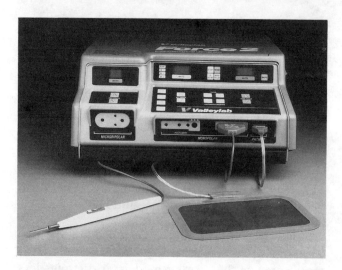

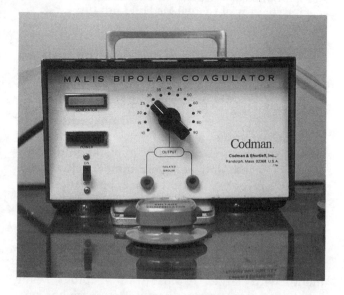

FIGURE 18.14.   Valleylab disposable hand-switching pencils, one featuring push-button activation and the other utilizing a rocker switch. The tip of the active electrode is small and the current density high. This tip may be a blade, ball, loop, or needle as the tip is removable and interchangeable. (Photograph courtesy of Valleylab, Inc., Boulder, CO 80301.)

FIGURE 18.15.   The Valleylab Force 2 Generator shown here with Valleylab's exclusive REM PolyHesive II Patient Return Electrode. (Photograph courtesy of Valleylab, Inc., Boulder, CO 80301.)

FIGURE 18.16.   The bipolar coagulation unit completely isolates the output of current between the tips of the cautery forceps. This allows the use of the coagulation current in close proximity to vital structures without damage to them.

cause the current returns to the unit through the tip of the electrode, a grounding pad is not needed for bipolar electrocautery.

The numbered dials on the unit represent the range of power, not the actual voltage delivered. If the surgeon is not obtaining the desired results and asks for a continued increase in power, the nurse should check the entire system for leaks. To continue to increase power is dangerous to the patient. Adequate training of personnel is the key to safe and effective use of electrosurgical units.

INSTRUMENTS

The patient has arrived and the monitors are in place. The circulating nurse has assisted the anesthesiologist with the induction of general anesthesia. Position has been established (Chapter 20), initial counts performed (Chapter 21), and skin prep completed (Chapter 19). The patient is draped, and the suction and electrocautery have been attached.

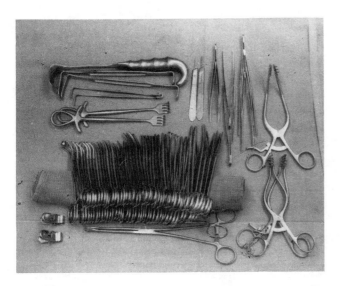

FIGURE 18.17.   A minor set contains numerous instruments. It is essential that the operating room nurse know them and their uses.

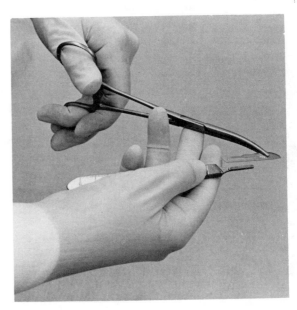

FIGURE 18.18.   A clamp is used to assemble the knife blade and handle, to prevent cuts.

At this point the focus is on the scrub person and the preparation necessary to provide the appropriate instruments and supplies to the surgeon.

Many different types of operations are performed. And the same procedure can be performed using different techniques, depending on the surgeon's preference. In the same operating room a particular operation may be performed in as many different modes as there are surgeons undertaking it. To assist with efficiency and organization, nurses have developed doctor's preference cards.

There should be a card for each procedure a surgeon performs. The process of developing and updating these cards is continuous to keep up with changes. Preference cards are basically standing orders of the surgeon and, combined with the plan of care formulated by the perioperative nurse, provide individualized care for the patient. The cards are necessary to gather the appropriate instruments and supplies the surgeon will use during surgery. They do not take the place of good professional nursing knowledge but assist with specific care that the surgeon will order. For the beginning practitioner or one not familiar with a particular surgeon, it is most helpful to have these cards posted in a convenient location for easy reference during the procedure.

Unfortunately, there is no standard nomenclature for the instruments used in surgery. The names change not only from region to region, but from hospital to hospital and manufacturer to manufacturer. What any particular operating room team may call their instruments depends greatly on the surgeons and where they were educated.

Instruments are constructed of a high-grade stainless steel with several special qualities. The 400 series is excellent for surgical instruments because it includes noncorrosive characteristics and good tensile strength. Surgical instruments are made by highly trained technicians. Although delicate, they can withstand innumerable sterilization cycles if handled and used properly.

Each instrument is designed to do a particular job and function in a particular fashion, and should be used only for that purpose. There are four basic types of instruments: cutting instruments (sharps), clamps, grasping instruments, and retractors.

Instruments must be assembled prior to the actual surgery. Even the instruments for a short, relatively simple procedure require preparation because a small set still has many components (Fig. 18.17). Disposable knife blades are placed on knife handles (Fig. 18.18). Sponges are placed on sponge sticks (Fig. 18.19). Peanuts (also called K-Ds, kittners, or pushers) are placed on clamps (Fig. 18.20); they are used in dissection of tissue. Sutures can also be placed on a clamp for use as a tie (Fig. 18.21). Sutures and needle packages are opened and the needles are placed on needle holders (Fig. 18.22). The preference card is checked to find out if the surgeon is right- or left-handed, and the needle is adjusted appropriately in the needle-holder (Fig. 18.23).

Many operating rooms have developed basic back table and Mayo stand setups for instruments. These basic setups can be helpful to the beginning practitioner in the operating room. Placing the in-

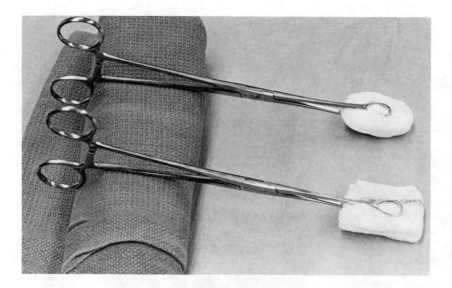

FIGURE 18.19. Sponges used on sponge sticks must be radiopaque and a part of the sponge count. The 4-×-4 is folded and placed in the sponge stick, which is then closed. Cherry sponges are positioned and used in the same manner. These sponges are used to absorb fluid or blood accumulations, or for blunt tissue dissection.

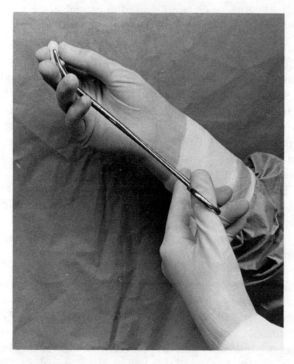

FIGURE 18.20.   A peanut is placed at the end of a Mayo (Kelly) clamp, with a small portion beyond the tip of the clamp. This is used to gently push and separate tissue during dissection.

struments on the back table in a specified manner will assist the scrub person in locating various instruments as they are needed. No specific design is better than another, but it is helpful to use only one basic setup during the learning process (Fig. 18.24). This basic setup can be adapted to accommodate all the instruments needed for surgical procedures.

Instrument counts necessitate the use of orga-nized basic back table and Mayo stand setups to fa-cilitate counting; therefore, standardized setups for both are recommended. If each person who scrubs has a different setup, counting time will be extended and disorganized. (See Chapter 21 for performing counts.)

Standardized basic setups are also helpful at those times when the circulating nurse and scrub person must be relieved, such as at shift changes. The individuals taking over will then know where instruments are on the setup and the transition will be smoother. There is nothing as frustrating to a sur-geon as having relieving scrub persons or circulating nurses be unable to find an instrument in the setup.

Each instrument must be checked prior to use. Today most instrument sets are probably assembled by someone other than the nursing team in the op-erating room. In hospitals using the modified Friesen concept, the instruments are put together in another department.

The instruments are checked at the time they are assembled, but it is still ultimately the responsibility of the nursing team in the operating room to per-form a final safety check on all instruments and equipment before they are used.

When the Mayo stand and back table are ready—and the patient and surgeon—the Mayo stand and back table are moved into place (Fig. 18.25). The Bo-vie cord and suction are put into position and at-tached. Sponges are up, and then the surgeon puts out a hand to receive the first instrument.

Scalpels

The first item to be passed is the instrument that makes the incision. A surgical knife, or scalpel, is

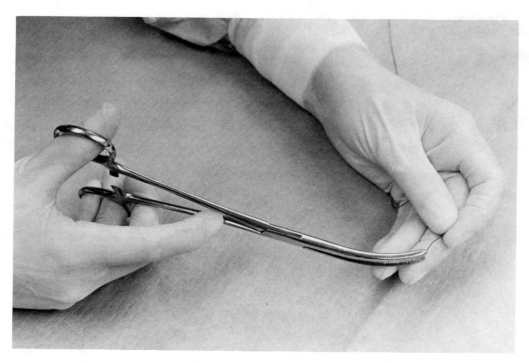

FIGURE 18.21.   One end of the suture is placed in the tip of the clamp, which is then closed. Different types of clamps may be used for this, such as Mayo, right-angled, or tonsil clamps.

needed. The scalpel has two parts: the handle and a disposable blade. There are several sizes and shapes of both blades and handles. Care must be observed whenever the knife is being handled by anyone on the team, as the blade is razor sharp. The nurse should always know where the scalpels are, whether on the back table, Mayo stand, or in use.

The nurse passes the scalpel, handle first and blade down, in position to make the incision. This move must be deliberate and made in a manner to avoid cutting the surgeon or oneself. The scrub person's hand should be above the cutting edge, as illustrated in Figure 18.26.

Clamps

At this same moment the assistant will need clamps to control bleeding. Hemostasis, that is, preventing and controlling loss of blood, is the fundamental job of all clamps. Clamps come in several shapes and lengths (Fig. 18.27). On the skin, subcutaneous tissue, and underlying tissues, shorter instruments are needed than those necessary for operating deeply within the patient, such as on kidneys or lungs.

The nurse places the clamp firmly into the assistant's hand in the position of use. The clamp should be closed, with the rings of the handle firmly yet lightly snapped into the palm, leaving the curve and point free to be applied to the tissue. The clamp is

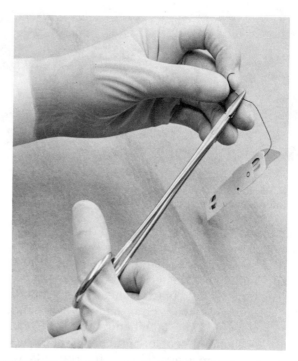

FIGURE 18.22.   The needle is placed in the tip of the needle holder approximately one-third of the way down the shaft from the junction where the suture is attached. The point of the needle is toward the scrub person.

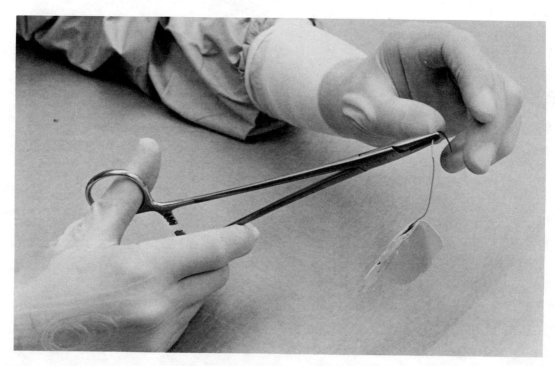

FIGURE 18.23. For the left-handed surgeon, the right-handed nurse can load the needle normally and then merely turn it over. The left-handed scrub nurse performs these maneuvers in reverse order.

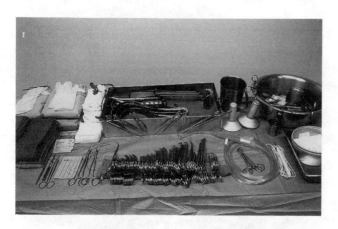

FIGURE 18.24. A basic back table setup after all the instruments have been prepared for surgery.

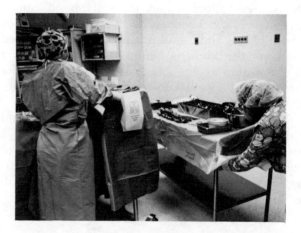

FIGURE 18.25. The scrub nurse slides the Mayo stand in over the patient's feet, being careful that the tray does not come in contact with them. The circulating nurse moves the back table and other equipment into place.

held by the box lock as it is passed (Fig. 18.28). This motion is the same for all clamps. The assistant may want a clamp in each hand and may need to use many clamps until the incision is completed.

The nurse should practice ahead of time handing the instruments with both hands. Left-handed people may find using both hands for passing easier than right-handed people. Scrubbing will be easier if the nurse can learn to pass instruments with either hand and at the same time—one to the surgeon and the other to the assistant. The surgeon may also wish to cauterize a bleeding vessel after it has been clamped (Fig. 18.29).

Scissors

If the surgeon ties a bleeding vessel that has been clamped, a strand of suture will be needed, and the ends of the suture must be cut (Fig. 18.30). Immediately after passing the tie, the nurse should have a suture scissor ready.

There are many types of scissors, each with a specific function and level of delicacy. The nurse should know the differences among them. A delicate scissor meant to cut tissue must never be used

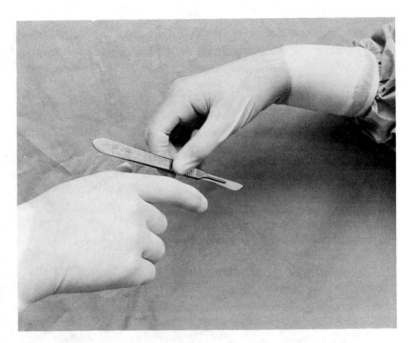

FIGURE 18.26. Hand the scalpel in position of use, with the blade edge down to come in contact with the patient's skin. Always use caution when handling the scalpel to avoid cutting anyone.

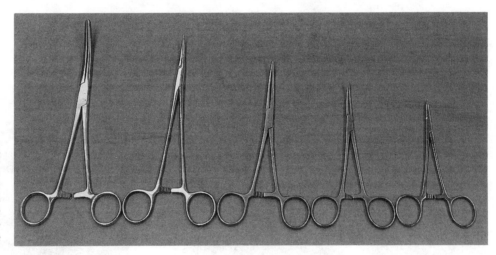

FIGURE 18.27. Basic clamps come in a variety of shapes (straight or curved) and lengths. They can have heavy or fine tips, as seen in the first two clamps on the left. They have ringed handles and box locks to secure the grasp.

as a suture scissor, and it is up to the scrub person to see that this rule is followed. Scissors are available with a variety of tips, blades, curves, and angles (Fig. 18.31).

The suture scissor is straight and can be seen at the 7 o'clock position in Figure 18.31. Scissors come in lengths ranging from 4 to 14 inches. The scrub person must select a length suitable to the immediate need. The surgeon working on subcutaneous tissue can use a 7¼-inch scissor, the most frequently used size. This clamp–tie–cut suture process may continue in series until all bleeding has been controlled.

Suture scissors should always be available, as they will be used throughout the procedure. It is also helpful to the scrub person to have a second pair available to cut and prepare sutures while the surgeon uses the first pair. Scissors are placed in the surgeon's hand with the same motion used for passing a clamp. A snap of the wrist at the moment of contact is helpful to let the surgeon know that the scissor is firmly in place (Fig. 18.32).

Forceps

Another instrument used when the incision is made may be a simple pick-up forceps with teeth, to grasp or pick up tissue as surgery proceeds. Tissue forceps are constructed with one and two teeth, multiple teeth, and no teeth. The types with one or two teeth

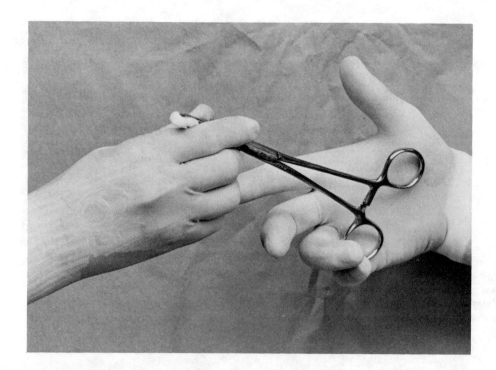

FIGURE 18.28. This clamp holds a peanut, but the basic motion for passing a clamp (whether curved, straight, angled, short, long, with or without sponges) remains the same.

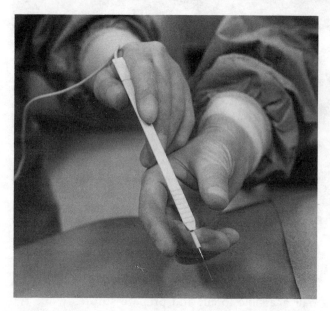

FIGURE 18.29. Pass the cautery pencil as the surgeon will use it.

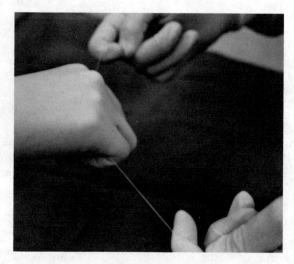

FIGURE 18.30. Hold the suture material out to the surgeon. Come in and under the surgeon's extended fingers, and up as he or she grasps the suture.

are used most frequently. Pick-ups come in various lengths, widths, and points (Fig. 18.33).

Retractors

As surgery proceeds, the subcutaneous tissue must be pushed or gently pulled aside. The assistant uses retractors for this. Retractors come in several shapes

and sizes and may be hand-held or self-retaining. Frequently used types include the Army–Navy retractor (Fig. 18.34) and the small Richardson retractor (Fig. 18.35). Other types of retractors available are rakes with either sharp or dull prongs (Fig. 18.36) and self-retaining retractors of many styles and sizes (Fig. 18.37).

Retractors should be handed to the surgeon in

Sutures and Needles

At this point in basic abdominal surgery, the fascia and muscle are penetrated and bypassed. This is done in the same manner as with the subcuticular layer. A suture may be necessary at any one of these points.

Use of sutures and needles is a vast subject. Several books have been published by suture manufacturers, covering the subject in great detail, and they should be read by serious students of perioperative nursing.

Basically, sutures are used to hold tissue together during wound healing or to control hemorrhage by tying off bleeding vessels. Surgical needles are designed to carry the suture through tissue with minimal trauma. Both sutures and needles are available presterilized in easy-to-open packages.

Numerous types of sutures are used at various times during surgery. Suture can be absorbable, such as chromic or plain catgut and some synthetic materials, or nonabsorbable, such as silk, cotton, and nylons of all types.

Most needles used today are disposable. They come in many sizes and shapes with various points and eyes, each with its own particular use. Needles and sutures are also available as one continuous unit. In the atraumatic needle the suture is attached to the eyeless needle by the manufacturer.

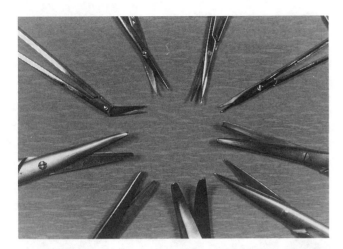

FIGURE 18.31. Scissors come with a variety of tips, blades, curves, and angles, each meant for a specific job. The four in the top of the picture are fine, delicate, and used for vascular, eye, ear, and plastic operations.

position for use. Some have handles and the operative portion is obvious; others, such as the Army–Navy retractor in Figure 18.34, are double-ended. The end to be inserted into the patient depends on the size of the job to be accomplished. Judgment is necessary; by watching what the surgeon is doing, the scrub person can anticipate the type of instrument that will be needed.

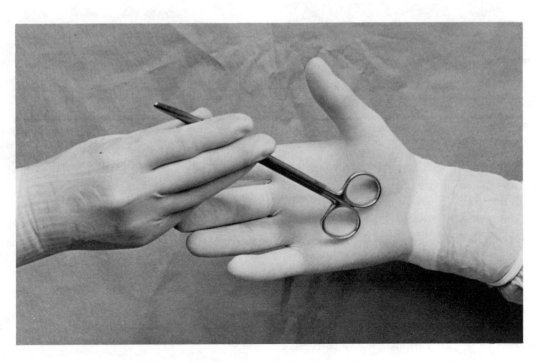

FIGURE 18.32. The scissor is placed in the hand as a hemostat is passed. A little snap or flip of the wrist, just at the moment of contact, is helpful. The scissor is firmly in place and the surgeon knows this without looking away from the surgical site.

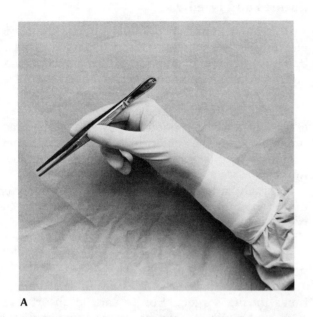

A

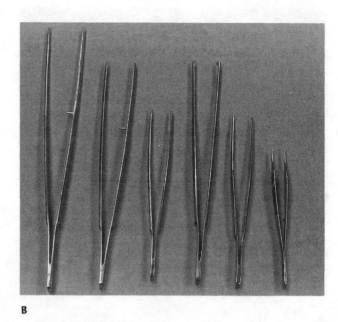

B

FIGURE 18.33. A. Pick-ups are passed to the surgeon in a position to be used. Remember this point about passing all instruments. B. Pick-ups come in several types and sizes. Some have teeth and others are plain. These tissue forceps provide an extension of thumb and finger for pinching-like actions.

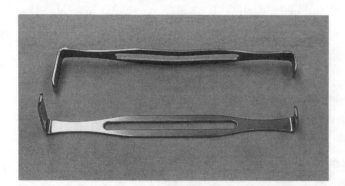

FIGURE 18.34. The Army–Navy retractor is hand-held and generally used in pairs. Notice that it is double-ended with different size blades.

There is a sequence of use for suture and needles, and each doctor has a personal preference. The surgeon's preference card should list what is to be used during incision and entry, the main portion of the procedure, and closure.

It takes time and practice to be able to assemble the correct suture with the appropriate needle and have it ready when needed. For the surgeon to use a combination suture and needle, a needle holder is necessary (Fig. 18.38). Needle holders come in many shapes and sizes for use at various times and types of operations.

The needle holder is passed into the surgeon's hand as any clamp would be, but attention must be paid to the direction of the needle. It must be in po-

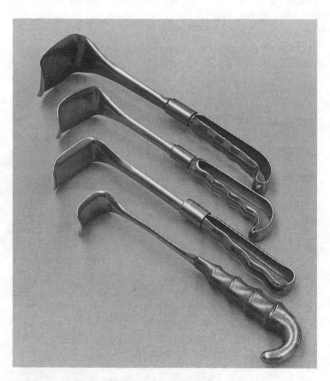

FIGURE 18.35. Richardson retractors come in a variety of sizes to hold back various depths of tissue. They can be used singly or in pairs.

sition for use, and the suture material should not be allowed to bunch up in the surgeon's hand (Fig. 18.39).

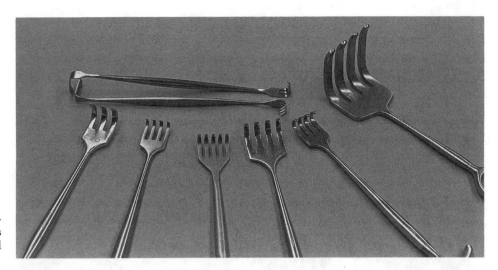

FIGURE 18.36. Rake retractors with sharp and dull prongs are generally used in pairs and are hand-held.

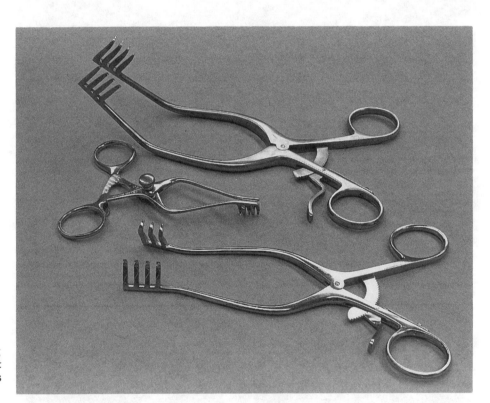

FIGURE 18.37. Self-retaining retractors are not hand-held but have ratchets, springs, or locks to hold them in position.

The peritoneum is the last layer to go through before entry into the abdominal cavity. Both surgeon and assistant may use a pick-up with teeth to lift the peritoneum so that it is not lying against an underlying organ. The surgeon uses a clean knife to nick this structure to make a hole. Then a Metzenbaum scissor, a delicate tissue scissor, is used to shear the peritoneum. At this point, the surgeon explores the cavity. Small, loose, 4 × 4″ sponges should be removed from the operative site at this point; sponges should now be used only on a sponge stick.

A self-retaining Balfour retractor is inserted (Fig.

18.40). Laparotomy sponges may be placed along the sides of the incision to protect the tissue. Once this entry has been completed, innumerable types of operations can be performed.

Instrument Care

The use of shortcuts in instrument care can lead to rust, corrosion, and stains. Corrosion will eventually disrupt the function of the instrument. Cleanliness, lubrication, and correct handling and storage procedures will ensure an instrument's proper

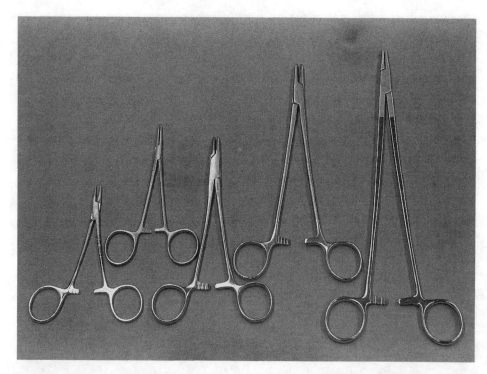

FIGURE 18.38. Needle holders have short, stubby jaws in comparison to clamps. They are made specifically to hold needles firmly. They come in many shapes and sizes to fit different needles as well as the procedures to be performed.

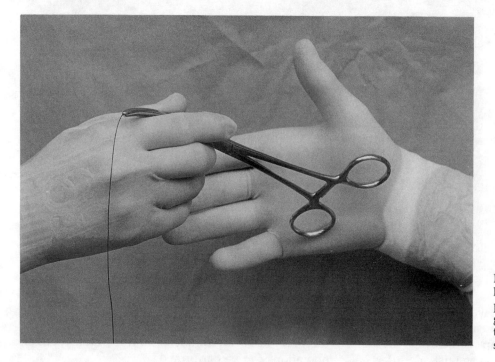

FIGURE 18.39. Needle holder loaded with atraumatic suture is passed to a right-handed surgeon. Notice that the suture material is hanging free over the scrub person's hand.

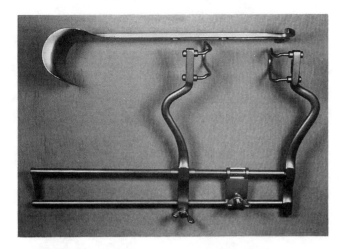

FIGURE 18.40. The Balfour retractor has two parts, retractor and blade. It is used to hold the abdominal wall open.

performance. Inspection, troubleshooting, and a professional instrument-maintenance program can lengthen the serviceable life of surgical instruments.

Cross-Specialty Innovations and Developments

Numerous high-technology innovations have been manufactured for use in multiple surgical specialties, including air-powered devices, operative microscopes, lasers, laparoscopes, and endoscopes.

Air-Powered Devices

Air-powered devices include a variety of drills and saws used for sculpting, cutting, and repairing bony tissue. In 1961 the first powered drills were developed by a dentist. Prior to this, these techniques were performed by hand, a tedious procedure (Fig. 18.41).

It was soon realized that powered equipment could dramatically reduce operative time and trauma to tissue. This also meant that the patient was under anesthesia for a shorter period. Today these drills are used in many specialties besides dentistry, for example orthopedics, neurosurgery, and maxillofacial microsurgery.

The power for such instruments is obtained from air or nitrogen under pressure. This compressed gas can be stored in large portable tanks. A pressure gauge controls the flow at a specified number of pounds per square inch (psi) (Fig. 18.42). Compressed air can also be piped into the operating suite though an extensive piping system that delivers suction vacuum, nitrous oxide, and oxygen. In this type of system, a wall unit acts as the pressure gauge and controls the flow, delivering specific pounds of pressure. Special high-power hoses connect the source of the power to the drill (Fig. 18.43).

The pounds of pressure needed to drive the motor change with the job expected of the equipment. For microdrills, such as those used in microsurgery on the ear, 80 to 90 psi is appropriate. For sculpting or cutting hard, large bones, a larger drill system of 110 psi with up to 20,000 rpm is used (Fig. 18.44).

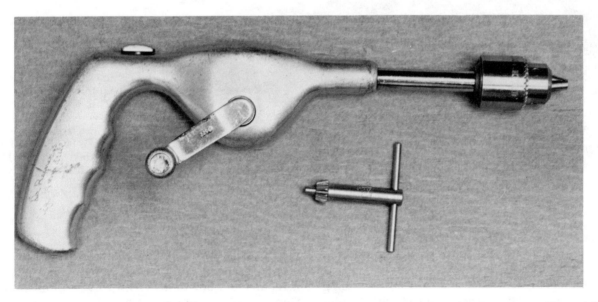

FIGURE 18.41.   Until 1961, only hand drills were available to the orthopedic surgeon and neurosurgeon. These drills are still available but seldom used.

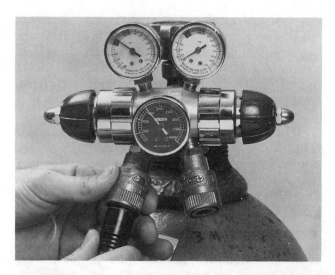

FIGURE 18.42. Air pressure determines the speed (rpm) of the air-powered equipment. When tanks of compressed air are used, they must be checked prior to surgery to make sure that they contain sufficient air to complete the procedure.

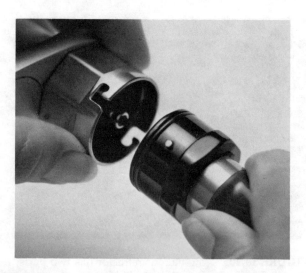

FIGURE 18.43. When attaching the air hose to the equipment, the fit should be snug. Grasp the handpiece connector in one hand, insert hose connector, and twist to lock. Reverse this process to remove. The equipment must be tested prior to use on the patient. (Photograph courtesy of 3M Surgical Products Division, St. Paul, MN 55144.)

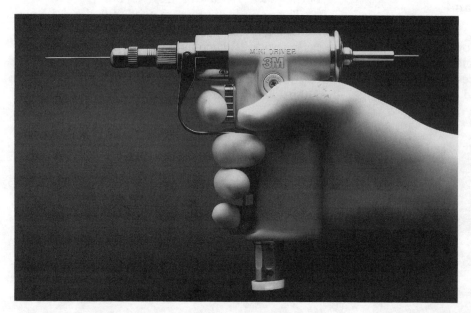

FIGURE 18.44. This 3M Mini-Driver is an example of modern air-powered equipment available to the surgeon. This is set up with the Swanson K-wire chuck attachment with K-wire in place. Normal operating pressure is 90 to 110 psi. (Photograph courtesy of 3M Health Care, St. Paul, MN 55144.)

These drills are precision instruments and should be handled as such. Care is necessary in putting them together correctly and cleaning and oiling them after a procedure. The manufacturer's recommendations must be followed for sterilization. This equipment is never immersed in any liquid. Fluid will penetrate the interior of the drill and cause extensive rusting and damage, necessitating expensive repairs and downtime. With rust accumulation, the motor will freeze up.

There are many attachments for air-powered drills, and they are used for a variety of jobs (Fig.

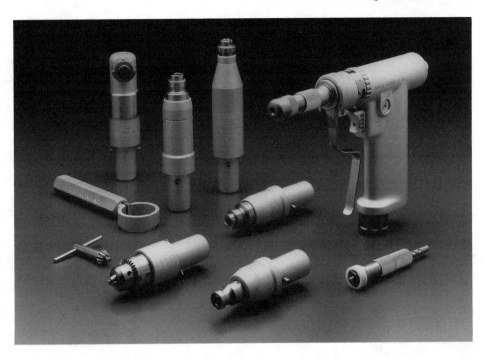

FIGURE 18.45. The Maxi-Driver II system is a versatile modular system powered by a durable vane motor. The handpiece provides speed and torque for large-bone orthopedic surgery, including drilling, pinning, sawing, reaming, and screwing. Each attachment is designed to automatically connect with the drive spindle, snapping onto the handpiece without tools. (Photograph and caption courtesy of 3M Surgical Products Division, St. Paul, MN 55144.)

18.45). When holes must be drilled for the placement of a metal plate to hold a fracture together, drill points, screw, and screwdriver are needed. Removing, reshaping, and reaming of bone at the knee or hip joint for placement of a total joint prosthesis require saws and blades of various sizes and shapes. Forward and reverse speeds are necessary for some of these activities. During a craniotomy, burr holes are drilled through the cranium and cut eventually to lift out a section of bone.

Three types of chucks can be placed on the main drill body (Fig. 18.46). Each chuck accepts different accessories, allowing for greater versatility overall. But the pieces must match the chuck on the drill in order to use the motor's drive power.

There are several manufacturers of air-powered drills. All have extensive inservice programs in the care, handling, and operation of their equipment. These programs should be presented frequently for initial instruction, to assist new staff members, and

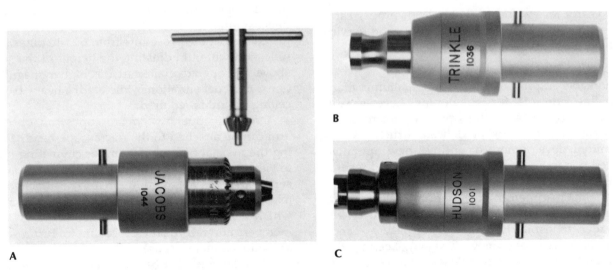

FIGURE 18.46. A. The L110 Jacobs chuck for the 3M Maxi-Driver is for use in driving up to one-quarter-inch pins, straight shank twist drills, to intramedullary reamers. Use the chuck key to loosen or tighten the chuck. B. The L112 trinkle chuck is used in driving twist drills with trinkle arbors, or in powering automatic screwdrivers with trinkle arbors. The sleeve is retracted to accept drill or screwdriver fully. C. The Hudson chuck is used during intramedullary reaming. The sleeve is retracted to accept a Hudson arbor or reamer. Release the sleeve to secure the attachment. (Photographs and caption courtesy of 3M Surgical Products Division, St. Paul, MN 55144.)

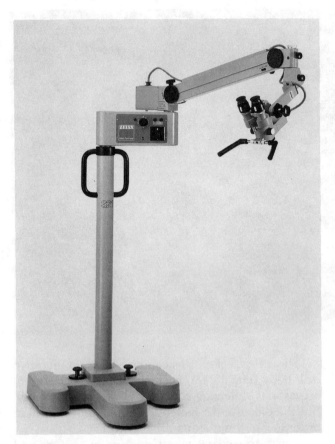

FIGURE 18.47. The Zeiss OPMII with movable floor stand permits easy and exact positioning of the microscope. The suspension arm is designed to ensure that the microscope remains in position. This particular setup is specially designed for use in otorhinolaryngology. (Photograph courtesy of Carl Zeiss, Inc., Thornwood, NY 10594.)

as a yearly review for everyone. With proper care, these precision instruments will give good service and last a long time.

Operative Microscopes

Remarkable improvements in optics, illumination, and fine controls for positioning have greatly expanded the role of the operative microscope. Improved visualization of delicate structures has permitted development of entirely new operative procedures in many surgical specialties and technical refinements in others.

The microscope can be either on a rolling stand or mounted on a ceiling rack (Figs. 18.47 and 18.48). In order to avoid tipping the top-heavy stand-mounted microscope, move it slowly, keeping the head and arms of the scope close to the center post, with the head over the longest arm of the footpiece. Touching the lens will cause smudging. The microscope lens should be cleaned only with lens paper and lens solution. A sterile, light-plastic drape can

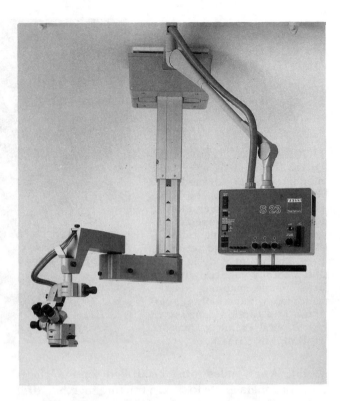

FIGURE 18.48. The low-vibration, motorized Zeiss S23 ceiling mount has been specially designed to meet the requirements of ophthalmic microsurgery. The mount consists of a telescope column, a lamp arm, an OPMI carrier arm, and an arm-mounted control panel. (Photograph courtesy of Carl Zeiss, Inc., Thornwood, NY 10594.)

be used to include the microscope in the operative field.

The microscope is used to illuminate and magnify the operative site, permitting the use of greater delicacy and finesse. The lens system can be adjusted during the procedure from 6 to 40 times magnification without adjusting the height of the scope above the operative site. At the higher magnifications, minimal vibration is tolerated; a heavy base or ceiling mount is required.

On many operative microscopes, an observer arm can be attached to the microscope head, allowing the assistant, scrub person, or circulating nurse to view the progress of the surgery. Instead of an observer arm, the microscope can also be attached to a television monitor and video-recording equipment, which displays the operative site to other team members and records the procedure for future study and educational purposes.

Developments in operative microscopy are being utilized by numerous specialties. Plastic surgery uses operative microscopes when dealing with traumatic loss of extremities, such as digits, ears, and composite tissue. Recent developments in operative

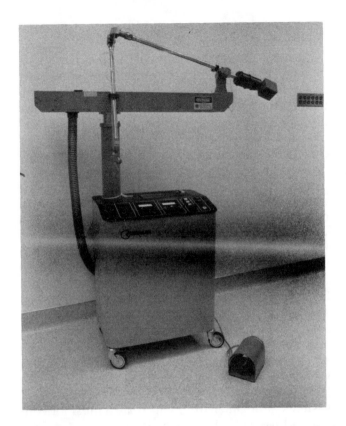

FIGURE 18.49.   The Sharplan 733 carbon dioxide (CO_2) laser with articulating arm and controlling foot pedal.

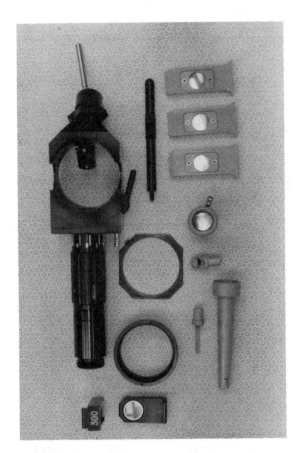

FIGURE 18.50.   The microslab and other pieces necessary to attach the Sharplan 733 CO_2 laser to the operative microscope.

microscopes have also facilitated new procedures in microvascular and nerve reconstruction and neurosurgery.

Some troubleshooting ability, such as knowledge of how to change light bulbs and fuses, is helpful. Refer to the manufacturer's manual for specific instructions on the model in use.

When not in use, the microscope should be covered to prevent dust from accumulating on the lens and other delicate parts. The ceiling-mounted scope should be removed from its mounting when not in use and placed in the padded box provided by the manufacturer.

Lasers

The term *laser* is an acronym for *l*ight *a*mplification by *s*timulated *e*mission *r*adiation, a process that converts electrical energy to a controlled beam of light energy. Lasers first appeared in perioperative patient care in the 1970s, and today they are used in many medical specialties, in both outpatient and general surgical settings.

Laser beams are delivered by either direct optics (mirror and lens) or fiberoptic systems. Only beams that are absorbed can affect tissue. As the light en-

ergy of the laser is converted into heat energy, it causes a thermal response that results in coagulation, cutting, vaporization, or welding of tissue.

Three types of lasers are commonly employed in surgery. They are referred to by the medium that creates the beam: carbon dioxide (CO_2), argon, or neodymium:yttrium–aluminum–garnet (Nd:YAG). Other medical lasers include excimer, tunable dye, and KTP.

The CO_2 laser (Fig. 18.49) has a self-contained cooling system and plugs into a regular wall outlet. In the past, the CO_2 beam could only be delivered via a direct optic system, but recent developments permit transmission via fiberoptics. This type of laser can be utilized in either a continuous or pulsed mode. If necessary, a pencil-like handpiece can be coupled with the operative microscope (Fig. 18.50). Because the CO_2 beam is invisible, it uses a red helium–neon laser to provide an aiming light. The beam penetrates to a depth of 0.1 to 0.2 mm and can be focused in a fine line for precise cutting effects. The CO_2 wavelength is absorbed by water; and since human cells have a high percentage of water, this

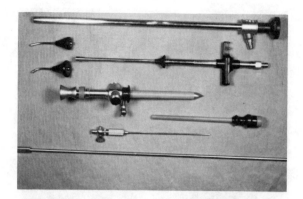

FIGURE 18.51. The laparoscope allows visualization of the abdominal cavity. As there are many pieces to a laparoscope, a checklist can be helpful to ensure the inclusion of all items and to check the total system during setup.

type of laser effectively vaporizes and denatures cellular protein when the beam comes in contact with it. The main applications for the CO_2 laser are in gynecology, otorhinolaryngology, neurosurgery, and plastic surgery.

The argon laser, another gas-based laser, emits a blue light that is readily picked up by red pigment, making it effective in coagulating small blood vessels and ablating superficial vascular lesions. The argon beam is easily transmitted through clear structures, such as the epidermis of nonpigmented skin and the clear vitreous body of the eye. This type of laser is used primarily in ophthalmology, gastroenterology, and dermatology.

The Nd:YAG laser uses 220-volt direct current to activate a bright flash lamp that strikes a solid crystal of yttrium–aluminum–garnet acting as a lattice for the neodymium. This type of laser beam can be transmitted over fiberoptic cable to a handpiece. It is used in endoscopy, pulmonology, urology, and gynecology. It can also be used with the operative microscope. The Nd:YAG laser beam is mainly absorbed by protein and partially absorbed by hemoglobin and water. It has the greatest penetration depth of all the lasers and is effective in coagulating larger vessels and ablating deep tissue. But the Nd:YAG beam scatters in tissue, making precise control difficult.

Lasers permit the surgeon to do fine dissection without disruption of the surrounding tissue. In skilled hands, the laser decreases surgical time, cuts and coagulates tissue while creating a relatively bloodless field, and reaches relatively inaccessible areas of the body with less trauma to the patient. Lasers have made it possible to convert numerous inpatient procedures to outpatient ones. They can be

used safely under local anesthesia, and at times with no anesthesia at all.

Despite these advantages, it is important to remember that lasers are powerful and potentially dangerous tools. The laser beam generates high temperatures and it can be reflected, scattered, transmitted, and absorbed by the patient, personnel, and others in the area. These characteristics create challenging safety hazards that must be addressed by the surgical team. Laser safety education is essential for all personnel. Everyone must be aware of the precautions necessary when a laser is in use, and personnel should be permitted to assist with laser procedures only after they have learned the necessary safety precautions. During the learning period, the new perioperative nurse must be under close supervision. In addition, well-formulated policies and procedures must be established and followed meticulously.

Laser equipment is sensitive and can present mechanical problems. Lasers must be tested immediately prior to use by a laser technician or a nurse trained in testing procedures. All laser companies have extensive educational programs and support systems for maintenance, which are a must for both OR and biomedical maintenance staffs.

The range of applications for which lasers are utilized is rapidly expanding as the technology is refined. Many procedures are now combining the elements of endoscopy, microscopy, and lasers. There are certainly many dynamic new treatment modes on the horizon for laser applications.

Laparoscopes and Accessories

One area of continued development is the use of the laparoscope (Fig. 18.51) to permit direct visualization of the abdominal cavity. For laparoscopic procedures, gas is instilled into the abdominal cavity to distend it and permit better visualization of anatomic structures. The gas most suited for this purpose is CO_2. In order to instill the CO_2, a sterile Verres needle is inserted abdominally and connected to sterile polyethylene tubing that is attached to the insufflator. The CO_2 flows into the patient at a rate of about 1 L/min; in an average-size adult about 3 liters are used. Gauges on the insufflator that indicate the amount of gas instilled into the cavity are carefully monitored by the surgeon and the circulating nurse. It is important that all pieces of the set fit snugly to prevent leakage of the gas during the procedure. All valves, needles, and gauges must be checked for workability before the patient is anesthetized.

Once the desired abdominal distention is reached, an incision is made through the abdominal

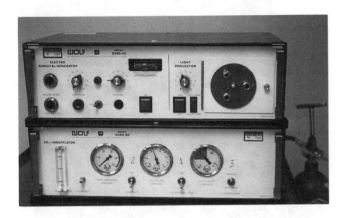

FIGURE 18.52.   The equipment on top is a generator that provides the light source for the fiberoptic illumination. The lower unit is the insufflator, which delivers carbon dioxide intraabdominally through sterile tubing and a Verres needle. Gauges on the panel indicate the amount of gas injected into the cavity.

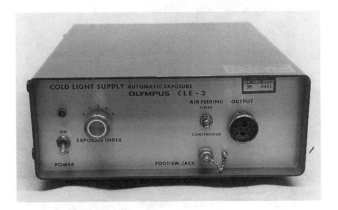

FIGURE 18.53.   Fiberoptic illumination is crucial in endoscopic procedures.

wall, using a puncture trocar to enter the abdominal cavity. This first incision is for insertion of the laparoscope. Using fiberoptic illumination (Fig. 18.52), the abdominal cavity is examined thoroughly. If the lens becomes fogged during the procedure, dipping it in warm, sterile water can keep fogging to a minimum. (Water is preferred; saline has adverse effect on the instrument.) After the initial inspection, additional small incisions are made to allow the insertion of probes, forceps, and/or biopsy instruments.

Video cameras have been adapted to attach to the lens of the scope, with the image produced on a monitor. In laparoscopic cholecystectomy, for example, the entire surgical procedure is done via the video screen. Two video screens are set up on opposite sides of the operating table: one for the primary surgeon and the other for the assistant. This allows each to visualize the operative site without changing position.

For laparoscopic cholecystectomy a heparinized solution (5,000 units of heparin to a liter of warm saline) under pressure is used to irrigate the operative site and retard clot formation. Automatic-loading, multiple-clip appliers designed for laparoscopic use are available to assist with hemostasis. Lasers may be used in this procedure for dissection and hemostasis.

Procedures that combine the use of laparoscopy, lasers, and video monitoring represent a significant breakthrough in surgical technique. Compared to conventional surgical approaches, laparoscopic and endoscopic procedures decrease the length of patients' hospitalizations, reduce care costs, and return the patient to normal activity more quickly.

Endoscopes and Accessories

Endoscopy permits visualization of the contents and walls of a body cavity or tube. Endoscopic procedures can be as simple as reviewing the eye grounds and ear canal during a basic physical examination; and as complex as intraoperative nephroscopy or endoscopic retrograde cholangiopancreatography (ERCP). Endoscopy is a major tool for ensuring diagnostic accuracy and, in combination with the laser, is becoming a method of treatment in many specialties.

The equipment used in this area has greatly changed since the first endoscope was developed in Germany in 1806. That instrument was a simple metal tube with candlelight reflecting off a hand mirror.

Great strides were made in endoscopy as the science of electricity became refined. Edison's light bulb allowed for the development of light carriers that could be placed in the scopes. Lamm's discovery of fiberoptics in 1930 brought further progress in lighting systems. Fiberoptics use multiple microscopic glass fibers wrapped in a sheath that allow light to travel through them without distortion (Fig. 18.53).

Advances in optics have also influenced endoscopy. In 1879 Nitze developed the first telescope to be used to visualize a deep internal cavity. This telescope used several small lenses separated by larger air spaces. Hopkins reversed this, using larger glass

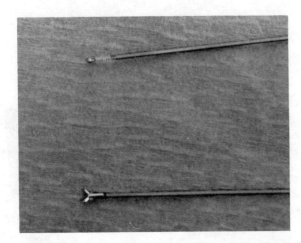

FIGURE 18.54.   The small biopsy cup and brush used in some endoscopic procedures to obtain tissue specimens.

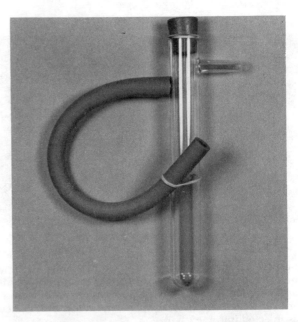

FIGURE 18.55.   A Luken's tube or a disposable specimen trap is attached to the suctioning system used in bronchoscopy to collect specimens for cytological examination. These tubes come in several styles and are available in sterile and disposable models.

rods and small air spaces, permitting greater resolution (clarity of detail) and magnification, with a wider field of vision.

Another important feature of endoscopic procedures is the ability to take still and motion pictures. Most endoscopes can be adapted with attachments for video monitoring systems, which allow the endoscopist to view the procedure via video screen instead of direct visualization. This adaptation also allows others to view the field and permits videotaping for clinical and educational purposes.

Many endoscopic procedures can be performed in the physician's office or on an outpatient basis in the hospital. Here, however, those procedures most likely to be performed in the operating room, under general or local anesthesia, are discussed. Some operating rooms have an area set aside for endoscopic procedures.

Some endoscopic procedures can be performed through natural openings, such as bronchoscopy, cystoscopy, and colonoscopy. Others are performed through small incisions, such as arthroscopy and laparoscopy. Still others are done during major surgical procedures, such as choledochoscopy and nephroscopy.

Bronchoscopy is used to inspect the trachea, main stem of the bronchus, and small bronchi. It can also be performed to remove a foreign body, such as a peanut or pin, or another type of obstruction to the airway. It is sometimes used for deep suctioning in patients with atelactasis.

Small biopsies, or brushings, can be taken of suspicious areas of the bronchial tree (Fig. 18.54), or bronchial washings can be performed by inserting 5 to 10 cc of saline followed by suctioning. A good suction flow is essential during this procedure. A Lu-

ken's tube (Fig. 18.55) can be attached to the suction tubing to gather specimens, which are then sent to the laboratory for cytological examination. Fractional studies of the bronchial tree require several specimens. The locations of these specimens must be carefully labeled and documented by the circulating nurse.

Bronchoscopy can be performed in many different modes: the patient may be under local or general anesthesia, the patient's position may be supine or sitting, the bronchoscope may be rigid or flexible. The combination used depends on the doctor's expertise with the equipment and the type of study to be performed.

The rigid bronchoscope (Fig. 18.56) is inserted as a laryngoscope would be, through the mouth and nasopharynx, then past the vocal cords into the trachea, and on into the bronchial tree. Inspection occurs as insertion takes place. The doctor views the area directly, without use of a telescope. The flexible bronchoscope may be inserted in the same manner, or through the nose. Nasal insertion is preferred by many doctors and patients. Vision is through a series of minute lenses (Fig. 18.57). Compared to the rigid bronchoscope, flexible scopes have a narrower diameter, are more comfortable for the patient, allow for greater maneuverability and depth of examination, and expose a far greater proportion of the tracheal bronchial tree. They have literally revolutionized this field of practice.

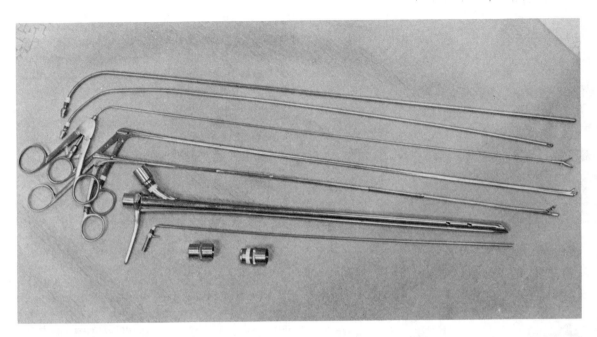

FIGURE 18.56.   The rigid bronchoscope comes in various sizes. It is basically a hollow tube that provides direct visualization of the area. Illumination is provided by fiberoptics. Long, rigid suction cannulas are essential to remove any secretions.

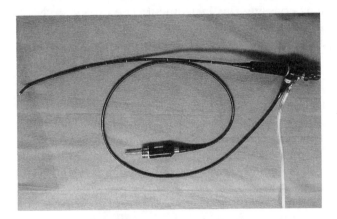

FIGURE 18.57.   This highly sophisticated, flexible, narrow-diameter bronchoscope with movable tip has greatly facilitated and extended the possible types of examinations of the bronchial tree. Tiny cables control movement of the tip. The scope has channels for water irrigation; suction removal of secretions, blood, and small particles; and passage of small brushes and biopsy forceps to obtain specimens for cytology and pathology.

Under local anesthesia, patient cooperation is necessary. Meticulous preoperative preparation of the patient can make the difference between a successful and unsuccessful procedure. As the patient's airway is involved, anxiety can be high. Reassurance throughout the procedure is necessary. Patients prefer the thin, flexible scopes, as they eliminate most of the discomfort.

At best, bronchoscopy is a clean procedure.

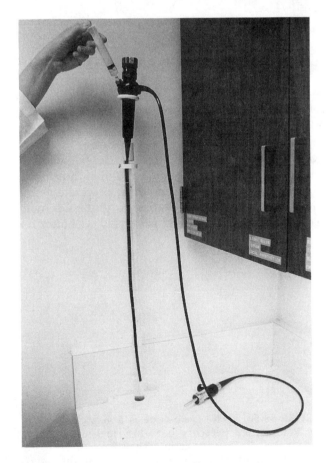

FIGURE 18.58.   Proper cleaning of the flexible scope between procedures is essential. A long test tube large enough to accommodate the flexible scope is helpful for cleaning.

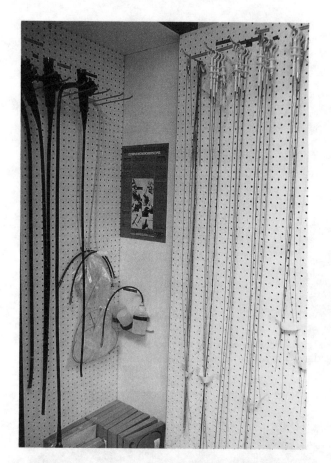

FIGURE 18.59.   Storage is greatly facilitated with a cabinet where flexible scopes and biopsy forceps can hang free.

Rigid scopes should be sterilized after each use. Flexible fiberoptic scopes should be thoroughly cleaned and disinfected with an appropriate germicide, such as povidone–iodine or glutaraldehyde. The scopes must be rinsed extremely well after use

of these solutions (Fig. 18.58). The manufacturer's instructions must be followed carefully. Storage of flexible scopes can be greatly facilitated by having a special cabinet that allows them to hang full length. This prevents bending and kinking of the scopes, possible breakage of the fiberoptic glass rods, and damage to the delicate lens system (Fig. 18.59).

Recent nasal sinus surgeries have combined the developments in both endoscopy and lasers, providing a new mode of treatment for patients with turbinate dysfunction or removal of nasal polyps. Laryngoscopes are being used with microscopes and lasers for treatment of patients with vocal cord and tracheal pathology.

Another frequently performed endoscopic procedure is cystoscopy. A cystoscope is composed of an interchangeable fiberoptic telescope with various sheaths (Fig. 18.60). A fiberoptic light source and cord activate the lighting system. The cystoscope also contains a system to instill an irrigation solution, which distends the bladder for visualization of the bladder wall. The cystoscope is introduced through the urethra. Lubrication on the sheath facilitates passing this instrument. The urologist visualizes the interior of the urinary bladder and adjacent structures to help diagnose urinary tract pathology. Simple cystoscopy takes only minutes to complete.

Cystoscopy can be performed on a standard operating room table with the patient in a modified lithotomy position, but most operating suites have a separate room that contains a special urology table. This table is adapted to contain and drain all the solution necessary during the procedure. The table also allows x-rays to be taken for retrograde and other studies.

Another urologic endoscopy procedure is the transurethral resection (TUR). TUR uses a resecto-

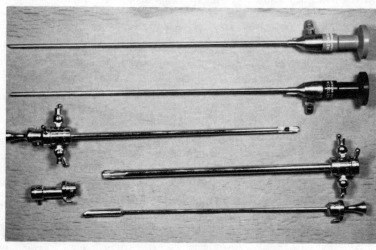

FIGURE 18.60.   The cystoscope is a very delicate, multilensed telescope used to visualize the bladder wall. It is available in several Foley sizes and angles to the lens. The lens at the top of the picture is 30 degrees, and the second one is straightforward. The sheaths and obdurator are displayed at the bottom of the picture.

scope and cutting electrodes to remove hypertrophic or malignant prostatic tissue or tumors of the bladder neck of slight to moderate size. Several types of scopes can be used, depending upon the surgeon's preference.

These scopes are complex and delicate, using the basic principles of cystoscopy. They are composed of telescope sheaths, obturators, cutting electrodes, and the working element, which provides the motion to the cutting loops.

An irrigating system runs solution into the bladder both to distend it and to wash out the tissue removed. Since water is hypotonic and saline disperses the coagulating current, glycine or sorbitol is generally used for TUR, although sterile distilled water may be used for cystoscopy.

High-frequency current is passed from the electrocautery unit to the insulated cutting loops for both cutting and coagulating tissue. All the precautions necessary for the use of the electrocautery unit must be followed meticulously because copious amounts of irrigating solution are used. The surgical team must also be aware of their own safety in this wet environment.

Catheter drainage is desirable postoperatively for most urologic procedures. The circulating nurse should be prepared for this with Foley catheters of several types and sizes.

Endoscopy is also being used in major operative procedures. In many of these procedures, the basic technique consists of threading a small fiber-optic telescope through another larger scope to look for pathology in very small internal, often tubular, structures, such as the common bile duct, ureter, or kidney pelvis. The small scope also has attached a cannula pathway for delivery and evacuation of an irrigating solution.

For visualization of retained common duct stones, a right-angled 40-mm choledochoscope is inserted through a small incision in the common bile duct and into the hollow viscus. Because the duct is so small, it must be expanded with irrigation under pressure. Normal saline in a plastic bag is preferred because a pressure cuff can be slipped over the bag and maintain a constant pressure of 300 mm Hg during the procedure. The choledochoscope is attached by sterile tubing to the irrigating solution, which is hung on an intravenous standard. The pressure exerted is sufficient to dilate the duct to visualize and flush out the area.

When a stone is spotted, it is grasped and removed with a Randall stone forceps. After removal, the area is visualized again with the scope. A full flushing with irrigating solution is then done to wash out any bits of calculi. This sounds simple, but it can be tedious and time-consuming.

If visualization farther than 40 mm is needed, 60-mm choledochoscopes are available, although seldom used. Some surgeons may use a Fogarty balloon catheter or Dormier stone basket to remove stones. Flushing is necessary after their use also. A biopsy forceps or brush can also be inserted through the choledochoscope to obtain tissue specimens for histological and cytological examination.

A separate sterile field should be set up for this procedure, in order to protect the telescope and other parts from inadvertent abuse, such as placing heavy instruments on top of them.

Another intraoperative use of endoscopy is angioscopy, which enables vascular surgeons to assess intraluminal pathology and directly view details of blood vessels during surgery. In these cases ultrafine endoscopes are utilized.

An individual checklist for endoscopic procedures is helpful, particularly when many small pieces are needed. These checklists will maintain everyone's sanity plus provide efficient, safe patient care. Gentleness is the key to handling all telescopes and fiberoptics.

Specialty Instruments and Equipment

Each specialty has equipment and instruments that are specific to that type of surgery. Instruments and equipment specific to gastrointestinal surgery, gynecologic surgery, plastic surgery, orthopedic surgery, arthroscopic surgery, neurosurgery, ophthalmic surgery, and otomicrosurgery are described below, followed by a discussion of cardiac pacemakers.

Gastrointestinal Surgery

One specialized technique used in gastrointestinal surgery is internal stapling, which was originally developed in Russia as a means of suturing tissue mechanically. In the past decade, internal stapling devices have been refined and are now used widely. As surgeons have gained experience in the use of stapling instruments, they have been widely adopted in procedures requiring ligation and division, anastomosis, resection, and closure (Figs. 18.61 to 18.65). The staples are made of a nonreactive metal that minimizes reaction and infection. The instruments come preloaded with staples, and cartridge refills are available.

Compared to conventional techniques, stapling reduces the amount of edema that occurs with the handling of tissue. The B-shape of the staple allows circulation to pass through the tissue at the staple

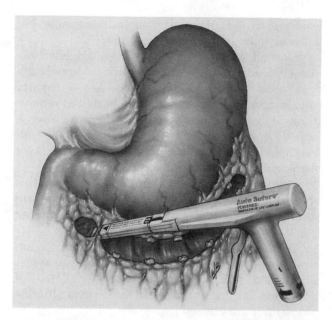

FIGURE 18.61. The LDS model is shown during a Billroth II gastrectomy. The stomach is mobilized using the LDS to ligate and divide the omental vessels. The jaws of the LDS are slipped around the vessel and fat to be divided and fired. Two staples ligate the vessel; simultaneously, a knife in the LDS divides the vessel between the staples. (Photograph and caption courtesy of United States Surgical Corporation © USSC 1974, 1980, 1988. We acknowledge the use in this work of certain copyrighted materials which have been reprinted with permission of United States Surgical Corporation as indicated by: © USSC 1988. These materials are copyrighted © United States Surgical Corporation 1981, All Rights Reserved, and may not be reproduced in any form or by any means.)

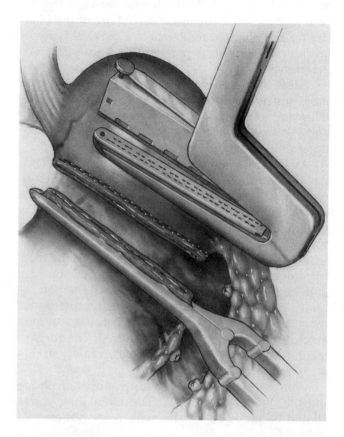

FIGURE 18.62. The TA 90 is shown as it is being used to close the gastric pouch during a Billroth II procedure. The jaws of the TA 90 are slipped around the stomach at the level of transection. Close the instrument and fire the staple. Before removing the instrument, a clamp is placed on the specimen side and transected using the TA 90 edge as a cutting guide. (© USSC 1974, 1980, 1988, Norwalk, CT)

line to the cut edge. Stapling devices have significantly reduced the amount of time necessary to perform anastomoses and resections, meaning less handling of tissue, less edema, and also a decrease in the length of time the patient is under the effects of anesthesia.

The devices shown in the figures are disposable, preloaded, one-time implements. They are supplied sterile, in convenient packaging. Similar implements have been developed for use in other specialties, such as thoracic surgery and gynecology.

Gynecologic Surgery

Gynecologists perform abdominal surgery on women of all ages. The procedure performed most frequently in this specialty is the D and C, or dilatation and curettage (Fig. 18.66), which is used for diagnostic studies of the lining of the uterus, removal of retained placenta after deliveries, and termination of pregnancy.

The specialized equipment used in gynecology includes stirrups, which are used to place the patient in the lithotomy position, with legs raised and abducted to expose the perineal region. (See again Fig. 18.4.) The stirrups must be level and at the proper height for the individual patient. The patient's back must be well supported, with the buttocks flush with the break in the table. In order to prevent stress and damage to the patient's hips, both legs and feet should go into the stirrups simultaneously. Ideally, two people help position the patient, each gently raising a leg and placing a foot into a stirrup strap. It is essential that the strap lie flat in all areas of contact with the foot. If the patient is to remain in the lithotomy position for any length of time, her feet must be padded, and her legs must be high enough to prevent limb compression and compartmental syndrome.

At the conclusion of the procedure, the patient's feet must be carefully removed from the stirrups and

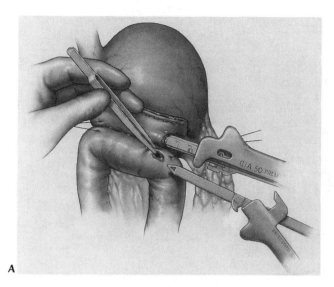

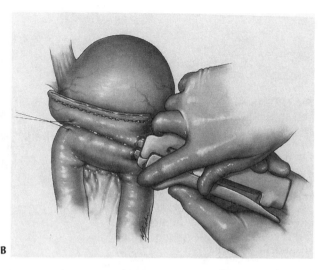

FIGURE 18.63.   A. The GIA model of Autosuture is used to incise the stomach and secure hemostasis of the cut edges in one application. A stab wound is made into the gastric wall at the level for the gastrostomy. One fork of the GIA is inserted into the lumen of the stomach and the other fork is placed on the serosal surface. B. The second step—closure of the GIA and firing of the staples. Two double-staggered hemostatic staple lines have now been placed in the gastric edges. (© USSC 1974, 1980, 1988, Norwalk, CT)

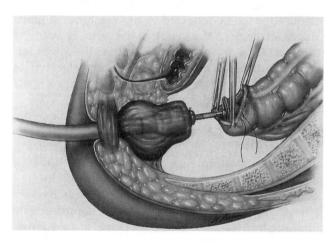

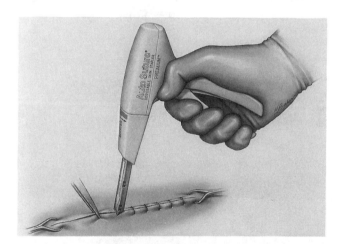

FIGURE 18.64.   In a low anterior resection EEA is used to perform the anastomosis. The EEA is introduced into the anus and advanced to the level of the purse-string suture. The EEA is opened and the anvil is introduced into the proximal colon with the rectal purse-string suture being tied. Ensure that the tissue is snug against the cartridge and anvil to reduce the possibility of bunching or overlapping as the tissue is approximated. Check that all tissue layers are incorporated within the loading unit prior to firing the staples. The EEA is closed and the staples fired. A circular, double-staggered row of staples joins the bowel, and simultaneously, the circular blade in the instrument cuts the stoma. (© USSC 1974, 1980, 1988.)

FIGURE 18.65.   A. The Premium model of Autosuture is used during skin closure. The cartridge tip rests lightly on the skin as the staples are placed by partially squeezing the handle. The staples are spaced at normal intervals for skin closure. B. The skin staples form and hold tissue. (© USSC 1974, 1980, 1988.)

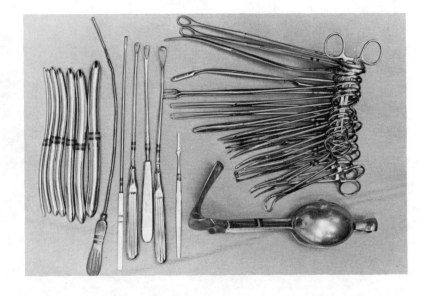

FIGURE 18.66. A basic D and C set. In the lower right-hand corner is the weighted vaginal speculum that is put into the vaginal vault. On the left, proceeding left to right, are Hegar's dilators used to dilate the cervix, uterine sounds used to measure the length of the uterine cavity, and four curettes of sizes used to scrape the wall of the uterine cavity to obtain a specimen for diagnostic studies.

the legs gently and slowly lowered together. Rapid lowering of the patient's legs could cause a sudden drop in the patient's blood pressure. Lowering her legs one at a time can place undue strain on her back and hips and possibly cause a dislocation.

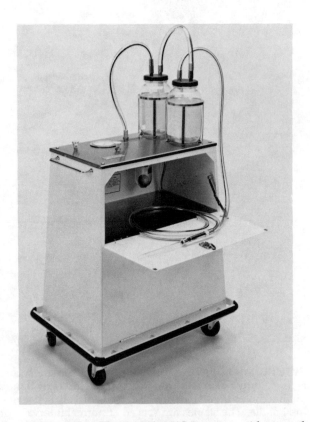

FIGURE 18.67. The Berkeley VC-2 system with two collection bottles. The tubing and cannula displayed on the open door are disposable and are available presterilized. (Photograph courtesy of Cooper Medical Devices Corp., Berkeley Bio-Engineering Division, San Leandro, CA.)

A vacuum curettage unit (Fig. 18.67) is used for aspirating the contents of the uterus. This has become an accepted, safe method of terminating early pregnancies. It is used in conjunction with a D and C instrument. Sterile, disposable cannulas and aspirating tubes are connected to the machine. A gauze sleeve attached to the inside of the primary bottle, at the end of the aspirating tube, collects the specimen. At the conclusion of the procedure, the sleeve is removed and the bottle contents emptied into a specimen container and sent to the laboratory.

Laparoscopy is commonly used in gynecology for direct visualization of the pelvic cavity. (See again Fig. 18.51.) An acorn cannula is inserted vaginally into the uterine cervix to permit manipulation of the uterus during the procedure. A small incision is made at the umbilicus. The telescope is inserted after the cannula and obturator have completed the opening into the cavity, and the pelvic organs are examined.

A second small incision is made in the right lower pelvic area for insertion of a probe for manipulation and use of other instruments.

Laparoscopy is used to biopsy suspicious tissue and to perform reproductive sterilization by incising and cauterizing the fallopian tubes. Many times it is performed to rule out suspected problems and thereby avoid unnecessary surgery.

Plastic Surgery

Plastic surgery deals with trauma patients, those with congenital problems or deforming diseases, and cosmetic procedures. It is not restricted to any particular anatomical area. It deals first with restoration of function and second with appearance.

During plastic surgery it is necessary to move

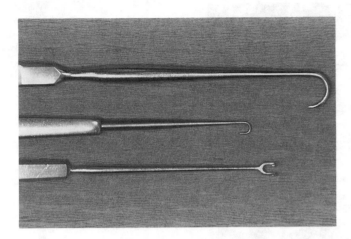

FIGURE 18.68.   Skin hooks of various sizes are used to gently retract or elevate the skin. Notice the extremely small and fine hooks on these instruments. Careful handling is necessary to prevent their piercing gloves and draping material and resultant contamination.

and handle tissue gently and with technical exactness. Thus the instruments used are fine and delicate (Fig. 18.68), as are the sutures and needles. Many of these procedures can be performed under local anesthesia.

Frequently used equipment in plastic surgery includes dermatomes for grafting tissue from one part of the patient to another (Fig. 18.69). These grafts can be removed by a simple razor or knife, but generally dermatomes are used. Dermatomes can be ad-

justed to acquire various thicknesses of skin. A split-thickness graft includes the entire epidermis and dermis.

Once a graft has been obtained, it should be kept in a moist, saline sponge or, if the edges tend to curl, placed on the bottom of a pan with a moist sponge over it. Every precaution should be taken to prevent dropping the graft out of the sterile field. A small graft can be expanded to cover a larger area by making multiple slits in it. This can be done automatically, by passing the graft on a carrier through a skin mesher that places the slits uniformly. The several sizes available determine the expansion of the graft.

Some practitioners in plastic surgery are now utilizing the laser in such procedures as reduction mammoplasty. In addition, they may use an operative microscope during hand surgery or repair of nerve or vascular tissue.

Seldom does the plastic surgeon have an assistant per se; the scrub person serves as the assistant. In this role, the nurse suctions, retracts tissue, cuts sutures, and uses cautery under the doctor's supervision. While performing these activities, arm or hand support prevents shaking motions.

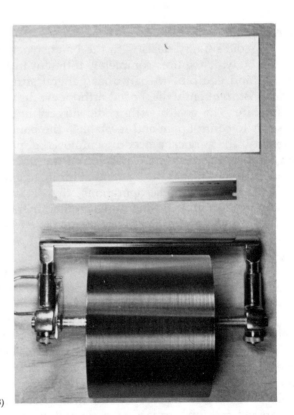

(A)   (B)

FIGURE 18.69.   A. The air-powered Brown dermatome is a popular type of dermatome used in obtaining skin grafts. Presterile, disposable, one-time-use blades are available. B. Padget dermatome is a manual instrument. The white tape is attached to the drum and used to receive the skin graft as it is cut. The blade comes presterilized and is disposable.

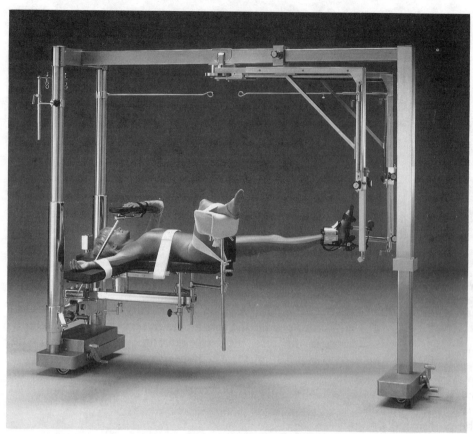

FIGURE 18.70. Chick-Langren table setup for left hip pinning procedure. Patient is supine, with the affected leg secured in traction and the nonaffected leg raised and abducted in the Well Leg Support Assembly. Cantilever table design and overhead suspension of leg spars allow easy access for mobile image intensifier placement. (Photograph courtesy of Midmark Corporation, Versailles, OH.)

Orthopedic Surgery

Orthopedic surgery deals with the bony structures of the body. It requires completely different instruments and equipment than does general surgery. The most frequently diagnosed orthopedic disorder is fracture. The goal of orthopedic surgery in such cases is to control pain and reestablish the patient's mobility. The surgical procedure employed depends on the patient's condition, position of the fracture, bone-healing capacity, and potential for infection.

For most orthopedic operations, the patient is placed in the supine position on a regular operating table. For hand and arm surgery, a side table extension or attachment can be slid into place on the regular table.

For patients with fractured hips or femurs, a specially designed orthopedic table can provide traction and good intraoperative alignment (Figs. 18.70 and 18.71). A fracture table is heavy and awkward; two people are required to move and assemble it. Once it is in position in the operating room, the nurse locks the table in place. This table can be used for many positions, each requiring different extensions. It is helpful to have each piece labeled and stored in an organized fashion for ease of accessibility and attachment.

These tables are equipped with x-ray shelves and cassette holders to allow for x-ray or fluoroscopic examination during the procedure (Fig. 18.72).

It is essential that members of the orthopedic surgical team have a full understanding of the fracture table prior to use. Team members must know what parts are needed, where they go, and how they are attached. The manufacturers of this equipment have brochures and extensive inservice programs available on the safe use of these tables.

As the electrocautery unit is used a great deal in orthopedic surgery, the metal parts of the fracture table that come in contact with the patient must be well padded to protect the patient from burns.

Pneumatic tourniquets are generally used for extremity surgery. They restrict venous blood flow, allowing a clearer view of the operative site (Fig. 18.73).

Care must be observed in the use of tourniquets. The cuff is applied far enough away from the incision site so that it will not be in the way, and the area where it is to be applied is padded with sheet cotton. The padding must be kept smooth, as a wrinkle can cause skin or nerve damage. In a correct-size cuff, the ends overlap by 2 to 3 inches. On male patients it is essential to check that the genitalia are not caught in the tourniquet when it is placed high on the leg. The patient and cuff should be protected

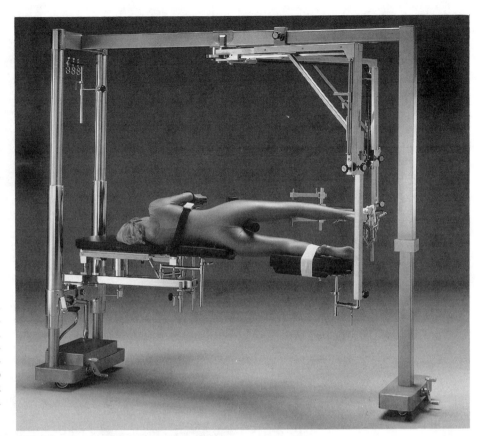

FIGURE 18.71. Chick-Langren table setup for closed/intramedullary nailing of the right femur. Patient is in the lateral decubitus position, with nonaffected leg resting on the foot board. The setup includes a 90-degree traction bow to accommodate either a Steinman pin or Kirschner wire. (Photograph courtesy of Midmark Corporation, Versailles, OH.)

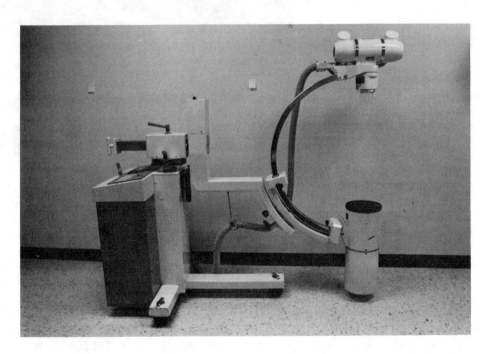

FIGURE 18.72. The C-arm is a fluoroscopic imaging system that presents real-time images on a television monitor. It is most frequently used intraoperatively during orthopedic procedures, particularly to repair fractured hips. Pacemaker insertions also require the C-arm.

from the prepping and procedural fluids by wrapping the tourniquet with an adherent plastic drape.

The nurse should check the tourniquet gauge prior to use to be sure it is working properly and accurately. The surgeon will determine the pressure setting. The time that the tourniquet goes up must be documented on either the perioperative nurse's notes or the anesthesia record. The surgeon should be informed at regular intervals of the length of time the tourniquet has been on during the surgery.

Instruments used in orthopedics include periosteal elevators, bone-holding clamps, bone-cutting instruments (osteotomes, rongeurs, curettes), and screwdrivers (Figs. 18.74 to 18.79). These instruments allow the surgeon to align bone fragments, cut and reshape bones, and drill holes for the application of hardware to be held by screws fixing the fracture in place for healing.

Basic to patient care in orthopedic surgery is the use of plaster of Paris as casting material. The purpose of casting is to immobilize the fracture site after bone alignment has been attained, by either closed or open reduction. Prior to application of the plaster, the incision site is dressed. The doctor then pads the extremity or the area to be casted with stockinette and sheet wadding to protect the patient's skin.

There are two types of plaster: slow-drying and fast-drying. The surgeon determines which type to use. The plaster comes in dry rolls or splints that are immersed in a small bucket of water for application. The plaster roll is dropped end-first into the water;

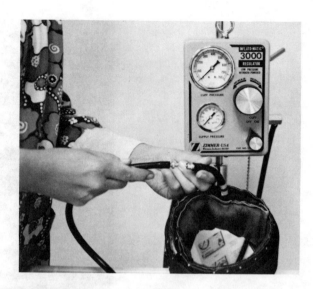

FIGURE 18.73.   A pneumatic tourniquet is frequently used in operations on the arms and legs. The cuff comes in a variety of sizes to match the extremity, larger for adult patients and surgery of the leg, smaller for children and surgery of the arm.

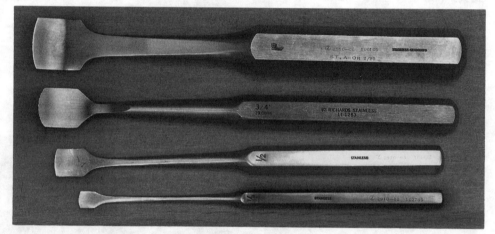

FIGURE 18.74.   Periosteal elevators, one-quarter inch to one inch wide, are used to scrape back the periosteal tissue, the outermost layer of bone.

when it stops bubbling, the roll is ready to be removed. The nurse squeezes the excess water from the roll by pushing both ends toward the middle. The nurse hands the roll to the doctor with the end pulled out so that the doctor can immediately begin to apply the cast, molding the pliable plaster to fit the patient. Drying occurs quickly, but the plaster does not solidify completely for several hours. Pillows under the extremity during the drying period help to prevent indentations of the soft material.

Orthopedic procedures can be complex and may require additional education and specialization. The nurse must be knowledgeable about prostheses and their highly specialized instrumentation, such as those used in total hip replacement and spinal operations using Harrington rods. Laminar air flow units may be used during these procedures.

Arthroscopic Surgery

Endoscopic examination of joints is being utilized more and more frequently in both ambulatory and inpatient surgeries. By far the most common of these procedures is arthroscopy of the knee. As a diagnostic tool, arthroscopy provides an almost complete view of the knee joint. It can confirm a diagnosis, rule out causes of patient symptoms, and determine followup care. Surgical procedures can also be performed arthroscopically, including removal of foreign bodies, lysis of adhesions, lavage of degenerated or septic knee, partial meniscectomy, patellar shaving, and anterior ligament repair.

The equipment employed in arthroscopic procedures is expensive. A high degree of skill is essential for the OR team to coordinate preparation and use of the instrumentation. The pneumatic tourniquet is

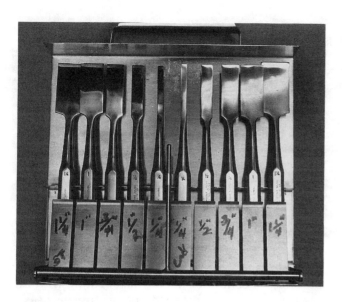

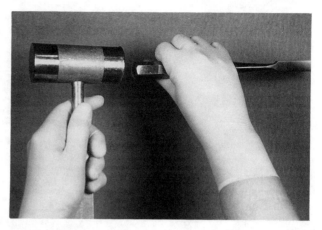

FIGURE 18.76. The osteotome is used with a mallet to cut into bone.

FIGURE 18.75. Osteotomes can be curved or straight and come in several widths. They are used to cut and shape bone. The rack in which they are held protects the cutting edges and keeps them organized for ease of selection and storage.

positioned. (See again Fig. 18.73). An arthroscopic leg holder is essential to stabilize the extremity and to allow for various positions of the knee during the procedure. Fiberoptic light cables and a light source are utilized. Warm irrigation with saline or Ringer's lactate is necessary to distend the joint for visualization and irrigation. This solution should never be allowed to run dry.

If the foot of the OR table is dropped, the circulating nurse wraps the nonoperative leg with elastic bandage and pads under the nonoperative thigh with foam.

Several portals of entry are necessary for passage of the telescope with camera attachment and sheath, and placement of the irrigation line and instruments. Arthroscopes are available with lenses at various angles, 30 and 70 degrees being the most common.

Arthroscopic instruments include biopsy punches of various types, scissors, pituitary rongeurs, grasping forceps, and various knives and probes.

The motorized intraarticular shaver with rotary cutting action trims torn meniscus, cartilage, and other soft tissue. It is essential that the field where this instrument is being used be well visualized.

FIGURE 18.77. Rongeurs are used for biting into bone. They are double- or single-action. Two single-action rongeurs are at the 4 and 6 o'clock positions; all the others are double-action. The biting cup also comes in various sizes and angles.

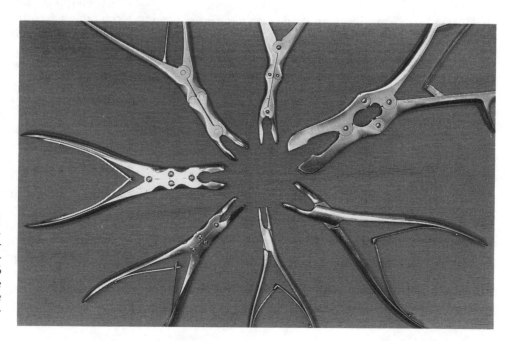

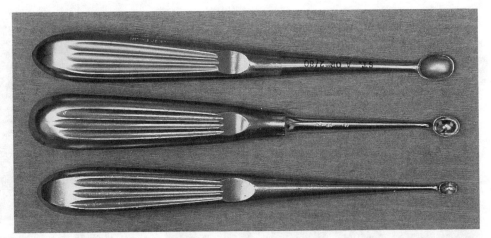

FIGURE 18.78. Curettes are used to scrape bone tissue; they have different size cups and are available in several angles and lengths.

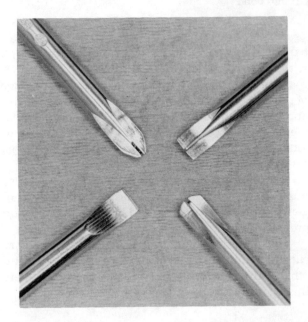

FIGURE 18.79. Screwdrivers are used to put the screws in place when fixing a fracture.

Neurosurgery

In neurosurgery, as in orthopedics, bony structures may need to be removed or penetrated to reach the main structures. To reach the brain, a flap of bone from the cranium has to be removed or burr holes made through it. To reach the spinal cord, vertebrae from the spinal column may be partially removed.

The standard operating table is used for neurosurgery, but numerous attachments are added, depending on the procedure. The microscope, laser, and video equipment may all be used. Nurses functioning in this area must have extensive knowledge of neuroanatomy and the use of highly specialized neurosurgical instruments. The beginning practitioner should be familiar with the basic equipment and instruments.

Basic to all types of neurosurgery is the cautery unit for the control of hemorrhage. Along with the regular cautery machine, the neurosurgeon uses a bipolar coagulation unit with forceps.

One of the most frequently performed neurosurgical procedures is the laminectomy, in which one or more of the vertebral laminae are removed. A laminectomy may be performed by either an orthopedist or a neurosurgeon, depending on the diagnosis, the patient's selection, and the surgeon's expertise. It is undertaken most frequently for a herniated disc and can be done at various levels of the spinal column, with lumbar laminectomy being the most common. The patient may be in the prone, sitting, or lateral position.

For a lumbar laminectomy, rubber rolls or a frame is used to maintain the patient's position yet allow for continued ventilation (Fig. 18.80). The type preferred by the surgeon should be listed on the doctor's preference card and be ready on the operating room table when the patient arrives.

The patient is anesthetized and intubated on the stretcher, and then turned and rolled over onto the operating room table and frame. Extra people are necessary to move the patient without injury to either patient or staff. Extra padding may be needed. The patient's arms and hands must be moved in a physiologically sound manner and placed on well-padded arm boards. For the male patient it is essential that the external genitalia are in no way compromised by the frame or table due to this position. Care must be taken to protect the breasts of female patients.

The instruments used for this procedure are a basic neurosurgical set plus special laminectomy instruments, which include curettes and rongeurs of various types, periosteal elevators, and nerve root retractors (Figs. 18.81 to 18.83).

For many neurological procedures on the cra-

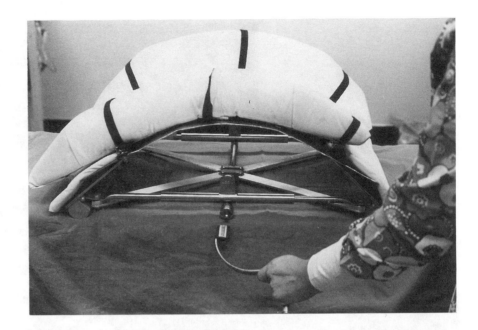

FIGURE 18.80. The Wilson convex frame is used for lumbar laminectomy, with the patient in a prone position. The frame can be raised or lowered using the handle shown.

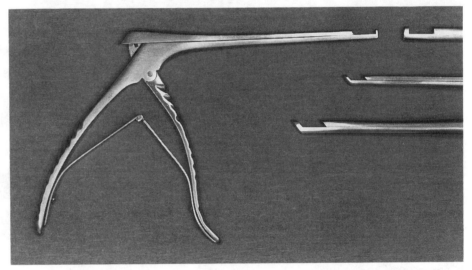

FIGURE 18.81. Kerrison rongeurs are specifically designed to facilitate the removal of lamina during a lumbar laminectomy. A variety of angled jaws are available.

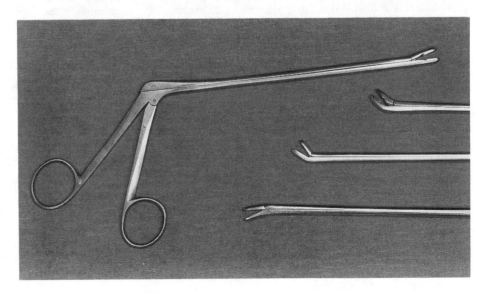

FIGURE 18.82. Pituitary rongeurs come in various cup sizes and angles. They can be used to remove herniated disc material during laminectomies, or to biopsy brain or tumor tissue. Depending on the cup size, they can be used for regular or microsurgery.

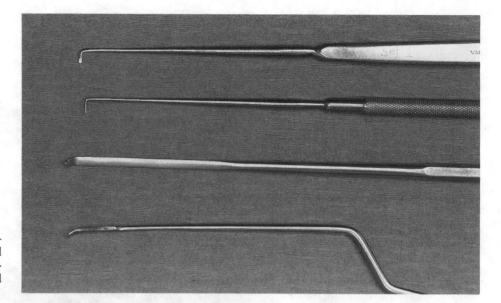

FIGURE 18.83. Nerve root retractors are specifically designed to gently move the nerves coming directly out of the spinal cord.

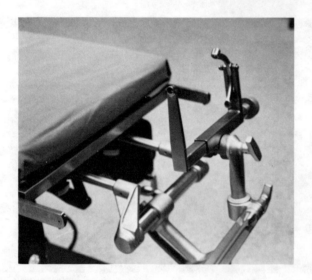

FIGURE 18.84. The Gardner head rest is a three-point skeletal traction device used in craniotomies to stabilize the patient's head.

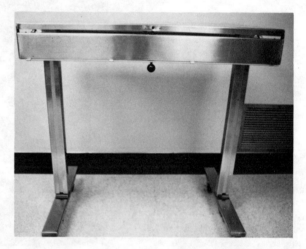

FIGURE 18.85. The Mayfield table is extra large to accommodate the numerous instruments necessary for intracranial procedures. The height of the table allows it to be placed over the patient, who is in a sitting position.

nium, a headrest is essential. Several types are available to be used in a variety of patient positions. To use the headrest, the head section of the standard surgery table must be removed; the prongs of the headrest fit into it (Fig. 18.84).

For operations on the head and neck, the standard Mayo stand is not large enough to hold the instruments needed. Special neurosurgical overhead tables have been developed, of which the Mayfield is one (Fig. 18.85). This is placed over the patient and draped to include it in the sterile field. In place, this table is much higher than the Mayo stand, and the scrub person must stand on a long, high lift to reach everything. Once this table has been draped, the scrub person moves the necessary instruments onto it.

Also basic to craniotomy is the air-powered equipment used to penetrate and remove parts of the cranium. The 3M craniotome illustrated in Figure 18.86 has numerous attachments, including the perforator that is used to penetrate the skull. The perforator can be replaced with a blade and dura guard to cut the bone flap. This is also interchangeable with a wire-pass drill bit, which is used when the bone flap is replaced at the closure and wired into place.

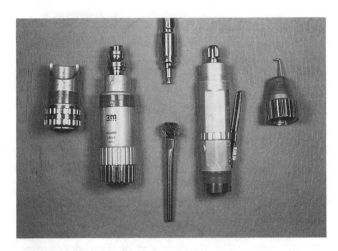

FIGURE 18.86. The 3M Craniotome can be used for burr holes when attached to the perforator. Remove the perforator, and to the remaining motor add the neurotome blade and dura guard, which can be used to carve out bone to facilitate exposure of the brain. (Photograph courtesy of 3M Surgical Products Division, St. Paul, MN 55144.)

These pieces of equipment are only a sample of the innumerable ones used in neurosurgery today. The nursing specialist learns to handle these instruments skillfully after many additional hours of study and practice.

Ophthalmic Surgery

The human eye is an extraordinary organ. It provides one of our most precious senses. A great deal of progress has been made in the last thirty years in eye surgery.

Think of its anatomy and remember how small and delicate the eye and all its parts are. The instruments used for surgery in this area match this anatomy and are small, fine, delicate—and expensive. Special care is needed in handling them (Fig. 18.87).

Before handling these instruments, the scrub person and surgeons should wash their gloved hands to remove any residual powder. Grains of powder could cause granulomas or other healing problems that are devastating to the eye.

At first glance, because they are so small and delicate, eye instruments appear different from basic surgical instruments. On closer examination, though, it can be seen that they are very similar. There are scalpels, clamps, forceps of various types, scissors, and needle holders.

Unlike other instruments, ophthalmic instruments should not be handled by the points or tips, but must still be handed to the surgeon in position for use. This is doubly important, as most procedures in ophthalmic surgery are performed through the operative microscope, and the surgeon generally does not look away from the scope to see what the scrub person is doing.

In using the small, fine instruments for eye surgery under the microscope, the surgeon must use equally fine, delicate motions on the minute anatomy. To aid the surgeon's concentration, the overhead lights are frequently turned out during some phase of these procedures. It is essential that the environment be quiet, including no phone calls or use of the intercommunication system. Talking and traffic must be kept to a minimum.

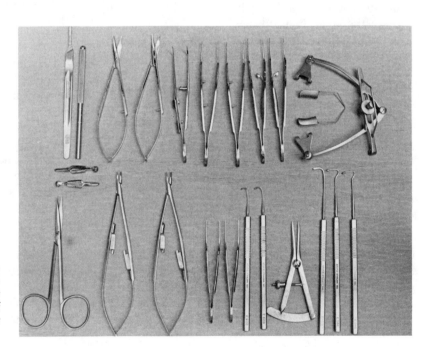

FIGURE 18.87. This basic set demonstrates the delicate design of ophthalmic instruments. They must be handled gently and carefully at all times. For comparison of size, the scissor in the lower left-hand corner is four inches long.

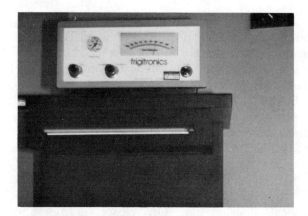

FIGURE 18.88. Frigitronic Cryoextractor is used in cataract extraction to remove the lens by freezing the tissue. Small probes are used to deliver the freezing nitrous oxide to the lens.

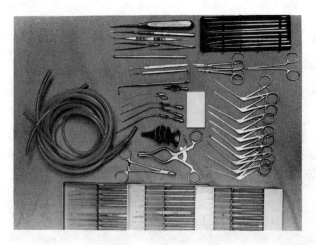

FIGURE 18.89. The development of these delicate instruments, coupled with the use of the operative microscope, allows the surgeon to perform numerous operations on the ear.

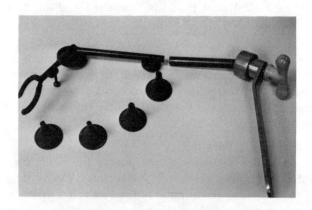

FIGURE 18.90. In performing ear surgery the surgeon works through an ear speculum. The Shea speculum holder secures the speculum in place and maintains its position, allowing the surgeon to use both hands to operate.

The operative microscope has made many new ophthalmic procedures possible and greatly facilitates the more common ones, including cataract extraction. Several techniques can be used for cataract: intracapsular extraction using the Cryoextractor, the extracapsular method, artificial lens implantation, or phacoemulsification using ultrasonic energy to fragment the inner lens material with aspiration.

Figure 18.88 shows the cryosurgical system. This is a nonelectrical system that uses nitrous oxide as a controlled, rapid-cooling agent, dropping to $-80\,°F$. The surgeon controls the flow of nitrous oxide with a foot pedal. Cryoprobes of various angles are used when the lens is ready to be delivered. The surgeon touches the lens with a cryoprobe, freezing it almost instantly. The solidified lens is then easily removed through the small incision.

Extracapsulary cataract extraction with placement of an intraocular lens in the posterior chamber is rapidly becoming the state of the art. The plastic lens is a permanent implant. Of all the artificial lenses used to correct vision, the implanted lens simulates natural vision most closely.

Ultrasonic measurements of the eye are taken preoperatively to determine the exact prescription of the lens needed. The lenses are available in various powers at one-half-diopter steps. The exact procedure for insertion depends on the type and style of lens used.

Otomicrosurgery
The anatomy and physiology of hearing are complex and principally contained within a small, bony anatomical area. The instruments and equipment used in this specialty reflect this anatomy and are even smaller than those for ophthalmic surgery (Fig. 18.89).

Part of the complexity in ear surgery is due to the tiny operative field, which is approached through an ear speculum (Fig. 18.90), and the use of the operative microscope for illumination and magnification.

Otomicrosurgery uses tiny, delicate instruments that tolerate very little abuse (Fig. 18.91). Great care must be taken to protect them. Several types of metal boxes are available in which these instruments should be stored and sterilized to protect them from damage. The same types of metal boxes are also useful in protecting delicate eye instruments (Fig. 18.92).

Great care must be taken with otomicrosurgery instruments so that they are not dropped, dumped together, or subjected to rough handling. Because of the fine picks, scalpels, and curettes, and the tiny cups on the alligator forceps, very little force is needed to fracture them.

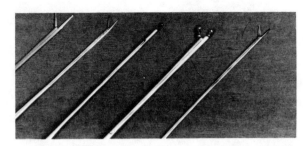

FIGURE 18.91. The tips of some of the ear instruments are very small and difficult for the scrub person to see. Notice the cups and scissors.

It is essential that the scrub person have good eyesight, as it is difficult to distinguish differences in the minute tips of the ear instruments. Some of the instruments may be engraved on the handle with distinctive marks to assist the scrub person. Special instrument-wipe material is available to clean them during surgery. A toothbrush is also helpful.

As in eye surgery, the atmosphere in the suite is an essential element. Close teamwork is required. All must be in readiness when the patient and surgeon arrive, to prevent unnecessary activity or noise. To avoid disturbing the surgeon in the middle of a delicate move, telephone and other intercom systems should be turned off. Each movement in this type of surgery must be precise, and unnecessary noise can cause an unwanted motion.

Also as with eye surgery, the gloves of the scrub person and surgeons must be washed prior to handling the sterilized instruments. Powder can act as a foreign body in the wound. If unwashed and washed gloves are compared under a microscope the amount of powder and lint that cling to the unwashed gloves can be seen. Both items can be transferred to the instrument and into the wound, causing problems for the patient.

The scrub person must hand the instruments in the method preferred by the surgeon. This can be difficult as the operative site is not readily visible. An observation arm on the microscope is helpful for both the circulating nurse and scrub person.

After the surgeon has received an instrument, the scrub person may guide the surgeon's hands back into the line of vision under the microscope. If the surgeon's eyes leave the scope, refocusing will be required.

Because the inner ear structures are surrounded by bone, it is often necessary to use drills of various sizes and shapes. The earliest drills used in the area were modifications of dental drills. Today microdrills designed for use on ear surgery are used for bone sculpting (Fig. 18.93). The tiny drill points are of various types and sizes, including diamond burrs, cross-cutting burrs, and polishing burrs.

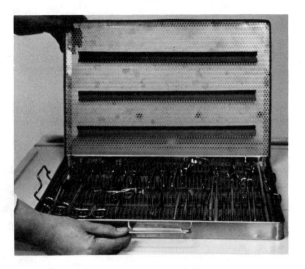

FIGURE 18.92. Microsurgical instrument trays are designed to safely position and secure the instrument. They are usually lined with posts constructed of polyfoam or Teflon to prevent direct contact between the instruments.

Pacemakers

Pacemakers were first implanted in the early 1950s. They are necessary when the heart can no longer sustain sufficient beats, as in heart block or arrhythmias with failure of the heart's conductive system. They can initiate atrial or ventricular contractions or both.

Today, three basic types of pacemakers are used for artificial ventricular stimulation: fixed-rate, demand-rate, and physiologic. The fixed-rate pacemaker is just that. It is set at a certain rate (e.g., 70 beats per minute) and stimulates every heartbeat. Demand-rate pacemakers fire off only when necessary, based on the heart's own ability to beat or not to beat. A major disadvantage of demand-rate pacing is competition between the natural heartbeat and that of the pacer, which could result in ventricular fibrillation. Physiologic pacemakers maintain atrioventricular synchrony, taking advantage of atrial systoli and enhancing cardiac output.

Initially, pacemakers must be inserted under fluoroscopy for correct placement of the electrode in the heart muscle (Fig. 18.94). Placement is crucial, as a common problem is displacement of the electrode. There are two types of electrodes: myocardial, which is attached under direct vision to the heart muscle, and endocardial, which is inserted transvenously under fluoroscopy.

Time must be taken during insertion for proper testing with a pacing systems analyzer (PSA). The PSA is a computer that assists in finding the best position for the electrode in the heart muscle. Is the myocardium at the point of contact appropriate? Is it sufficiently sensitive to the stimulation? Testing also

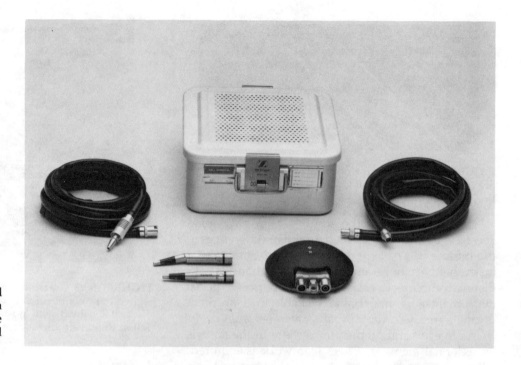

FIGURE 18.93. The Hall Osteon Drill System drives a variety of burrs for bone sculpting and was designed for use in ear surgery.

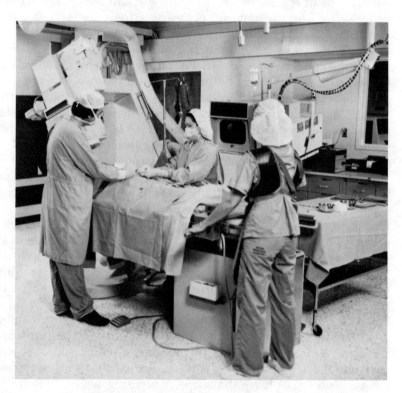

FIGURE 18.94. The Fluoricon intensifier imaging system used during pacemaker insertion for proper placement of cardiac leads. (Photograph courtesy of General Electric Medical Systems Division, Milwaukee, WI 53201.)

assists in determining the specific type of generator appropriate for the patient. The circulating nurse may be asked to use the PSA. In this case, complete knowledge of and familiarity with the device is necessary before attempting its use. Pacemaker companies offer detailed demonstrations of their equipment. When the patient is scheduled for a battery change only, fluoroscopy is not necessary, as the electrode is already in place, although placement may again be tested.

Today's pacemakers are multiply programmable (Fig. 18.95). Functions can be tailored to each patient's specific needs, and the established program can be changed as the patient's condition changes.

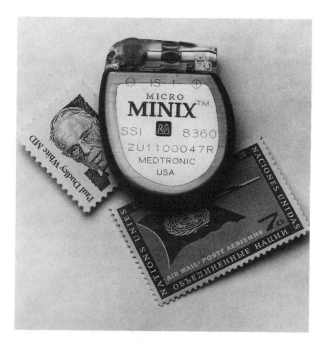

FIGURE 18.95. The Medtronic Micro Minix implantable cardiac pacemaker is the smallest in the world. Only 1⁹/₁₆ inches high and 1¹/₄ inches wide, the pulse generator weighs 0.6 of an ounce. It is designed for full programmability via telemetry and for pacing either the atrium or ventricle of the heart. (Photograph courtesy of Medtronic, Inc., Minneapolis, MN 55432.)

This decreases the need for additional operative procedures to change the pacemaker. The new lithium-powered units last five to ten years, decreasing the number of procedures necessary to sustain the patient.

More recent developments have made it possible to insert a second lead into the ventricle for additional pacing controls. This may be performed in either the operating room or a special room in the radiology department. Most of the time these procedures are done under local anesthesia. The emergency cart with defibrillator and drugs must be readily available. The ECG should be in place, an IV solution running, and oxygen available.

All pacemakers eventually fail due to battery depletion, and the patient must return to surgery for periodic replacement.

Another recent development in this area is the automatic implantable cardioverter defibrillator (ACID). This device is able to sense, charge, and defibrillate malignant ventricular arrhythmias and tachycardia. It has been shown that direct defibrillation needs much less electrical energy than was previously believed. The ACID system consists of a pulse generator and two leads. The leads are sewn directly onto the heart, thus requiring a thoracotomy. The main generator is the size of a cigarette

package and has a lithium battery that lasts up to three years. Patients treated with this device have usually experienced at least one cardiac arrest or been on medication for dysrhythmias. Further developments in this area are on the horizon.

CONCLUSIONS

In addition to the instruments and equipment covered in this chapter, the perioperative nurse will encounter many others. This is an immense area of knowledge, to which this chapter presents only an introduction.

Perioperative nursing has been tremendously affected by the technology explosion of the past several decades. Continued investigation throughout one's experience in the operating room is necessary, whether that experience is for one month or twenty years. Innovative procedures are constantly being developed, and there are always improvements and advancements in the instruments and equipment used in the operating room.

SUGGESTED READINGS

Aielo, D. H. "Arthroscopy of the knee: A perioperative nursing challenge." *AORN J* 43:824, 1986.

American Heart Association. *Textbook of Advanced Cardiac Life Support* 2nd ed. Dallas: AHA, 1987.

Atkinson, L. J., and Kohn, M. L. *Berry and Kohn's Introduction to Operating Room Technique* 6th ed. New York: McGraw-Hill, 1986.

Baxter Healthcare Corporation, V. Mueller Division. *Atlas of Surgical Instrument Care.* McGaw Park, IL: Baxter Healthcare Corporation, 1990.

Bland, D. S. "Pulse oximetry: Monitoring arterial hemoglobin oxygen saturation." *AORN J* 45:964, 1987.

Borgini, L., and Almgren, C. C. "Peripheral vascular angioscopy: Performance, equipment, technique." *AORN J* 52:543, 1990.

Bunn, J. C., and Becker, D. W. "Reduction mammoplasty: The laser deepithelialization technique." *AORN J* 48:50, 1988.

Culbertson, J. H., Rand, R. P., and Jurkiewicz, M. J. "Advances in microsurgery." *Adv in Surgery* 23:57, 1990.

Groah, L. K. *Operating Room Nursing: Perioperative Practice* 2nd ed. San Mateo, CA: Appleton and Lange, 1990.

Huth-Meeker, M., and Rothrock, J. C. *Alexander's Care of the Patient in Surgery* 9th ed. St. Louis, MO: C. V. Mosby, 1991.

Jackson, D. C., Martin, T., Evans, M. M., and Rubio, P. A. "Endoscopic laser cholecystectomy." *AORN J* 51:1546, 1990.

Krug, P. J., and Speelman, J. A. "Tonsillectomy and adenoidectomy laser procedure." *AORN J* 50:990, 1989.

LeBlanc, K. A., and LeBlanc, Z. Z. "Gastrointestinal end-to-end anastomosis." *AORN J* 51:986, 1990.

Lee, B. L., and Mirabal, G. "Automatic implantable cardioverter defibrillation." *AORN J* 50:1218, 1989.

Lehr, P. S. "Surgical lasers: How they work, current application." *AORN J* 50:972, 1989.

Lin, T. Y., Siemens, M. A., and Lam, K. W. "The effects of YAG laser anterior capsulotomy on aqueous humor." *Ann Ophthalmology* 20(3):95–99, 1988.

McConnell, E. A. *Clinical Considerations in Perioperative Nursing: Preventive Aspects of Care.* Philadelphia: J. B. Lippincott, 1987.

Moak, E. "Electrosurgical unit safety: The role of the perioperative nurse." *AORN J* 53:744, 1991.

Moses, H. W., Taylor, G. J., Schneider, J. A., and Dove, J. T. *A Practical Guide to Cardiac Pacing* 2nd ed. Boston: Little, Brown, 1987.

Pfister, J. "A guide to lasers in the operating room." *Surgical Technology: Principles and Practice* 2nd ed. Philadelphia: W. B. Saunders, 1986.

Phillips, W. J., Long, B. C., Woods, N. F., and Cassmeyer, V. L. *Medical Surgical Nursing: Concepts and Clinical Practice* 4th ed. St. Louis, MO: Mosby Year Book, 1991.

Rippe, J. M., Irwin, R. S., Alpert, J. S., and Fink, M. P. *Intensive Care Medicine* 2nd ed. Boston: Little, Brown, 1991.

Rothrock, J. C. *The RN First Assistant and An Expanded Perioperative Nursing Role.* Philadelphia: J. B. Lippincott, 1987.

Saver, C. L., and Hurray, J. M. "Electrocardiogram monitoring: Interpreting normal cardiac rhythm." *AORN J* 52:264, 1990.

Swazuk, J. J., Mueller, B. J., and Daly, C. J., "Laser cholecystectomy: A perioperative nursing view." *AORN J* 50:998, 1989.

U.S. Surgical Corp. *Stapling Techniques: General Surgery with Autosuture Instruments* 3rd ed. Norwalk, CT: USSC, 1988.

Zichefoose, S. "Nasal surgery using laser with endoscopy surgery." *AORN J* 50:979, 1989.

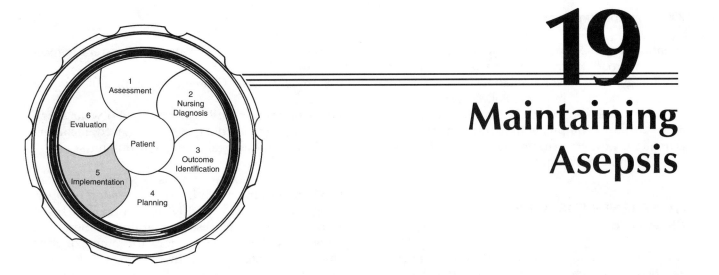

19

Maintaining Asepsis

The nurse assures an aseptic environment for the patient.

As a patient advocate, one of the most important functions of the perioperative nurse is establishing and maintaining asepsis during the intraoperative phase of surgical intervention. It is important to recognize that the intraoperative phase may occur in traditional or nontraditional operating room settings. The increasing number of nontraditional settings are a result of recent increases in the number and locations of noninvasive surgical interventions.

SURGICAL CONSCIENCE

Regardless of location, it is imperative for perioperative nurses to develop a surgical conscience that permits no compromises in the principles of asepsis and sterile technique. Anything less than strict attention to these principles increases the potential for postoperative infection.

A surgical conscience means attention to aseptic principles during the perioperative period. It involves constant inspection, monitoring, and regulation of the patient, environment, personnel, and equipment. The nurse anticipates the needs of the patient, and the surgical team and gives unselfish, vigilant care to the patient.

A surgical conscience can be considered fully developed when the perioperative nurse's attention to sterile technique and aseptic practices becomes automatic. In addition, the perioperative nurse will have developed an awareness of what is occurring at all times during the perioperative period, even when attention is directed to other priorities.

Developing a surgical conscience requires:

1. Knowledge of principles of asepsis
2. Self-discipline in inspecting and regulating one's own hygiene, dress, and nursing practice, with attention to breaks in technique
3. Ability to anticipate the need for supplies and services based on knowledge of the patient, the procedure being performed, the preferences of the surgical team, and where and how to obtain the supplies
4. Good communication skills to determine the needs of patient and team members and to identify and correct breaks in technique
5. Maturity to overcome personal preference and prejudice to provide optimal patient care, regardless of the operative procedure, the patient's circumstances, or other perioperative personnel

Each member of the operative team assumes not only individual responsibility but responsibility for the surgical conscience of the group. Monitoring others' activities and calling attention to their errors should be seen as positive steps in providing the best patient care. Correcting others or being corrected is often stressful for inexperienced perioperative personnel and requires the development of communication and assertiveness skills as well as maturity (1).

The scope of a surgical conscience includes continuing evaluation of the patient, environment, personnel, and equipment. Continuous, simultaneous attention to these four areas may be difficult. It requires a broad knowledge base in anatomy and physiology, interpersonal relationships, and environmental safety. It relies on skilled observation using each of the senses. Although the perioperative nurse also uses equipment to monitor the patient, it is frequently experience and the senses that first signal a potential problem.

GUIDELINES FOR ASEPTIC PRACTICE

Knowledge of and adherence to the guidelines of aseptic practice are essential to the safe practice of nursing in the perioperative setting. Aseptic practices are carried out during every phase of the perioperative period: preoperatively in establishing the aseptic environment and sterile field; intraoperatively in maintaining the sterile field, and confining and containing contamination; and postoperatively in terminal cleaning of the room and sterilizing supplies.

Why have we established guidelines for aseptic practices? Consider the many sources of wound contamination: shedding of resident and transient flora from the skin and hair of patients and perioperative personnel; droplets expelled from the respiratory tracts of patients and perioperative personnel; inadvertent and unknowing use of unsterile equipment or supplies; airborne bacteria or particles; and endogenous bacteria from the patient's gastrointestinal tract or blood. Consider the cost to the patient of wound infection. Time and money are lost due to the increased length of hospital stay. Skin integrity is lost, and there are possible threats to body image and even possible loss of life. Infection is costly to hospitals due to the need for increased staff and extended hospital stays. Because of the many sources of wound infection and the costs of treating it, each member of the operative team must be aware of and practice good aseptic technique.

In order to understand aseptic practices, a few terms must be defined:

Asepsis: The condition of being free from disease-causing microorganisms.
Aseptic technique: The methods used to maintain asepsis.
Scrubbed personnel: Personnel who are scrubbed, gowned, and gloved, including the surgeon, the scrub nurse or technician, and assisting physicians.
Sterile: Free from microorganisms.
Sterile field: The area immediately around the pa-

tient that has been prepared for a sterile procedure.
Surgically clean: Cleaned mechanically but not sterile.
Unscrubbed personnel: Personnel who wear surgical attire but are not gowned or gloved, including the anesthesiologist and circulating nurse.

The overall goal in asepsis is to minimize contamination of the wound. The Association of Operating Room Nurses (AORN) has developed seven recommended practices for aseptic technique (2). They are well-accepted methods for minimizing the chances of contamination. In adhering to each practice, nurses should realize the purpose behind it. They should also realize that a break in aseptic technique will not automatically cause microbial contamination but will increase the probability of its occurring.

AORN's guidelines cover: (1) wearing sterile gowns and gloves; (2) use of sterile drapes; (3) sterility of items introduced into the sterile field; (4) maintenance of sterility and integrity of items within the sterile field; (5) monitoring and maintaining the sterile field; (6) traffic patterns in the sterile field; and (7) policies and procedures for basic aseptic technique.

Taking into account guidelines issued by AORN and other government and voluntary agencies, each institution establishes and documents its own policies and procedures for aseptic practices. In the ever-changing perioperative environment, provision must be made for periodic review and refinement of these policies. In any institution, however, the basic objective of policies and procedures related to aseptic technique remains the same—protection of patients and perioperative personnel.

SURGICAL ATTIRE

Surgical attire minimizes cross-contamination between the patient and surgical personnel. Head and body coverings decrease shedding from the skin and hair of surgical personnel and protect them from contact with bloodborne pathogens that may be present in the patient.

When personnel move from unrestricted to semirestricted or restricted areas, they must wear appropriate clothing, as follows:

- The unrestricted area around the central desk and lounges provides limited access for communication among hospital personnel and families. Street clothes are permitted in the unrestricted area.

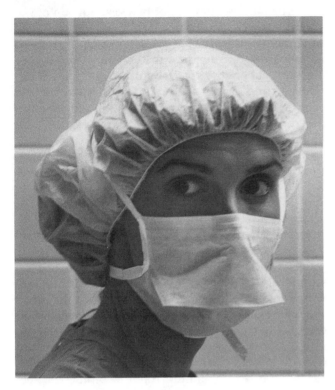

FIGURE 19.1.   The surgical cap should cover all hair and be of a style to keep the hair contained.

- In the semirestricted area, which includes the operating rooms, peripheral support areas, and hallways, appropriate attire, hair covers (caps or hoods), and shoe covers are required.
- Restricted areas are areas where sterile procedures are performed. Masks are required in restricted areas. All personnel who enter the surgical suite must be appropriately attired according to institutional guidelines.

Surgical attire should be laundered between wearings in institutional settings rather than at home.

Donning surgical attire proceeds from head to toe. The surgical cap or hood is put on first. This eliminates possible contamination of scrub clothes by falling hair. All hair should be covered and contained within the head covering (Fig. 19.1). Materials used for caps and hoods should be lint-free. Head coverings should be comfortable and allow for ventilation. Most are disposable, but nondisposable caps should be laundered in a facility used for laundering other hospital textiles. Personnel with facial hair should use hoods to cover all hair. Head and facial hair should be covered at all times in the restricted and semirestricted areas.

Scrub suits are put on after covering the hair. They should be made of materials that meet or exceed the National Fire Protection Association stan-

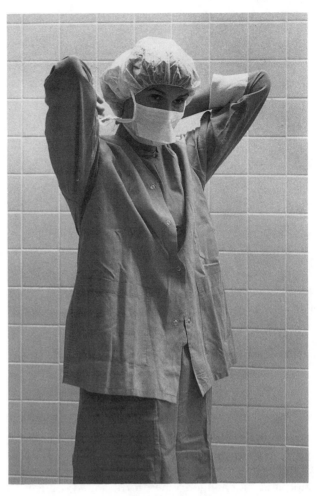

FIGURE 19.2.   Unscrubbed personnel should wear a warmup jacket with stockinette cuffs on the sleeves and fasteners that keep the jacket close to the wearer's body.

dards. Scrub suits are considered more effective barriers to contamination than scrub dresses. Scrub shirts should be secured at the waist or tucked into scrub pants to reduce shedding. Loose shirttails and baggy scrub clothing should be avoided. Scrub pants and one-piece suits should have ankle closures. The attire chosen depends on the policies of the institution.

Garments should fit the body closely and be comfortable and easy to put on. Scrub clothes should be laundered daily and remain clean and dry. They should be changed when soiled.

When wearing surgical apparel with short sleeves, unscrubbed personnel should wear warm-up jackets with stockinette cuffs or unsterile long-sleeved gowns to avoid possible contamination by shedding from the arms. Warm-up jackets should remain snapped to prevent flapping of the jacket tails (Fig. 19.2).

Shoe covers are put on after the scrub suit. Dis-

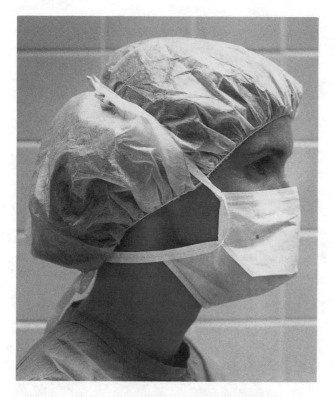

FIGURE 19.3. Masks must cover both the nose and the mouth. The sides should conform close to the face to minimize venting.

posable shoe covers should completely cover the shoe and be changed when torn, soiled, or wet to avoid possible cross-contamination. In the interest of safety, clogs, sandals, and tennis shoes should not be worn in the operating room. Shoes should provide some protection from foot injury.

When personnel enter the restricted area of the surgical suite, masks remain in place to avoid contamination by respiratory droplets. Disposable masks of high-filtration efficiency should be used. Cloth and gauze masks are unacceptable because of their ineffective filtration and rapid wetting from expired moisture.

Masks should cover both the nose and mouth, and venting at the sides should be minimized by proper positioning. Strings should be tied snugly and should not be crossed because this prevents the mask from conforming to the face (Fig. 19.3).

Once a mask is taken off it should be discarded. Masks are changed between procedures. Some disposable masks may be efficient for eight or more hours. When removing a mask, personnel should take care to avoid touching the mask itself. It should be removed by untying the strings or touching only the elastic band and disposed of properly. Hands must be washed after removing the mask.

Scrub clothes should not be worn outside of the surgical environment. If it is necessary to leave the suite, personnel can wear laboratory coats, but these are not an effective barrier to contamination. If they are worn, laboratory coats should be buttoned, long-sleeved, and of an adequate length to cover the scrub suit to the knees. Ideally, they should be laundered after each use. Wraparound cover gowns that tie in the back are also acceptable.

Attire worn outside the suite should be changed upon returning. Since masks, caps, and shoe covers will have already been removed before leaving the suite, all the proper attire must be redonned in the correct sequence. Scrub clothes should also be changed whenever they become wet or soiled.

Questions are often asked about jewelry, such as earrings and watches, and other accessories. Jewelry should not be worn in the operating room. If it is worn, it should be totally confined within scrub clothes or caps and hoods; for example, small stud earrings completely covered by the cap. Necklaces, rings, and watches are sources of contamination and difficult to keep clean. Wearing nail polish and artificial nails in the operating room is prohibited, because bacteria breed in and around chipped polish, and polish inhibits inspection for dirt under and around nails. Artificial nails, including bondings, tips, tapes, and wraps, contribute to increased gram-negative microorganisms and can contribute to increased infections.

Each institution chooses its own OR apparel and standards according to cost constraints and other factors. Within these constraints, each OR suite maintains the highest standards possible.

In order to reduce the risk of exposure to blood-borne pathogens such as the human immunodeficiency virus (HIV) and hepatitis B virus, additional rules have been promulgated by the Occupational Safety and Health Administration (OSHA). For example, OSHA requires that protective barriers, including gloves, eyewear, and fluid-resistant apparel, be available to all employees who may anticipate contact with blood and body fluids.

When handling potentially infective materials, all perioperative personnel should wear gloves. Gloves are required to be sterile only when the practitioner is involved in a sterile procedure. Unsterile gloves are more accessible and cost-effective for most activities carried out by unscrubbed personnel. Gloves should be changed, not washed, between uses to avoid leakage of contaminated fluids through undetected holes.

Protective eyewear and face shields must be worn by all scrubbed personnel, and by unscrubbed personnel when indicated. Eyewear and face shields should provide adequate protection to mucous membranes. Eyewear and shields should be changed or washed when soiled.

PERSONAL HEALTH, HYGIENE, AND GROOMING

Operating room personnel must be aware of possible contaminants they bring into the environment. Good hygiene practices, including daily bathing and frequent hair washing, will help minimize the number of pathogens brought into the operating room. The skin should be clean. Makeup should be used judiciously. Persons with draining wounds or other infections should not work in the operating room. Those with hand wounds or dermatitis should not scrub because of the high number of bacteria on the hands.

Upper respiratory and other infections should be carefully monitored. Personnel with untreated rhinorrhea or productive coughs should be restricted from scrubbing. If they do circulate, they should change masks frequently during the procedure. Personnel with infections should be cleared by a physician before they return to work. Each institution should have an established policy regarding employee health and instances when work in the surgical suite is prohibited. Policies should also address when personnel with infections are permitted within the suite and the guidelines for any precautions.

SURGICALLY CLEAN SKIN

Skin preparation of the patient and surgical personnel is of equal importance. Surgically clean skin serves to prevent infection. Skin preparation of the patient includes removing hair and scrubbing the incisional area. Skin preparation of surgical personnel includes good handwashing techniques and surgical hand scrubs. The objectives of skin preparation include removing skin oil, dirt, and microbial deposits; decreasing the microbial count as much as possible; and leaving a film of antimicrobial residue on the skin.

The dermis, or lower layer of the skin, contains sebaceous glands, connective tissue, hair follicles, and blood and lymph vessels. The epidermis, or outer layer of the skin, acts as a protective barrier and constantly sheds cells. Resident flora in the dermis are shed with the movement of old cells and skin secretions from the dermal layer to the epidermal layer. Shedding of resident flora is a source of

wound contamination. Transient flora that reside on the epidermis are usually only loosely attached to the skin surface and can be removed by cleansing the skin with soap or detergent.

Providing for surgically clean skin includes mechanical and chemical actions. Mechanical actions use friction to remove soil and the transient flora of the epidermis. Chemical actions reduce the flora. Types of chemical antimicrobial agents used for hand scrubs and preoperative skin preps include povidone–iodine solutions, chlorhexidines, and hexachlorophenes.

- Povidone–iodine solutions, or iodophors, are effective against gram-negative and gram-positive organisms. Iodophors are not as irritating as tincture of iodine solutions but have a persistent effect if not rinsed off.
- The chlorhexidine group is effective against gram-positive and gram-negative organisms and has a persistent effect.
- Hexachlorophenes are most active against gram-positive organisms and least active against fungi and gram-negative organisms. Hexachlorophene has a long-lasting, cumulative, bacteriostatic effect, but it is soluble in alcohol, and washing with alcohol reduces its persistent action. Hexachlorophene can be toxic when absorbed through the skin. It is not recommended for surgical site preparation and should not be used for routine bathing of infants or by pregnant women.
- Alcohol in a 70 to 90% solution is used as an antiseptic but should not be applied to mucous membranes because it is inactivated by coagulating protein.
- Iodine compounds may be irritating for handwashing but are excellent for surgical skin preparation.

Those responsible for choosing among commercially marketed antimicrobial surgical hand scrubs can obtain information on these products from the Food and Drug Administration.

SURGICAL HAND SCRUB

The scrub itself differs among institutions, but within an institution, the procedure should be standardized for all personnel. It should be a written policy, available to everyone who scrubs within the perioperative area, and a part of the procedure manual.

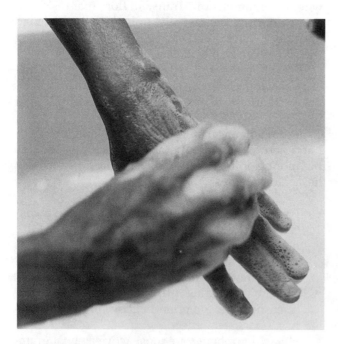

FIGURE 19.4. During the surgical scrub, each aspect of the fingers, palm, back of the hand, and wrist are subject to light friction with a sudsed antimicrobial agent.

All scrub personnel must meet certain criteria before beginning the surgical scrub. Nails must be short, clean, and free of polish or artificial nails. Cuticles should be in good condition. Hands and arms should be free of cuts and any other skin problems. The head covering should be in place, covering and containing all hair. The surgical mask should be properly positioned, tied securely, and venting minimized. Surgical attire should be worn, with ties and shirttails properly controlled. Rings, watches, and bracelets should be removed.

The institution's infection control committee should approve the antimicrobial agent selected for surgical hand scrubs. The antimicrobial agent selected should (1) be capable of significantly reducing the number of microorganisms on intact skin; (2) be nonirritating; (3) be broad-spectrum; (4) be fast-acting; (5) contain an effective detergent; and (6) have a residual effect.

Staff and patients are sometimes sensitive to antimicrobial agents. In those instances, a liquid nonmedicated soap can be used for the scrub, followed by application of an alcohol-based cleanser. The cleanser should be applied for 5 minutes; multiple applications should be rubbed dry after each application.

Scrub agents should be stored in clean, closed containers. Disposable containers should not be refilled but be discarded when empty. Reusable containers should be thoroughly cleaned and dried between refills.

There are two types of surgical hand scrubs, the timed scrub and the stroke-count scrub. Initial procedures for both techniques are the same and proceed from hands to arms. Hands and arms are wetted and washed with the antimicrobial agent to remove transient flora and gross contamination. Nails are cleaned under running water, using disposable or metal nail cleaners. Wooden sticks are not used for this purpose. After rinsing, the selected scrub procedure is carried out, using either a terminally sterilized, nondisposable brush or a disposable sponge brush.

The timed scrub usually takes at least five to ten minutes to complete. Each anatomical area is scrubbed for a specified length of time, with special attention to the fingers and hands. Each aspect of the fingers, between the digits, palms, and backs of the hands, must be subjected to light friction with sudsed antimicrobial agent (Fig. 19.4). Once hands are scrubbed, the procedure is extended to arms, scrubbing with a circular motion to two inches above the elbow. Hands should be held higher than the elbows to allow water to run from the cleanest area down the arm (Fig. 19.5). Care should be taken during scrubbing to prevent water from splashing onto the scrub clothes. At the completion of the timed scrub, the hands and arms are rinsed. The water is turned off using a foot pedal or knee or elbow handle, being careful not to contaminate the hands. The brush is properly disposed of. With hands still held higher than arms, the scrubbed person proceeds into the operating room.

The stroke-count scrub also takes five to ten minutes to complete. It differs from the timed scrub in that all aspects are scrubbed using a specific number of strokes rather than a specified length of time. There are a number of formulas for stroke-count scrubbing. A documented procedure should be specified for each institution. Rinsing, disposing of brushes, and entering the operating room are the same as for the timed scrub procedure.

Rescrubbing procedures are the same as the initial method. Rescrubbing should last five to ten minutes, because bacteria can multiply rapidly in the warm, moist environment of a gloved hand.

A sterile towel is used for drying the hands. Towels should be removed from the sterile field carefully to avoid dripping water onto the field. Grasping the towel with one hand, the person lifts it from the sterile field and allows it to unfold to its full length. Ideally, the towel, gown, and gloves should be on a separate table from other supplies. Scrub personnel should lean slightly forward so the towel hangs away from the body and does not contact the body or the scrub personnel's clothing. Hands must be

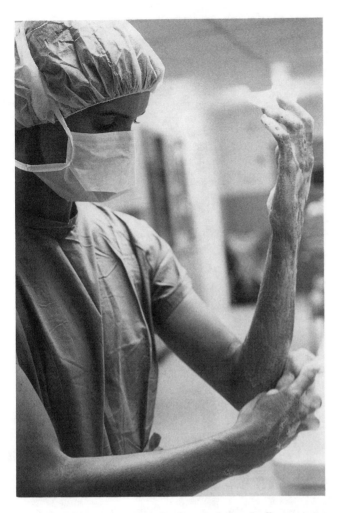

FIGURE 19.5.   Keeping the hand elevated allows water to run off, the scrub proceeds in a circular motion to two inches above the elbow.

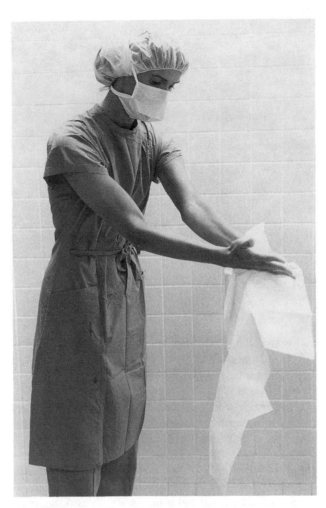

FIGURE 19.6.   Drying hands after the scrub. The towel is carefully removed from the sterile field to avoid dripping, the arms are fully extended to prevent touching attire with the towel as drying the first hand begins. The towel is reversed after the first hand and arm are completely dried. Arms are dried with a rotating motion, and care is taken not to retrace an area.

dried thoroughly, using one hand with the towel to dry the opposite hand. Dry hands make gloving easier and prevent moisture strike-through to the gown sleeve. The towel is then advanced up the arm, drying each subsequent area with a rotating motion and taking care not to retrace an area. The towel is reversed, bringing the dry end up to the still wet hand and arm, and the opposite hand and arm are completely dried in a similar manner. The towel is then discarded without manipulation (Fig. 19.6).

STERILE GOWNS AND GLOVES

Gloves and gowns worn by scrubbed surgical personnel are barriers to the transfer of microorganisms from personnel to patient and vice versa. The materials used for gowns and drapes should have similar characteristics, whether reusable or disposable. Most important, the material must be an effec-

tive barrier to the transfer of microorganisms. It should prevent liquid penetration and must be resistant to abrasion, tears, and punctures, and free of toxic ingredients and nonfast dyes. Materials should be nonglare and of a color that minimizes distortion from reflected lights. Reusable materials must be able to withstand multiple launderings and sterilizations. Disposable materials should not be resterilized unless written instructions for reprocessing are provided by the manufacturer. The material should also meet the safety guidelines of the National Fire Protection Association and be lint-free and porous, allowing steam penetration and eliminating excessive heat buildup. Finally, the material should be memory-free and highly drapable.

Surgical gowns should be comfortable to wear, allowing ease of movement without being bulky or

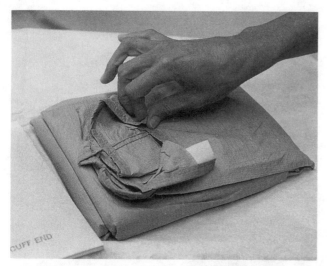

FIGURE 19.7. The gown is grasped firmly at the neckline.

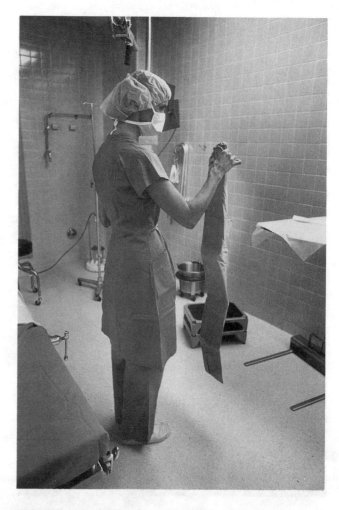

FIGURE 19.8. The gown is allowed to unfold completely, without touching unsterile objects.

awkward. They should be wraparound, with impervious material in front from waist to shoulders and sleeves below the elbow. The stockinette cuffs should fit snugly.

Surgical gloves are usually disposable. They are made of latex or neoprene rubber. Processing reusable gloves is difficult and time consuming and may not be cost-effective. Gloves should meet the surgical glove standards of the Food and Drug Administration.

Scrubbed personnel who establish and organize the sterile field are responsible for gowning and gloving themselves with assistance from circulating personnel. Gowns and gloves for these initial scrubbed personnel are individually packaged.

Gowning

All gowns are packaged and folded inside-out. This allows scrubbed personnel to grasp the gown and put it on without contaminating the sterile front. The gown should be grasped firmly at the neckline (Fig. 19.7) and allowed to unfold completely (Fig. 19.8). Keeping the hands on the inside of the gown, the scrubbed person identifies the armholes and inserts both arms simultaneously (Fig. 19.9). Haphazard donning of the gown may flip ties from sterile to unsterile areas. Next the circulator assists by pulling the gown up over the shoulders of the scrubbed person and securing it at the neck and waist (Fig. 19.10). Unscrubbed personnel should touch only the unsterile inside of the gown.

If scrub personnel are using the closed-glove technique, they should not extend their hands through the cuff of the gown but wait until gloves

have been put on. With the closed-glove technique, it may be necessary to don gloves before tying the back of the gown to allow enough arm length to manipulate the gloves.

Once donned, gowns are considered sterile on the front from chest to the level of the sterile field and on the sleeves from the cuff to two inches above the elbow. Wraparound gowns are not considered sterile in the back because it is not possible to keep a constant eye on that area. The cuffs of the gown, the neckline, the shoulders, and the underarm areas are also considered unsterile. Stockinette cuffs must be completely covered by sterile gloves. To avoid the possibility of contamination, gowns and gloves should be donned in a sterile auxiliary field and not at the main instrument table.

Gloving

Closed and open gloving have been shown to be equally effective (3). The closed-glove technique be-

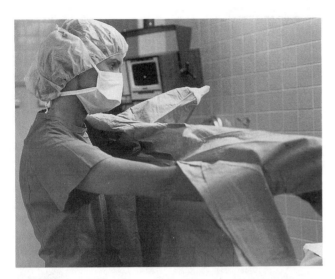

FIGURE 19.9. Keeping the hands on the inside of the gown, the person identifies the armholes and inserts both arms simultaneously.

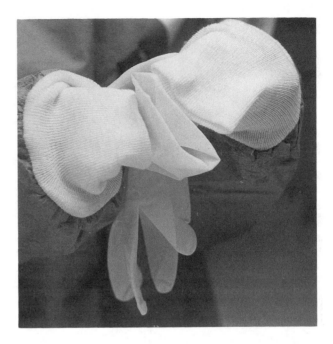

FIGURE 19.11. Closed-glove technique begins with the hands remaining in the gown sleeves. The glove is grasped through the stockinette.

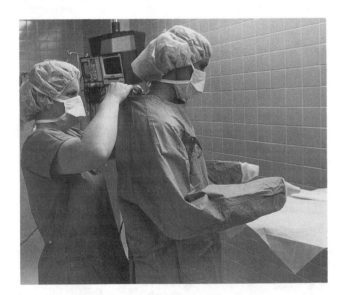

FIGURE 19.10. The circulator assists by pulling the gown over the shoulders and securing it at the neck and waist, taking care not to touch any other outer areas.

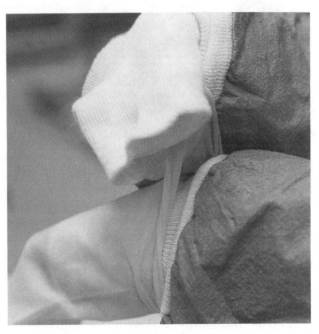

FIGURE 19.12. The cuff of the glove is stretched up and over the cuff of the sleeve.

gins with the hands remaining in the gown sleeves. The enclosed hand grasps the folded cuff of the glove. The glove is placed on the upturned, gown-enclosed hand, with glove fingers extending toward the body and the glove thumb on the appropriate side. The inferior glove cuff should be grasped by the enclosed thumb. Using the opposing gown-enclosed hand, the glove is stretched up and over the stockinette cuff of the sleeve. The hand is then advanced through the cuff into the glove, being careful to keep the entire stockinette cuff enclosed in the glove. The other hand is gloved in a similar manner. Using the already gloved hand, the remaining glove is placed with fingers extended toward the body,

thumb over thumb, on top of the up-turned gown-enclosed hand (Figs. 19.11 to 19.13).

When using the open-glove technique, the hands are extended through the cuffs of the sterile gown. The exposed hands should never come in contact with the glove exterior. The glove is grasped

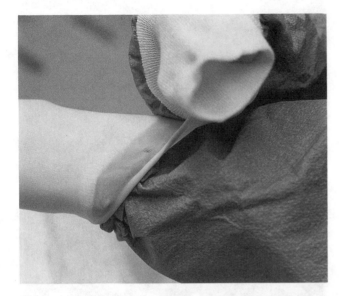

FIGURE 19.13.   Care is taken to enclose the entire stockinette cuff in the glove.

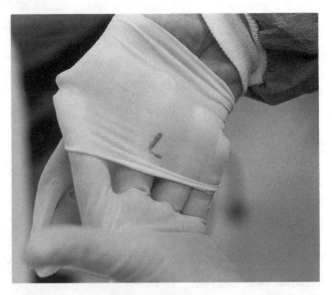

FIGURE 19.15.   The gloved right hand is used to pick up the left glove under the cuff, the left hand is inserted, and the glove cuff is pulled up over the stockinette cuff.

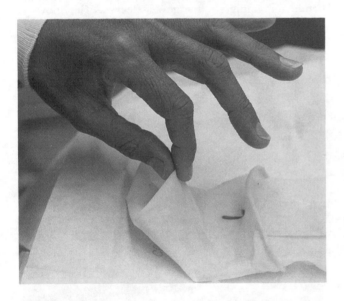

FIGURE 19.14.   Open-glove technique. The right glove is grasped at the cuff, on the fold, by the left hand.

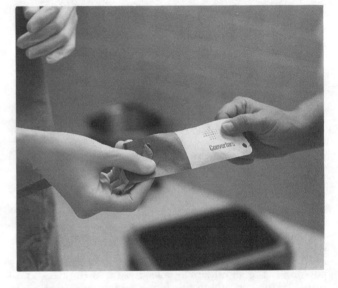

FIGURE 19.16.   A scrubbed person hands the prepackaged card or a sterile instrument to the circulator, who holds the apparatus securely.

at the cuff, on the fold (Fig. 19.14). The opposing hand is inserted into the glove without turning the cuff back (Fig. 19.15). The gloved hand, cuff still unturned, is then used to pick up the remaining glove, keeping the sterile glove under the cuff, glove to glove. The hand is inserted into the glove, and the cuff is then pulled up over the stockinette cuff to cover it completely. The sterile gloved hand can then be placed under the opposite cuff, glove to glove, and the cuff stretched up to cover the stockinette cuff of the sleeve completely. Gloves should be in-

spected after they are donned to assess for pinholes and other compromises to integrity. In some instances, institutional policies call for double gloving (donning of two pairs of gloves) by the scrubbed team.

To wrap the gown once gloving is completed, scrubbed personnel can use the prepackaged cards attached to disposable gowns, or attach a sterile instrument or glove wrapper to the end of the tie. Carefully handing the card or instrument to the circulator (Fig. 19.16), the scrub person then pivots

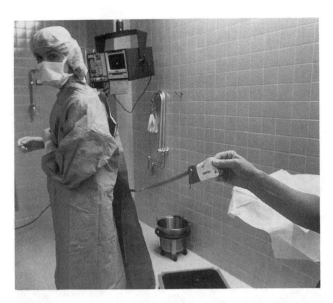

FIGURE 19.17.   The scrub person pivots away from the circulator. The belt is then pulled free and tied while the circulator retains the card or instrument.

away from the circulator. The belt is then grasped and tied by the scrubbed member, and the circulator retains the card or instrument (Fig. 19.17). If other scrubbed personnel are present, they can assist, grasping the tie with a sterile gloved hand.

Occasionally, the sterile gown becomes contaminated before donning the gloves. When this happens, the scrub personnel should complete the gowning and gloving procedure using aseptic technique. Then, the gown should be removed first, pulling the more contaminated upper aspect of the sleeve down over the arms and the still-gloved hands while everting the gown sleeve. The gloves protect the hands. The gloves should then be removed using skin-to skin, glove-to-glove technique. Or the circulator may remove the glove without touching the skin of hand or arm. If no further contamination occurs, the scrub personnel can then regown and reglove. If any contamination of the arms or hands occurs, however, the entire scrubbing procedure should be repeated, just as it would be if contamination occurred during the initial scrub.

If a glove is contaminated after the initial donning, it is preferred that another member of the scrubbed team assist with regloving. If no other scrubbed person can assist in regloving, the open glove technique should be utilized. The scrubbed personnel should be careful that the gown cuff does not extend down over the hand during the glove changes. This prevents contact of a clean hand by the more contaminated surface of the stockinette cuff edge. (Stockinette is a moisture-collecting fabric and not an effective microbial barrier. The cuff

should be considered contaminated once the gloves are donned and should not be exposed to the sterile field.)

At the termination of the surgical procedure, the gown and gloves should be removed; they should not be worn outside the operating room. Proper removal of the gown minimizes contamination of the clothes and arms of personnel. An unscrubbed person should untie the gown in the back. The scrub person then grasps the gown's shoulders on the outside and pulls them down over the arms, everting the sleeves in the process. The gown is pulled completely down over the hands, folded outside-in without undue handling, and discarded. Gloves are then removed, again avoiding gross contamination by using skin-to-skin, glove-to-glove technique. Gloves are discarded in the appropriate waste container.

Once the initial member of the team has scrubbed, gowned, and gloved, other personnel can be dressed similarly. Gowning others uses the same skills as gowning oneself but an opposite approach. The scrubbed team member passes a towel to a newly scrubbed member's outstretched hand, without touching it. The unfolded sterile towel should be held by the upper end and carefully laid over the extended newly scrubbed team member's hand. The newly scrubbed team member then dries the hands/arms and disposes of the towel. The scrubbed team member can then proceed to gown the newly scrubbed person. The gown should be grasped at the neck and held away from the sterile field to unfold. The armholes are located and turned toward the newly scrubbed member. The scrubbed person's hands are positioned on the exterior of the gown at shoulder level, with the neck area draped over the hands, acting as a cuff to protect the gloves from possible contamination (Fig. 19.18). The gown is placed on the outstretched hands of the newly scrubbed team member. Scrubbed personnel then release the gown and allow the newly scrubbed member to advance hands and arms into the gown with assistance from unscrubbed personnel.

Once the gown is secured by circulating personnel, the newly scrubbed member is ready to don gloves. Hands should be extended through the gown cuff. Scrubbed personnel assist in gloving others. The sterile glove should be grasped under the everted cuff and turned with the palm facing the newly scrubbed member, glove thumb in opposition to thumb. The cuff is stretched open, with special attention to keeping the sterile thumbs away from the glove interior (Fig. 19.19). The newly gowned member then advances a hand into the glove, while a slight upward pressure is exerted by the scrubbed

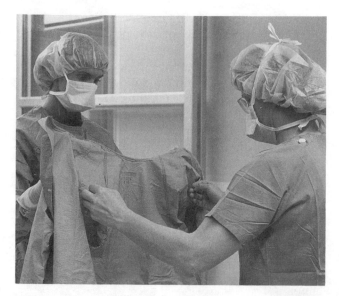

FIGURE 19.18. Gowning other team members. The gown is opened carefully, the scrubbed person's hands are positioned on the exterior of the gown at shoulder level, with the neck area draped over the hands acting as a cuff to protect the gloves from possible contamination.

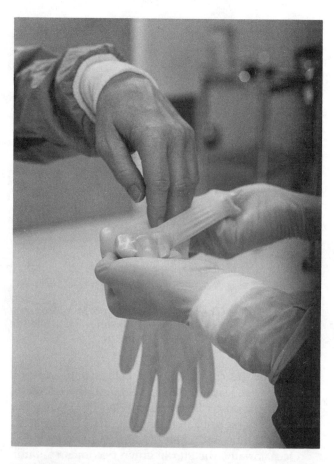

FIGURE 19.20. The newly gowned member advances a hand into the glove, while slight upward pressure is exerted by the scrubbed person.

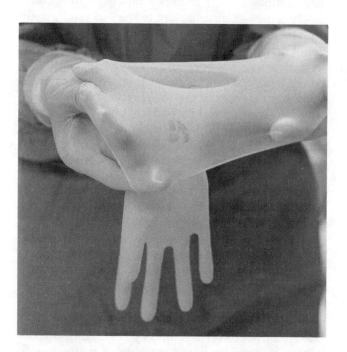

FIGURE 19.19. Gloving other team members. The cuff is stretched open, with special attention to keeping the sterile thumbs away from the glove interior.

person (Fig. 19.20). The cuff should be extended to cover the stockinette cuff entirely. The second glove is then donned in a similar manner.

If contamination occurs during the procedure, the glove should be removed without pulling the gown cuff down over the hand. A new glove is applied using the procedure described above or the open-glove technique.

Unscrubbed personnel can remove the gowns and gloves of others. After the gown is untied, the scrubbed person faces the unscrubbed person. The gown shoulders are grasped by the unscrubbed person, who withdraws the gown, everting the sleeves, and pulling it completely off. Gloves can also be removed by unsterile personnel. Since no part of the scrubbed person's skin should be touched, the unscrubbed person grasps the previously sterile, external side of the glove and removes it in a smooth, single action. Regowning can then take place if necessary. Circulating nurses should wear unsterile disposable gloves and wash their hands after touching others' gowns or gloves because these may be contaminated.

At the conclusion of gowning and gloving procedures or after glove changes, scrub personnel should remove the glove powder from newly donned gloves. Powder residue has been associated with granulomas and peritonitis. It can be removed with moistened towels and sponges or splash basins. Use of a splash basin is discouraged, however, because of the potential for contaminating the sterile

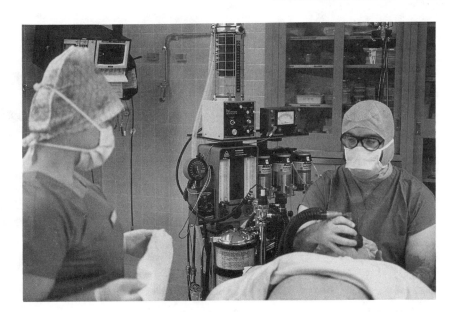

FIGURE 19.21. The circulator should be aware of the activities of the anesthesiologist and should not proceed with the prep until the patient is fully anesthetized.

field with water droplets. Whatever method is used, the towel, sponge, or splash basin and its contents should be removed from the sterile field immediately after use.

PATIENT'S SKIN PREPARATION

The boundaries of the skin area to be prepared are identified by both the written policies of each institution and surgeons' preferences. Generally, a wide area around the incision site is prepared, to provide a margin of safety during draping and in the event that the incision is extended.

Prior to beginning the surgical skin prep, the patient's skin should be inspected for cleanliness, hair, and intactness. Gross soil and debris should be removed from the area to be prepped through patient showers, cleansing the site on the surgical unit or in the perioperative holding area, and cleansing in the operating room immediately prior to beginning the surgical prep.

Hair is removed from the operative site only if it would interfere with the surgical procedure. If hair removal is necessary, it should be accomplished using a depilatory, clippers, or wet shaving with a sharp razor. Depilatories should be tested for patient sensitivity prior to use. Clippers should be disposable; if not, the removable head should be sterilized between patients. Razors used for shaving should be disposable or terminally sterilized. Shaving should be done by gloved personnel, as close as possible to the time of the incision. The gloves may be sterile or nonsterile, depending upon the operative site and the location of the patient when the shave is performed.

After hair removal and immediately prior to draping, the patient's skin is scrubbed at and around the incision site with an antimicrobial agent. Antimicrobial agents used for this purpose should be selected based on the following considerations: (1) patient sensitivity, skin condition, and operative site; (2) broad spectrum of action; (3) lack of toxicity; (4) long-acting residual action; and (5) inclusion on the Food and Drug Administration (FDA) list of approved antimicrobial skin preparation products.

Before beginning the prep, all equipment and supplies should be assembled on a sterile field. Most often, a small, movable table is used as a prep table. The prep set is disposable or nondisposable, depending upon the institution. It should include containers for the prep solutions, sponges for prepping, sterile gloves, and extra containers for depositing used sponges. Occasionally included are cotton applicators for cleaning out small areas, such as the umbilicus, ears, and nose. Solutions used vary depending on effectiveness, institutional preference, cost, and availability.

The circulating nurse or, in a teaching hospital, a resident or medical student is usually responsible for the skin preparation. This person assembles the supplies and proceeds with the scrub prep when agreeable to both surgeon and anesthetist. Circulating nurses should be aware of the activities of the anesthetist and should not proceed with the prep until the patient is fully anesthetized and the nurse's assistance is not immediately required by other team members (Fig. 19.21). Preparation of the incision site requires at least a 5-minute scrub with an effective antimicrobial agent.

Taking care to protect the patient's privacy, the incision site should be assessed for skin integrity; cleanliness; presence of denuded tissue, mucous

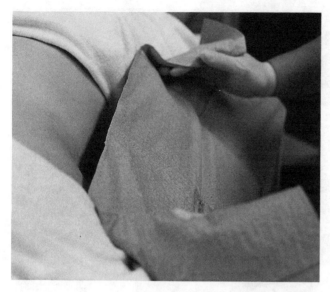

FIGURE 19.22.   Towels are placed on either side of the area to be prepped to prevent pooling of fluids and undue wetting of bed linens.

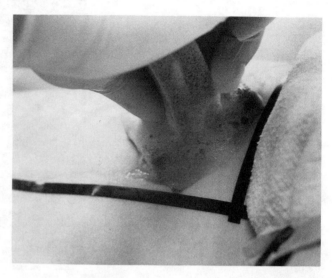

FIGURE 19.24.   The nurse begins the prep at the site of incision and works toward the periphery in a circular motion.

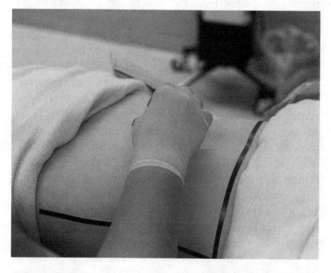

FIGURE 19.23.   The prep should be extended as far as is necessary to ensure a wide margin of safety around the incision.

membrane, or bowel; and the anatomy involved. The proposed procedure and the size of prepped area must also be considered.

The procedure for doing the skin preparation is essentially the same for any area of the body. First, sterile gloves are donned and the prep set is arranged for most efficient use. Sponges should be folded, if necessary, and placed in appropriate containers to avoid undue handling later. Any draping

with sterile towels should be done before scrubbing of the skin. This includes placing sterile towels on either side of the patient's body at the table's edge to prevent pooling of the antiseptic solution under the patient, or placing sterile, impervious drapes under extremities to avoid undue wetting of bed linens (Fig. 19.22).

Prepping intact skin begins at the site of the incision. Using friction and an effective antimicrobial agent, the prep is extended in a circular motion away from the incision site as far as is necessary to ensure a wide margin of safety (Figs. 19.23 and 19.24). Once the sponge has been used and the periphery prepped, that sponge should be discarded in a manner that prevents strike-through. Subsequent sponges are used in the same manner, proceeding from the incision site to the periphery.

Occasionally, the prepping procedure is modified, usually when the prep area includes an open, draining wound or a body orifice. Modifications are based on the basic principle that washing should proceed from clean to dirty areas. The most contaminated area, whether or not it is the site of incision, should be scrubbed last. For instance, the operative area around a colostomy would be prepped first, the stoma itself would be prepped last, and then the sponge discarded. Vaginal preps proceed from the mons and perineum to the vagina itself. The anus should be washed last. The umbilicus should be scrubbed just before disposal of the sponge.

The prep solution is usually allowed to dry by itself prior to draping, but some surgeons prefer that the prepped area be dried. If drying of the incision site is requested, a sterile towel should be laid upon the area. After blotting away any remaining solution, the edges of the towel farthest away from the prepper should be grasped, and the towel should be lifted up and away from the skin, avoiding contamination of the area with the towel edges.

Flammable prep solutions should never be used for laser procedures. If an electrosurgery unit (ESU) will be utilized, prep solutions should be allowed to dry or evaporate prior to activating the unit.

During the prep, care should be taken to prevent pooling of the prep solution under the patient, around a tourniquet or ESU grounding pad sites, or near electrodes.

Once the prep has been carried out, sponges are discarded in an appropriate manner, depending on institutional policy. Prep sponges should be of a different size and shape than those used during the operative procedure. This allows for a much easier sponge count during the procedure and avoids confusion as to what types of sponges are to be counted. Sponges should be contained in a defined area until the end of the operative procedure. Prep solution, once used, should be considered contaminated and disposed of in the same manner as suction container contents or other liquid from the operative field in accordance with institutional policy.

Documentation of the surgical prep should include the name of the person performing the prep; the skin condition before and after prepping; a notation about hair removal, if any; and the type of prep solution used.

DRAPING

Draping establishes a sterile field around the operative site. Isolating the operative field with drapes prevents cross-contamination among perioperative personnel, the patient's wound, and unprepared areas of the patient. Disposable or reusable sterile towels and sheets are used.

Desirable characteristics of draping materials are the same as for OR apparel. Drapes must be resistant to moisture strike-through, safe, and easily drapable. Materials should be free of toxic agents or dyes. Reusable draping materials should maintain their barrier properties through multiple laundering and use cycles. Disposable materials should maintain their barrier qualities throughout the operative procedure and should not be resterilized without written instructions from the manufacturer.

Reusable textiles must be resistant to damage by sharp objects, towel clips, or needles. If holes occur, heat-sealed fabric patches may be used. Reusable material is easily handled, memory-free, and has excellent drapability, but it is more prone to shed lint particles than some nonwovens. Patches do not significantly inhibit sterilization in prevacuum or ethylene oxide sterilizers (4).

Disposable drape materials are also resistant to fluid and bacterial penetration. They are manufactured to meet a variety of draping specifications for special procedures. Disposables are soft and nonirritating. As with reusable drapes, care should be taken to prevent damage from sharp objects. Disposables take up less storage space than reusables, but may require a larger inventory. Maintaining adequate supplies may be costly. Disposal according to community environmental standards is sometimes a problem.

Plastic incisional drapes may be used in conjunction with other draping materials. They decrease the need for skin clips, prevent the migration of microorganisms, stabilize other drapes, and isolate gross sources of contamination such as stomas and fistulas. Their use, which is controversial, depends on physician preference. If plastic drapes are not used properly, bacterial growth at the edges can be increased. Studies support both views.

When selecting draping materials, the most important factors are maintenance of sterility and cost-effectiveness. Packaging, presentation to the sterile field, and draping of the operative site should not compromise sterility. Cost should be studied in relation to the institutional setting, availability and need for supplies, and staff preferences.

The surgeon is responsible for delineating the area to be draped and the type of drape to be used. The entire surgical team is responsible for maintaining asepsis during the procedure. Scrub personnel should be adept at handling drapes and draping the patient (Figs. 19.25 and 19.26). Circulating nurses should be aware of the limits of the sterile field.

Draped tables are considered sterile only at the table level. All drapes, supplies, and equipment extending over or dropping below table level must be considered unsterile because they are out of sight and their sterility cannot be monitored. Before draping, tables must be checked to ensure they are clean and dry, and they must be monitored once the sterile field is established to prevent strike-through. Strike-through occurs when moisture soaks through unsterile layers to sterile layers or vice versa. Many styles, shapes, and sizes of drapes are available.

For general surgery, the following draping procedure is used:

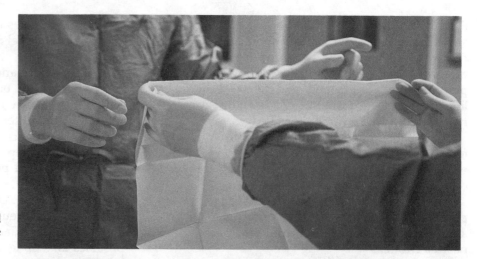

FIGURE 19.25. Scrub personnel should know how to handle the drapes correctly.

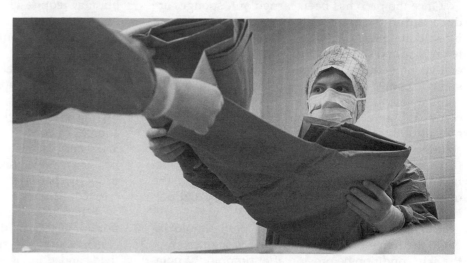

FIGURE 19.26. The drape is kept above the patient until it is placed over the site of incision.

1. Two to four sterile towels, placed with a folded edge toward the operative site, are used to outline the operative site.
2. Nonperforating towel clips are used to prevent displacement of the towels.
3. A laparotomy sheet, often called a lap sheet, with a fenestration or window, is placed on the operative site, slit side down (Fig. 19.27).
4. The sheet is unfolded to cover the patient completely, with adequate length and width for draping the anesthesia screen and both arms (Figs. 19.28).

The general dimensions of a lap sheet are 9 feet by 6 feet, with a longitudinal fenestration of 10 by 4 inches located approximately 4 feet from the top. Standard-sized single sheets, 9 by 6 feet and folded in half, can be used in conjunction with lap sheets to provide a larger sterile area.

Certain procedures may require sheets with fenestrations in different locations. For instance, thyroid drape fenestrations are located closer to the head of the sheet and are transverse, whereas breast and chest drape fenestrations are larger and square. Perineal drapes, used for patients in the lithotomy position, may have two leggings located on either side of a fenestration. When in place, the drape covers the patient's legs, abdomen, and the lower end of the operating table. Split U-shaped sheets are frequently used to drape extremities but are the same overall size as other lap sheets. Sterile drapes are also available for special equipment and supplies that cannot be sterilized, such as microscopes, eyepieces, and magnets.

Drapes should be applied from the incision area to the periphery. When draping is complete, the incision site should be the only exposed area. All other unprepared areas of the patient must be covered by sterile drapes (Fig. 19.29).

Draping materials should be handled as little as possible. They are kept in a specific area of the sterile table to avoid undue handling and disturbances of air currents or other sterile supplies. They should never be passed over an unsterile area or held below the waist. During transfer from the sterile field to

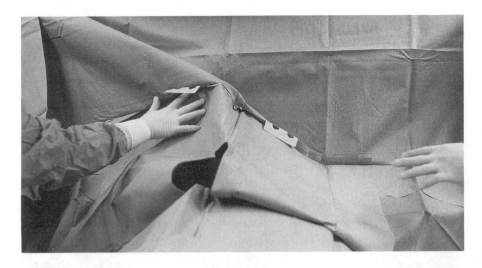

FIGURE 19.27. In abdominal surgery, a lap sheet with fenestration is placed on the operative site.

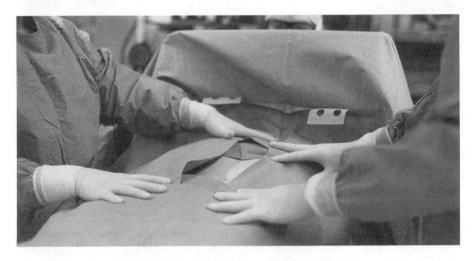

FIGURE 19.28. The sheet is unfolded completely to cover the patient.

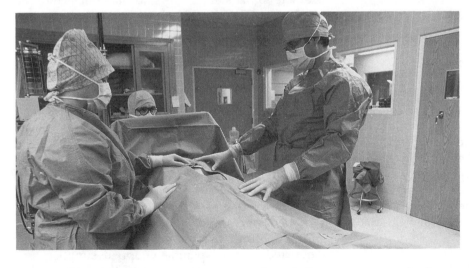

FIGURE 19.29. All unprepared areas of the patient must be covered by sterile drapes.

the patient, they should be held in a compact position, avoiding fanning or haphazard unfolding.

To avoid contamination, scrubbed personnel must not touch the patient's skin, and their gloved hands should always be protected by cuffing the draping material back over the hands.

Once drapes are positioned, they should not be adjusted, as shifting or moving the drapes can contaminate the sterile field.

Needles and other sharp instruments occasionally perforate the draping material, leading to contamination. Scrubbed personnel are responsible for

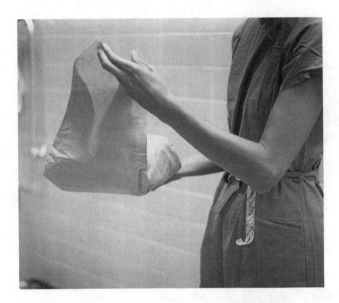

FIGURE 19.30.   Opening sterile supplies. The circulator opens the flap farthest away first.

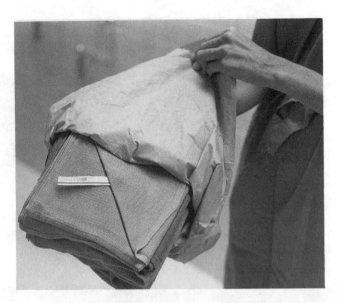

FIGURE 19.31.   All wrapper tails are secured before presenting the item to the sterile field.

avoiding such perforation. If it does occur, the area should be isolated by covering it with new draping material and the instrument removed from the sterile field.

Blood, other serous drainage, and irrigation solutions can become sources of contamination if strikethrough occurs. Once an area becomes wet, it must be considered contaminated. The area should be isolated, either by adding extra waterproof drapes or by redraping the area.

DISPENSING STERILE ITEMS

All items used within a sterile field should be sterile. Any items of questionable sterility should be considered unsterile. All items presented to the sterile field should be checked for proper packaging, processing, expiration date, and handling. All packages should be checked for moisture, seal integrity, possible penetration of the sterile barrier (e.g., pinholes or tears), and the appearance of the sterilizer indicator. When items are delivered to the sterile field, the integrity of the contents and the sterile field must be maintained.

Packages should not delaminate during opening, should not reseal once opened, and must permit aseptic presentation of the contents to the sterile field. The inner edge of a peel package seal is considered the sterile boundary. Wrappers must be free

of holes. They should be memory-free, to facilitate opening on flat surfaces. Once opened, wrappers are considered sterile to within one inch of the edge.

Packaging materials should be compatible with the method of sterilization. Reusable materials require laundering between uses to maintain fiber hydration. To prevent rupture during sterilization, peel pouches should have as little air present as possible. Packaging materials selected for sterilization should promote initial sterilization and maintenance of the sterile contents through storage and opening.

Sterility and integrity must be maintained when opening, dispensing, and transferring sterile items to the sterile field. Sterile items should not be tossed onto the sterile field; instead, they should be handed to the scrubbed person or placed on the sterile field. Tossed items may roll off the sterile field or dislodge other items already placed there. Sharp items (e.g., knife blades, rakes, or trocars) should be presented to scrubbed personnel to allow them to take the items safely. Sharps may be placed on a separate surface. Items that are coiled or prone to flailing when opened should be presented to the scrubbed person to prevent the contents from springing from the package and becoming contaminated. When opening wrapped supplies, unscrubbed personnel should open the wrapper flap farthest away from them first and the nearest wrapper flap last (Fig. 19.30). All wrapper tails should be secured when supplies are presented to the sterile field to prevent the wrapper from flipping back to its original position and thus contaminating the package contents (Fig. 19.31). Scrubbed personnel opening wrapped supplies proceed in an opposite manner, opening the nearest wrapper flap first and the farthest flap last. All personnel should avoid undue handling and fanning of wrappers.

Connecting ends of drill cords, electrosurgery cords, suction tubing, and the like must be handed off the sterile field for attachment to their power source, using the principles of asepsis. Scrub personnel should extend enough length off the sterile field to allow the circulating nurse to connect the equipment without contaminating the field. Once connected, the cords should be secured with nonperforating devices and should not be repositioned. Any suture, instruments, or cords that extend beyond the edge of the sterile field should be considered contaminated.

When dispensing sterile liquids, personnel should take care to prevent contents from splashing onto the sterile field or onto an unsterile area that might then drip onto the sterile field. Bottle contents should all be poured at one time or the unused portion discarded. Reuse of opened bottles can contaminate solutions, due to drops contacting unsterile areas and then running back over sterile bottle lips. Bottle caps should not be replaced, as the edges are considered unsterile once the container is opened.

Sterile items dropped on the floor should be considered unsterile. Any items of questionable sterility should be considered unsterile. The adage, "when in doubt, consider it unsterile," prevails when opening sterile supplies and maintaining the sterile field.

A sterile field should be set up as closely as possible to the time of use. Once sterile supplies have been opened, they should not be left unattended. The length of time sterile supplies can be opened and still be considered sterile depends on the type of procedure to be performed and the patient's status. Each institution must have an established policy regarding this practice; however, the practice of maintaining opened sterile supplies for more than one hour should be questioned.

Sterile supplies should never be opened and then covered, because it is virtually impossible to uncover the sterile field without contaminating it. Once a patient has entered a room where sterile supplies have been opened, those supplies may only be used on that patient. In the event of case cancellation, supplies must be discarded to prevent cross-contamination.

The setup is maintained until the patient leaves the room. This assures that if supplies are needed in an emergency, their integrity has been maintained.

TRAFFIC PATTERNS

Maintenance of the integrity of the sterile field is the responsibility of all personnel who move within or around it. Once gowned and gloved, scrubbed personnel should remain near the sterile field and should not leave the room.

During the procedure, scrubbed team members must be alert to maintaining gown sterility at table level during adjustments in table height. Scrubbed personnel should never lean or sit on unsterile areas. Sitting is permitted only when the entire procedure will be done in that position. Hands and arms must be kept between table and shoulder level.

Scrubbed personnel move only in the areas of similar preparation. All personnel moving within or around a sterile field should do so in a manner consistent with maintaining the sterility of that field. That is, scrubbed personnel only come in contact with and reach over sterile areas; unscrubbed personnel only come in contact with and reach over unsterile areas.

In delivering supplies to the sterile field, unscrubbed personnel must always be aware of the distance between themselves and the sterile field. Single-use transfer forceps may be used as an extension of the unsterile hand, ensuring a safe distance. Transfer forceps stored in solution should not be used because maintenance of sterility is questionable.

In pouring solutions, scrubbed personnel should hold sterile containers away from the sterile field or set them near the edge of the sterile field so unscrubbed personnel do not lean over the field while pouring. Unscrubbed personnel should maintain at least a one-foot distance between themselves and the sterile area. Unscrubbed persons should not pass between two sterile areas that are close together.

Scrubbed personnel must remain close to the sterile field and never turn their backs to it. Scrubbed personnel should not walk in traffic pathways. When changing positions and passing other scrubbed personnel, they should turn face-to-face (Fig. 19.32) or back-to-back (Fig. 19.33). In draping unsterile areas, scrubbed personnel must drape those areas nearest to them first. This ensures that when they drape areas farther away, they will be leaning over a sterile field to do so.

Observers of surgery can be a threat to the sterile field. Both new and veteran personnel may be eager to see surgical procedures being carried out. They must occasionally be reminded that they should not lean over the sterile field. This includes the anesthetist who leans over the anesthesia screen.

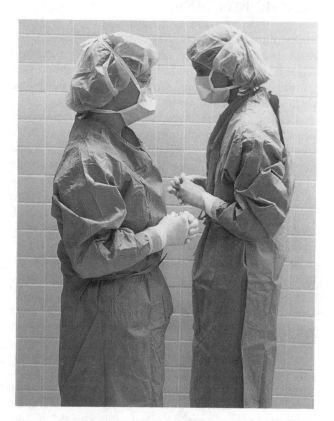

FIGURE 19.32. In keeping with the principle sterile to sterile and unsterile to unsterile, scrubbed personnel pass face to face.

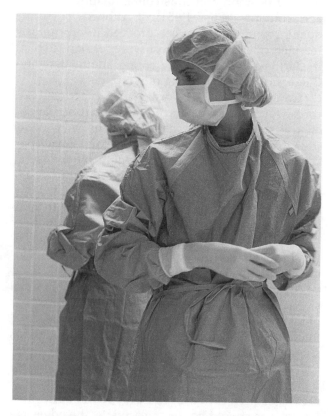

FIGURE 19.33. Scrubbed personnel pass back to back.

OTHER INTRAOPERATIVE PRECAUTIONS

Once the skin has been incised, constant monitoring and maintenance of the sterile field is required. Each team member must be alert to potential and actual breaks in sterile technique and take corrective action if necessary. Conversation should be kept to a minimum.

Blood should be removed from instruments each time they are passed from the incision back to the instrument stand. They can be wiped with damp sponges or towels, or carefully submerged in sterile water. Blood remaining on the instruments can be a source of wound contamination and corrode the stainless steel finish. And blood can be difficult to remove during terminal cleaning.

Repositioning overhead lights is discouraged because it requires the scrubbed person to reach above the level of the shoulders and out of the line of sight. In addition, blood- and serum-coated gloves can leave a residue on the light handles; when dry, this can be a source of airborne contamination.

Soiled sponges should be discarded from the

sterile field to avoid contamination, maintain clear visibility of the wound site, prevent an increase in the number of airborne contaminants, and assist the circulating nurse to confine and contain contamination.

During procedures that involve opening unsterile body cavities, such as in vaginal closures during abdominal hysterectomy, bowel resection, and bronchus transection, some authorities believe extra care should be taken in handling instruments. According to this practice, once instruments have been in contact with a contaminated area, they are isolated by scrubbed personnel and no longer used. Other authorities believe that these precautions are necessary only for colon resection when the patient has not had a cleansing enema or gastrointestinal-specific antibiotics. Except in cases of ruptured viscus or unprepared large bowel, copious irrigation may have the same effect in limiting the spread of contaminants.

Instruments used for cancerous lesions may also be segregated, because they can be sources of seeding of malignant cells to other parts of the body.

Another danger is insects. Any insect found on

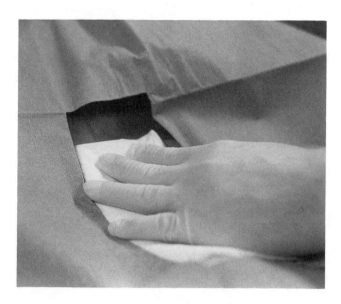

FIGURE 19.34. Sterile dressings are applied before removal of the drapes to avoid contamination of the incision.

the sterile field should be removed, and any portion of the sterile field that might have been contaminated should be isolated. If there is doubt about whether an insect landed on a sterile field, it should be considered contaminated and either isolated or struck and set up again.

Other possible sources of contamination are perspiration, contact lenses, and loose hair. If perspiration becomes a problem, the scrubbed person should turn away from the sterile field to mop the damp area. Perspiration should not be allowed to fall onto the sterile field. Contact lenses worn by the surgical team must also be monitored. Loose hair should not be a problem if the surgical team is dressed appropriately.

After closure of the incision, sterile dressings are usually applied before removing the drapes (Fig. 19.34). The dressing is completed and secured by

the circulating nurse or the ungloved surgeon after drape removal. Drapes should be removed in an orderly manner and disposed of in an appropriate container. Suction tubing and other drainage devices should also be discarded in appropriate containers.

The surgical team is the patient's advocate. Team members must be alert in establishing and maintaining asepsis. Each member should have developed a surgical conscience that allows for no breaks in technique and no less than excellent practice.

REFERENCES

1. Gruendemann, B. J., Casterton, S., Hesterly, S., Minckley, B., and Shetler, M. *The Surgical Patient: Behavioral Concepts for the Operating Room Nurse* 2nd ed. St. Louis, MO: C. V. Mosby, 1977.
2. Association of Operating Room Nurses. "Recommended practices for aseptic technique." *AORN Standards and Recommended Practices for Perioperative Nursing—1992.* Denver: AORN, 1992.
3. Schroder, Elinor S. (Ed.). "Glove study shows both open and closed techniques appropriate." *AORN J* 34(September):390, 1981.
4. Green, V. W., Borling, G. M., and Nelson, E. "Effects of patching on sterilization of surgical textiles." *AORN J* 33(June):1249–1261, 1981.

SUGGESTED READINGS

Association of Operating Room Nurses. *AORN Standards and Recommended Practices for Perioperative Nursing—1992.* Denver: AORN, 1992.

Cruse, J. E., and Foord R. "A five-year prospective study of 23,649 surgical wounds." *Arch Surg* 107(August):206, 1973.

Dineen, P. "An evaluation of the duration of the surgical scrub." *Surg Gynecol Obstet* 129(December):1181–1184, 1969.

Garner, Julia S. *Guideline for Prevention of Surgical Wound Infections.* Atlanta: Centers for Disease Control, 1985.

Garner, Julia S., and Favero, Martin S. *Guideline for Handwashing and Hospital Environmental Control.* Atlanta: Centers for Disease Control, 1985.

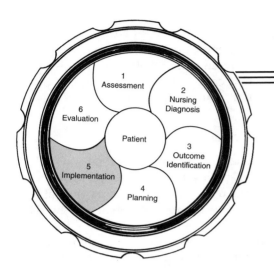

20

Positioning the Patient

The surgical team positions the patient.

Positioning is an interdependent nursing–medical task performed by all professional members of the surgical team. Perioperative nurses share responsibility and legal accountability for positioning with the surgeon and the anesthesiologist (1). Every institution should have policies and procedures related to positioning that include, but are not limited to, assessment criteria, anatomical and physiological considerations, safety and security measures, patient monitoring, and documentation of position and devices used (2).

Proper positioning for surgery requires knowledge of anatomy and physiological principles, as well as familiarity with the equipment required. The ideal surgical position provides optimal exposure for the surgeon while allowing access to the patient's airway, intravenous lines, and monitoring devices. At the same time, the position should not compromise integumentary, circulatory, respiratory, musculoskeletal, or neurological structures. The comfort and dignity of the patient should also be considered, especially for conscious patients (2).

Planning and preparation begin with the assessment process. From the patient history and preoperative interview, the nurse identifies any potential problems with the anticipated surgical position. Factors that can influence a patient's ability to cope with the surgical position include:

- Age and physical limitations. Under anesthesia, the central nerve reflexes are obtunded and skeletal muscles are relaxed, permitting a patient's normal physical limitations to be exceeded.

- Height. Positioning devices should be of appropriate size to prevent patient injury (e.g., a tall patient needs a padded table extension).
- Weight. Obese patients are more likely to trap moisture in skin folds and adipose tissue if not well perfused. Both overweight and underweight patients experience greater than normal pressure on bony surfaces.
- Skin condition. Patients with previously damaged tissue and tissue receiving decreased circulation are at increased risk for pressure ulcers.
- Central and peripheral nerve function and cardiopulmonary status.
- Nutritional status. Patients with poor nutrition are at greater risk for tissue damage.
- Preexisting disorders, such as arthritis, diabetes, or general debilitation. Hypothermia, hypotension, and prolonged procedures without position change are examples of conditions that can lead to decreased tissue perfusion.
- Type and length of procedure.

If possible, the preoperative nursing assessment should include having the patient assume the position required during surgery (e.g., extension of the legs of an arthritic patient for the lithotomy position). The expected outcome of positioning is that the patient will be free from positioning-related injury. In order to achieve this outcome, any physical limitations should be carefully described in the plan of care and communicated to anesthesia and other surgical personnel.

The surgical procedure and the patient's anatom-

319

ical and physical limitations dictate the types of positioning devices that will be needed intraoperatively. The surgeon's preference card should identify the position that will be used for the procedure. This card can be used as a guide in selecting the necessary equipment and positioning aids, and determining the number of personnel required to achieve the position (3). Before placing the patient on the OR bed, the bed itself and any necessary positioning aids should be inspected. They should be in good working order, clean, free of sharp edges, and padded where applicable. Depending on the position to be used, such equipment may include stirrups, armboards, footboards, lumbar supports, kidney rests, various types of doughnuts, foam padding for pressure points, pillows, sheet rolls, and securing devices such as tape and/or safety belts.

Usually, the patient is placed in the supine position, anesthetized, and then positioned for surgery. Exceptions are patients who experience pain upon moving (such as accident or trauma victims) and children, who are frequently held during the induction phase and then placed on the OR bed.

A team of at least four personnel are recommended to lift an unconscious adult patient (2). Having adequate personnel available avoids sliding or pulling the patient across the bed and consequent dislodgement of indwelling catheters, tubes, or cannulas. The patient should always be moved slowly, avoiding movements outside of the normal range of motion. If possible, the head should be kept in a neutral axis and turned as little as possible (4).

During positioning, exposure should be limited, to both protect the dignity of the patient and maintain proper body temperature. Warm blankets can also help to provide a comfortable environment.

Once the desired position has been achieved, reassessment of the respiratory, circulatory, musculoskeletal, neurological, and integumentary systems is needed. Body parts should never be touching each other, and the patient should not be touching any metal part of the OR bed. If the patient, the OR bed, or any positioning device is repositioned intraoperatively, the patient should be reassessed for body alignment and tissue integrity.

PHYSIOLOGICAL CHANGES DURING POSITIONING

Harmful physiological effects that can result from improper positioning include ineffective breathing patterns, impaired gas exchange, alterations in cardiac output, impaired mobility, alterations in kinesthetic and tactile sensory perception, impaired tissue perfusion, and impaired skin integrity (5). It may be helpful to remember that there are three primary forces that can result in such injuries: pressure, obstruction, and stretching (6).

Respiratory System

Position influences respiration in several ways. Perhaps the most significant factor affecting respiration is the mechanical restriction of lung expansion at the ribs or sternum and the reduced ability of the diaphragm to push down against abdominal retractors. Normally, the thoracic cage expands in all directions except posteriorly. Interference with any of these movements reduces respiratory function.

At the same time, the ventilation:perfusion ratio is disturbed. That is, the pulmonary capillary blood volume and consequently the amount of blood available for oxygenation are altered by gravity. In addition, the inspired air in the lungs is redistributed, affecting the air available to oxygenate blood. For example, patients with unilateral lung disease have an increase in arterial oxygen pressure when lying with the "good lung down" because the best-oxygenated lung also receives the greatest amount of blood (7, 8).

Another position effect on respiration is that the compliance or stretchability of the lung tissue is decreased by ventilators or changes in blood volume, reducing the amount of air that can be taken in for gas exchange.

Preoperatively, the nurse can evaluate respiratory function through the patient history. Such factors as smoking, obesity, or preexisting pulmonary disease should alert the nurse to look further for medical evaluation of respiratory status. Arterial blood gases or pulmonary function tests can help the nurse determine the patient's ability to cope with transport as well as the surgical position. The nurse should also keep in mind that patients with reduced pulmonary function may suffer respiratory difficulties with heavy premedication and must be observed closely.

Circulatory System

Anesthesia causes circulatory changes. With both general and regional anesthesia, peripheral blood vessels tend to dilate, resulting in a drop in blood pressure. The dilated vascular beds allow venous blood to pool in dependent areas, reducing the amount of blood returned to the heart and lungs for oxygenation and redistribution. Both general and spinal anesthesia obtund normal compensatory mechanisms for maintaining blood pressure. General anesthesia depresses the cerebral medulla, which normally maintains cardiac output and peripheral vascular constriction. Muscle relaxants used during general anesthesia reduce the milking action of normal muscle tone that aids in venous return. Reduced respiratory effort as well as ventilator-assisted positive respiration diminish the negative thoracic pressure that aids in pulling venous blood back to the heart. Spinal or epidural anesthesia directly blocks autonomic output from the spinal cord, bringing about extreme vasodilation and venous pooling below the areas of the block.

Any patient with poor cardiac status, hypovolemia, or arteriosclerotic vascular disease will be at greater risk under anesthesia in most positions. Again, the severely obese individual (100 pounds overweight) exhibits marked deviations from normal circulatory function even without the additional stress of anesthesia and compromising positions.

Peripheral Nerves and Vessels

The most evident changes seen as a result of poor positioning are damage to peripheral nerves and vessels. This problem is usually due to direct mechanical pressure, as from the weight of surgical instruments or personnel leaning on the patient. Pressure for even a few minutes can bring about impaired nerve function, resulting in sensory and/or motor loss. Preexisting conditions such as alcoholism, diabetes, peripheral neuropathies, and hypothermia can contribute to nerve damage. Most postoperative palsies are thought to result from malposition on the operating table (2). Generally, the longer the peripheral nerve and the more superficial its position, the greater the possibility for injury. The most vulnerable time is during anesthesia, when muscle tone is reduced. Damage to nerves and vessels is not usually discovered until recovery from anesthesia is complete, and may be masked for days by postoperative sedation as well.

Peripheral vascular damage occurs with occlusion of the vessels. The most frequent cause is external pressure such as a tight restraint or crossed legs. Vessels may also occlude by hyperextending or twisting a limb, thereby obliterating flow by compressing the vessel against the body's bone structure. Even normal, awake people can obliterate a radial pulse by simply hyperabducting an arm over their head.

Skin Pressure

Another important perioperative responsibility is skin pressure. Decubitus ulcers can develop as a consequence of poor positioning and poor pro-

tection during surgery. One study found a 13% frequency of pressure sores in patients having operations lasting longer than two hours (9). The highest frequency was in the elderly and those in poor general condition.

The critical factor in the formation of pressure sores is tissue perfusion. Pressure sores can develop if capillary pressure is lowered, as with low blood pressure; if blood flow is obstructed by compression of vessels or torsion of tissue; or if external pressure increases, as with a hard surface or tissue edema. Body weight is unevenly distributed when a person is lying on a hard surface. The concentration of weight is on the bony prominences and surrounding tissue. If blood pressure is normal, capillary pressure will remain in the range of 32 to 40 mm Hg (10). Therefore, if external pressures are higher than this, ischemia could result. With a lower blood pressure, even less pressure could produce ischemia.

Duration of pressure is thought to be a more important factor than pressure intensity. Healthy individuals can tolerate external pressures up to 100 mm Hg on bony prominences without tissue ischemia for short periods of time. Tourniquet pressures over nonbony portions of limbs are indeed much higher for even an hour or more. But low, constant pressures on bony prominences of even 70 mm Hg have been shown to cause microscopic changes in healthy individuals after two hours (11). Intermittent pressures of high intensity are also tolerated better than low, constant pressure. The significant factors in pressure sore formation are a bony prominence and constant pressure. Patients with diabetes, peripheral vascular disease, a debilitated state, or hypotension are particularly vulnerable.

Comfort

Surgical positioning should not alter the patient's perception of comfort during the intraoperative or postoperative phases of the surgical experience. This becomes even more important when positioning conscious patients. Maintenance of the patient's comfort level requires application of the principles of positioning, familiarity with positioning equipment, and preoperative assessment of the patient's individual needs.

POSITIONS

The positions used most often in operative procedures are the supine, Trendelenburg, reverse Trendelenburg, lithotomy, sitting, lateral, prone, and jackknife positions.

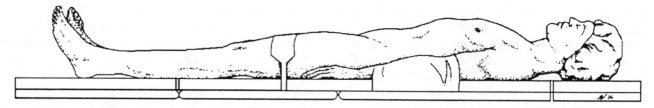

FIGURE 20.1. Supine (dorsal) position.

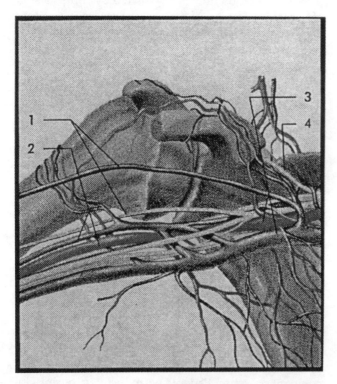

FIGURE 20.2. Anatomical structure of the upper arm and shoulder.

Supine (Dorsal Recumbent)

The supine position is the most common surgical position. The patient reclines on his or her back, with the arms extended at the sides. The supine position is used for any anterior approach, such as abdominal surgery, most extremity procedures, some thoracic procedures, and head and neck surgery.

Positioning

The most common supine position is with the table flat. The head should be on a small pillow, flexing the neck slightly. Arms are either at the sides, palms down, or extended on armboards (Fig. 20.1).

As an alternative, Martin has recommended placing the OR bed in the so-called lawn chair position, with the back of the OR bed elevated and the foot section lowered (12). If the OR bed is adjusted in this manner, the patient's weight is distributed along the full length of the dorsal body surface. In addition, gentle flexion occurs at the hips and knees, allowing these joints to be placed in a more neutral position. The lawn-chair position is especially useful for patients having a regional or local anesthetic, because lying flat on the OR bed can be distressful and uncomfortable for the conscious patient (5). This position has been advocated for all but abdominal surgery.

As with all surgical positions, careful placement of extremities is important to prevent peripheral nerve and vessel damage. Damage is most likely to occur in areas exposed to hard surfaces or in misaligned limbs. Brachial plexus injury is considered the most common nerve injury. In the supine position, most patients with reported injuries had an arm extended. The extended arm must be kept at less than a 90° angle from the body, to decrease the length of stretch to the brachial plexus. Having the head and neck turned in the opposite direction from the arm and extension, and suspension of the arm straight from the wrist also places undue pressure on the brachial plexus. Damage to the brachial plexus results in motor and sensory loss to the arm and shoulder girdle. Also, subclavian and axillary arteries may be compressed or occluded with hyperabduction of the arm (Fig. 20.2). If the arm is abducted on an armboard, radial or brachial pulses should be checked periodically.

Misplacement of the arm or compression against the side of the table can result in radial (wrist drop), median (ape hand), or ulnar nerve (claw hand) damage. Ulnar nerve paralysis has occurred in thin or emaciated patients because an elbow or arm was pressing against a hard surface (Fig. 20.3)

The leg strap should be placed at least two inches above the knee. No direct pressure should be placed on the popliteal space, as might be seen with a pillow and a tight leg strap. Compression in this area can result in venous thrombosis. Although less common, tibial or sural nerve damage can occur and cause numbness on the plantar surface of the foot. Lumbar support may decrease the incidence of posterior back pain.

Physiological Effects

Although the supine position is thought to be the least harmful, significant physiological changes have

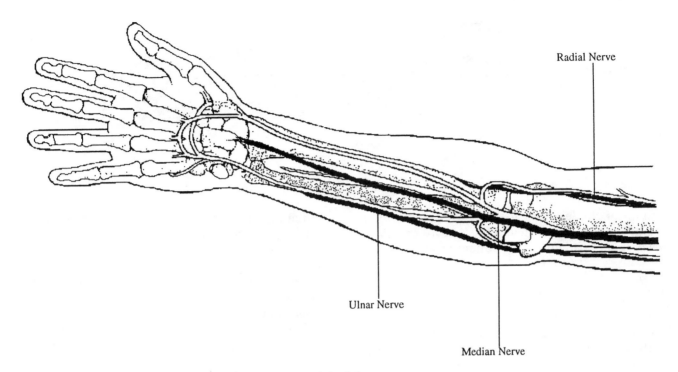

Radial Nerve

Ulnar Nerve

Median Nerve

FIGURE 20.3.   Anatomical structure of inner aspect of the left arm.

been measured. Lung tissue compliance has been shown to decrease, compared to the sitting position. This decrease is probably due to increased pulmonary blood volume and small airway closure (13). Vital capacity decreases because of restricted posterolateral chest movement. A gallbladder rest arches the patient's back and, if it is up, vital capacity is further reduced due to additional diaphragmatic restriction. Tidal volume decreases from the upright position during anesthesia and even more so with the gallbladder rest. Without adequate respiratory assistance, a patient may easily become hypoxic when the gallbladder rest is used. Instead, an extended or elevated thorax position has been recommended for upper abdominal surgery (14). Healthy individuals have been found to have much less adverse cardiovascular and respiratory effects with this position than with an extended gallbladder rest.

When supine, obese patients (100% over normal weight) have as much as 40 to 50% increase in the mechanical work of breathing. At the same time, oxygen consumption also increases. Therefore supplemental oxygen should be considered in an obese patient who must remain supine for extended periods of time. If the patient is awake, respirations should be assessed periodically.

Circulatory changes in the supine position are usually less pronounced than in other positions. Both regional and general anesthesia, however, decrease mean arterial pressure. Abdominal retractors,

packs, or a large intraabdominal mass can markedly obstruct venous return to the heart. A person with such a mass may become normotensive when placed in a left lateral position, reducing the direct pressure on the vena cava.

Even in the supine position, obese patients are at greater risk for cardiovascular deficiencies. Blood volume in the heart and lungs is increased. Cardiac output increases over sitting, and pulmonary artery wedge pressure can increase dramatically, presenting a risk of heart failure. Therefore continuous cardiac and blood pressure monitoring is necessary, even in the awake obese patient.

Skin pressure areas occur most frequently in the supine position. Underweight as well as obese individuals are vulnerable to pressure areas. Underweight individuals have greater intensities of pressure in smaller areas, while obese individuals have more extensive moderate pressure areas. Patients having surgery of two or more hours' duration, or those who are diabetic, hypotensive, hypothermic, underweight, or obese should have protective padding under heels, elbows, sacrum, and occiput. Sheepskin, foam rubber, or alternating pressure pads have been used successfully.

If the patient is pregnant, the weight of the gravid uterus can compress the vena cava to cause transient hypotension and even fetal hypoxia. To alleviate compression of the vena cava, the gravid uterus can be displaced to the left by laying a folded sheet or towels under the patient's right side at her waist. El-

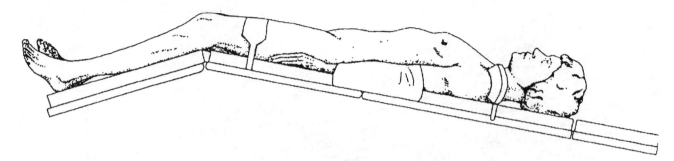

FIGURE 20.4. Trendelenburg's position.

evation of the legs and use of elastic stockings or elastic bandage wraps should be standard procedure for pregnant patients in the supine position (15).

Trendelenburg's Position

Trendelenburg's position is named after a German urologist. It is a variant of the basic supine position, with the body tilted head-down. Trendelenburg's has been used for lower abdominal surgery and whenever better exposure of abdominal organs is needed, as with obese patients. It has been shown to decrease bleeding and facilitate central venous cannulation.

Positioning

With the patient in the supine position, the OR bed is tilted downward at the patient's head. The legs are lowered parallel to the floor to maintain the position and to allow more room for the Mayo stand above the toes. Care must always be taken to prevent pressure on the toes once the position is attained.

As in the supine position, arms may be extended on armboards or tucked at the side, palm down or toward the body. Shoulder braces may be used for maintaining the position with extreme angles of Trendelenburg (Fig. 20.4). If the shoulder brace is misplaced over soft tissue, however, the brachial plexus can be damaged.

When returning to the horizontal position, the leg section should be raised first, and slowly.

Physiological Changes

Despite its advantages, Trendelenburg's position may have adverse effects on the heart, vessels, and lungs. The head-down position immediately reduces respiratory compliance and increases the work of breathing, hinders cardiac filling and performance, increases intracranial pressure, and heightens the risk of passive regurgitation of gastric contents (4).

Respiratory changes are more pronounced than in the supine position. Vital capacity falls compared to that in the sitting position, and tidal volume decreases progressively with the degree of Trendelenburg. Respiratory depression is due to limitation of diaphragm expansion and maldistribution of blood to ventilation. The apex of the lung receives the greatest blood supply in this position but has less alveolar tissue than the base of the lung. In addition, Trendelenburg's position increases intrathoracic pressure, which could be undesirable in patients with cardiac decompensation or those in whom increased intracranial pressure may be hazardous.

The possibilities of nerve and vessel injuries are similar to the basic supine position.

Reverse Trendelenburg

The reverse Trendelenburg position is another variation of the basic supine position, with the entire table slanted feet-down (Fig. 20.5). It is used for head and neck surgery, because it decreases the blood supply to that area. It may also be used to facilitate respiration in obese patients.

Positioning

In the reverse Trendelenburg position, the OR bed is tilted toward the patient's feet. For extreme angles, a well padded footboard may be needed to support the patient's body. A roll, bolster, or sandbag may be placed under the shoulders for better access and stabilization in operations such as thyroid, radical neck, tracheostomy, or jaw and mouth surgery. The head may be turned to one side in carotid surgery.

Physiological Changes

Respiratory and circulatory problems are nearly the opposite of those of Trendelenburg's position. Respiration is less affected, but circulation can be greatly compromised. The reverse Trendelenburg position permits considerable peripheral pooling of as much as several hundred milliliters of blood in the lower extremities. As expected, mean arterial pressure decreases. Moving the anesthetized patient from both Trendelenburg's and reverse Trendelen-

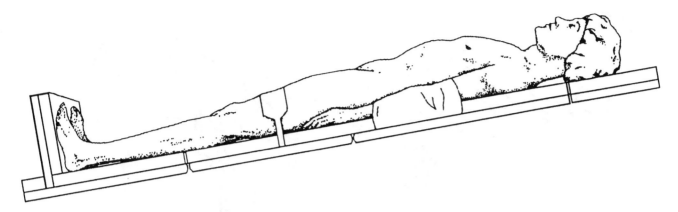

FIGURE 20.5.   Reverse Trendelenburg's position.

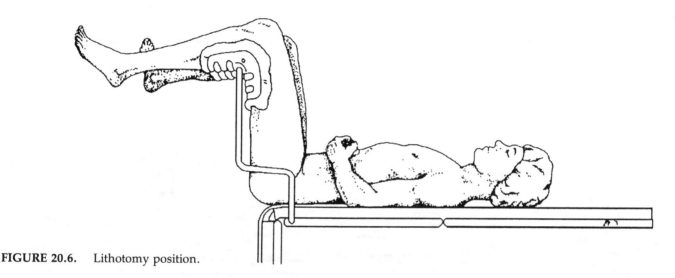

FIGURE 20.6.   Lithotomy position.

burg positions must be done slowly to allow the heart time to adjust to the great changes in blood volume.

Lithotomy Position

In the lithotomy position the patient is supine, with the legs suspended in stirrups; the foot section of the table is lowered (Fig. 20.6). This position is used for perineal surgery, including procedures on the vulva, vagina, prostate, and rectum. It is the second most common position used in surgery.

Positioning

Special considerations are necessary to prevent peripheral nerve damage from the lithotomy position. If the arms are allowed to remain at the sides, pressure injuries or even crushing injury to the hand can occur when the end of the table is raised or lowered. The hands should not extend beyond the break in the table. If the arms are to be placed at the patient's sides, they should be crossed over the patient's

chest prior to raising the end of the table. The arms may be folded across the chest loosely at the beginning of the procedure and held by the patient's gown or a sheet. Respiratory effort is restricted in this position, however, and ulnar damage can result from pressure on the inner aspect of the elbow against the table. Armboards placed parallel, against the table are ideal. Patients with a history of carpal tunnel syndrome or ulnar nerve sleep palsy should have their arms extended at the elbows (16). Patients with no such history can tolerate elbow flexion to 45° without interference of ulnar nerve conduction (17).

The patient's buttocks must not extend beyond the break in the table in the lithotomy position or undue stress will be placed on the back when the legs are lowered. Instead, the patient should be positioned with the buttocks just above the break in the table. Since most of the patient's body weight rests on the sacrum, additional padding may be needed to prevent a pressure area.

Correct placement of the legs in the stirrups is ex-

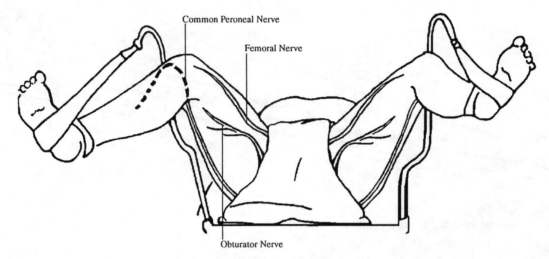

FIGURE 20.7.   Location of these anatomical structures must be known so as to prevent pressure on the groin and popliteal area. Pressure on the peroneal nerve has the potential of causing foot drop. Calves are not shown parallel to bed for illustrative purposes.

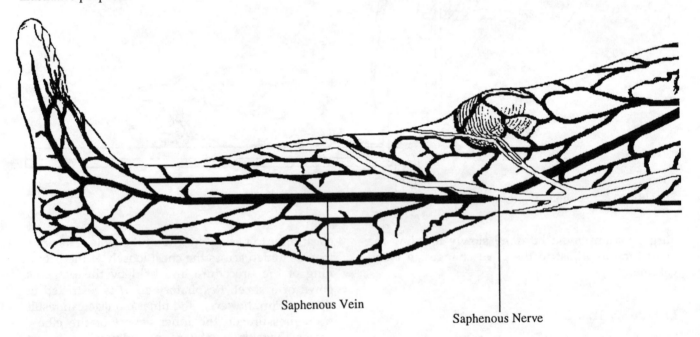

FIGURE 20.8.   The saphenous vein and nerve.

tremely important. To avoid straining the lumbosacral muscles, two people should simultaneously raise the legs and place the feet in stirrups while supporting the lower legs. Hips should be symmetrical. Calves should be parallel to the table. If more abduction is needed for greater exposure, flexion or external rotation should be done at the hip and not the knee. Extreme abduction of thighs with external rotation at the hip can result in femoral neuropathy caused by kinking of the femoral nerve beneath the tough inguinal ligaments (18). If the patient has had a prior hip pinning, total hip replacement, or is arthritic, the hip should be supported by one hand as the leg and foot are gently extended.

In the groin, damage can occur to the femoral and obturator nerves from undue pressure (Fig. 20.7). Such an injury might be caused by misplacement of instruments. The obese patient is particularly at risk, as extra effort is frequently needed for adequate retraction. Damage to the femoral or obturator nerve can result in sensory disturbances to the inner aspect of the leg and the abductor muscles of the inner thigh.

Unpadded or misplaced stirrups can damage the saphenous vessels and nerves on the medial aspect of the knee (Fig. 20.8). The most prevalent problem, however, is peroneal nerve damage on the lateral aspect of the knee, which can produce foot drop. Stirrup holders should be placed well on the outside of the leg, allowing no contact between the leg and the holder. If necessary, additional foam padding around the knee and under the calf may be used.

When the legs are lowered from the lithotomy position, 500 to 600 ml of blood may drain into the legs from the trunk, resulting in severe hypotension. Elastic stockings may prevent some of this large influx by increasing venous pressure. Slow and smooth movement when lowering the legs is extremely important. Optimally, the legs should be lowered and the hips/knees extended simultaneously by two people over a period of not less than two minutes.

Physiological Changes

The lithotomy position carries the potential for a variety of injuries. Systemic changes that occur with this position can be significant. Respiratory effectiveness is reduced by marked restriction of diaphragmatic movement caused by increased abdominal pressure from the thighs. Pulmonary blood volume is increased, resulting in engorgement of lung tissue, reducing its compliance. Vital capacity and tidal volume decrease compared to a sitting posture. With an addition of 10° Trendelenburg, tidal volume can decrease even more. Circulatory pooling occurs in the lumbar region in the lithotomy position. Venous flow can be reduced by interference with lung expansion, which normally provides a negative "thoracic pump," aiding in venous return.

Nerve damage and secondary muscle damage are the primary complications arising from use of the lithotomy position. Most nerve injuries related to use of this position occur with the standard ankle-strap stirrup, which does not control abduction of the thigh.

Compartment syndrome of the calf is a rare but potentially serious complication of lengthy urologic and gynecologic procedures (19). Any acute increase in pressure in a limited anatomic space which compromises both circulation and neurologic function can result in a compartment syndrome. Typical symptoms are severe pain, hypesthesia, muscle weakness, pain on passive stretch of the muscles, and tenseness of the compartment. It carries the risk of permanent neuromuscular and kidney damage. Attention to postoperative symptoms and timely intervention are of prime importance in reducing complications (19).

In order to reduce the risk of compartment syndrome, it is recommended that the foot be neutral or slightly plantar-flexed when in the lithotomy position (20) so that circulation to the feet can be examined frequently using distal pulses or color changes as indexes; and so that the use of calf-support devices (which support the entire weight of the leg in the area of greatest risk for compartment syndrome) can be avoided.

The ideal lithotomy positioning system would avoid contact with the popliteal space and the calf, while controlling rotation and abduction of the hip and extension of the leg to avoid injuries such as femoral nerve entrapment beneath the inguinal ligament. A boot stirrup is one possible alternative (19).

Increasing the time in the lithotomy position may prolong compression, obstruction, and pressure factors, which clinically increases the risk of nerve, muscle, and vascular injuries. Thus it is recommended that use of the lithotomy position in which the knees are in fixed holders be limited to six hours (21).

Sitting Position

The sitting, or high Fowler's, position is used primarily in neurosurgical procedures, such as posterior fossa craniotomy or posterior cervical spine procedures. It may also be used for facial operations and breast reconstruction.

Positioning

Placing the patient in the sitting position is a carefully planned, step-by-step process. The novice is encouraged to do a dry run to gain confidence and familiarity with the equipment prior to positioning the anesthetized patient. All equipment—head holder, pillows, tape—should be in the room before positioning is started. If an antigravity suit is used, it should be placed on the table before the patient is. For cervical procedures, one or two pillows are placed on the thigh section of the table, which help elevate the patient. In the final position, the patient's second or third thoracic vertebra is at the elevated table edge when the head platform is removed (22).

To put the patient in the sitting position, the nurse first loosens the thigh straps, then flexes the table fully and lowers one foot section at least 45°. Slowly, the nurse elevates the back section and at the same time tilts the table chassis in steep Trendelenburg. The foot section is kept horizontal. The patient's blood pressure is carefully monitored with each table manipulation; the patient may require vasopressors before additional back elevation. The nurse continues to elevate the back section until the desired position is obtained, with the patient's legs horizontal and at about the level of the heart.

The head is manually supported as the head portion of the table is removed. Then the head can be

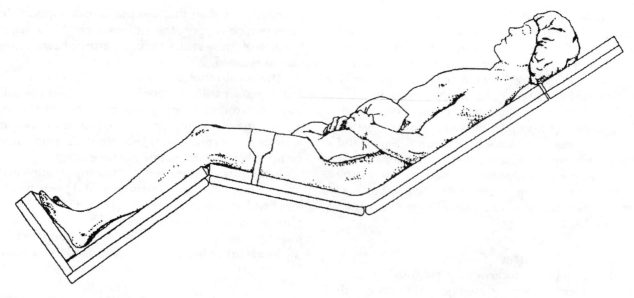

FIGURE 20.9.   Sitting position.

stabilized with a horseshoe headrest or, preferably, with a head holder or pin (Mayfield) holder. All head holder units can become partially or completely dislodged, causing either eye injury (more common with horseshoe holder) or neck injury. The neck should be neutral or slightly flexed. Extreme neck flexion can result in edema of the face, tongue, and soft tissue of the mouth. Scrupulous attention must be paid to stabilizing the head and neck position prior to draping. Arms are usually crossed on a pillow in the patient's lap and secured with wide adhesive tape to the table frame. Elbows should be supported on pillows to prevent ulnar nerve damage (Fig. 20.9).

Physiological Changes

Physiologically, the sitting position is the best possible position for respiration; there is practically no abnormal restriction of chest expansion. But the sitting position can greatly compromise systemic circulation. Hypotension and loss of consciousness have occurred even in unanesthetized individuals when placed in the sitting position from a supine position. Antigravity suits (G-suits) have been used to reduce venous pooling in the dependent legs. It is recommended that a G-suit, elastic stockings or, preferably, Ace leg wraps to the groin be applied to all patients in this position. In addition, the craniotomy patient is at further risk to develop vascular air emboli, and a central venous pressure (CVP) monitor and precordial Doppler are almost always standard anesthesia equipment for such procedures.

In this position most of the body weight rests on

the ischial tuberosities. Unless the table is well padded, skin pressure areas can develop here, as can sciatic nerve damage, particularly in thin or diabetic individuals. Supporting the feet at near right-angle alignment to the legs will reduce sacral pressure and prevent foot injuries.

Lateral Position

The lateral position is used for hip, thoracic, or kidney procedures. The patient is anesthetized while supine and then turned onto the unoperated side.

Positioning

Teamwork is essential; four people are needed for a smooth and gentle turn. The anesthetist guides the head and shoulders, one person is on each side, and one is at the feet. The break of the table should be at the level of the iliac crest instead of under the flank or lower ribs. The patient is first moved close to the edge of the table, keeping good alignment. The "down" arm is brought forward to reduce direct pressure, then the patient is gently turned with the operated side up. The head should be neutral, midline supported with a headrest, and the back in straight alignment. A pillow is placed between the legs with the lower leg flexed to 90° and the upper leg straight, or vice versa (Fig. 20.10). The upper arm is supported with an over-bed arm support. An axillary roll should be under the down axilla, with the lower shoulder forward. The down arm is slightly or fully flexed. Radial pulse should be

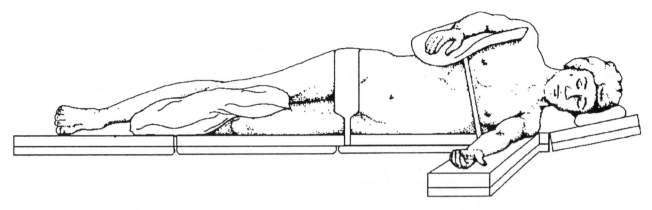

FIGURE 20.10.   Lateral position.

checked often to ensure circulatory adequacy in the down arm. Wide adhesive tape is used over the hips and frequently over the shoulders to stabilize the position.

There are a number of variations on the lateral position:

- For hip procedures, stabilization is maintained with a suction bean bag that is covered with a bath blanket or towel to reduce skin friction and pressure. The anesthetized patient is turned on the device, the ends correctly placed, and the air evacuated to hold the patient in position.
- For thoracotomy, the back torso is stabilized with a sandbag or pillow at the back and another in front of the chest. The suction bean bag can also be used, instead of these devices, to maintain positioning in chest procedures.
- For kidney procedures, the table is flexed, with the patient's head and feet down. In addition, the table's kidney rest may be raised for better access.
- If the patient is pregnant, an armboard may be placed parallel to the bed at waist level to help support the patient's protruding abdomen (15).

Physiologic Changes
A simple lateral position reduces vital capacity and tidal volume. The kidney position decreases vital capacity even more, due to restriction of chest expansion as well as a change in blood ratio:gas exchange ratio in each lung.

Blood pools in dependent limbs. Blood pressure measurements are lower than the actual arterial pressure. The pressure in the upper arm is measured above the level of the heart, and in the down arm it is measured on a partially compressed axillary artery. Direct arterial pressure measurements, however, are known to drop. It is postulated that more

obstruction to vena caval flow occurs on the right side, and there may also be actual interference with heart action; that is, a possible shift in heart position.

Skin pressure areas can develop between the legs from the weight of the upper leg on the lower but may be minimized with proper placement of pillows. Pressure under the trochanter major of the femur has been measured as high as 110 mm Hg when using only standard operating room table pads (11).

Peripheral injuries to the brachial plexus and the median, radial, and ulnar nerves can occur if the upper arm is not properly supported on the overhead armboard. But the most common nerve damage with the lateral position is to the peroneal nerve, from compression of the down knee against a hard surface. Extra padding should be provided under the down knee, particularly in thin individuals.

Prone Position

The prone position is used for any procedure requiring a dorsal approach. It is used most often for spinal surgery, such as laminectomies and fusions. It may also be used for posterior cervical and occasionally occipital procedures when a sitting position is not preferred. If the patient has had a recent spinal cord injury requiring immediate decompression or stabilization, special precautions are taken.

Positioning
In most cases, the patient is anesthetized in the supine position, usually on the transport vehicle, and then turned prone onto the OR bed. If the patient is unusually large, however, it may be better to anesthetize him or her on the OR bed rather than trying to turn an anesthetized patient from the transport vehicle to the OR bed.

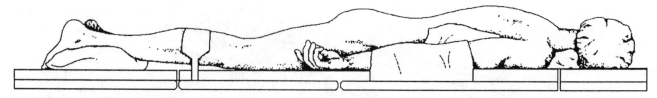

FIGURE 20.11. Prone position.

The anesthesiologist coordinates the turn because he or she is responsible for head and airway management. Movements should not be made until the anesthesiologist is ready. One or two people (if the patient is large) stand on both sides of the patient, on the outside of the stretcher and the table. It is preferable to have one person at the foot. The patient's arms are either straight down at the sides or straight above the head (usually for the awake patient). The patient is moved to the side of the stretcher and then, as the anesthesiologist holds the head, is gently rotated onto the side and then onto the abdomen. The team members on the opposite side of the stretcher receive the patient with their arms under abdomen, chest, and shoulders. If the arms are to be placed on armboards, it is critical that the elbows be bent and the palms of the hand face inward before the arms are extended. Dislocations can occur very easily during this maneuver. If the patient has had a recent cervical trauma, the head must remain in a neutral position throughout positioning. Traction may be needed prior to intubation or turning to stabilize the neck. An additional person must be available to assist anesthesia. If there is no recent cervical injury, slight flexion is preferred when moving the head.

Once the patient is prone, restrictions on the chest and abdomen are reduced by either a preplaced laminectomy frame or body rolls extending from shoulders to iliac crest on either side (Fig. 20.11). Breasts should be free, and male genitalia protected by an additional towel or small pillow at the pubis. Feet should be supported in a 30° to 45° angle to the legs by pillows or rolls with no pressure on the toes. With the head turned to one side, a head donut or small towel will help prevent pressure on the ear and eye. Doughnuts are also placed under the knees and ankles.

If the patient is pregnant, rolled-up bath blankets or bolsters may be placed under the sides of the patient, from the nipple line to the iliac crest. Their purpose is to prevent vena caval compression, provide stability, and allow for adequate chest expansion. If possible, the knee–chest position should be used, because it provides for better circulatory and respiratory functioning (15).

Physiologic Changes

Blood pressure always drops in the prone position. With the use of chest rolls, however, mean arterial pressure may drop less. Chest rolls or a laminectomy frame relieves the mechanical restriction on chest movement, which can reduce vital capacity and tidal volume. The improvement of respiratory effectiveness facilitates venous flow and assists blood pressure. Skin pressure areas are greatest on the chest, knees, and ankles, but also occur on the shoulders and iliac crests in thin individuals. Because many procedures done in the prone position are of long duration, sheepskin or additional padding placed under these pressure areas is helpful.

Jackknife or Kraske Position

In this variation of the prone position, the patient's head and feet are both lower than the hips. The jackknife position is used most frequently for proctologic procedures.

Positioning

The patient is either anesthetized supine and turned prone, or is placed in position before spinal anesthetic is administered. The hips are on a pillow or towel directly over the table break, and the table is flexed 90°, with the head and legs down. The patient's arms are on armboards with hands toward the head (Fig. 20.12). The buttocks may be separated by wide tape placed at the level of the anus on both sides and secured to the table. The patient is taken out of the position by first flattening the table and then reversing the order of movements into the prone position. Arms are usually positioned over the head for turning.

Physiologic Changes

The jackknife position has been described as the most precarious of surgical positions. Both respiration and circulation can be most adversely affected. Vital capacity is reduced due to restricted diaphragmatic movement and increased blood volume in the lungs, reducing lung compliance.

With blood pooling in both the chest and feet, mean arterial pressure drops significantly. A most severe drop in blood pressure can occur when a lat-

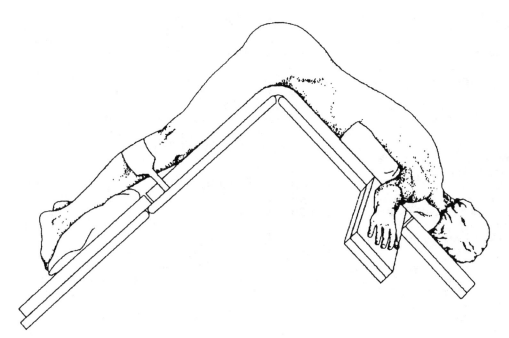

FIGURE 20.12. Jackknife position.

eral tilt is added to the jackknife. A 38-mm Hg drop has been recorded in a right lateral jackknife and a 27-mm Hg drop in a left lateral jackknife position. Although lateral tilt is not often used, the additive effect should be known (22). In addition to dependent pooling, venous return may also be seriously limited by mechanical obstruction at the point of the table break as well as by the reduced negative intrathoracic pressure. The slowed venous return of blood in combination with obtunded compensatory mechanisms by anesthesia can produce a decrease in stroke volume affecting cardiac output. A drop in blood pressure may be accompanied by bradycardia. Continuous cardiac and blood pressure monitoring is recommended, even in patients under local anesthetic. An intravenous line should also be open. Blood pressure may be maintained with the use of fluid volume, and intravenous medications such as atropine may be needed.

Skin pressure areas are similar to those in the prone position, with greater pressure on the pubis at the table break if no protection is used.

DOCUMENTATION OF POSITIONING DATA

The circulating nurse records the position of the patient, and any special equipment used, in the perioperative nursing notes. For example, the circulator might record:

Patient in supine position with right arm tucked under drawsheet at side, palm up, left

arm abducted approximately 75° on padded armboard, safety belt across thighs, padded footboard supporting feet.

Documentation serves both legal purposes and quality improvement purposes. It may be used to evaluate or identify any patient complications that are attributable to positioning and aid in making necessary corrections to ensure quality care (6).

EVALUATION

The final step in positioning is to evaluate attainment of the expected outcome, "Patient will be free from injury related to positioning." The nurse has a responsibility to determine whether the planned interventions were effective in preventing positioning-related injury (5). In order to evaluate implementation of the plan of care, the patient must be observed during surgery, immediately after surgery, and a day or two postoperatively. If necessary, the plan of care must be revised to reflect identification of any new problems.

REFERENCES
1. Bargagliotti, L. Antoinette. "Critical analysis: 'Sequelae of the intraoperative lithotomy position.' " *AORN J* 50(4):832–837, 1989.
2. Association of Operating Room Nurses. "Recommended practices for positioning the surgical patient." *AORN Standards and Recommended Practices—1992*, pp. III:14–1 to III:14–5. Denver: AORN, 1992.

3. Groah, Linda K. "Positioning and draping." *Operating Room Nursing: The Perioperative Role*, pp. 259–280. Reston, VA: Reston Publishing, 1983.

4. Biddle, Chuck, and Cannady, Melinda Joan. "Surgical positions: Their effects on cardiovascular, respiratory systems." *AORN J* 52(2):350–359, 1990.

5. Phippen, Mark L. "Positioning the patient for surgery." Jane C. Rothrock, ed. *The RN First Assistant: An Expanded Perioperative Nursing Role*, pp. 245–295. Philadelphia: J. B. Lippincott, 1987.

6. Smith, Kimberly A. "Positioning principles: An anatomical review." *AORN J* 52(6):1196–1208, 1990.

7. Remolina, C., Khan, A. U., Santiago, T. V., and Edelman, N. H. "Positional hypoxemia in unilateral lung disease." *N Engl J Med* 26(304):523–525, 1981.

8. Grosmaire, E. K. "Use of patient position to improve PaO_2: A review." *Heart Lung* 12(6):650–653, 1983.

9. Hicks, D. J. "An incidence study of pressure sores following surgery." *ANA Clin Sess* 49–54, 1970.

10. Bennett, L., Kavner, D., Lee, B. Y., et al. "Skin stress and blood flow in sitting paraplegic patients." *Arch Phys Med Rehabil* 65(4):186–190, 1984.

11. Souther, S., Carr, S., and Vistnes, L. "Pressure tissue ischemia and operating table pads." *Arch Surg* 107:544–547, 1973.

12. Martin, J. "General requirements of safe positioning of the surgical patient." J. Martin, ed. *Positioning in Anesthesia and Surgery*, pp. 1–5. Philadelphia: W. B. Saunders, 1978.

13. Behrakis, P. K., Baydur, A., Jaeger, M. J., and Milic-Emili, J. "Lung mechanics in sitting and horizontal body positions." *Chest* 4:643–646, 1983.

14. Videbek, F. "Posture with elevated and extended thorax." *Acta Anaesthes Scand* 24:458–461, 1980.

15. Kovacs, Rebecca Ramirez. "When your patient is also pregnant." *AORN J* 36(4):559–565, 1982.

16. Walpin, L. "The flexed elbow and sleep." *Arch Phys Med Rehabil* 65:51, 1984.

17. Harding, C., and Halar, E. "Motor and sensory ulnar nerve conduction velocities: Effect of elbow position." *Arch Phys Med Rehabil* 64:227–231, 1983.

18. Tondare, A. S. "Femoral neuropathy: A complication of lithotomy position under spinal anesthesia." *Can Anaesth Soc J* 30(1):84–86, 1983.

19. Adler, Lisa M., Loughlin, Jacquelyn S., Morin, Christopher J., and Haning, Ray V., Jr. "Bilateral compartment syndrome after a long gynecologic operation in the lithotomy position." *Am J Obstet Gynecol* 162(May):1271–1272, 1990.

20. Gershuni, D. H., Yaru, N. C., Hargens, A. R., et al. "Ankle and knee position as a factor modifying intracompartmental pressure in the human leg." *J Bone Joint Surg* 66(9):1415–1420, 1984.

21. Graling, Paula R., and Colvin, Donald B. "The lithotomy position in colon surgery." *AORN J* 55(4):1029–1039, 1992.

22. Martin, J. "The head-elevated positions." J. Martin, ed. *Positioning in Anesthesia and Surgery*. Philadelphia: W. B. Saunders, 1978.

Suggested Readings

Atkinson, Lucy Jo, and Kohn, Mary Louise. "Positions." *Berry and Kohn's Introduction to Operating Room Technique* 6th ed., pp. 295–305. New York: McGraw-Hill, 1986.

Cantin, Joyce E. "Proper positioning eliminates patient injury." *Today's OR Nurse* 11(4):18–21, 1989.

Ethicon. "Importance of patient position." *Nursing Care of the Patient in the OR* 2nd ed., pp. 27–32. Summerville, NJ: Ethicon, 1987.

Gregory, Brenda. "Position the patient." Julia A. Kneedler, ed. *CNOR Study Guide*, pp. 101–114. Denver: National Certification Board: Perioperative Nursing, 1990.

Groom, Linda E., and Frisch, Sara R. "Sequelae of the intraoperative lithotomy position." *AORN J* 50(4):826–831, 1989.

Gruendemann, Barbara J. *Positioning Plus*. Chatsworth, CA: Devon Industries, May 1987.

McConnell, Edwina A. "Patient positioning." *Clinical Considerations in Perioperative Nursing*, pp. 103–114. Philadelphia: J. B. Lippincott, 1987.

Meeker, Margaret Huth, and Rothrock, Jane C. "Positioning the patient for surgery." *Alexander's Care of the Patient in Surgery* 9th ed., pp. 103–113. St. Louis, MO: C. V. Mosby, 1991.

Merrill, Sunny. "A teaching plan for positioning." *AORN J* 35(1):63–66, 1982.

Miner, Dennis. "Patient positioning: Applying the nursing process." *AORN J* 45(5):1117–1127, 1987.

Murphy, Ellen K. "Liability for injury resulting from poor patient positioning." *AORN J* 53(6):1361–1365.

Paschal, Charles R., Jr., and Strzelecki, Lorna R. "Lithotomy positioning devices: Factors that contribute to patient injury." *AORN J* 55(4):1011–1022, 1992.

Rothrock, Jane C., ed. *Perioperative Nursing Care Planning*. St. Louis, MO: C. V. Mosby, 1990.

21
Performing Counts

The nurse is responsible for sponge, needle, and instrument counts.

The number of foreign bodies left in surgical patients has increased in recent years. In 1984, St. Paul Fire and Marine Insurance Company reported fifty-two cases in which sponges, instruments, or needles were left in surgical patients. The average settlement in these cases was $13,096. In 1990, the same company reported ninety-five such claims filed, with an average settlement cost per incident of $30,349 (1).

A few examples of such incidents include the following:

- A sponge was left in the gallbladder bed of a patient who had a gastroplasty. The patient was brought back to surgery and the sponge removed. In this case, the circulating nurse did not follow the hospital procedure of bagging the laparotomy sponges in sets of 5 and the small sponges in groups of 10. Also, the scrub nurse and circulating nurse did not do a joint count. Rather, the circulating nurse had someone from the anesthesia department validate the count.
- A patient had a cesarean section. The scrub nurse and circulating nurse did only one count and reported it as correct. The patient came back to the hospital 6 weeks after delivery with an abscess and complained of pain. Before the patient could be brought to surgery, the abscess broke.
- A laparotomy sponge was left in a patient who had had a cesarean section, with the sponge count reported as correct. A mass with the lap sponge was found by x-ray one year later, when

the patient came back to the hospital for an elective procedure.

- A needle broke off during an anterior and posterior repair. Informed of the needle's location, the patient elected to have it left in rather than undergo surgery to retrieve it. One year later the patient reported no ill effects.

Sponge, needle, and instrument counts help to prevent these problems. Sponge counts are well established, yet a number of institutions still do not count needles and instruments. Some argue that such counts are not justified; however, all three types of counts should be part of daily practice in every operating room.

The Association of Operating Room Nurses (AORN) first published guidelines for counts in 1976. Continuous revisions and updates have resulted in the current recommended practices that provide guidelines for counting sponges, sharps, and instruments (2). These recommendations represent an optimal level of practice; each institution is encouraged to develop policies and procedures that can be implemented in its specific clinical environment.

Having a policy is the key to a successful count program. The policy should be developed jointly by medical and nursing staffs and approved by the institution's administration. It should become a part of the healthcare facility's standard operating procedure. Once these ground rules have been established, every member of the OR team will know

Sponge count policies
- A sponge count will be taken on all operating procedures except cystoscopies, transurethral resection of the prostate, or when a particular surgeon has given the associate director of nursing service a written letter stating she does not want a count of sponges taken on her case and she is assuming full responsibility for sponges used on her patients.
- Sponges are counted in the operating room by scrub and circulating personnel: (1) prior to the beginning of the operation; (2) as closure of the wound begins; and (3) as closure of the skin begins.
- The count is carried out audibly. The scrub person audibly counts the sponges on the sterile field. The circulating nurse audibly counts the sponges off the sterile field.
- Additional counts will be done before any part of a cavity or a cavity within a cavity is closed, as in a cesarean section, a gastrointestinal anastomosis, and the retroperitoneal space.
- Additional counts will be taken at any other time judged necessary, for example, if two incisions are made, as in a bilateral hernia repair.
- The count is recorded on the operating room counting sheet immediately after it is taken. Additional sponges added to the case are recorded.
- A registered nurse must participate in every count and sign the operative record accordingly.
- Incorrectly numbered packages of sponges are isolated. They are *not* removed from the room. These sponges should not be added to the count and should be labeled appropriately and initialed by the RN isolating them.
- Counts omitted due to an extreme patient emergency must be documented by the circulating nurse on the nurse's notes in the chart.
- All personnel must comply with the procedure of the hospital. If there is any deviation from this policy, the circulating nurse reports it to the operating room associate director of nursing service or to the head nurse, who documents it on the operating room record and initiates an incident report.
- Counted sponges are not taken from the operating room for any reason while a count is in effect.
- X-ray-detectable sponges will not be used for dressings. All sponges are packaged in groups of 5 or 10, including dental rolls and cottonoids.
- Soiled sponges are handled as little as possible, using forceps or gloved hands if necessary.
- The ongoing tally is recorded on the count sheet.
- If a sponge cannot be located, an incident report will be filled out.
- When a sponge cannot be located, an x-ray will be taken before the patient leaves the operating room. If the surgeon refuses to have the x-ray taken in the operating room, this must always be documented on the incident report and signed by the surgeon. An incident report will be completed whether the x-ray is negative or reveals a sponge.

Needle and knife blade counting policies
Policies are the same as for counting sponges, with these additions:
- Needle and knife blade counts are done for all procedures.
- Scrub personnel count needles and blades continually during the procedure and should hand them to the surgeon only on an exchange basis.
- Needles broken during a procedure are accounted for in their entirety.
- Used needles are kept on a needle count pad to ensure their containment in the sterile field.

Instrument counts
Policies are the same as for counting sponges, with these differences:
- Instruments are counted on all surgical procedures when the abdominal, thoracic, pelvic, and retroperitoneal cavities are opened. This includes all hernia repairs.
- Standardization of instrument sets is established for ease in counting, based on the minimum number and types of instruments in the set.
- Instruments broken or disassembled during a procedure are accounted for in their entirety.

FIGURE 21.1   Sample policies for sponge, needle, and instrument counts. These policies are those of the operating room at the University of Colorado Hospital, Denver.

what is expected. The time for debate about counts is while the policy is being written, not during a case when the surgeon is ready to close the wound. When a facility has a policy, perioperative nurses have an obligation to uphold it.

What should such a policy require? Sponge, needle, and instrument counting policies at the University of Colorado Hospital are based on the AORN recommended practices (Fig. 21.1). Under such poli-

cies, the counts are carried out as indicated in this chapter.

SPONGE COUNTS

Before surgery, the scrub person and circulating nurse count the sponges aloud. The scrub person should hold the sponges up off the table, and each sponge should be separated and checked closely by both persons. Both are responsible for verifying that all sponges have x-ray detectable strips. The circulating nurse records the number and type of sponges in units of 5 or 10 on a count sheet or board.

Nurses should never take for granted that the count on prepackaged sterilized sponges is accurate. If a package does not contain the right number of sponges, the sponges should be bagged and the bag marked with the actual number, initialed, and isolated from the rest of the sponges. Some institutions require that inaccurately numbered sponges be returned immediately to central supply. It is unwise to attempt to compensate for an incorrectly numbered package during the operation.

During surgery, the scrub nurse's responsibilities are as follows:

1. Discard soiled 4×4 and laparotomy sponges into one kick basin lined with a plastic bag.
2. Keep small soiled sponges contained on the field, grouping them in 5s or 10s, according to the way they were originally packaged.
3. Replace 4×4s with laparotomy sponges as the body cavity is opened.
4. Account for all free 4×4s or sponge sticks used.
5. Notify the circulating nurse if a 4×4 is to remain temporarily in the wound, such as when a sponge is placed in the vagina during a hysterectomy.

During surgery, the circulating nurse's responsibilities are as follows:

1. Discard prep sponges into trash as the prep is being done, to avoid mixing them with the counted sponges.
2. Use two plastic-lined kick buckets for handling sponges. The first is for soiled sponges thrown off the field by the scrub person, and the second is for counting. Take sponges from the first bucket and lay them around the rim of the second bucket for counting. Weigh the sponges for blood loss as they are being transferred if the anesthesiologist requests it.
3. When a unit of 5 or 10 sponges is on the rim of the second bucket, count these aloud with the scrub person prior to bagging and check for the x-ray-detectable strips. Then place the sponges in separate plastic bags and close. Always handle sponges with forceps or gloves, never with bare hands.
4. Place bagged sponges away from sterile sup-

plies in view of the anesthesiologist so that he or she can estimate blood loss.
5. Mark off a unit on the count sheet or board as each unit is bagged to keep the count accurate.

As wound closure begins, the scrub person and circulating nurse count aloud all the sponges on the sterile field, the Mayo stand, and the back table. Then they count the sponges discarded in the kick buckets. The circulator should add the total of bagged sponges to the current total at this time to verify that all sponges are accounted for. The circulator reports the results to the surgeon.

As closure of the skin begins, the final count is done in the same manner, with the circulator reporting the results to the surgeon.

In order to prevent sponges from being left in patients in the operating room or delivery room, all sponges (except for prep sponges) should be x-ray detectable. All used sponges should be placed in the kick bucket's plastic bag. The bag should be closed and placed on top of the laundry hamper. All linen and supplies should be left in the OR until the patient leaves the room.

When the count is complete, the professional licensed nurse who participated in the count must sign the operative record that it is correct. Many facilities have both the scrub person and the circulating nurse sign the record.

If a count is incorrect, the nurse notifies the surgeon immediately and initiates a search. If a sponge is not accounted for in the search, the nurse fills out an incident report and makes arrangements for an x-ray. If the surgeon refuses to have an x-ray taken, the nurse notifies the charge nurse, documents this on the incident report, has the surgeon sign the incident report, and documents the event on the nurse's notes in the patient's chart. The risk management department/person is then notified.

When a scrub person or circulator is relieved for any reason, the name of the relief person is added to the operative record, followed by the word *relief.* A complete count of sponges must be made between shift changes. If this is impossible because of the nature of the procedure, attempts to do a count are documented on the operating room record.

Figure 21.2 is an example of one type of device used to count sponges. It was invented by an OR nurse. One busy operating room that was leaving sponges in patients started to use the Keep-A-Count. A retrospective audit was done after 3000 surgical procedures and not one sponge had been left in a patient. The Keep-A-Count gives the nurs-

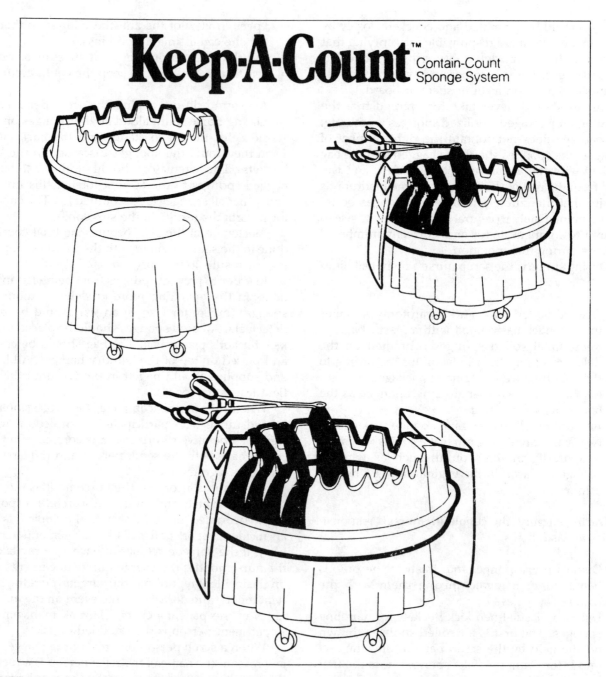

FIGURE 21.2.   One of the devices currently used to assure correct sponge counts.

ing team an additional count, for it is an accurate, uniform method for counting and containing surgical sponges.

NEEDLE COUNTS, INCLUDING KNIFE BLADES AND OTHER SMALL OBJECTS

Before surgery, the scrub person counts the total number of needles in the packs to be used, and the circulator records the number on a count sheet.

During surgery, as each needle package is opened, the scrub person verifies that it contains the correct number of needles. If the number is not correct, the package is handed to the circulator, who isolates it from the field and subtracts the number from the count sheet.

Open needle packages are kept in a basin separate from other items to aid checking if a count is incorrect. The scrub person retains broken needles and blades in their entirety. If a needle or blade is flipped off the field, the circulator retrieves it and isolates it off the field. Used needles are kept on a needle-disposal pad. When a pad is full, the scrub person may hand it to the circulator, who counts the needles on the pad, verifies the count with the scrub person, and subtracts it from the total remaining on the sterile field.

As with sponges, closing counts are taken first when closure of the incision begins, and again when skin closure begins. Results are reported to the surgeon.

If a count is incorrect, the team follows the same procedure as for an incorrect sponge count. If the tally has too many needles, the scrub nurse hands the circulator the basin of open needle packages. The scrub person and circulator then count the unopened packages together. These two numbers plus the number of needles used should match the number recorded on the count sheet. The count is entered in the operative record and signed by the circulator. Used needles are disposed of properly to prevent injury to hospital personnel.

As with sponge counts, names of relief personnel are entered in the operative record.

INSTRUMENT COUNTS

Before surgery, the sterile instrument set is placed on the back table. The top rack of instruments is removed from the pan and placed on a rolled towel. Knife handles, towel clips, suction tips, tissue forceps, and sponge sticks are removed and placed on the back table.

The scrub nurse and circulator count the instruments. The circulator calls off the instruments from the count sheet. The scrub person points to each instrument and counts aloud. The circulator records the number on the count sheet.

During surgery, instruments added to the field are counted aloud by the scrub person, observed by the circulator, and recorded on the count sheet. If an instrument falls off the sterile field, the circulator retrieves it, shows it to the scrub nurse, and isolates it from the field. Then he or she records it on the sheet as being off the field.

The closing count is taken when closure begins. Results are reported to the surgeon. If the count is incorrect, personnel follow the same procedure as for incorrect sponge and needle counts.

THE NURSE'S LEGAL RESPONSIBILITY

Recent data from healthcare associations indicate a significant rise in frequency and severity of liability claims (3). As malpractice and liability suits have grown in number, courts have tended to assign liability to individuals both directly and indirectly involved with surgical procedures (4). Leaving a sponge or other foreign object inside a patient has been taken as virtual proof of negligence or malpractice (3). Since means for keeping count of sponges, sharps, and other surgical items are readily available, there is little or no justification for operating room procedures that omit such precautions.

Counting is part of the professional nurse's responsibility for patient safety; moreover, it is an area of legal accountability. Nurses can no longer take the attitude that the surgeon bears total responsibility for their actions as "captain of the ship." Under this traditional operating room doctrine, nurses were considered "borrowed servants." That is, while the operation was in progress, the surgeon was considered in command, and the nurses, although hospital employees, were temporarily under the surgeon's sole authority. Courts now recognize that nurses have independent areas of responsibility in the operating room. The "captain-of-the-ship" doctrine has weakened, especially in the area of counts. Nurses and hospitals are being held liable.

When a patient sues in a surgical case, a judge or jury decides whether there has been negligence on the part of the personnel involved. In reaching a decision, they examine what is considered to be the standard of care for healthcare facilities and for the professions involved. One test of negligence is whether the professionals involved exercised the degree of care that other reasonable professionals would have exercised. The same would be considered for institutions. When a foreign body is left in a patient and the patient sues, the courts are likely to examine, first, whether the hospital had a counting policy and, second, whether the nurses followed the policy. When negligence is found in such a case, the hospital, not the surgeon, will probably be held liable, as the employer of the nurses, whose duty it is to executive a correct count.

A 1977 ruling by the Texas Supreme Court illustrates how the captain-of-the-ship doctrine is breaking down. The decision came in *Sparger* v *Worley Hospital et al. Texas* (547 SW 2d 582). A sponge was left in a patient's abdominal cavity. The count, performed by the scrub nurse and circulating nurse, did not show a missing sponge. The nurses were employees of the institution, not of the surgeon performing the operation. The institution had written policies and procedures for the duties of scrub nurse and circulator, which included sponge counts.

The original trial court held that the hospital, as the nurses' employer, was liable. The hospital appealed, saying the surgeon should be held responsible as captain of the ship. The state supreme court turned down the appeal, saying the doctrine was a false rule of law. The court found instead that, as hospital employees, the nurses were obligated to follow the institution's policies, which specified a sponge count (5). The decision, as Regan pointed out, does not mean that surgeons are never liable for the actions of nurses. When nurses are employed directly by the surgeon instead of the hospital, they still are considered "borrowed servants" (5). Nevertheless, the case did emphasize that nurses can be held liable for their own actions and that they do have a legal duty to follow hospital policy.

Professional standards are used by courts to measure whether personnel have been negligent. Standards provide a guideline for what is considered a reasonable degree of care within the field. The AORN-recommended practices for sponge, needle, and instrument counts, although voluntary, are considered the standard for when and how counts should be performed in the operating room. They are a way that perioperative nurses indicate to society that they are self-regulating professionals. In turn, the recommended practices may be used by those who are attempting to determine whether nurses have met the expected standards of conduct.

WHY NEEDLE AND INSTRUMENT COUNTS?

Nurses often ask if needle and instrument counts are necessary, because some operating rooms do not require them. Both counts, however, should be part of the routine in every operating room because of the principles of patient safety.

Some nurses object to needle counts as time consuming and complex. Hundreds of needles may be used on a case, and needle packages of different types do not contain a standard number of needles. These nurses believe the probability of an incorrect count is high, even though a needle may not, in fact, be missing. Their objections do not outweigh the merits of doing needle counts. The process need not be time consuming, because the scrub person and circulator should be counting needles continuously throughout the case. A well-organized count, using the system described, should keep incorrect counts to a minimum.

Instrument counts are the most controversial. The principal argument against them is that they are too time consuming, extending the time of the pa-

tient's anesthesia. Some argue that the occurrence of instruments left in wounds is so rare that counts are not justified.

But what happens when an instrument remains in the body? In one case, a patient had had a cholecystectomy. The procedure was uneventful, but six days later the bowel obstructed because a loop of the bowl had slipped through a ring of a Kelly clamp that had been left in the wound. The patient was taken back to surgery, given general anesthesia once again, and the clamp was removed. He died several days later of acute hepatitis. Given the seriousness of such an incident, developing an instrument count procedure is well worth it, even if such cases are uncommon.

As with other types of counts, organization and efficiency are the keys to preventing delays. Instrument counts cannot be done properly until instrument sets are standardized. Generally, instrument sets should contain only the minimum number of instruments required for the typical case. Extra instruments that the surgeon requests can be counted and added separately. Having an instrument-counting sheet such as that in Figure 21.3 expedites the process. The circulating nurse need write in only the number of those instruments used on the case.

After instrument sets are standardized, instrument counting should not begin until the staff has had a chance to practice and become thoroughly familiar with the procedure. Staff may wish to visit other hospitals where instrument counts are done to see how they mastered the process. In addition, staff may practice with mock setups so that they become accustomed to counting in the proper sequence. Nurses who have implemented their system gradually and deliberately report that they do not have problems with delays.

Some institutions believe it is acceptable to take x-rays of every surgical patient rather than to perform counts. This is inappropriate. Counting *can* be done efficiently. And it is not necessary or wise to expose patients to extra radiation.

Nurses should not underestimate their role in developing count policies and carrying them out. Counts are not a trivial matter. They are a crucial aspect of assuring the patient's safety while he or she is under their care in the operating room. A well-developed policy is the backbone of an enforceable and consistent system. If a hospital does not have a count policy, one should be instituted. If an institution does have a policy, nurses should be aware that it is their legal and professional responsibility to abide by it.

INSTRUMENT COUNT SHEET OPERATING ROOM

NAME _____

DATE _____

Instruments	First Count	Add	Off Field	FINAL		Needle	Umb Tape	Clips	Blades
Knife Handles									
Scissors									
Pickups									
Needleholders									
Mosquitoes - CVD									
Mosquitoes - ST									
Criles - CVD									
Criles - ST									
Crawfords									
Allis									
Kockers									
Peans									
Babcocks									
Penningtons									
Tonsils									
Rt. Angles									
Metal Suctions & Parts									
Sponge Sticks						Laps	Raytec	Peanuts	Cotton oids
Kidney Pedicle									
Lung Clamps									
Towel Clips									
Balfour Sidewall Blades & Screw									
G.I. SPECS									
Doyans ST & CVD Rubber Pieces									
Shoe Strings									
Colostomy Rod									
DeMartel Clamps & Pts.									
Allen Kochers									
Glassman Bowel Clamps									
Debakey Bowel Clamps									
G.B. INSTRUMENTS									
Dilators									
Probes									
Stone Forceps									
Trochar									
GYN SPECS									
Heaneys									
Tenaculums									
C.V. TRAY									
C.V. Clamps									
Bulldogs									
Rummel Tourniquet & rubber pieces									
Nerve Hook									
Freer Elevator									
Penfield									
Clip Appliers									
Chest Retractor & Parts									

FIGURE 21.3. Instrument count sheet. (Permission given by University of Colorado Health Sciences Center.)

REFERENCES

1. St. Paul Fire and Marine Insurance Company. *Hospital Update Yearly Report.* Wichita, KS: St. Paul Fire and Marine,' 1990.

2. Association of Operating Room Nurses. *AORN Standards and Recommended Practices for Perioperative Nursing—1992,* pp. III:19-1. Denver: AORN, 1992.

3. Lile, Barbara A. "Instrument counts: Juries won't buy excuses." *OR Manager* 1(7):3, 1985.

4. Murphy, Ellen K. "Incorrect counts: Surgeon's negligence does not absolve nurses from liability." *AORN J* 43(4):918–924, 1986.

5. Regan, W. A. "Texas court holds OR nurses agents of hospitals." *AORN J* 26:458, 1977.

Suggested Readings

"Can doctor rely on your sponge count?" *Legal Lesson of the Month, Seminars on Nursing Law.* Providence, RI: Medica Press, 1989.

Fogg, Dorothy M. "Recommendations for instrument counts; testing sterilizers with biological indicators;

organizational structure of OR." *AORN J* 49(6):1667–1672, 1989.

Murphy, Ellen K. "Liability for waived OR inaccurate instrument counts." *AORN J* 50(1):14–19, 1989.

Murphy, Ellen K. "Nurses' liability for inaccurate counts." *AORN J* 51(4):1067–1069, 1990.

22

Documenting Patient Care

The nurse records and reports nursing care.

The care patients receive during the perioperative period must be recorded to provide other members of the healthcare team with that information and details of the patient's response during surgery. This chapter examines documentation as a process that starts with the decision to have surgery and in some cases continues after the patient has returned home. Documentation includes followup after hospital discharge. The rationale for communicating important information by way of medical records and reports is discussed, as well as the responsibilities involved in keeping an accurate picture of the patient on permanent file. The sources of data, types of information that should be retained, and how to record the data are included.

DOCUMENTATION: A PROCESS

A surgical patient's record begins at the physician's office or in the hospital clinic. The record is kept up to date by the physician and nurse, who include the patient's medical, social, and psychologic status during visits to the office. When the patient decides to have surgery, personnel at the office or clinic call the operating room to schedule the procedure. This is usually the first contact with the hospital or ambulatory care setting.

Data recorded in the OR scheduling book include the patient's name, sex, surgical procedure, surgeon, and anesthesiologist. Other pertinent comments may also be written, such as weight, height,

or physical disabilities. The data entered in the scheduling book for all patients are used to produce the surgery schedule. The surgery schedule is likely to be the first place the perioperative nurse will look in planning for the surgical patient.

The record begins when the patient is admitted to the facility or is seen in preadmission testing (PAT). Patients scheduled for outpatient or ambulatory surgery and those admitted the morning of surgery have diagnostic tests completed at a prescheduled time prior to the operation. Data about the patient may be obtained during the preadmission visit or when the patient arrives in the outpatient department. Ambulatory surgery centers have established admission protocols that are communicated to the patient by telephone or by the physician's office. Admission data include information about the date, time, and mode of admission plus nursing observations and examination, habits of daily living, and medical history. The nursing observation admission note, under physical status and general appearance, might state "Elderly man showing no signs of shortness of breath, has slight edema in both ankles." Under emotional status and behavior the nurse might record, "Mild anxiety stated by patient. He does understand why he is hospitalized." Other chart forms might be the progress record for nurses and allied health personnel, and the problem list. In the record the nurse states the mode of admission and begins identifying problems using the format that is standard in the particular institution.

TABLE 22.1. Information Documented on the Intraoperative Plan of Care

Nursing Diagnosis	Outcome	Plan	Implementation	Evaluation
1. Potential for respiratory problems secondary to chronic COPD and emphysema.	1. The patient will maintain present respiratory status.	1. Explain coughing, deep breathing, give rationale for postop implementation.	1. Explained rationale and demonstrated exercises with patient.	1. Postop: patient doing exercises with encouragement.
2. Potential for neuromuscular problems secondary to osteoporosis, steroids, and T7-T12 fracture.	2. The patient will maintain current neuromuscular comfort.	2. Have several people available for positioning. Use care when moving patient. Use padding.	2. Assistance available when moving. Foam padding used.	2. Postop: patient not experiencing neuromuscular problems.

In some instances, patients will have had preadmission laboratory tests, radiologic studies, or other diagnostic studies, and the results are made available at admission.

When admitted, the patient is assigned a bed on a surgical unit or received in a short-stay unit. At this time, members of the healthcare team begin to record information on the patient record. Nurses on the surgical unit or in the short-stay area complete nursing interview forms with information about daily routines at home, allergies, likes and dislikes, and health problems, including present illness. A nursing history is taken, covering such subjects as functional and dysfunctional health patterns. This is different from the medical history, which includes the medical diagnosis; physician's history and physical examination, including history of the present illness and previous medical and surgical history; and findings of laboratory examinations. In contrast, the nursing history covers not only the patient's health problems but factors such as emotional and social states, which may have a bearing on surgery and recovery. A nursing history may take a variety of forms, depending on the institution. With the pressures of cost containment, nurses are attempting to develop standardized forms. The nurse documents the patient's reason for being admitted to the facility, the history of the current problem, previous hospitalizations and illnesses, observations of the patient's condition, mental status, allergies, medications, and any prosthesis the patient might use. A review of systems, health patterns, and a typical-day profile may also be included, depending on hospital procedure.

The surgical consent form is completed by the patient and surgeon and validated by the nurse. Physician's orders are in the record and provide data about the patient's diet, diagnostic tests, medica-

tions, and preoperative preparation. All information in the record is later used to evaluate the care provided and determine its effectiveness. Each health team member has the responsibility for recording complete and accurate facts.

In performing the preoperative assessment, the perioperative nurse analyzes all the data obtained thus far. These data provide clues to what further information is needed from the patient during the assessment to complete a plan of care that will meet the patient's individual needs. The intraoperative plan of care is the major contribution the perioperative nurse makes to the patient's record because it describes nursing diagnoses, expected outcomes, and activities to be implemented during surgery. On it, the nurse notes skin condition, neurologic status, allergies, anxiety, emotional distress, physical disabilities, and preexisting disease processes. In some institutions, the form used for the plan of care incorporates information about the surgeon, procedure, previous surgery, preoperative diagnosis, and vital signs.

Consider, for example, a patient who is scheduled for implantation of a Harrington rod. The patient has a fracture at T7-T12. In addition, he is hypertensive and has chronic obstructive pulmonary disease, arthritis, and osteoporosis. Two potential problems the perioperative nurse has identified, treated, and documented are illustrated in Table 22.1. Information for completing the intraoperative plan of care is obtained from the unit nurses, the patient record, the patient, and family members.

The purpose of the plan of care is to provide a guide for those involved in actually giving care. Keep in mind these five points: (1) the plan should be consistent with the overall medical regimen; (2) human and material resources called for in the plan must be available; (3) the plan is based on the immediate needs of this patient; (4) the plan reflects participation of the patient, family, and other members of the healthcare team; and (5) the plan includes the nursing diagnosis, patient outcomes, and activities to meet the established outcomes. The format of the perioperative plan of care should be as close as possible to the one used in other areas of the facility so that all personnel will understand the entries fully. This will also aid in planning postoperative care and may help promote continuity of care.

During the patient's admission to the surgical or short-stay unit, personnel review a preoperative checklist to verify that prerequisites have been met. This summary sheet is an addition to the plan of care and is completed by nursing personnel preparing the patient and verified by the nurse in the operating room. It assists the perioperative nurse because vital signs, allergies, and information from the history, physical, and laboratory tests are in one place, so the nurse does not have to look on many forms to find all these data.

In the operating room, other forms are introduced to document activities that take place during surgery:

- The anesthesia record specifies the time anesthesia begins and ends, the operative procedure, preoperative and postoperative diagnoses, and a record of the anesthetic agents used and the patient's physiologic response.
- Operating room nurses make their notes in another record, sometimes called the operative nursing record. Focusing on nursing care during the surgical procedure, this form may include sponge, needle, and instrument counts; grounding location for the electrosurgical units; monitors used; tourniquet location, times, and pressure set; implants and lot numbers; dressings; drains; specimens; cultures; medications; patient position on the operating room table; and types of safety devices such as hand restraints, heel protectors, and safety belt. The record usually allows space for nurses' comments.
- A third record, called the progress notes, completed by the surgeon after the procedure, gives a detailed account of the surgical technique.
- When the patient is transferred from the operating room to the postanesthesia care unit, another record is initiated that documents the patient's condition during emergence from anesthesia.

With properly kept OR records, other personnel can readily determine what happened to the patient during the surgical procedure. They can see the patient's physiologic as well as emotional responses to surgery. The operative documentation of activities and patient responses shows a continuous picture of the patient's condition. Thus there is no interruption in the documentation process while the patient is in surgery.

The perioperative nurse completes the documentation at the time of postoperative followup. This report includes observations of the wound site, evaluation of the patient's response to surgery, and the patient's perception of his or her care. The patient's and family's perception of care should be solicited in an effort to measure outcome attainment from their point of view. The documentation process is congruent with the nursing process in that the patient record depicts application of the nursing process throughout. During the postoperative followup interview and evaluation of the patient, the perioperative nurse records the patient's progress based on the preoperative nursing diagnosis and established outcomes. Documentation at this point reflects effectiveness of nursing care and the patient's response.

Nurses in postoperative units continue to document care throughout the patient's stay. The final recording is the discharge summary, which includes plans for the patient at home. Plans for discharge start at admission and are considered throughout the patient's stay. For patients who are discharged directly from the postanesthesia care unit, outpatient department, or ambulatory surgery center, the nurse provides postoperative instructions and documents that these instructions have been reviewed with the patient and family. In some instances nurses do postoperative telephone interviews to determine patient outcomes.

SOURCES OF DATA

The documentation of nursing activities furnishes information about what the nurse does for the patient and about the patient's condition and response to care. Data are obtained and recorded through observation, written records, and asking about the patient's perception of care.

Observation

As a guide to observation, the nurse should:

1. know what to look for when observing and inspecting the patient
2. conduct a systematic inspection

3. never jump to conclusions, but ask what contributing factors might exist and what else could be going on

4. never make judgments based on preconceived ideas

5. examine personal feelings about the patient and the patient's problems

6. use touch, when appropriate, during observation and inspection

7. follow up on hunches; be certain to obtain all the facts

8. continue to observe and inspect throughout the patient's hospital stay

9. identify the patient's problem first, then gather additional supporting data that will assist in writing the plan of care, and

10. understand why observing and inspecting are so important and how they relate to the total nursing process.

Written Records

Written records or reports are another source of data. As discussed earlier, the perioperative nurse bases documentation on a variety of other written records, beginning with the surgery schedule and including notes from the unit nurse, physician, and other health team members. It is crucial that documentation be in writing so that it can be communicated easily to other members of the healthcare team. Sharing information promotes continuity of care because at each stage of care, personnel will know what has been done before. They will not be planning care in a vacuum.

The perioperative nurse who records the facts in writing is also demonstrating accountability. Documented care is a legal record of the nurse's actions and the patient's response to those actions. A written record can be compared with the institution's standards of practice to evaluate the quality of care. Still another reason for writing the information down is so it can be retrieved for research and other uses, which will ultimately improve care.

Many nurses ask what they should record. In general, all basic facts are documented. Specifically, the nurse should write

1. what is seen: bleeding, color, amount of fluid, type of drainage

2. what is heard: chest rales, moaning, patient complaints

3. what is smelled: acetone breath, feces, malodorous drainage

4. what is felt: body heat, distended stomach, motion at a fracture site

5. what he or she does for the patient and the patient's response to treatment (e.g., "45 minutes after meperidine hydrochloride 100 mg is given for pain in the right ankle, the patient states he still has had no relief.")

6. what he or she does to protect the patient: place foam pads under heels, secure safety belt, place on egg crate mattress

7. what he or she did to the patient's private property to protect it from loss (e.g., "Gave hearing aid to wife, placed dentures in bedside stand.")

Patient Perception

The patient's perception is as important as observation when documenting. The patient can furnish information about his or her physical and emotional condition that is available from no other source. Careful observation and questioning assist the nurse in gathering pertinent data. In evaluating care, for example, the nurse should ask simple questions such as, "Did your family know where to wait during your surgery?" "Did your doctor explain the surgery to you?" "Did anyone communicate to you the reason the surgery took longer than expected?" The patient's and family's perceptions indicate their degree of satisfaction with the care given. Each time the nurse visits the patient, additional data are obtained for reporting the patient's response to surgery on the nurse's notes, progress notes, or other forms in the patient record.

CHARTING FORMATS

Every hospital has its own format for charting. It varies depending on the philosophy of nursing and the methods chosen. Some types of nursing documentation are source-oriented recording, problem-oriented recording, the SOAP format (Fig. 22.1), baseline recording, and the APIE format.

Source-Oriented Recording

Source-oriented recording is a description of what happens to the patient in narrative format. It depicts a sequence of nursing activities performed and is written chronologically. The forms generally used with this type of documentation are operating room nurse's notes, surgery worksheets, flow sheets, and the operative record. For example, the operating room nurse's notes might say the following:

DATE	TIME	PROB #	PHYS PROB#	PROBLEM TITLE AND S.O.A.P. FORMAT (S-Subjective O-Objective A-Analysis P-Plan)
10/7/92	1530			Admitted ambulatory an elderly appearing gentleman
		1		S: "I'm here to find out what's wrong with me."
				O: Admitted for surgical removal of recurrent
				carcinoma of Ⓛ lateral tongue and
				alveolar ridge
				A: Patient with jaw mass scheduled for
				surgery
				P: ① Encourage patient to express concerns.
				② Explain hospital routines.
				③ Include family in information and
				instruction.
				④ Validate understanding of surgical
				procedure. G. Hodge, RN

Allied Health Personnel
PROGRESS RECORD

(Addressograph)

FIGURE 22.1. SOAP format.

5/4/93 4:30 A.M.
Mr. Clark admitted to OR from unit. placed in supine position on operating room table. Foam pads placed under both heels. Heels slightly reddened due to pressure of hard mattress.

Karen Crawford, RN

Problem-Oriented Recording

Problem-oriented medical recording (POMR) is a popular method. All the patient's problems are recorded, as well as the extent to which they are resolved (Fig. 22.2). This system usually incorporates the nurse's notes, physician record, and documentation by other members of the healthcare team. For example:

5/4/93 7:30 A.M.
1. Anxiety. Expresses fear of anesthesia. States, "I am afraid I will not wake up after my surgery." Eyes blink, perspires while expressing feelings. Continue to allow patient to express feelings. Encourage him to walk up and down the hall and see other patients who have had surgery.

Karen Crawford, RN

SOAP and APIE

Another type of recording is the SOAP or SOAPIE (subjective, objective, analysis, and planning). The IE stand for implementation and evaluation. Similar to this is the APIE (assessment, planning, implementation, and evaluation). Both approaches are variations of the POMR method. They reflect the nursing process and provide a good framework for documentation. For example:

5/4/93 7/30 A.M.

A: Anxiety. Patient states he is afraid he will not wake up after surgery. Perspires and blinks eyes excessively.

P. Encourage patient to express feelings of fear and walk in hall to observe postoperative patients.

I. Nurse from OR talked with patient. Anesthesiologist reviewed type of anesthesia and explained what would happen during his anesthesia.

E: Patient states he is confident that he will return from the OR.

Karen Crawford, RN

Whatever the system, the general principles are the same. Documentation must include time and date care was given; the signature of the person giving or observing care; notations placed in chronologic order; use of uniform abbreviations; and notes that are clear, concise, unambiguous, and accurate. Above all, notes must be legible. If a patient refuses treatment, the nurse has a responsibility to encourage compliance with the medical regimen. If the patient chooses not to have the treatment after the nurse has provided adequate rationale, the nurse must record what the patient refused and why (1).

Dos and Don'ts of Charting

The following dos and don'ts of charting for the perioperative nurse are taken from *Reporting and Documenting Patient Care* (2).

Dos: When charting patient care given in the operative period the nurse should:

- read previous nurse's notes before giving care
- imprint name, identification number, date, and time on every sheet
- always use ink for recording data
- write legibly
- use the appropriate form for charting
- describe symptoms or patient conditions accurately and completely
- use patient's own words if possible
- use acceptable, hospital-approved abbreviations whenever possible
- use concise, descriptive terms
- be definite in descriptions and wording
- begin each phrase with a capital
- begin each new entry on a separate line
- document the need for nursing action
- record all nursing care provided before surgery, in the operating room, and afterward, and
- sign the completed record.

Don'ts: When documenting patient care given, the nurse should not:

- record without checking the name on the record
- record on blank forms
- use ordinary paper
- use pencil
- back-date entry
- tamper with or add to previous charting
- skip lines or leave spaces
- erase

DATE	PROB #	PHYS PROB#	DATE OF ONSET	ACTIVE PROBLEMS	DATE RESOLVED	INACTIVE OR RESOLVED PROBLEMS
10/7/92	A-1			Mild Anxiety Related to		
	A-			Jaw mass		
	A-2			Lack of Knowledge About	10/7/92	
	A-			Surgical procedure		7/6/85 Circulatory
	A-					problem due to
	A-					phlebitis
	A-					
	A-					
	A-					
	A-					
	A-					
	A-					
	A-					
	A-					
	A-					
	A-					
	A-					
	A-					

Name	Init.	Name	Init.	Name	Init.	Name	Init.
G. Dodge	gD						

(Addressograph)

FIGURE 22.2.   Problem-oriented medical record.

- chart in advance of nursing actions
- use broad, nonspecific terms (e.g., "good condition," "tolerated well")
- use medical terminology unless absolutely sure of meaning
- rely on memory (should chart immediately)
- discard nurse's notes or records with errors (should use specific error-correction format)
- repeat in narrative what is recorded in other parts in chart, or
- use imprecise terms (e.g., "appears to," "seems to," or "apparently").

Computerized Documentation

The operative record shown in Figure 22.3 has been designed to obtain data that are then keyed into a computer. These data create a patient record and store that information for future uses. Nursing documentation is retained and can be recalled when needed.

Computers can even be used to complete nursing documentation forms and the operative record while in the operating room (3). Instead of written documentation, nursing documentation is completed by using a computer during the procedure. Advantages of using such a system are improved legibility, greater precision, easier data retrieval, and facilitation of quality improvement activities and other studies.

RECOMMENDED PRACTICES FOR DOCUMENTATION

Perioperative nurses have a responsibility to the patient to record observations and nursing care provided. This responsibility is reinforced by the Association of Operating Room Nurses (AORN) and the Joint Commission on Accreditation of Healthcare Organizations (JCAHO).

AORN's "Competency Statements in Perioperative Nursing" (4) identify communication/documentation of various types of data as criteria for demonstrating competency in perioperative nursing. The data to be documented include the patient's physical and psychosocial health status, nursing diagnosis, goals, plan of care, transfer, patient teaching, intraoperative care, and postoperative followup. Intraoperative care includes maintenance of the sterile field, provision of equipment and supplies, counts, administration of drugs, monitoring the patient's physiologic response to surgery, environmental control measures, provisions for the protection of

the patient's rights, and nursing actions. Postoperatively, patient outcomes must be documented as a means of determining goal achievement; the results of nursing care are documented; and the reassessment process is communicated.

"Recommended Practices for Documentation of Perioperative Nursing Care" were developed by AORN as guidelines for documenting nursing care for each surgical procedure (5). AORN recommends that the patient's record reflect assessment, planning, implementation, evaluation, and expected outcomes. Table 22.2 lists items that AORN recommends for inclusion in perioperative documentation (5).

These are very broad recommendations. Each institution should establish documentation policies that meet these recommendations. In addition, these policies and procedures should be reviewed annually and be readily available in the practice setting.

Perioperative nurses are finding that documentation requirements are being incorporated into operative nursing records, in order to meet standards set

TABLE 22.2. Items to Be Included in Perioperative Documentation

- Name, title, and signature of persons providing care
- Evidence of a patient assessment upon arrival to the perioperative suite
- Skin condition on arrival and discharge from the suite
- Presence/disposition of sensory aids and prosthetic devices
- Patient's position and supports, and/or restraints used during the procedure
- Placement of the dispersive electrode pad and identification of the electrosurgical unit and settings
- Placement of electrocardiogram or other monitoring electrodes
- Medications, irrigations, and solutions administered or dispensed
- Specimens and cultures taken during the procedure
- Skin prep solutions, area prepared, and any reactions
- Placement of drains, catheters, packing, and dressings
- Placement of tourniquet cuff and person applying the cuff, pressure, time, and identification of the unit
- Urinary output and estimated blood loss (as appropriate)
- Placement of implants (i.e., tissue, inert or radioactive material inserted into a body cavity or grafted onto the tissue of the recipient), manufacturer, lot number, type, size, and other identifying information
- Occurrence and results of surgical item counts
- Time of discharge, disposition of patient, method of transfer, and patient status
- Intraoperative x-rays and fluoroscopy
- Wound classification
- Other direct patient care issues pertinent to patient outcomes

Date _____ Second Floor OR# □ 1 □ 2 □ 3 □ 4 □ 5 □ 6 □ 7 □ 8 □ 9 □ 10 □ 11
                                Third Floor OR# □ 1 □ 2 □ 3

PRE-SURGICAL PATIENT CONDITION	SURGERY CLASSIFICATION	TIME	
□ ALERT □ AGITATED	□ SCHEDULED □ EMERGENCY □ TRAUMA	ANESTHESIA START	ANESTHESIA STOP
□ DROWSY □ APPREHENSIVE	□ NON SCHEDULED □ OPEN HEART		
□ CONFUSED □ NON-RESPONSIVE	CALL CLASS □ YES □ NO	SURGERY START	SURGERY STOP
□ OTHER _____	ALLERGIES		

PROCEDURE _____
_____
_____
_____

Preop Diagnosis _____
_____

Postop Diagnosis _____
_____

LOCAL ANESTHESIA DEVICES	POSITION	POSITIONING DEVICES	
□ CARDIAC MONITOR □ YES □ NO	□ SUPINE □ JACKKNIFE	□ Eggcrate □ Knees Padded □ Chest Rolls	
□ OXYGEN □ YES □ NO	□ PRONE □ LITHOTOMY	□ Heels Padded □ Lam Rest Padded □ Bean Bag	
□ OXIMETER □ YES □ NO	□ KNEE-CHEST	□ Elbows Padded □ Axillary Roll □ Pad Between Legs	
ANESTHESIA TYPE	□ LAT □ L □ R □ TILT	□ Other _____	
□ GENERAL □ REGIONAL □ LOCAL □ STANDBY □ NONE	□ OTHER _____	□ Safety Strap Applied	

ANESTHESIOLOGIST _____ CRNA _____

RESIDENT _____ MED. STUDENT _____

Team	1	2	3
Surgeon			
First Assistant			
Second Assistant			
Third Assistant			
Fourth Assistant			
Teaching Assistant			
Dictation			
Time Started			
Time Ended			
Duration			

SKIN PREP
□ IODOPHOR □ NONE □ OTHER _____

COUNTS
SPONGE: □ CORRECT   □ INCORRECT   □ N/A

NEEDLE: □ CORRECT   □ INCORRECT   □ N/A

FINAL COUNT: Scrub Nurse _____

CIRCULATING NURSE: (Signature) _____

X-RAY TAKEN □ YES □ NO

EQUIPMENT USED	
ELECTRO SURGICAL CLINICAL ENGINEERING UNIT # _____	

READ BY _____ □ NEG □ POS
SURGEON NOTIFIED _____

GROUND PLATE PLACED BY _____
SITE _____ POST OP SKIN □ POS □ NEG
K-THERMIA CLINICAL ENGINEERING UNIT # _____
TEMP _____ POST OP SKIN □ POS □ NEG
TOURNIQUET CLINICAL ENGINEERING UNIT # _____
SITE _____ PRESSURE _____ POST OP SKIN □ POS □ NEG
OTHER _____
_____

SPECIMENS
□ PATHOLOGY □ RFS   □ OTHER
□ BACTI-LAB □ CORD BLD   _____
□ CYTOLOGY   □ NONE   _____

DRAINS/PACKS	URINARY CATHETER
□ Chest Tube □ Jackson Pratt	Type & Size _____
□ Hemovac □ Penrose □ None	Color _____
□ Gastrostomy _____	Character _____
□ Packing _____	Inserted By _____
□ Other _____	□ From Nursing Unit □ None

IRRIGATION / MEDICATIONS
_____
_____
_____
_____
_____

IMPLANTS / GRAFTS	OUT-PT. INSTRUCTIONS GIVEN
□ YES □ NO	WRITTEN □ YES □ NO

DISPOSITION OF PATIENT
□ ICU □ PACU □ PT ROOM □ MORGUE □ DISCH HOME
□ OUT-PT SURG ED □ OTHER _____

NURSING PROGRESS NOTES | _____
_____
_____
_____

SCRUB NURSE: _____
CIRCULATING NURSE: _____

ADMINISTRATIVE CONTROL | A B C D E F G H I J O N | 1 2 3 4 5 6 7 8 9 10 11 12 | WD CLASS □ 1 □ 2 □ 3 □ 4 □ 5 □ 6

LOMA LINDA UNIVERSITY MEDICAL CENTER   PATIENT IDENTIFICATION

OPERATIVE NURSING RECORD

04-0378 (7-86)   White- Chart   Yellow - Operating Room   Pink - Medical Records

FIGURE 22.3.   Operative nursing record records pertinent information pertaining to each surgical procedure in such a way that it can be inserted into the computer for storage and retrieval.

forth by JCAHO and other agencies that license healthcare institutions.

LEGAL PROTECTION

The patient care record is a legal document that may be used in case of a lawsuit. It shows the series of events leading up to the patient's complaint about care and aids in determining if anyone is to blame. The courts may use the record to prove what information the staff had available in giving care. Records are also used to show if important information was transferred from one department to another.

Good documentation provides protection for both patients and nurses. Nurses can protect themselves by reporting specific facts and avoiding generalities. Instead of writing "Feet swollen," they should write, "Feet swollen; warmth, color, and movement satisfactory." This makes it clear that the nurse is aware the swelling is not dangerous. Noting that the patient is in "good condition" could mean anything. Rather, the nurse should ask, "What facts about the patient led me to the conclusion that he or she was in good condition?"

The patient record should show continuity of care. Flow sheets depict all activities, the times each activity is performed, and the patient's response on a continuing basis.

Each healthcare facility should have a written policy and procedure for documenting care. The policy will vary from institution to institution, but should include:

1. what to do when the nurse cannot reach the doctor when needed, and how and where this action should be recorded
2. what and where to report when the nurse has given a medication or fluids inappropriate for a patient
3. what to do when the doctor gives an oral order or unclear written order not to resuscitate a terminally ill patient
4. when and where to record when a patient refuses medication or other prescribed treatment, and
5. what to do when the nurse believes standing orders are no longer valid for medication or treatment being given.

The nurse's documentation should reflect that he or she followed established institution policy and what the result was. These should be recorded in proper time sequence.

Another way to protect him- or herself legally is to chart at various times throughout the patient's stay or the shift the nurse is working. Chronologic entries show that the nurse has recorded care and patient responses. In the operating room, if the procedure is long, the nurse should chart continuous monitoring of physiologic responses to surgery, position on the operating room table, and other nursing measures. The nurse's full name—not just an initial—should be placed on each form.

In order to correct an entry in the patient record, the nurse should simply put one line through it. The nurse should not try to cross out the entire notation and should not try to cover up mistakes. If a computerized documentation system is used, provisions must be made that define who will have access to the data, how corrections in the records will be made, who will make the corrections, what security mechanisms are built into the system to prevent unauthorized access, and what mechanism prevents erasing all or part of the record (4).

The focus of documentation should be on communicating important data about the patient from one member of the healthcare team to another. If the nurse describes nursing actions and how the patient responded as objectively as possible, documentation will be accurate and complete.

REFERENCES

1. Eggland, E. T. "Charting: How and why to document your care daily—and fully." *Nurs 80* 10 (February):38–43, 1980.
2. Manuel, B. J. *Reporting and Documenting Patient Care: OR Modular Independent Learning Systems.* Denver: AORN, 1980.
3. Latz, Paula Anne. "Computerized nursing documentation systems: Development, implementation." *AORN J* 56(2):300–311, 1992.
4. Association of Operating Room Nurses. "Competency statements in perioperative nursing." *AORN Standards and Recommended Practices for Perioperative Nursing—1992.* pp. I:2–1 to I:2–12. Denver: AORN, 1992.
5. Association of Operating Room Nurses. "Recommended Practices for Documentation of perioperative nursing care." *AORN Standards and Recommended Practices for Perioperative Nursing—1992.* pp. III:4–1 to III:4–4. Denver: AORN, 1992.

SUGGESTED READINGS

Joint Commission on Accreditation of Healthcare Organizations. "Nursing care standards." *Accreditation Manual for Hospitals.* Oakbrook Terrace, IL: JCAHO, 1991.
Pobojewski, Barbara J., Neper, Nancy, Guzzo, Patricia M., and Beadle, Patricia K. "Documenting nursing process in the perioperative setting: Continuity of care, patient evaluation." *AORN J* 56(1):98–112, 1992.
Poss, Carol. "Outpatient surgery documentation: Incorporating nursing diagnoses." *AORN J* 53(1):81–92, 1991.

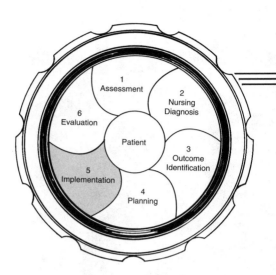

23

Postanesthesia Care

The nurse monitors the patient's emergence from anesthesia.

The origin of postanesthesia care dates back to 1846, when ether was introduced as an anesthetic agent. And as early as 1863, Florence Nightingale recognized the need for an area near the operating room where patients could be observed until they recovered from the immediate effects of surgery. In 1923, a three-bed neurosurgical recovery room was created at Johns Hopkins Hospital to monitor patients following neurosurgery.

During the 1940s, the need for more intense postoperative monitoring surfaced. The advent of major surgeries, a developing knowledge base of postanesthesia complications, and a nursing shortage during World War II are credited with the founding of postanesthesia care units (PACUs). At the end of the 1940s, an eleven-year Anesthesia Study Commission reported that approximately one-half of the deaths occurring during the first twenty-four hours after surgery could have been prevented. Following this report, PACUs were viewed as a necessity (1).

By 1970, invasive monitoring equipment such as arterial lines and pulmonary artery pressure catheters were introduced, along with the trend to provide postoperative ventilatory support and oxygenation. This increased the necessity for skilled PACU nurses who could manage the more routine patients recovering from anesthesia, as well as the recovery of critically ill patients requiring intensive monitoring.

The importance of postanesthesia care has been recognized at both state and national levels. In 1980, the American Society of Post Anesthesia Nurses

(ASPAN) was organized, recognizing postanesthesia care as a nursing specialty.

The postanesthesia recovery period may be the most dangerous period of the patient's hospital stay, due to the stress of both the surgical procedure and the anesthetics; therefore, the immediate postanesthetic phase places multifaceted demands on the PACU nurse. The PACU nurse is challenged with the goal of returning the patient to his or her preoperative physiological state.

A trial judge stated the functions and responsibilities of a PACU and its staff as follows (2):

> The function of this room is to provide highly specialized care, frequent and careful observation of patients who are under the influence of anesthesia. . . . Respiratory arrest is not an uncommon occurrence in the PAR [post anesthesia recovery] room and therefore the personnel in this room must be watchful and alert at all times in order to protect the patients in this labile and vulnerable stage. . . . [T]his is the most important room in the hospital and the one in which the patient requires the greatest attention because it is fraught with the greatest potential dangers to the patient. This known hazard carries with it, in my opinion, a high degree of duty owed by the hospital to the patient. As the dangers of risk are ever-present, there should be no relaxing of vigilance if one is to comply with the standard of care required in this room

The role of the PACU nurse will continue to change and expand, reflecting emerging trends toward less-invasive and outpatient surgery, same-day admissions, shorter hospital stays, and in-home postsurgical care, as well as healthcare cost-containment efforts. PACU nurses in hospital-based and free-standing ambulatory centers are becoming more involved with families. As hospital stays become shorter, family members become integral components of the caregiving team. It is not uncommon to send patients home on various types of medical treatments that used to be performed in the hospital setting. Patient and family education and counseling are becoming prominent aspects of the PACU nurse's role. Based on research findings showing that a patient's postanesthesia anxiety is reduced if family members visit the PACU, family members are now being allowed into this unit. More and more, healthcare providers are recognizing the important role of the patient's support system in the recovery process.

Inpatient and outpatient PACU designs must accommodate both Phase I and Phase II recovery of patients. Phase I areas, the critical recovery phase areas, should assure a patient's privacy while maintaining continual observation of all patients by all nursing staff. Phase II areas, less acute care areas, should assure ongoing protection of privacy and observation while accommodating a family support system and teaching.

In Fresno, California, a group of physicians have implemented an innovative network of postsurgical recovery centers. If necessary, these centers provide overnight care for patients who have undergone elective surgery and require nursing care and pain management for an extended period of time. The centers have been successful because most surgical procedures can be performed in a recovery care facility at lower cost and greater comfort to the patient than would be possible in a hospital setting (3).

Ambulatory surgery continues to be the wave of the future. As patient mix and acuity increase, nurses will be challenged to deliver quality care and teaching to patients who may be recovering at home. One thing remains evident: change is inevitable, and those who are adaptable will have the greatest success and satisfaction in PACU nursing now and in the future.

ASSESSMENT

The PACU is a critical care area. Most PACU patients are emerging from general anesthesia, which depresses their respiratory, circulatory, and central ner-

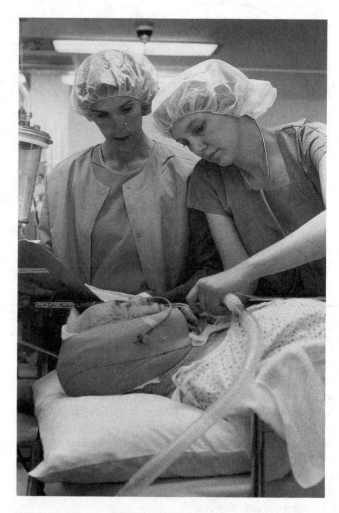

FIGURE 23.1.   When the patient is admitted to the postanesthesia care unit, the perioperative nurse reports his or her status, the type and extent of the surgical procedure, and other information pertinent to care in the PACU.

vous systems. Patients may have preexisting cardiovascular, respiratory, renal, or metabolic conditions which, with the added stress of surgery, further jeopardize their stability. In addition, the populations of many units include everyone from elderly patients to pediatric patients. Thus, PACU nurses must be proficient in patient assessment for all ages and disease entities.

When the patient arrives in the unit following surgery, the perioperative nurse and anesthesiologist provide relevant data to the PACU nurse (Fig. 23.1). The recovery process really begins in the OR, when the anesthesiologist initiates the reversal of the anesthetic agents. Clear communication between the PACU nurse and the anesthesiologist is imperative for adequate postoperative assessment, planning, and care of the patient.

The information to be obtained by the PACU nurse from the perioperative team is listed in Table 23.1.

TABLE 23.1.   Data to Ascertain from Perioperative Team

- Surgical procedure performed
- Urine output
- Estimated blood loss
- Complications related to the procedure
- Sensory or motor limitations
- Presence of a prosthesis
- History of present illness
- History of chronic illness
- Allergies
- Relevant preoperative laboratory tests and vital signs
- Type of anesthesia administered, including reversal agents, antibiotics, narcotics, etc.
- Duration of anesthesia
- Fluid replacement and type
- Invasive monitoring lines

TABLE 23.2.   Initial Assessment of the PACU Patient

A. Airway/Adequate Gas Exchange
1. Symmetry of chest expansion
2. Breath sounds and adequate air exchange
3. Adequate oxygen saturation (use pulse oximetry)
4. Rate and depth of respirations
5. Color of skin and mucous membranes
6. Presence of stridor or air hunger
7. Use of accessory muscles
8. Patency of mechanical airways such as nasal, oral, and endotracheal tubes
9. Need to position the jaw, head, or neck to facilitate air exchange

B. Circulatory
1. Rate and rhythm apically and from the monitor
2. Arterial blood pressure through noninvasive and invasive techniques if arterial line is present
3. If present, connect, calibrate, and record central venous pressure, arterial and pulmonary artery pressure
4. Temperature

C. Central Nervous System
1. Determine level of consciousness
    a. Responds to painful stimuli
    b. Responds to verbal stimuli but drifts off to sleep
    c. Awake and alert; oriented to person, place, and time

Initial assessment begins as soon as the patient arrives in the PACU. This first assessment covers the patient's respiratory, circulatory, and central nervous systems, as detailed in Table 23.2. Status of the surgical dressing is noted. Oxygen and/or ventilatory support is initiated, as well as cardiac monitoring and oximetry. All catheters, drains, and tubes are connected as ordered and are checked for proper functioning. Excessive drainage is emptied and recorded. Baseline pressure readings and waveforms are obtained and documented. Based on admission temperature, appropriate cooling or warming techniques are initiated.

The patient is positioned to maximize ventilation and prevent complications. The unconscious patient should be placed in a side lying position unless contraindicated due to the surgical procedure. This position facilitates airway patency, enhances drainage of secretions, and prevents aspiration. The side-lying position is also considered the safest for transfer from the OR to the PACU. Patients may benefit from elevating the head of the bed 30 to 45°, to facilitate chest expansion and improve ventilation. Patients who have had spinal anesthesia and/or hypotension should remain flat until the spinal recedes and/or blood pressure returns to their baseline. Positioning for safety includes good body alignment to prevent foot drop, stretch injuries, and pressure injury.

ASPAN standards recommend that the nurse:patient ratio for patients requiring life support systems include one nurse per patient, with a second nurse available. This nurse:patient ratio is critical upon admission to the PACU, when patient assessment and stabilization occur. Ideally, the nurse accepting the patient should take a report from the perioperative team and conduct the initial assessment, while the second nurse assists with airway management, con-

nects the equipment, and initiates physician's orders appropriate to the PACU. Most PACU patients require a minimum 2:1 nurse:patient ratio while the patient is unconscious and during emergence.

After determining stability of the respiratory and circulatory systems and level of consciousness, the nurse begins a more thorough assessment utilizing a systematic approach. The techniques of inspection, palpation, percussion, and auscultation are used to obtain objective data. These data are then compared with the preoperative data in order to determine deviations from baseline parameters.

Respiratory Assessment

The priorities of respiratory assessment are adequate gas exchange and patency of the airway, which are established immediately upon arrival to the PACU. Airway obstruction, hypoxemia, and hypercapnia are respiratory complications requiring prompt corrective action. Aspiration, another major respiratory complication, is best prevented by proper positioning and timely clearance of airways.

The chest should be inspected for size, shape, and symmetry of expansion during respirations.

Asymmetrical expansion may be due to pneumothorax, consolidation, or splinting due to pain at the incisional site. Breath sounds are auscultated to check for the presence of rales or rhonchi, which may indicate fluid overload or poor mobilization of secretions. Diminished or absent breath sounds may indicate obstruction, pneumothorax, or misplacement of the endotracheal tube.

It is also important that the patient demonstrate adequate muscle tone to accommodate breathing. Further reversal of muscle relaxants given intraoperatively may be required upon arrival to the PACU. Muscle function is checked in the conscious patient by asking him or her to perform a head lift from a supine position, unless the surgical procedure contraindicates this type of movement (e.g., following a cervical laminectomy).

Respirations should also be assessed for rate, depth, and pattern. A decreased respiratory rate may be related to the administration of narcotics or inhalation anesthetics, or it could be indicative of a neurological disease. An increased respiratory rate is often seen in patients who are anxious, febrile, or have a metabolic imbalance, or it may be due to respiratory insufficiency. Shallow respirations may be a sign of continuing depression from anesthesia, or may be related to incisional pain, a tight dressing restricting expansion of the chest cavity, or even abdominal distention. Assessment of the respiratory system is ongoing throughout the patient's stay in the PACU, and a final assessment is conducted prior to discharge from the unit.

Laryngospasm is defined as a partial or complete closure of the vocal cords; it is a reflex response that can occur especially during the emergent phase of anesthesia. It is essential that all PACU nurses comprehend the pathophysiology and possible resulting complications of laryngospasm, such as hypoxemia and noncardiac pulmonary edema. Laryngospasm may occur in an anxious patient who manifests an inspiratory stridor, with or without paradoxical chest movement, depending on the severity of airway obstruction. In the anesthetized patient, paradoxical chest movements may signal a laryngospasm. The PACU nurse must assess the patient closely for signs and symptoms of hypoxemia and hypercapnia secondary to the spasm. After laryngospasm, the patient must be assessed for the development of noncardiogenic pulmonary edema.

Circulatory Assessment

The focus of the circulatory assessment is on cardiac output and tissue perfusion. Rate and rhythm are documented upon admission to the PACU and monitored throughout the postoperative course. Cardiac arrhythmias are quite common in the PACU.

Bradycardias are often seen in patients who are hypothermic or have increased vagus nerve stimulation. Cholinergic drugs, such as neostigmine (Prostigmin) and the narcotics fentanyl (Sublimaze) and morphine, may also cause slowing of the pulse.

Tachycardia may be associated with increased anxiety, pain, fever, hypovolemia, or hypoxemia. Anticholinergic drugs, such as atropine and glycopyrrolate (Robinul) are vagalytic; even meperidine (Demerol) may cause a tachycardia. Treatment will depend upon the etiology of the cardiac arrhythmia; often, ectopic beats can be treated by giving or increasing supplemental oxygen.

Heart sounds are auscultated to determine if a murmur or extra heart sounds are present, referred to as S_3 and S_4. Extra heart sounds are often present in patients with fluid overload and/or heart disease.

Blood pressure is monitored very closely, because labile pressures are very common in postoperative patients, and blood pressure monitoring assists with identifying volume status and hemostasis. Anesthetic agents and other drugs used in the perioperative period tend to relax the vessel walls, resulting in hypotension. Patients, especially those with spinal anesthesia, are encouraged to move very slowly to eliminate drastic falls in blood pressure.

Neck veins are inspected; flat veins could indicate hypovolemia, while distended veins may be a result of fluid overload. Invasive monitoring by means of a central venous pressure (CVP) or Swan-Ganz line helps determine fluid status and cardiac function.

Peripheral pulses are palpated to determine adequate perfusion to all extremities. Nail beds are assessed to determine capillary refill.

The surgical dressing is continuously monitored for signs of hemorrhaging, and all drainage is recorded. Drainage tubes are continuously monitored for patency, as well as nature and amount of output.

Temperature and Postanesthesia Shakes

Despite improved heat-loss prevention during surgery, many patients are hypothermic upon arrival to the PACU. The nurse assesses the patient's need for warmth, because adequate body warmth speeds recovery by increasing the patient's redistribution, metabolism, and excretion of anesthetic agents. A variety of rewarming techniques are currently in use or being researched for effectiveness.

Approximately 67% of patients recovering from anesthesia develop spontaneous, involuntary, and unpredictable muscle spasms. The etiology of postanesthesia shaking (PS) remains unknown, yet most nurses believe it is related to hypothermia or to the patient's sensation of being cold. Studies conducted to determine the cause of PS indicate that patient temperature on admission to the PACU does not necessarily determine which patients will develop PS.

Further research is needed to differentiate hypothermic shivering from postanesthesia shaking in order to initiate effective nursing interventions for each condition (4). The treatment for hypothermia consists of warming the patient, whereas the treatment for severe PS may include the use of butorphanol (Stadol) or meperidine.

The excessive muscle activity of shivering or shaking may increase oxygen consumption and result in excess carbon dioxide and heat production. These patients must be watched for development of hypoxemia, hypercapnia, sepsis, and malignant hyperthermia.

Central Nervous System and Musculoskeletal Assessment

Level of consciousness is assessed initially and throughout the postoperative course.

Delayed Return to Consciousness
Delayed return to consciousness may be the result of a synergistic effect of perioperative drugs, metabolic abnormalities such as hypoglycemia, and delayed elimination of drugs, as in renal failure. Hypothermia, cardiopulmonary dysfunction, or neurologic injury as the result of surgery or cerebral ischemia may also be reasons for a patient's delayed recovery. In response to the excessive stimuli that occur upon admission, patients may appear oriented at first and then regress, resulting in dangerous respiratory depression. This may be due to the continued effects of the anesthetic agents, to drugs known to have a second peak phase (e.g., fentanyl), or to renarcotization after naloxone (Narcan) reversal. Obese patients, especially following a long anesthetic course, may be slower to awaken due to storage of fat-soluble agents in their excess adipose tissue.

The mental status examination should include the patient's orientation to person, place, and time. Communication is often difficult in postanesthetized patients due to altered levels of consciousness and drug-induced amnesia.

Pupil reaction should be checked in any patient who has had cranial surgery. Motor and sensory function are continuously monitored in patients who have undergone spinal anesthesia, regional blocks, or neurological and orthopedic surgeries.

Motor function and muscle strength are assessed by hand grips and pedal pushes. The level of recession of a spinal anesthesia (i.e., T_{12}) is recorded, along with vital signs. The PACU closely assesses respiratory function in patients with high levels (T_2) of spinal anesthesia.

The central nervous system is assessed very closely in patients receiving regional anesthetics such as Bier blocks. Assessment is essential due to the rapid release of anesthetic agents such as lidocaine (Xylocaine) into the circulatory system when the tourniquet is released postoperatively. Patients may complain of dizziness, numbness, and tingling and could exhibit seizure activity.

Pain
Assessment of pain is a challenge in postoperative patients, due to barriers to communication such as artificial airways and altered levels of consciousness. The PACU nurse must assess all parameters in order to determine a patient's need for pain management. For example, clues that relate to pain, such as restlessness, may also be a sign of hypoxia or an extrapyramidal reaction to phenothiazines. Increased or decreased blood pressure may be a sign of pain, or compromised cardiovascular status. Vasovagal responses, such as hypotension, bradycardia, pallor, sweating, and nausea, are often seen in patients who are experiencing pain. Pain may also produce irregular, shallow breathing patterns and dilated pupils.

Severity of pain is difficult to assess since pain is a personal experience. Pain perception is influenced by previous surgical experiences, culture, education, and attitudes about pain and pain relief, as well as by fear and anxiety. Feelings of helplessness and powerlessness may increase anxiety and enhance the perception of pain. The patient's expectations, fears, and coping mechanisms with respect to pain should be explored during the preoperative interview.

Other factors impacting pain include the type of operation, the site of incision, and environmental noise and temperatures. The type of anesthetic agent delivered intraoperatively will also be a factor in pain. The anesthesiologist's report should include all anesthetic agents administered, including narcotics. The anesthesiologist may have administered minimal narcotics during surgery, or reversed the narcotics with naloxone. Narcotic antagonists are short-acting; therefore, administration of additional narcotics may or may not be appropriate. Nurses must collaborate with the anesthesiologist to determine the appropriate method for treating pain.

The nurse should be aware of two additional factors that affect pain management during the post-anesthesia phase: the patient's age and body weight. Age is important because elderly patients' metabolism is often slowed, causing drugs to remain in the body longer than usual. Barbiturates often cause severe agitation in the elderly, which can lead to accidental trauma. Propoxyphene (Darvon) can cause confusion with or without hallucinations. Body weight is an important factor when calculating dosages.

Determining the etiology of pain may influence the patient's treatment, so it is important to assess the nature of the pain. Pain may present as sharp and localized from the incision, or dull and aching from visceral damage. There may be muscle spasm or ischemic pain from vasospasm, clot, or a restrictive bandage. In the awakening patient, a postoperative delirium or excitement may be caused by pain, a full bladder, or anxiety. All require very different treatment approaches.

Children under three years of age may not understand the word *pain*; therefore, the nurse must communicate by using familiar words such as *owie* or *hurt* instead (5). Other tools have been developed, such as the Face Scale, which presents six faces to the pediatric patient. The first face depicts a happy expression with no pain, and the others progress to faces that reflect pain. This method may or may not be effective, depending upon the child's level of consciousness and willingness to participate.

The nurse must monitor the physiological changes along with the behavior manifested by the child. Often a test dose of pain medication is delivered and the patient's response evaluated closely to determine if pain is the cause of behavior and physiological changes.

It is imperative to remember that different age groups, cultural backgrounds, past experiences, and expectations all affect the patient's perception and response to pain. Therefore, assessment of pain in the postanesthetic patient presents a challenge to all PACU nurses.

Genitourinary System

Urine output is an important indicator of kidney perfusion; therefore, it is monitored closely during the PACU stay. Color, amount, and characteristics of the patient's urine are evaluated and recorded. Catheters are checked for patency. Patients who have undergone a spinal anesthetic are assessed for bladder distention because they may be unaware of a full bladder. A distended bladder can lead to physiological responses such as hypotension, hypertension, restlessness, or even emergence delirium.

Gastrointestinal System

Patients often complain of a sore throat due to the use of an endotracheal tube, and they need to be reassured that this symptom will subside. The mouth and throat should be inspected for any blisters, swelling, and intactness of teeth. The presence of loose teeth needs to be documented during the preoperative assessment.

Nausea and vomiting are common during postoperative recovery. Potential causes include dehydration and a response to drugs, pain, and the surgical procedure. Patients who are nauseated and unable to handle secretions must be placed on their side to avoid aspiration. Medication may be necessary to control nausea and vomiting in some patients.

Paralytic ileus can occur after abdominal surgery; therefore, the abdomen should be monitored for distention and the return of bowel sounds.

Integumentary System

The skin is assessed for color, turgor, moisture, and temperature, as well as the presence of redness, rashes, or burns. Assessment and care of the skin in the elderly is essential, since aging causes a thinning of all layers of skin and a general loss of adipose tissue.

Assessment Documentation

Data on the patient's condition are recorded at least every fifteen minutes at first, with the frequency of documentation declining as the patient stabilizes or progresses to Phase II recovery. Some units utilize postanesthesia scoring systems to assess the condition of the patient upon arrival and discharge. (See Fig. 23.2). The scoring method used in the figure includes respiratory status, blood pressure, level of consciousness, skin color, and muscular response.

Patient classification systems, such as the one detailed in Table 23.3, have been developed to assist units with staffing. An additional incentive to develop some type of patient classification system is to satisfy the requirements of the Joint Commission for Accreditation of Healthcare Organizations (JCAHO), which requires that nursing assignments meet the nursing care needs of patients (6).

NURSING DIAGNOSES/OUTCOMES

Documentation of nursing care provides physicians and nurses with information that is essential to the

VITAL SIGN RECORD

POST ANESTHESIA RECOVERY SCORE

Able to Deep Breath &/Or Cough	=2
Asleep - Adequate Airway	=1
Dyspnea or Limited Breathing or Apneic	=0
BP + 20% of Preanesthetic Level Pre-Op	=2
BP + 20%-30% of Preanesthetic Level BP	=1
BP + 50% of Preanesthetic Level	=0
Oriented and/or Awake	=2
Arousable on Calling	=1
Non-Responsive	=0
Normal Skin Color	=2
Pale, Dusky, Blotchy, Other	=1
Cyanotic	=0
Moving Extremities-	3 or 4	=2
If Chronic Deficit-	1 or 2	=1
Explain		=0
Post Anesthesia	TOTALS
Score Upon Transfer	

TIME

220
200
180
160
140
120
100
80
60
40
P
R

MEDICATIONS AND TREATMENTS

HOUR

TOTAL IV in OR:
Crystalloid _____ cc
Blood _____ cc
Colloid _____ cc

IV INFUSING:
Crystalloid _____ cc
Blood _____ cc
Colloid _____ cc

TOTAL INTAKE OR and RR
Crystalloid _____ cc
P.O. _____
Blood _____ cc
Colloid _____ cc

IV Added In RR

Output EBL: OR _____ cc
Urine: OR _____ cc RR
NG: OR _____ cc RR
Emesis: OR _____ cc RR
Other: OR _____ cc RR
TOTAL OUTPUT OR _____ cc RR

Type of Airway _____
Time Out _____
☐ O₂ Not Given O₂ _____ TIME STARTED _____ TIME DC'D _____ O₂ Liters/Min. _____ Temp. _____
Surgical Procedure: _____
Anesthetic Agent: _____
Angiocath Gauge: _____

HOUR   NOTES

Pertinent Health Information _____
Allergies _____
Report Given To: _____ Accompanied by: _____
Discharge Time _____ To _____ (Responsible Person)
Mode of Discharge _____
Discharge Nurse _____
Post-Op Instructions _____

PORTER MEMORIAL HOSPITAL

7211-023-81C Revised (6-85)

357

FIGURE 23.2.   Nursing postanesthesia assessment record. (Reprinted with permission of Porter Memorial Hospital, Denver.)

TABLE 23.3.   Postanesthesia Patient Classification System

Level I: Minimal nursing involvement	Taking vital signs every 15 minutes Reviewing patient's chart Assessing patient continuously Checking dressings Monitoring IV fluids Supplying oxygen as needed Applying basic nursing procedures and/or treatments
Level II: Requires moderate nursing involvement; includes all Level I criteria plus one or more Level II	Administration of medications Changing dressings Obtaining laboratory work and calling physicians with results Monitoring electrocardiogram Monitoring urinary output and catheter care Administering blood or blood components Managing airway and respiratory care, including insertion of airways, obstruction, extubation Treatment of hypotension or hypertension Checking neurological signs Monitoring drainage tubes Assisting with central or IV line insertion Closely observing patients receiving reversal agents Frequent bed changing due to incontinence Using hypothermia or hyperthermia unit
Level III: Requires highest level of nursing involvement; patient needs at least 1:1 nurse:patient ratio; includes all criteria in Level I and a greater degree of involvement than Level II	Managing long-term airway or ventilator Handling emergency delirium and combative patients Invasive pressure monitoring Closely monitoring newly placed fistulas or shunts Isolation cases requiring registered nurse at all times Treating and recognizing malignant hyperthermia, life-threatening hypotension or hypertension, hemorrhage, and complications requiring return to surgery Treating infections, burn, reverse isolation and infection, or ketamine cases

Copyright © AORN, Inc., 10170 E. Mississippi Avenue, Denver, CO 80231. Adapted with permission.

provision of quality care and maintenance of continuity of care. In the fast-paced PACU it may not seem realistic to formulate nursing diagnoses, but it is indeed possible to deliver care in the PACU that is based on nursing diagnoses. Some units have incorporated nursing diagnoses into their records, because there are a number of diagnoses that frequently pertain to postanesthesia patients. (See Fig. 23.2 and Table 23.4.) For example, hypothermia related to environmental heat loss, as manifested by temperature reading 96° rectally, is a common nursing diagnosis used in the PACU. Including nursing diagnoses on the PACU record saves time and provides a system for implementing the nursing process and continuity of care.

Once nursing diagnoses have been determined, the nurse and client can focus on the desired outcomes to be achieved in the PACU. For example, one outcome may be that the patient's blood pressure will return to the preoperative baseline level.

PLANNING

Once outcomes have been identified, the nurse must determine and implement the nursing care measures necessary to achieve them. Expected outcomes specific to the postanesthesia patient always include respiratory and cardiovascular maintenance or improvement, stabilization of fluid and electrolyte balance, protection from infection, management of pain and nausea, environmental safety, privacy, and emotional support.

The PACU nurse must continue to assess and modify the plan of care based on the patient's changing needs. For example, an outpatient undergoing general anesthesia may arrive in the PACU not responding to stimuli and requiring chin support for adequate gas exchange. This patient requires total support from the nurse. As the patient emerges from the anesthesia, the nurse is no longer needed to physically maintain an adequate airway. At this

TABLE 23.4.   Sample PACU Record of Nursing Diagnoses

Normal Health Status

A. Potential for alteration in patient's normal health status as related to anesthesia/surgical procedure.

B. Potential for alteration in body temperature as related to anesthesia/surgical procedure.

C. Potential for alteration in cardiac output as related to anesthesia/surgical procedure.

D. Potential for urinary retention as related to anesthesia/surgical procedure.

E. Potential for impairment of skin integrity as related to anesthesia/surgical procedure.

Respiratory Status

F. Potential for ineffective airway clearance as related to anesthesia/surgical procedure.

G. Potential for ineffective breathing patterns as related to anesthesia or surgical procedures.

H. Potential for impaired gas exchange as related to anesthesia or surgical procedures.

Fluid Status

I. Potential for alteration in fluid volume, excess, or deficit related to anesthesia/surgical procedure.

Injury

J. Potential for physical injury related to sensory–perceptual alteration (including decreased level of consciousness) from anesthesia/surgical procedure.

K. Potential for physical injury related to impaired physical mobility (including muscle strength) from anesthesia/surgical procedure.

Communication

L. Potential for impaired verbal communication, related to intubation, surgical procedure, language barrier, or underlying physical defect.

Comfort

M. Potential for alteration in comfort related to anesthesia/surgical procedure and/or operative positioning.

N. Potential for anxiety/fear as related to emergence from anesthesia, surgical procedure, diagnosis, separation from significant other or parent.

Reprinted with permission of the University of Colorado Health Sciences Center, Denver, CO.

stage of recovery, the patient may require only monitoring and pain management. As the patient continues to recover from anesthesia, the nurse's role changes from caregiver to educator. The nurse now may diagnose that there is a knowledge deficit regarding the postoperative care to be implemented in the home setting. At this point, plans would be developed for implementing patient and family teaching.

This example demonstrates how quickly the needs of the PACU patient change, thus impacting the role of the nurse. The *Standards of Postanesthesia Nursing Practice* describe postanesthesia nursing as multidimensional because of the three different phases the patient undergoes. The *Standards* define the Preanesthesia, Postanesthesia I, and Postanesthesia II phases of postanesthesia nursing as follows:

- The Preanesthesia Phase consists of assessing, teaching, and planning for the operative experience.
- Postanesthesia Phase I focuses on providing a smooth transition from a totally anesthetized state to one requiring less acute interventions.
- In Postanesthesia Phase II, the role of the nurse changes; the focus is now on preparing the patient for self-care or care by others outside the PACU.

PACU managers are challenged with planning and providing adequate staffing. Staffing requirements are often difficult to predict because of patients' different acuity levels and postoperative phases. The patient:staff ratio will vary according to patient classifications. The *Standards of Postanesthesia Nursing Practice* recommend the following nurse:patient ratios:

1:3 Class I patients: stable and awake, uncomplicated adult patients, or pediatric patients who are awake and stable in Phase II with a parent or guardian present.

1:2 Class II patients: stable, unconscious adult patients; patients who have undergone major surgery and whose systems are stabilized; uncomplicated pediatric patients in Phase I with a family member or support staff present; unconscious, stable, uncomplicated patients aged eleven to seventeen years.

1:1 Class III patients: patients newly arrived to the PACU, patients requiring life support, unconscious pediatric patients less than eleven years old.

Some postanesthesia units are incorporating the use of standard plans of care, which can guide nurses in planning care. It is important that nurses individualize care based on each patient's specific needs. There are, however, some basic needs that are prevalent in the majority of postanesthesia patients. Therefore, a standard plan of care can be useful in planning nursing interventions. A sample standard of care for the general anesthesia adult patient is provided in Table 23.5.

Same-Day Surgery

Due to the fast pace and frequent turnover of same-day surgical patients, time for planning care is limited. In some instances, patients are not seen until the day of surgery, making planning extremely difficult. Since the patient will be going home the same day, discharge planning must be initiated during the preoperative phase in order to allow the patient and family time to plan and make arrangements for care at home.

Nurses working with same-day patients can identify with the lack of time allotted for the nursing process. Many units have developed time-saving formats for documenting nursing diagnoses and plans of care.

IMPLEMENTATION OF CARE

Nursing interventions are multidisciplinary and require scientific knowledge, clinical skill, and decision making based on assessment and planning. Nurses also implement physicians' orders such as administration of medications, laboratory tests, and specific treatments (e.g., irrigation of catheters)

Respiratory Interventions

All PACU nurses must be experienced in airway management and oxygenation techniques. Respiratory care is essential in the PACU due to the use of narcotics, anesthetic agents, and other perioperative drugs that depress the respiratory system. Inadequate air exchange may be due to a number of causes, and the nurse must determine the etiology of the symptoms assessed and implement the appropriate intervention.

If inadequate air exchange is due to the tongue obstructing the airway, the nursing intervention in this circumstance would be to reposition the jaw, head, and neck to relieve the airway obstruction.

Backward tilt of the head and slight elevation of the mandible prevent the tongue from obstructing the airway. (See Fig. 23.3.) Pressure applied at the notch of the angle of the jaw may stimulate the patient and improve respirations. (See Fig. 23.4).

If the airway obstruction is due to an increased amount of secretions, the nurse would intervene with suctioning if the patient is unable to clear the secretions. (See Fig. 23.5.)

Guided by pulse oximetry, oxygen is provided via cannula, catheter, mist, or respirator, depending upon each patient's need. Arterial blood gases may be an essential intervention with patients on mechanical ventilation in order to set the parameters on the respirator. These interventions would be a collaborative effort between the nurse, the physician, and the respiratory therapist.

PACU protocols may include giving naloxone to reverse narcotic-induced respiratory depression. The anesthesiologist may request that doxapram (Dopram) be administered to increase rate and depth of respiration and help eliminate the inhalation anesthetic. Administration of more cholinergic agent or prolonged assisted ventilation may be required for surgical patients with myasthenia gravis. Oversedation and respiratory depression caused by midazolam (Versed) or diazepam (Valium) may be reversed by flumazenil (Mazicon).

Proper anatomical body positioning should be implemented at all times to maximize respirations. The nurse should frequently encourage coughing and deep breathing. This regimen prevents patchy atelectasis and speeds alveolar reexpansion. It also facilitates the excretion of inhalation anesthetics via the lungs.

If an endotracheal tube is present, nursing interventions include stabilizing the tube with tape to prevent it from slipping into the right mainstem bronchus or being removed accidentally. Auscultating the chest for bilateral breath sounds is an essential step in assessment.

Extubation of the patient is an intervention that nurses in many PACUs implement after determining that the patient has an adequate tidal volume, muscle strength, oxygenation, and ability to mobilize secretions. After extubation the patient is monitored carefully for any sign of respiratory distress and aspiration of vomitus, which may occur any time after the cuff of the endotracheal tube is deflated.

Postanesthesia laryngospasm requires immediate diagnosis and intervention. Laryngospasm is often secondary to edema, postsurgical trauma, and foreign-object irritation (i.e., endotracheal and oral

TABLE 23.5.   Standard of Care: Postanesthesia Care: General Anesthesia for the Adult Patient

Nursing Diagnosis

A/P Pt. Care Problem	Patient Outcomes	Date/Time Met	Nursing Intervention	Time
1. Potential for alteration in respiratory function: • Ineffective airway clearance (IAC) • Ineffective breathing pattern (IBP) Related to: • Anesthetic agents • Medications, i.e.: muscle relaxants, reversals, narcotics, sedatives, barbiturates	Demonstrates adequate respiratory function as evidenced by: • Respirations spontaneous, regular, quiet, nonlabored 12–28 min. without airway assistance or adventitious noises • Breath sounds clear, equal bilaterally, without adventitious noises • Symmetrical chest expansion	Upon discharge from PACU	• Determine types, amounts administration times of anesthetic agents and medications. • Assess airway for patency, secretions. Assist with airway maintenance and secretion removal if needed. Utilize position, chinlift, jaw thrust, oral or nasopharyngeal airways for ineffective airway.	Adm. Adm; q 15 min × 2 hrs; q 30–60 mins/prn
• Intubation: irritation, edema (IAC) • Excessive/thick secretions (IAC) • Temperature alterations/shivering (IBP) • Pain/anxiety (IBP) • Position/restrictive dressings/surgical site (IBP) • Preoperative factors (IBP), i.e.: COPD, obesity	• Pulse oximeter reading ≥ 94% or preanesthetic value • BP ± 20 beats/min. of baseline • Absence of dysrhythmias/EKG changes • Absence of restlessness, agitation, apprehension, lethargy • Adequate muscle strength • Ability to cough (IAC) • Skin warm, dry; absence of duskiness from nailbeds/mucosa • Temperature (oral, axillary, rectal, tympanic) 96.0°–101.0°F (35.5°–38.3°C) (IBP) • Oriented to person, place, situation, time (IBP)		• Assess respiratory rate, depth, rhythm, use of accessory muscles/intercostal retractions, adventitious noises. Observe chest movement and symmetry; feel for air exchange. • Auscultate breath sounds for equality, intensity, and adventitious noises. • Initiate protocols for airway compromise unresolved by above measures (i.e. laryngospasm) and notify anesthesiologist (IAC). • Obtain pulse oximeter reading. Follow oxygen therapy protocol. • Assess B/P. Initiate hypotensive protocol if systolic < 90 mm/Hg. Notify anesthesiologist if B/P > 180/90. Initiate hypertensive protocol as indicated. • Assess pulse rate. Notify anesthesiologist of consistent rate < 48, > 120 beats/min. • Monitor cardiac rhythm. Initiate emergency orders for cardiac dysrhythmias according to standing PACU orders (ACLS protocol). Notify anesthesiologist of dysrhythmias/EKG changes. • Assess skin for warmth, dryness. Assess color of nailbeds and/or mucosa.	Adm; q 15 min × 2 hrs; q 30–60 mins/prn Adm/prn Prn Adm; per protocol. Adm; q 15 min. × 2 hr; q 30–60 min/prn. ″ ″ Continuous; document on adm; q 1 hr; discharge. Adm; q 30 min x 2 hr; q 30–60 min/prn.

(continued)

TABLE 23.5.   *(continued)*

Nursing Diagnosis

A/P Pt. Care Problem	Patient Outcomes	Date/Time Met	Nursing Intervention	Time
Potential for alteration in respiratory function *(cont.)*			• Assess muscle strength as defined by PACU discharge criteria.	Adm/prn
			• Maintain pharyngeal airways (oral, nasal) until demonstrates return of swallow and gag reflex. Upon return of reflexes remove airway to avoid prolonged gag reflex stimulation.	Adm/prn.
			• Extubate according to extubation protocol.	Adm/prn.
			• Assess ability to cough (IAC).	Prn.
			• Assess for restlessness, agitation, apprehension, lethargy.	Adm/prn.
			• Assess orientation to person, place, situation, time.	Adm; q 30 min/prn.
			• Observe for shivering. Obtain temperature on admission. Use hypothermia/hyperthermia protocols (IBP)	Adm; q 30 min; prn.
			• Assess for restriction of chest expansion due to tight dressings, binders, etc. (IBP).	Adm/prn
			• Identify preexisting conditions that may result in ineffective breathing patterns and integrate into nursing care.	Adm/prn
			• Position for maximum lung expansion unless contraindicated (IBP).	Adm/prn
			• Assess and intervene for pain and anxiety using potential alteration in comfort care plan (IBP).	Adm/prn
			• Obtain ABGs, chest x-ray per standing orders (IBP).	Prn
2. Potential for alteration in cardiac output Related to: • Anesthetic agents • Medications, i.e.: muscle relaxants and reversal agents, barbiturates, sedatives	Demonstrates adequate cardiac output as evidenced by: • BP ± 20 mmHg of baseline with absence of narrowing pulse pressure, systolic 90–180; diastolic < 90.	Upon discharge from PACU	• Determine types, amounts, administration times of anesthetic agents and medication.	Adm.
			• Identify preoperative factors that may result in altered cardiac output.	Adm.

TABLE 23.5. *(continued)*

Nursing Diagnosis

A/P Pt. Care Problem	Patient Outcomes	Date/Time Met	Nursing Intervention	Time
Potential for alteration in cardiac output (*cont.*) • Impaired respiratory function • Fluid and/or electrolyte imbalances • Dysrhythmias • Temperature alterations/ shivering • Surgical procedure • Pain/anxiety • Preoperative factors, i.e.: coronary artery disease, peripheral artery disease	• Heart rate 60–100 min or ± of baseline • Absence of dysrhythmias/EKG changes • Pulse oximeter reading ≥ 94% of preanesthetic value • Respirations spontaneous, regular, quiet, nonlabored 12–28/min. • Breath sounds clear, equal bilaterally without adventitious noises • Temperature (oral, axillary, rectal or tympanic) 96.0°–101.0°F (25.5°–38.3°C) • Urine output ≥ 30 cc/hr (if Foley in place) • Skin warm, dry; absence of duskiness from nailbeds, mucosa • Extremities warm, dry, capillary refill ≤ 5 sec. • Dressings/drains—absence of drainage excessive for surgical procedure • Absence of restlessness, agitation • Oriented to person, place, situation, time • Pulmonary artery catheter readings (if in place): Systolic 15–30 Diastolic 8–15 Mean 10–20; PCWP 4–12 C.O. 4–8 • CVP 3–15 (if in place)		• Determine baseline requirement for fluid replacement since NPO status; initiate standing orders for fluid replacement, monitoring oral and IV intake. • Determine estimated blood loss (EBL) and surgery fluid replacement. • Assess B/P, heart rate, respirations, breath sounds, cardiac rhythm, and temperature according to nursing interventions under Potential for alteration in respiratory function. • Assess extremities for warmth, color, dryness, peripheral pulse volume and equality, capillary refill. • Assess skin for warmth, dryness. Assess color of nailbeds and/or mucosa. • Monitor all dressings and drainage tubes for type and amount of drainage. See care plan specific to type of surgery for excessive amounts of drainage. • Assess LOC and orientation to person, place, situation, time. Assess for restlessness, agitation. • Monitor urine output (if Foley in place). Catheterize for bladder distention if indicated. • Monitor pulmonary artery pressure and CVP readings. • Monitor lab results (i.e., Hgb, Hct, electrolytes, ABGs). • Initiate appropriate protocols/guidelines for any abnormal findings.	Adm.; continuous Adm. Adm; q 15 × 2 hr.; q 30–60 min prn Adm; q 30 min/prn Adm; q 30 min × 2 hr; q 30–60 min/prn Adm; q 30 min × 2 hr; q 30–60 min prn Adm; q 15 min × 2 hr; q 30–60 min/prn Adm; q 1 hr/prn Adm; PAP q 30 min; PCWP & CVP q 1 hr × 2, then q 4 hr/prn, CO as ordered Prn Prn

(continued)

TABLE 23.5.   (*continued*)

Nursing Diagnosis

A/P Pt. Care Problem	Patient Outcomes	Date/Time Met	Nursing Intervention	Time

3. Potential for alteration of fluid and electrolyte balance
 	
Related to:
• NPO status
• Fluid loss
• Fluid replacement
• Type/length of surgery
• Stress response
• Administration of blood products
• Preoperative factors, i.e.,
    Fever
    Renal disease
    Diuretic therapy
    Burns
    Dehydration
	Demonstrates normovolemic state and electrolyte balance as evidenced by:
	• B/P ± 20mmHg of baseline, with absence of narrowing pulse pressure; systolic 90–180; diastolic < 90
	• Heart rate 60–100 or ± 20 beats/min of baseline
	• Respirations spontaneous, regular, quiet, nonlabored 12–28 min.
	• Breath sounds clear, equal bilaterally, without adventitious noises
	• Absence of dysrhythmias/EKG changes
	• Dressings/drains—absence of drainage excessive for surgical procedure
	• Temperature (oral, axillary, rectal, or tympanic) 96.0°–101.0°F, (35.5°–38.3°C)
	• Absence of vomiting for minimum 30 min.
	• Skin warm, dry; absence of duskiness from nailbeds/mucosa
		Upon discharge from PACU	• Assess B/P, heart rate, respirations, breath sounds, cardiac rhythm, and temperature according to nursing interventions under potential for alteration in respiratory function.	Adm; q 15 min × 2 hr, q 30–60 min/prn

			• Assess for narrowing pulse pressure; notify anesthesiologist if < 15.	Adm; q 15 min × 2 hr; q 30–60 min/prn
			• Assess skin for warmth, dryness. Assess color of nailbeds and/or mucosa.	Adm; q 30 min/prn
			• Palpate for bladder distention. Catheterize per standing orders.	Adm: q 1 hr prn
			• Determine urinary output (if Foley in place). Assess characteristics of urine (i.e.: concentration).	Adm; q 1 hr/prn
			• Assess type and amount of drainage from tubes, dressings.	Adm; q 30 min/prn
			• Assess LOC and orientation to person, place, situation, time. Assess for restlessness, agitation.	Adm; q 15 min × 2 hr, q 30–60 min/prn
			• Assess IV site for infiltration/inflammation, type, amount, rate of infusion.	Adm; q 30 min/prn
			• Monitor pulmonary artery pressures and CVP readings.	Adm; PAP q 30 min; PCWP & CVP q 1 hr × 2 q. 4 hr/prn; CO as ordered
			• Determine EBL and fluid replacement in OR.	Adm.
			• Identify preexisting conditions that may result in fluid and/or electrolyte imbalances (i.e.: burns, diuretics, renal disease, fever.	Adm.
			• Determine baseline requirements for fluid replacement since NPO status; initiate standing orders for fluid replacement, monitoring oral and IV intake.	Adm.

TABLE 23.5.   (*continued*)

Nursing Diagnosis

A/P Pt. Care Problem	Patient Outcomes	Date/Time Met	Nursing Intervention	Time
Potential for alteration of fluid and electrolyte balance (*cont.*)			• Assess for bowel sounds. Withhold oral fluids if absent. • Obtain Hgb, Hct, electrolytes, ABGs per standing orders.	Adm/prn Prn

4. Potential for alteration in body temperature
Related to:
• Anesthetic agents
• Medications, i.e.:
  Muscle relaxants
  Narcotics
  Sedatives
  Phenothiazines
• Body surface exposure/ ambient air temperatures
• Intraoperative events, i.e.:
  Irrigations
  Fluid replacement
• Surgical procedure
• Preoperative factors, i.e.:
  Alcohol intoxication
  Burns
  Infection
  Multiple trauma
  Age
	Demonstrates normal body temperature as evidenced by:
	• Temperature (oral, axillary, rectal, tympanic) 96.0°–101.0°F (35.5°–38.3°C)
	• Respirations spontaneous, regular, quiet, without airway assistance
	• Pulse oximeter reading ≥ 94% of preanesthetic value
	• B/P ± 20mmHg of baseline: systolic 90–180; diastolic 90
	• Heart rate 60–100 min or ± of baseline
	• Adequate muscle strength
	• Skin warm, dry
	• Capillary refill ≤ 5 secs
	• Absence of shivering
	• Absence of lethargy, restlessness, agitation
	• Oriented to person, place, situation, time
	• Urine output 30 cc/hr. (if Foley in place)
		Upon discharge from PACU	• Obtain temperature. Use hypothermia/hyperthermia protocols.
			• Assess B/P, heart rate, respiration, breath sounds, and cardiac rhythm according to nursing interventions under potential for alteration in respiratory function.
			• Obtain pulse oximeter reading; follow oxygen therapy protocol.
			• Assess muscle strength as defined by PACU discharge criteria.
			• Assess peripheral circulation (i.e.: skin color, warmth, dryness, peripheral pulses, capillary refill).
			• Observe for shivering. Maintain oxygen therapy if shivering. Utilize medications/warming methods as needed.
			• Assess level of consciousness.
			
			• Monitor intake and output.
			• Maintain PACU room air temperature between 70°–74°F; humidity 50%.
			• Utilize methods to maintain normothermia (i.e.: warm blankets).
				Adm; q 30 min/prn
				
				Adm; 1 15 min for 2 hr; q 30–60 min/prn
				
				Adm/per protocol
				
				Adm/prn
				
				Adm; q 30 min/prn
				
				Adm/prn
				
				Adm; q 15 min for 2 hrs; q 30–60 min/ prn.
				Adm; q 1 hr/prn
				Continuous
				
				Continuous

5. Potential for injury Related to: • Altered level of consciousness • Sensory/perceptual/ motor deficits • Lack of awareness of	Demonstrate ability to protect self from injury as evidenced by: • Oriented to person, place, situation • Answers questions appropriately	Upon discharge from PACU.	• Determine types, amounts, administration times of anesthetic agents and medications. • Determine preoperative mental status. • Assess LOC—provide	Adm. Adm. Adm/prn

(continued)

TABLE 23.5.   *(continued)*

Nursing Diagnosis

A/P Pt. Care Problem	Patient Outcomes	Date/Time Met	Nursing Intervention	Time
Potential for injury*(cont.)*			continuous observation until patient reaches State I anesthesia.	
environmental hazards	• Follows verbal commands appropriately		• Evaluate airway patency per respiratory function interventions.	Continuous
• Surgical procedure	• Absence of restlessness or agitation		• Evaluation oxygenation status per respiratory function interventions.	Continuous
• Anesthetic agents/medications, i.e.: narcotics, barbiturates, anticholinergics, muscle relaxants	• Purposeful, controlled movement of all extremities or preoperative status		• Position to avoid aspiration until gag and cough reflexes present; notify anesthesiologist if aspiration suspected.	Prn
• Emergence delirium	• Adequate muscle strength and ability to cough		• Assess muscle strength as defined by PACU discharge criteria.	Adm/prn
			• Have suction equipment readily available and functional for use.	Continuous
			• Maintain siderails in upright position with cart wheels locked.	Continuous
			• Restrain patient/pad siderails.	Prn
			• Orient to person, place, time, situation. Assess for restlessness, agitation.	Adm/prn
			• Approach in calm, quiet manner; use touch; avoid startling; reassure when needed; explain care procedures.	Continuous
			• Avoid use of painful stimuli whenever possible. Utilize pain relief measures.	Continuous
			• Provide calm, quiet environment.	Continuous
			• Position in proper alignment; reposition with attention to all drains, IV lines, ventilatory equipment, etc. Change position slowly to avoid initiating/potentiating N/V.	Adm/prn
			• Palpate for bladder distention—straight catheterization per standing order.	Adm/prn
			• Maintain body substance isolation precautions.	Continuous
			• Utilize preexisting sensory deficit equipment as soon as appropriate (i.e.: glasses, hearing aids).	Prn

TABLE 23.5.   (*continued*)

Nursing Diagnosis

A/P Pt. Care Problem	Patient Outcomes	Date/Time Met	Nursing Intervention	Time
Potential for injury(*cont.*)			• Evaluate type of surgery for related potential injuries and intervene with nursing actions (see specific surgical procedure care plans).	Adm.

6. Potential for alteration in comfort
 	
Related to:
• Psychological/physical responses to surgical event
• Positioning/immobility
• Environmental factors, i.e.:
    Cold drafts
    Bright lights
    Loud noises
    Noxious odors
	Demonstrates satisfactory level of comfort as evidenced by:
	• B/P ± 20mmHg of baseline, systolic 90–180, diastolic < 90
	• Heart rate 60–100/min or ± of baseline
	• Respirations—regular, quiet, nonlabored 12–28 min.
	• Skin warm, dry
	• Absence of nausea/vomiting
	• Absence of nonverbal communication suggestive of anxiety/discomfort (i.e.: restlessness, crying, moaning, muscle tension).
		Upon discharge from PACU	• Assess type, amount, administration times of anesthetic agents and medications.
			• Assess physical responses to discomfort (i.e.: changes in B/P, heart rate, respiratory rate, skin).
			• Assess verbal and nonverbal communication suggestive of discomfort, nausea, anxiety.
			• Palpate for bladder distention. Catheterization per standing orders.
			• Administer pain medications/sedative/antiemetics judiciously and evaluate response.
			• Position for comfort, avoiding stress on surgical site and enhancing adequate ventilation. Change position slowly to avoid initiating/potentiating N/V.
			• Decrease sensory stimulation (i.e.: dim lights, eliminate noxious environmental stimuli).
			• Change saturated or restrictive dressings if not contraindicated.
			• Keep linens next to skin dry. Utilize nursing interventions to attain desirable sensation of warmth.
			• Orient to place, situation. Explain procedures using simple, factual statements in calm voice. Use touch.
			• Assure privacy whenever possible (i.e.: minimal skin exposure, use of curtains).
			• Include family/significant other involvement as appropriate.
				Adm.
				
				Adm/prn
				
				Adm/prn
				
				Adm/prn
				
				Prn
				
				Continuous
				
				Prn
				
				Prn
				
				Prn
				
				Prn
				
				Prn
				
				Prn

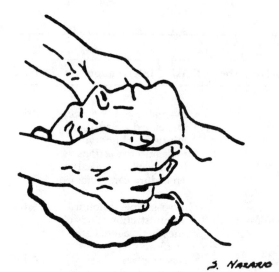

FIGURE 23.3. Elevation of the mandible. Approach from the head of the patient. Head should be pulled back as above, the nurse's fourth finger at the notch of the mandible and forefinger on side of the mandible.

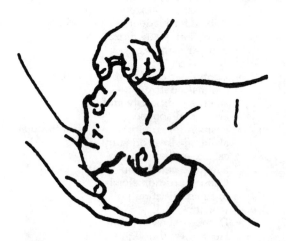

FIGURE 23.4. Elevation of the mandible. Approach from side of the patient. A combination of backward head tilt and anterior mandibular elevation is most effective to relieve airway obstruction.

pharyngeal airways). Laryngospasm can also occur from excess secretions that irritate the vocal cord tissue or pharynx. Nursing intervention consists of notifying the anesthesiologist at once; treatment varies with the severity of the spasm, but may require managing the patient's airway and oxygenation with the use of a bag mask valve apparatus that delivers 100% oxygen.

The PACU nurse must be prepared to treat nausea and vomiting in order to prevent the patient from aspirating vomitus into the airway. Nursing interventions include positioning the patient in a side-

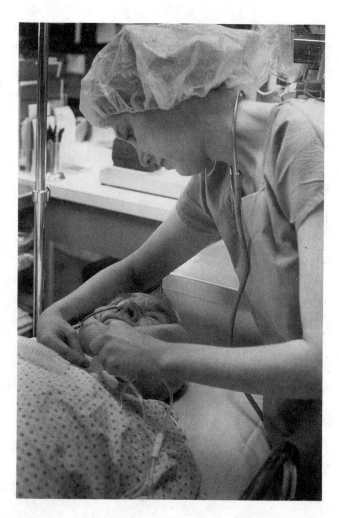

FIGURE 23.5. The postanesthesia nurse removes secretions with a catheter through the tracheostomy tube.

lying position and administering antiemetics as ordered.

Cardiovascular Interventions

Cardiovascular status is monitored throughout the postoperative phase. Vital signs are measured and recorded every 15 minutes.

If the heart rate rises above 110 beats per minute, reasons for the increase should be determined. Tachycardia often responds to nursing interventions for pain control and anxiety relief. Bradycardias are seen frequently in the PACU. The nurse must intervene if the heart rate falls below 45 or if the patient becomes symptomatic. Intervention usually involves a collaborative approach with the anesthesiologist and includes administering atropine or glycopyrrolate.

If cardiac arrhythmias are present, the nurse must determine if they are due to hypoxia, drugs, electrolyte imbalance, anxiety, or a history of cardiac arrhythmias. In most instances, arrhythmias are self-limiting, but treatment measures should be implemented if they alter the patient's condition or become life-threatening. The PACU nurse must be skilled in reading rhythm strips and implementing advanced cardiac life support measures.

Anesthetic agents tend to cause hypotension; therefore, blood pressure is monitored very closely throughout the postoperative phase. Hypotension can also be caused by hypovolemia or impaired venous return to the heart, as in mechanical ventilation (i.e., positive end expiratory pressure, or PEEP).

The nurse must first determine the etiology of the hypotension and then implement treatment based on the cause. For example, if the drop in pressure is due to hypovolemia caused by excessive blood loss, then the nurse would consult with the anesthesiologist to determine the type of fluid replacement to implement. Nursing interventions in shock states (i.e., hypovolemic or septic shock) may include increasing fluid administration, placing the patient in a Trendelenburg position, implementing oxygen therapy, if not already in progress, and notifying the anesthesiologist and surgeon.

Medical treatment for hypotension may include insertion of additional monitoring lines, such as a CVP or Swan-Ganz line, and restoration of blood pressure with the use of IV medication drips (e.g., dopamine). Bicarbonate may be needed to combat metabolic acidosis if pH falls to 7.2. Nursing measures would then include constant observation to prevent complications from the medical therapy instituted.

Postoperative hypertension (systolic pressure > 160 mm Hg and/or diastolic pressure > 90 mm Hg) can be caused by anxiety, intraoperative medications (e.g., epinephrine), a full bladder, or pain. Labile hypertension may occur as a result of specific procedures such as carotid endarterectomy. Hypertension may also develop as a result of increased PCO_2, hypervolemia, and/or postanesthesia shivering. Patients with undiagnosed pheochromocytomas may present with a sudden rise in blood pressure and pulse rate as the result of the stress of surgery.

The nurse and physician must collaborate to determine the etiology of the hypertension and the type of intervention to be implemented. If the hypertension is related to hypervolemia, measures would be taken to reduce the IV infusion rate; diuretics may be administered in some instances. Hydralazine, labetalol, nifedipine, sodium nitroprusside (Nipride), or a nitroglycerin drip may also be used to lower blood pressure in the PACU.

The patient's temperature is also monitored.

Body temperature can be anticipated to be lower during the immediate postoperative period. The nurse intervenes by placing warm blankets on the patient, hanging warm IVs, and using overhead warmers until body temperature approaches the normal range.

The nurse also monitors temperature to watch for signs of malignant hyperthermia (MH). MH is a critical complication that most often commences during the intraoperative period when a patient receives general anesthesia, but it can also occur in the PACU. MH is a pharmacogenetic disease of the musculoskeletal system characterized by one or more of the following: muscle rigidity, tachycardia, tachypnea, respiratory and metabolic acidosis, and a rapid rise in temperature. Body temperature may rise to 108°F or more. The condition is precipitated by certain inhalation anesthetics, depolarizing neuromuscular blocking agents, and possibly stress (7).

People who are susceptible to MH sometimes have a history of muscle weakness and/or muscle cramps, but the most definitive test for MH is skeletal muscle biopsy. The muscle is exposed to halothane (Fluothane) or caffeine in a laboratory setting to look for signs of increased isometric tension.

In MH patients, a trigger such as succinylcholine causes an excess of calcium ions in the myoplasm, which causes a continuous skeletal muscle contraction. This prolonged muscle contraction leads to a hypermetabolic state of acid and heat production, which causes the rise in temperature, acidosis, release of catecholamines, and hyperkalemia. This, in turn, results in cardiac arrhythmias, alterations in cardiac output, decreased level of consciousness and, if untreated, death (7).

MH must be diagnosed and treated quickly in order to prevent death; a team approach is essential. Dantrolene sodium (Dantrium) is the only known pharmacological agent effective in the treatment of MH; it relaxes the skeletal muscles by interfering with the release of calcium and stops the cascading events. In addition, the nurse administers cooled crystalloids intravenously, packs the patient in ice, and uses iced gastric lavages to return the patient's core body temperature to normal. Sodium bicarbonate may be given to correct acidosis while continuing to monitor both the end tidal CO_2 and pH of the patient. Vital signs are monitored, and cardiac arrhythmias not corrected by dantrolene administration may be treated with procainamide hydrochloride (Pronestyl). Level of consciousness is assessed and the nurse implements seizure precautions.

Malignant hyperthermia patients present a challenge to the perioperative team. The patient's survival depends upon early diagnosis and immediate intervention.

Fluid Replacement

The main goals for parenteral fluid therapy in the PACU are to correct past deficits; replace concurrent losses from drainage tubes, such as nasogastric tubes; and maintain satisfactory blood pressure and hemostasis.

Fluid replacement cannot be determined without monitoring output. The nurse must continually monitor and record output from all drainage tubes, obtain blood-loss estimates from the perioperative team, and monitor invasive line pressures if present. Once all fluid output data are collected, the nurse collaborates with the anesthesiologist to determine the amount and type of fluid replacement needed. For example, a plasma expander or blood transfusion may be necessary in patients who have had excessive fluid and blood loss during surgery.

Pain Management

The goal of pain management is to achieve and maintain safe analgesia while avoiding toxicity. Postanesthesia pain management is influenced by the many variables that can alter the patient's perception of pain (e.g., age, environmental temperature, and noise). A variety of new methods of postoperative pain control offer alternatives to administration of analgesics, including patient-controlled analgesia and epidural analgesia.

Patient-controlled analgesia (PCA) allows the patient to self-administer predetermined doses of intravenous narcotics as needed. These devices are programmed to provide appropriate time intervals between doses and a timed maximum dose, protecting the patient from an accidental overdose. Patients appear to benefit from PCA, because it gives them the satisfaction of having some control over their pain (8). PCA may be implemented in the postoperative recovery phase as soon as patients are awake and able to push the button for self-administration.

Success in implementing this type of pain management requires preoperative patient teaching, as well as additional instruction for the PACU staff. One factor in the success of PCA is the administration of an adequate loading dose of narcotic prior to implementing the PCA. The PACU nurse stabilizes the patient's comfort level and connects the PCA device only when the patient is oriented. The usual PCA prescription for the average adult patient is 1 mg morphine with an interval of 6 to 10 minutes. The dosage and lockout interval may be calculated

based on age and weight, then adjusted to provide adequate pain relief.

Another alternative to postoperative pain management is epidural analgesia. Disposition of the analgesic at the site of action would prove most beneficial; however, this is not possible with the drugs and techniques available. Administration of spinal opiates is the closest to the receptor site that an analgesic drug can be given (9). The epidural catheter is placed preoperatively, and the initial dose of medication is given by the anesthesiologist. Morphine has been the most popular opiate because it can be given in doses of 2 to 10 mg diluted in 10 ml 5% glucose or normal saline. It also provides pain relief without producing anesthesia, paralysis, or sympathetic block (10). Other epidural analgesic agents include hydromorphone hydrochloride (Dilaudid) and fentanyl. A combination of fentanyl and bupivicaine (Marcaine) may reduce the required amount of each drug and also the side effects. Administering a local anesthetic, however, may produce sympathetic and motor block.

The advantages of the epidural method of administration of analgesics are a consistent level of pain control without depression of the central nervous system and level of consciousness; and the ability to use a decreased amount of medications as compared to intramuscular injections. The disadvantages of epidural narcotic administration are the possibilities of delayed respiratory depression, itching, nausea and vomiting, and urinary retention, which can occur with all narcotics regardless of the route of administration. Naloxone can be used to control these complications without antagonizing the analgesic effects of the narcotic.

PCA and epidural infusion are proving to be effective options for postanesthesia pain management, as is the use of nonsteroidal antiinflammatory drugs (NSAIDs). In order to efficiently monitor patients receiving medications, PACU nurses must be knowledgeable about these drugs and their side effects, as well as how to potentiate their action. All patients receiving narcotics, regardless of the route of administration, must be observed closely for hypotension, respiratory depression, and/or adverse allergic reactions.

Once the presence and nature of pain is diagnosed, the type, route, and dosage of medication to be administered must be determined in a timely fashion. Inadequate intervention can initiate escalating pain, which increases the patient's anxiety and retards the recovery process. (See Fig. 23.6.)

If alleviation of pain by analgesics must be postponed (e.g., when narcotic antagonists have been given to reverse respiratory depression), the nurse

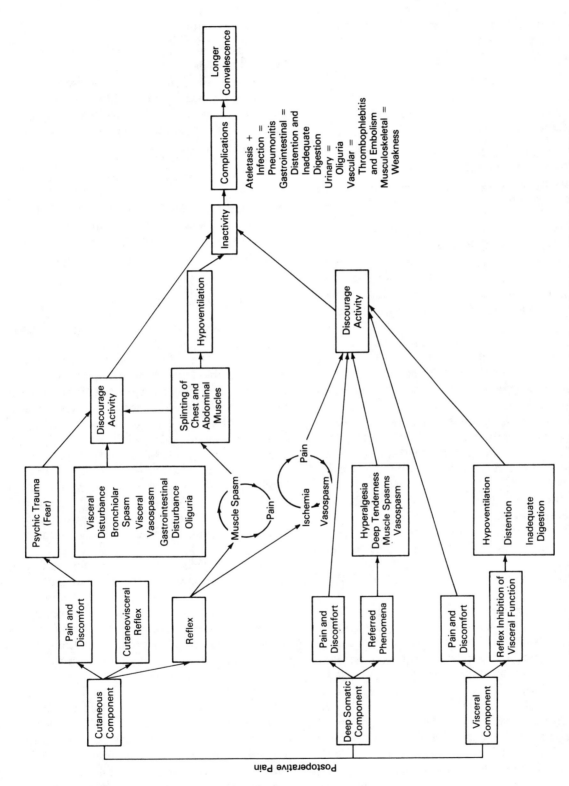

FIGURE 23.6. Possible effects of postoperative pain. (Reprinted by permission from J.J. Bonica. *The Management of Pain,* p. 1241. Copyright © 1953 by Lea & Febiger, Philadelphia.)

371

must implement other measures. Changing the patient's position, giving back rubs, or providing warm blankets can offer some relief. If the patient is able to concentrate, focusing on breathing techniques can be effective. Research continues to be conducted on control of acute pain without use of drugs, and the nurse should stay informed about these new techniques.

Pediatric Patients

Infants and small children are not "little adults"; they are physiologically different. Pediatric patients are more prone to hypoxia, hypoglycemia, hypovolemia, and hyper- or hypothermia. The primary intervention for children in the postanesthesia phase is prevention and/or correction of these four potential physiological problems.

In order to prevent hypoxia and provide optimal ventilation in the pediatric patient, the PACU nurse must be aware that a child's airway differs from that of an adult. A child's airway is soft and much more reactive; therefore, the child's head should be in a neutral position when the nurse is repositioning the airway to improve ventilation. Hyperextension of the neck could cause airway obstruction. Placing a small towel under the shoulders may help ensure proper alignment.

Pediatric patients' decreased vital capacity also leaves them more prone to respiratory compromise. Suctioning should be performed quickly and smoothly to prevent interruption of ventilation and laryngospasm.

Due to high energy levels and low energy reserves, infants and small children are at a greater risk for hypoglycemia. The added stress of surgery and keeping the patient NPO prior to the operation increase this risk. Prevention includes the administration of intravenous therapy as prescribed by the physician until the patient is able to take oral fluids.

The pediatric patient is closely monitored for hypovolemia; infants can lose up to 25% of circulating blood volume before exhibiting signs of hypovolemia (11). The body compensates by increasing the heart rate; therefore, tachycardia must be diagnosed in a timely fashion. Hypovolemia is prevented and corrected by administering fluids.

Infants and smaller children are especially prone to heat loss, due to the large ratio of surface area to body mass, increased body water content, and an immature central nervous system (11). Nursing intervention consists of maintaining a neutral thermal environment, which decreases the amount of oxygen and glucose required and promotes recovery.

Careful monitoring and prevention are the best measures for ensuring a neutral thermal environment.

Elderly Patients

Elderly patients require special consideration in the PACU. Their decreased ability to metabolize and eliminate medications may result in a delayed response and an extended half-life. Patients aged sixty or older may require lower dosages and longer dosing intervals. Medications such as midazolam hydrochloride (Versed) have specific prescribing information for the elderly.

Elderly patients also experience cardiovascular deterioration, are more prone to respiratory fatigue, and experience slowing of neurological transmissions. In addition, extra care must be taken in the elderly to protect the integumentary system, since aging causes a thinning of all layers of skin.

General Considerations

Each surgical procedure requires implementation of measures specific or unique to that particular procedure. The PACU nurse must be knowledgeable about possible complications and expected outcomes for specific surgeries. For example, surgical intervention for a meningioma requires frequent assessment of the patient's neurological status and vital signs to detect subtle changes. The nurse must also be aware of potential complications (e.g., sinus thrombosis, intracranial hemorrhage, aseptic meningitis, and seizure) and must be familiar with interventions to manage these complications. The PACU nurse also must be skilled in monitoring for increased intracranial pressure and decreased cerebral blood flow.

Vascular procedures, such as femoral popliteal bypass surgeries, require that the nurse pay particular attention to the extremity or extremities that may be affected postoperatively. Such monitoring would consist of checking for the absence of peripheral pulses, loss of movement or sensation, decreased temperature, and/or change of color in the affected extremity.

Surgery on the spinal column requires that the nurse be knowledgeable regarding the anatomy of the spine, because the spinal level at which the surgery is performed affects the patient's needs and complications that could occur in the PACU. The nurse must take care in positioning the patient by "log rolling" in order to maintain proper alignment of the spine, thus minimizing stress on the operative site and reducing pain. The patient's pain is usually due to muscle spasm, but excessive pain and restlessness may be the first sign of bleeding. An abnormal neurological assessment should prompt the nurse to report the changes immediately, since hematoma compression of the cord may very quickly cause irreversible neurological deficits below the level of surgery.

Nursing care for thoracic surgery patients would include interventions such as coughing, deep breathing, turning, suctioning, postural drainage and, if necessary, mechanical ventilation to promote oxygenation and ventilation.

Less-invasive surgical approaches such as laparoscopy, thoracoscopy, and arthroscopy are commonplace today. The PACU nurse must be knowledgeable about such endoscopic procedures and their possible complications. For example, these patients require a thorough assessment prior to discharge for any signs or symptoms of internal hemorrhage and visceral perforation.

Nursing considerations for less-invasive procedures are similar to the considerations in conventional procedures. There may be less surgical pain with less-invasive surgery; however, patients who have undergone laparoscopy may experience shoulder pain when they sit up. This referred shoulder pain is due to residual carbon dioxide in the abdomen, which rises when the patient sits up, causing pressure on the diaphragm. Nursing interventions consist of keeping the patient flat as long as possible in order to allow time for the gas to dissipate. Patients are instructed to stay flat at home until the pain subsides. These patients also have a high incidence of nausea and vomiting. Nursing interventions consist of maintaining adequate fluid intake by administering intravenous fluids; having the patient recline as much as possible and move slowly; and administering antiemetics. Antiemetics such as the scopolamine patch and ephedrine used for motion sickness may be most effective in counteracting nausea in these patients. The advantages include little sedation and drop in blood pressure. They may also prevent vagal slowing of the pulse.

Less-invasive same-day surgery is on the rise, and nurses will continue to be challenged with providing healthcare during a short time span. Special emphasis must be placed on educating patients and their families so that they can provide effective care at home.

EVALUATION

All patients must be discharged from the PACU in accordance with the written policies and discharge criteria set forth by the Department of Anesthesia. Discharge from the PACU is based on the accomplishment of established goals. This requires thorough patient assessment to evaluate the effectiveness of implemented nursing care. The minimum expected patient outcomes in order for inpatients to return to their rooms are stable vital signs within the patient's normal limits, normal thermic state, orientation to surroundings, absence of surgical and anesthetic complications, a minimum of pain and nausea, controlled wound drainage, adequate urine output (30 cc/hr), fluid and electrolyte balance, and adequate pulmonary status. The patient's postanesthesia score on the discharge scale should be high, if one is used. Table 23.6 provides an example of one discharge criteria scoring system.

The documentation of data collected through the use of the nursing process should reveal the patient's achievement of the discharge criteria. If a numerical scoring system is used, the discharge score will be recorded to reflect the patient's status and meet the facility's written policy (12). Evaluation by an anesthesiologist should be required if a patient fails to meet the established criteria for discharge.

Patients who are being discharged directly home must meet the discharge criteria, plus demonstrate the ability to take nourishment by mouth, ambulate, and void. They also are required to have written discharge instructions regarding their specific postoperative care.

Evaluation of the effectiveness of nursing care should be an ongoing process, along with patient assessment. The discharge criteria scoring system is one method of evaluating attainment of patient outcomes. If the score is acceptable, then most of the predetermined outcomes should have been attained.

Another effective way of evaluating patient care is to develop indicators. Indicators are essential in measuring and providing continuous quality improvement.

Standards of care for the PACU provide an avenue for evaluating patient care outcomes. A comparison of the nursing orders prescribed in the *Standards* with those in the plan of care should reveal consistency. To demonstrate professional as well as legal accountability, the PACU nurse must implement the standards of care established by the institution.

The trend toward performing more complex procedures on an outpatient basis continues. In the last few years, even certain American Society of Anesthesiologists (ASA) Class III anesthesia risk patients, defined as having severe systemic disease

TABLE 23.6.   Wohrle Discharge Criteria Scoring System

LEVEL OF CONSCIOUSNESS

1. Infant awake (cries; has startle reflex; moves freely)	2
2. Adult awake (answers simple questions; follows two-step commands)	2
3. Patient very sleepy (requires light tactile or verbal stimulation to arouse; attempts to follow commands; falls back to sleep easily)	1
4. Patient requires deep painful stimuli to awaken; does not respond to other stimuli	0

CIRCULATORY STATUS

1. Urinary output	
1 cc/kg/hour	2
0.5 cc/kg/hour	1
Less than 0.5 cc/kg/hour	0
2. Capillary activity	
Capillary beds bilaterally are equally pink, warm, blanche rapidly	2
Capillary beds are not equal in response or blanche sluggishly, skin cool	1
Capillary beds fail to blanche, skin cold and pale	0
3. Dressings	
Dressing did not require reinforcement; no evidence of bright red bleeding within last hour	2
Dressing required reinforcement due to serosanguineous drainage within last hour	1
New bright red bleeding noticed on dressing within last 15 minutes	0
4. Vital signs stable × 30 minutes	
Systolic blood pressure	
± 10 mm Hg of preop value	2
± 20 mm Hg of preop value	1
± greater than 20 mm Hg of preop value	0
Pulse	
± 20/min of preop rate	2
± 30/min of preop rate	1
± greater than 30/min or preop rate	0
Respirations	
± 5/min of preop rate	2
± greater than 5/min of preop rate	0
Temperature	
± 1 degree of oral/rectal preop temp	2
± 2 degrees of oral/rectal preop temp	1
± greater than 2 degrees oral/rectal preop temp	0
5. Drains, tubes	
Tubes are patent with less than 100 cc/h drainage; no bright red bleeding in last hour	2
Drainage in excess of 100 cc/h but not bright red	1
Bright red bleeding within last hour	0
6. Edema	
Edema of extremities, sacrum, and surgical site not in excess of initial postop assessment	2
Edema in excess of initial assessment but no moist basilar lung rales auscultated	1
Edema in excess of initial assessment and rales developing in lung bases	0

AIRWAY PATENCY

1. Airway assistance	
Requires no assistance	2
Requires oral/nasal airway or chin lift	1
Requires endotracheal tube	0
2. Breath sounds (auscultation)	
Bilateral exchange with no abnormal breath sounds	2
Bilateral exchange with rhonchi and/or faint rales	1
Absent or diminished breath sounds in any part of lungs and/or coarse rales; wheezes; stridor	0
3. Able to cough and swallow on command	2
Requires external tracheal irritation to cough; drooling	1
Requires suctioning and side-lying position	0
4. Has not retched or gagged; no nausea or emesis within last 30 minutes	2
Required antiemetic within last 30 minutes	1
Has vomited within last 30 minutes	0
5. Has had no bright red bleeding from nose or throat in last hour	2
Has had copious dark bloody secretions requiring suctioning in last 30 minutes	1
Is having bright red bleeding or copious dark secretions requiring suctioning in last 15 minutes	0

Printed with permission of Carmen Brochu, RN, MSN, CNAA; Product Line Director, Empire Health Services, Spokane, Washington.

status, can be safely cared for outside the traditional inpatient setting (13). Providing quality care for these patients presents additional challenges to the PACU nurse; discharge teaching and followup are essential components of PACU nurses' responsibilities to these patients.

Most healthcare organizations that provide outpatient services have implemented a system for calling patients twenty-four hours postoperatively to ascertain how they are recovering. The nurse asks questions regarding the patient's ability to take nourishment, void, and ambulate. The interview should also assess the patient's ability to care for the wound and manage postoperative pain. It is important to evaluate how patients feel they are coping with their recovery and to answer any questions. It is difficult to fully assess a patient over the telephone. If there is a concern that the patient or significant other is unable to provide appropriate care, the nurse may need to advise the patient to seek medical assistance and refer the call to the patient's physician or the anesthesiologist. A repeat phone call is then needed to ascertain the patient's condition and determine the effectiveness of any recommended intervention.

The postoperative phone call is also an excellent opportunity to evaluate the patient's perception of services received. It is imperative that these postoperative phone calls be documented and that provisions be made for followup to be initiated, if needed. A number of ambulatory surgery centers have standardized forms that facilitate the documentation process.

As the trend of less-invasive surgery and ambulatory services continues, PACU nurses will be challenged with developing innovative methods and models for providing quality care. Postanesthesia nursing is multidimensional and requires a broad knowledge base and the ability to adapt to an ever-changing environment.

REFERENCES

1. Miller, Ronald D., ed. *Anesthesia. Volume 2* 3rd ed. New York: Churchill Livingstone, 1990.
2. Carr, T., and Wester, C. S. "Recovery care centers: An innovative approach to caring for healthy surgical patients." *AORN J* 53(4):986–995, 1991.
3. Creighton, Helen. *Law Every Nurse Should Know* 5th ed. Philadelphia: W. B. Saunders, 1986.
4. Vogelsang, J. "Patients who develop postanesthesia shaking show no difference in postoperative temperature from those who do not develop shaking." *J Postanesthesia Nursing* 6:231–237, 1991.
5. Rivera, W. B. "Practical points in the assessment and management of postoperative pediatric pain." *J Postanesthesia Nursing* 6(1):40–42, 1991.
6. Allen, J. "Patient classification in the postanesthesia care unit." *J Postanesthesia Nursing* 5(4):228–238, 1990.
7. Ashby, D. "Malignant hyperthermia: A potential crisis in the postanesthesia care unit." *J Postanesthesia Nursing* 5(4):279–281, 1990.
8. Hylka, S. C., and Shaw, C. F. "Implementation of a pain controlled analgesia program under the direction of the nursing department." *J Postanesthesia Nursing* 6(3):170–175, 1991.
9. Frost, E. *Postanesthesia Care*. Norwalk, CT: Appleton and Lange, 1990.
10. Fuk, C., and Hadley, J. D. "Something for pain: New trends in epidural analgesia." *J Postanesthesia Nursing* 5(4):247–253, 1990.
11. Hedman-Dennis, S. "Stabilization of the sick infant or child." *J Postanesthesia Nursing* 6(3):165–169, 1991.
12. American Society of Postanesthesia Nurses. *Standards of Postanesthesia Nursing Practice*. Richmond, VA: ASPAN, 1991.
13. Young, C. M. "The postoperative followup phone call: An essential part of the ambulatory surgery nurse's job." *J Postanesthesia Nursing* 5(August):273–275, 1990.

SUGGESTED READINGS

Allen, A. "New horizons in PACU Practice." *J Postanesthesia Nursing* 4(4):268–270, 1989.
Esberger, K. K., and Hughes, S. T., Jr. *Nursing Care of the Aged*. Norwalk, CT: Appleton and Lange, 1989.
Fetzer-Flower, S., and Mullen, C. A. "Laryngospasm—Induced pulmonary edema: Case report." *J Postanesthesia Nursing* 5(4):222–227, 1990.
Hill, J. M. "Time-saving formats for patient care planning in outpatient surgery units." *J Postanesthesia Nursing* 6(3):181–184, 1991.
Luczun, M. E. *Postanesthesia Nursing: A Comprehensive Guide*. Rockville, MD: Aspen Publications, 1984.
Luczun, M. E. "Postanesthesia nursing: Past, present, and future." *J Postanesthesia Nursing* 5(4):282–285, 1990.
Miller, K. M., and Taylor, B. J. "Standard care plans for the postanesthesia care unit." *J Postanesthesia Nursing* 6(1):26–32, 1991.
Murray, S. E. "Patient assessment in the postanesthesia care unit: A critical care approach." *J Postanesthesia Nursing* 4(4):232–238, 1989.
Noonan, A. T., Anderson, P., Newton, P., Patrin, T., Weber, K. L., and Winstead-Fry, P. "Family-centered nursing in the postanesthesia care unit: The evaluation of practice." *J Postanesthesia Nursing* 6:13–16, 1991.
Partyka, M. B. "Practical points in the care of the post-lumbar spine surgery patient." *J Postanesthesia Nursing* 6(3):185–187, 1991.
Stewart-Amidei, C. "Meningioma: Nursing care considerations." *J Postanesthesia Nursing* 6(4):269–278, 1991.
Summers, S. "Using nursing diagnosis to document nursing care in the postanesthesia care unit." *J Postanesthesia Nursing* 4(5):306–311, 1989.

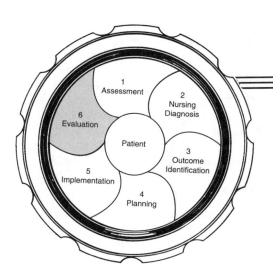

24

Evaluating Outcome Attainment

The degree of outcome achievement is determined.

Evaluation is a process for determining worth, value, or effectiveness. To make an evaluation, the evaluator assesses data and compares the findings to established criteria (1).

Evaluation is the final phase of the nursing process (Fig. 24.1). It follows implementation of the nursing actions identified in the plan of care and reflects how the patient responded to those actions. As the final component of the plan of care, it allows the nurse to make an objective and measurable judgment regarding the resolution of the problem or the patient's progress toward achieving the desired outcome. It indicates the completion of one cycle of interventions, and may begin another one based on current data and changing patient responses. Evaluation is a continuous process. The sixth standard in AORN's *Standards of Perioperative Clinical Practice* states, "The perioperative nurse evaluates the patient's progress toward attainment of outcomes" (2). It directs the nurse to measure the effectiveness of interventions in relation to outcomes through the ongoing assessment of data (2).

In 1984 the Association of Operating Room Nurses (AORN) developed and published *Patient Outcome Standards for Perioperative Nursing.* Later, these were retitled *Patient Outcomes: Standards of Perioperative Care* (3). The six outcome standards focus on aggregate patient outcomes for all surgical patients. They are general statements that reflect the outcome statements in Standard III: Outcome Identification in the *Standards of Perioperative Clinical Practice.* They represent guidelines for nurses as the

evaluation process is individualized, very specifically, for each patient according to the nursing diagnosis. (See Fig. 24.2.)

The patient plan of care forms the framework for evaluation. It clearly states the patient's diagnosis, projected outcomes, planned interventions, and criteria for measuring outcome achievement. The plan integrates the nurse's intellectual, interpersonal, and technical interactions to best meet the needs of the patient (Fig. 24.3).

STEPS IN THE EVALUATION PROCESS

Evaluation consists of three steps: (1) selecting criteria for judging outcome attainment, (2) collecting outcome data, and (3) comparing data with the criteria to determine whether projected outcomes have been attained. The process requires continuous systematic assessment of the patient during and after interventions by the nurse (4).

Selecting Clients

Criteria are supporting evidence the nurse uses to determine whether a projected outcome has been achieved. A criterion states a desired or normal condition to compare with the actual condition. Outcome criteria are used to evaluate the nursing interventions selected to assist the patient in achieving the projected outcomes.

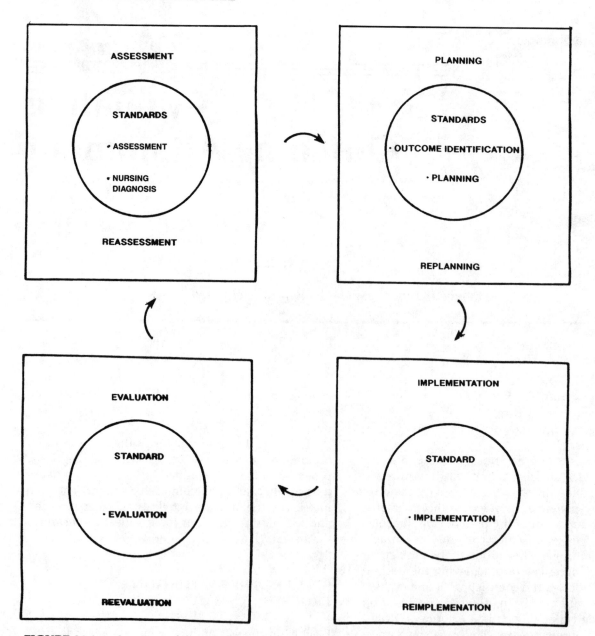

FIGURE 24.1. As a part of the nursing process, evaluation marks the completion of one cycle of interventions and the beginning of another. Evaluation leads to reassessment, replanning, reimplementation, and reevaluation. The phases of the nursing process correlate with the *Standards of Perioperative Clinical Practice.*

Outcome criteria should include applicable components of the outcome standards shown in Figure 24.2, and should be individualized for each patient, specific, and measurable. For example, one criterion for blood pressure might state, "48 hours postoperatively the patient's systolic pressure is no greater than ±20 mm Hg, compared with the preoperative value." The criterion would not have been individualized or realistic if it had stated, "48 hours postoperatively, the systolic pressure is no greater than 120 mm Hg," because this is an average value for middle-aged adults.

Criteria can be stated in many ways: as signs and symptoms, data from diagnostic or laboratory tests, statements from the patient, or patient responses (Fig. 24.4).

The number of criteria for each expected outcome varies. They should be sufficient in number and precise enough to measure change in the patient's status. For example, two patients may undergo the same surgical procedure, such as a bowel resection, but not follow the same postoperative regimen. The first patient may have a nasogastric tube after surgery, but the second may not. The expected

Standard I

The patient demonstrates knowledge of the physiological and psychological responses to surgical intervention.

Interpretive statement

The patient has a right to information regarding the operative procedure and potential physical and psychological effects. The information is shared with the patient's family or significant others. The patient has the right to expect the assurance of privacy, confidentiality, and maintenance of personal dignity. This standard is most relevant in the preoperative phase but may also be used for postoperative evaluation.

Criteria

Dependent upon the physical and psychological status, the patient

- confirms, verbally or in writing, consent to the operative procedure.
- describes the sequence of events during the perioperative period.
- states outcome expectations in realistic terms.
- expresses feelings about surgical experience.

Standard II

The patient is free from infection.

Interpretive statement

Prevention of infection requires the application of the principles of microbiology and aseptic practice. Preexisting patient conditions can increase susceptibility to infection. Other factors independent of nursing care can contribute to the development of infections. Examples of these factors are

- type of operative procedure
- systems transected
- tissue trauma
- wound classification (clean, clean contaminated, contaminated, dirty)
- length of procedure
- implants
- presence of devices, i.e., urinary catheters, IVs, endotracheal tubes

Criteria

Dependent upon the physical and psychological status, the patient will be free from infection following the operative procedure.

Standard III

The patient's skin integrity is maintained.

Interpretive statement

Skin integrity is assessed preoperatively. Existing conditions such as diabetes and obesity may compromise skin integrity. No anticipated alteration to skin occurs during the intraoperative phase.

Criteria

Dependent upon the physical and psychological status, the patient is free from evidence of skin breakdown or altered state.

Standard IV

The patient is free from injury related to positioning, extraneous objects, or chemical, physical, and electrical hazards.

Interpretive statement

Prevention of injury requires application of the principles of positioning, knowledge of instrumentation and equipment, and the proper use of chemical agents.

Criteria

Dependent upon the physical and psychological status, the patient is free from injury during the intraoperative phase and any sequela during the postoperative phase.

Standard V

The patient's fluid and electrolyte balance is maintained.

Interpretive statement

Continual monitoring of fluid losses and replacement therapy occurs during the intraoperative phase. Decisions relating to replacement therapy are generally not within the scope of practice of the OR nurse.

Criteria

Dependent upon the physical and psychological status, the patient's

- mental orientation is consistent with the preoperative level.
- elimination processes correlate with activities related to the operative procedure.
- fluid and electrolyte balance is consistent with preoperative status.

Standard VI

The patient participates in the rehabilitation process.

Interpretive statement

The patient should be able to participate in own care, decision making, and discharge planning, and expect a reasonable continuity of care.

Criteria

Dependent upon the physical and psychological status, the patient

- describes responsibilities resulting in optimal benefit of surgical intervention.
- identifies problem areas related to surgical experience.
- performs activities related to care.

FIGURE 24.2. Patient Outcomes: Standards of Perioperative Care. (Reprinted by permission from AORN, Inc. 10170 East Mississippi Ave., Denver CO 80231. All rights reserved.)

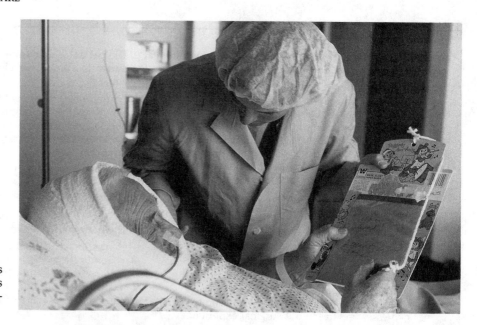

FIGURE 24.3. The nurse follows through to evaluate the patient's ability to attain the desired outcome.

Expected Outcome: The patient with history of chronic bronchitis will demonstrate adequate pulmonary ventilation throughout a surgical procedure performed under local anesthesia with heavy sedation.

Criteria	Sources of Data
No rales or rhonchi heard on chest auscultation	Signs and symptoms
$PaCO_2$ consistent with patient's preoperative value of 40 mm Hg	Laboratory data
No abnormalities identified on intraoperative chest x-ray	Diagnostic data
No statements of shortness of breath	Patient's responses, expressions
No flaring of nostrils or facial grimacing	
Compliance with deep-breathing instructions when requested	Demonstration

FIGURE 24.4. Examples of criteria statements.

outcome for both patients may be the same, but the outcome criteria would indicate different measurements for evaluation. An outcome applicable to both patients might be, "The patient demonstrates no evidence of fluid and electrolyte imbalance." Criteria for the first patient might include, "No loss of electrolytes through drainage from the nasogastric tube." This would not be a criterion for the second patient, who has no nasogastric tube.

The criteria specify when a patient is expected to attain the projected outcome. Each outcome statement should indicate whether the outcome is immediate, intermediate, or long-term. Immediate and intermediate outcome statements usually have a specific interval for checking the patient's progress. Long-term projected outcomes may not include a final date and not be measurable until after the patient is discharged to the home or community. If the outcome statement is, "The patient's skin integrity is maintained," a criterion for immediate evaluation could read, "No evidence of skin abrasion." An intermediate evaluation criterion could be, "No evidence of wound dehiscence within 48 hours after surgery." Long-term evaluation could be indicated with, "Evidence of intact skin and closure after removal of suture from incision site." Regardless of the time and conditions identified in the outcome statement and criteria, nursing activities must be appropriate to the statement so evaluation can be done and a judgment made (4).

Collecting Data

In the evaluation process, the nurse gathers data identified in the criteria. This is an assessment of the patient during or after the implementation of the nursing activities in the plan of care.

The nurse must gather and report data in a manner that will allow quantitative and qualitative measurement. Measurement should be reliable so each observer following the patient's plan of care will record the data consistently (5). For example, one projected outcome statement might read:

- Outcome: The patient will be free from injury caused by improper safety measures during intraoperative period.
- Criteria
  1. The skin is free from abrasions.
  2. There is no edema from positioning devices.
  3. There are no fractures or dislocated bones.

In this example, each nurse following the plan of care would collect the same data, assessing the patient's skin for abrasions, tissue for edema caused by positioning devices, and the bony structure for dislocations. Data gathered by two or more nurses could be compared because the same criteria were used. The criteria are individualized for the patient. Of course the third criterion, "no fractures or dislocated bones," would not be valid for measurement purposes if the patient's preoperative condition included fractures or dislocated bones.

Comparing Data

The final step of evaluation requires the nurse to compare the data to the criteria. This enables him or her to determine the degree of outcome attainment and record it as a problem that is either resolved or requires further action (5).

The nurse can use a variety of methods to determine relationships between the criteria and patient responses (6). The criterion itself identifies the means for gathering the data; for example, "No rales or rhonchi heard on chest auscultation." Methods of data collection include observation of signs and symptoms; review of laboratory and diagnostic data; intervention with technical skills or teaching techniques; or use of interpersonal skills through communication with the patient, family, or significant others. For example, in evaluating a patient's response during local anesthesia, a nurse might ask the following questions:

1. Were rales or rhonchi auscultated during the surgical procedure?
2. If arterial blood gases were measured during the procedure, what was the relationship of that value to the preoperative value of 40 mm Hg?
3. Did the intraoperative x-ray reveal any abnormalities in the lung field?
4. Did the patient complain of shortness of breath during the procedure?

5. Did the patient flare his or her nostrils or grimace?
6. Did the patient take deep breaths when instructed to during the procedure?

One tool used in evaluation is a patient outcome scale, which requires assigning a numerical value to a number of factors. An example is the Glasgow coma scale, an assessment tool that numerically describes level of consciousness. It is a means for a quick and accurate evaluation of the patient's neurological status, as noted in eyes open, verbal responses, and motor responses. The patient's responses in these categories are objectively scored and plotted on a graph. This scale is widely used for admitting and discharging patients from neurological and postoperative care units. The perioperative nurse could adapt the Glasgow coma scale for intraoperative patient care by using it to determine the patient's level of consciousness and as a principal component of preoperative assessment and postoperative evaluation data. Other assessment tools include those that evaluate outcome according to patient classification scales or level of activity in addition to numerical rating (7).

As the nurse compares the data with the patient's response to the criteria, a judgment can be made regarding outcome attainment, the validity of the nursing activities, or the circumstances under which the activities were performed. A relationship can be defined among the projected outcome, the nursing action, and the evaluation. Results may be any one or a combination of the following (8):

1. The patient's response was as expected and the problem was resolved. There is no need for further nursing actions, and those used were appropriate.
2. The patient's response indicated that the entire problem was not resolved. Evidence indicated that immediate projected outcomes were achieved, but intermediate and long-range outcomes were not. Complete problem resolution may be slow, and nursing actions should be directed at solving intermediate and long-range outcomes. Reevaluation will be necessary.
3. The patient's response revealed little evidence that the problem is being resolved. Immediate intervention and long-range outcomes were not reached and, in some instances, not even approached. Reassessment and replanning are required.
4. The patient's response indicated that new prob-

lems exist. Assessment and planning for these must be coordinated with planning for the original problems. Evaluation will follow implementation for new problems.

The nurse puts the evaluation data into one of these categories, then examines factors that may have affected the evaluation process. These can include internal or external factors that control or alter the patient's response to the nursing actions. These factors might be economic (low income), cultural (adherence to a vegetarian diet), sociological (no family or friends), and religious (refusal of blood) aspects of the patient's lifestyle, or physical or psychosocial factors external to the patient's environment. The effect of these factors on the patient or the surroundings where the nursing actions took place may directly correlate with the patient's responses to nursing intervention.

Once the nurse has analyzed evaluation data and considered the influencing factors, he or she plans further actions appropriate to the situation, such as reassessment, replanning, changes in implementation, and reevaluation.

REASSESSMENT

Reassessment is a necessary sequel to evaluation. It involves reassessing the patient's health status, reconsidering the identified problems, resetting expected outcomes, and reorganizing the plan of care. The new plan is activated, evaluated, and judged again based on the patient's changing needs. Thus the nursing process continues with changes in the patient's status until the targeted health problems are resolved.

For example, for the patient who underwent a surgical procedure under local anesthesia, one outcome statement was that the patient would demonstrate adequate pulmonary ventilation throughout the surgical procedure. A criterion for the outcome was, "No statements of shortness of breath." If at some time during the procedure the patient complained of shortness of breath, the projected outcome would not have been met based on evaluation of that particular criterion. The nurse would reassess the data, reevaluate the projected outcome, and alter the plan of care to assist the patient toward adequate pulmonary ventilation. Once the new plan is implemented, the patient is reevaluated based on reassessment of the data at hand.

DOCUMENTATION

Throughout implementation of the plan of care, the nurse evaluates the patient's response and records this information in the patient record. The patient record is then used to validate nursing actions and continuity of care. By evaluating and recording nursing actions and patient outcomes, the nurse assumes accountability for the care given. If the nurse does not record nursing actions or the patient's response, measuring outcome attainment becomes very difficult.

Intraoperative care is documented on the operative record. Operative nursing records are a valued addition to the patient record, both for legal purposes and as a method for evaluating the quality of care provided. Figure 24.5 provides an example of an intraoperative nursing record that incorporates expected outcomes, followed by checklists of criteria by which to determine the appropriateness of the intraoperative nursing care to each outcome. One section of this form covers three outcome statements: "The patient's skin integrity is maintained," "The patient is free from infection," and "The patient is free from injury related to positioning, extraneous objects, or chemical, physical, and electrical hazards." The evaluation criteria used by one hospital to measure the extent of achievement of these outcomes are:

1. Preoperative condition and turgor of skin
2. Operative position and positioning aids used
3. Eye-care measures taken
4. Skin preparatory solution used and area prepped
5. Comments

The criteria used on the form illustrated in Figure 24.5 can be adapted to any intraoperative record. Similar criteria could also be used to review and evaluate indicators that have been identified for the unit's quality improvement program.

This chapter demonstrates how to measure the effectiveness of nursing care and the patient's response to that care. It shows how to use an outcome statement to reflect desired patient outcomes, and how to develop criteria that can be used to evaluate an individual patient's care. The actual results of care are then compared to projected outcome statements, to measure the degree of outcome attainment. All persons who are involved in the patient's care—the patient, healthcare personnel, and fam-

Surgeon:		Date	OR:

Assistants:	Building: ☐ MOR ☐ FBOR ☐ GYN ☐ NSC ☐ NSA ☐ ASU

Case Priority: ☐ 10 Elective ☐ 20 Emergency

Patient Acuity:　　　　Time Scheduled:

Patient Admit Type: ☐ 01 IN/P ☐ 02 OP ☐ 03 SDA

Other:

Patient Discharge Type: ☐ 01 IN/P ☐ 02 OP ☐ 03 SDA

TMF #'s

Anesthesiologist:

Anesthesia ☐ 00 None ☐ 11 General ☐ 20 Regional
☐ 21 Bier Blk ☐ 22 Spinal ☐ 23 Epi/Caudal ☐ 24 IV Block

CRNA

☐ 25 Axillary ☐ 30 Local (No Anes.) ☐ 31 MAC

Pre-Operative Diagnosis

Operations

Post-Operative Diagnosis

Cormis Codes:

The Patient Demonstrates Knowledge of the Physiological and Psychological Response to Surgical Intervention

Pre Op Assessment:　　Patient Arrival Status: ☐ Alert ☐ Oriented ☐ Anxious ☐ Drowsy ☐ Crying ☐ Confused ☐ Comatose

ID Bracelet: ☐ Yes ☐ No　　Location:　　　　NPO Since　　　　Consent ☐ Yes ☐ No

Chart Checked for Lab/EKG/X-Ray ☐ Yes ☐ No　　　　Patient Verbalizes Correct Procedure ☐ Yes ☐ No

Pre-op Teaching ☐ Yes ☐ No　　Comment:

ALLERGIES　　　　　　　　　　☐ Interviewed By:

The Patient's Skin Integrity is Maintained/The Patient is Free From Infection/The Patient is Free From Injury Related to Positioning, Extraneous Objects, or Chemical, Physical, and Electrical Hazards.*

Skin Pre Op: ☐ Warm ☐ Cool ☐ Dry ☐ Moist ☐ Intact ☐ Open ☐ Denuded ☐ Abrasions ☐ Bruises

Turgor: ☐ Good ☐ Fair ☐ Poor　　Comment:

Operative Position and Aids: ☐ Supine ☐ Prone ☐ Rt. Lateral ☐ Lt. Lateral ☐ Sitting ☐ Lithotomy ☐ Rotating Bed

Arms: ☐ Tucked ☐ Padded Arm Boards　**Aids:** ☐ Safety Strap ☐ Headrest ☐ Chest Roll ☐ Egg Crate ☐ Gel Pad

☐ Shoulder Roll ☐ Pillows ☐ Bean Bag ☐ Bony Prominence Padded　By:

Eye Care: ☐ Lacrilube ☐ Moist Cotton Balls ☐ Eye Occluders ☐ Taped ☐ Rt Eye ☐ Lt Eye　By:

Prep: ☐ Scrub ☐ Alcohol ☐ Other　　Area

Betadine ☐ Paint ☐ Phisohex ☐ Shave Prep

Comments:

The Patient's Fluid and Electrolyte Balance is Maintained

NG Tube Pre Op:	NG Tube Intra Op
Indwelling Catheter Pre Op	Wound Packing
Indwelling Catheter Intra Op: Size:　　cc Balloon　By:	☐ Urimeter ☐ Closed Drainage　　　cc Urine
Drugs on Field	Drug
Drug	Drug
Drug	Drug
Drug	Drug
Drug	Drug
Drug	Drug
Wound Drains: ☐ Penrose ☐ Hemovac ☐ Davol ☐ Other____	☐ Nacl 1000 ccX____ ☐ Tis-U-Sol 1000 ccX____
Size:　　Location:	☐ Nacl 3000 ccX____ ☐ St H$_2$O 1000 ccX____

Methodist

Otorhinolaryngology/Hand Intraoperative Report

The Methodist Hospital 6565 Fannin Houston, Texas 77030

(continued)

FIGURE 24.5.　Intraoperative nursing record. By recording nursing actions, the nurse becomes accountable for the actions and demonstrates responsibility in patient involvement.

Service:

☐ 10 Anesthesia	☐ 01 Obstetrics	☐ 20 Plastics	☐ 27 CV
☐ 03 Dental	☐ 08 Ophthalmology	☐ 22 Procto	☐ 33 Urology
☐ 25 General	☐ 14 Orthopedics	☐ 29 Thoracic	☐ 31 Organ/Transp
☐ 10 GYN	☐ 06 OTO/Rhino	☐ 35 Radiology	☐ Other
☐ 50 Pathology	☐ 18 Neurosurgery		

Time Patient Arrives:

IN OR	Anesthesia Start
Incision 1.	Closure 1.
2.	2.
3.	3.
Dressing Comp	Room Departure:

Scrub Nurse	To	Circulating Nurse	To
	To		To
	To		To
	To		To
	To		To
	To		To
	To		To

Sponge Count: Initial _____ Closing _____

By: _____ By: _____

Change of Shift By _____ Cor/Incor/NA   Additional By: _____ Cor/Incor/NA

Lap	Raytex	Peanuts	Cottonoids	Blades	Needles	Inj. Needles	Bulldogs	Tonsil	

Electrosurgical Units: Type: _____ ECN # _____ Setting: _____ Grounding Site: _____

Type: _____ ECN # _____ Setting: _____ Grounding Site: _____

Tourniquet(s) ☐ Do-Nut ☐ Penrose ☐ Nitrogen ☐ Kiddie   Padded: ☐ Yes ☐ No   Cuff: ☐ Single ☐ Double

Checked By: _____ Location: _____ Pressure: _____ Up: _____ Down: _____

Checked By: _____ Location: _____ Pressure: _____ Up: _____ Down: _____

SKIN CONDITION: ☐ Intact ☐ Redness ☐ Bruises ☐ Dry ☐ Swelling   Up: _____ Down: _____

☐ Laser ECN: _____ Setting: _____ ☐ Microscope ECN: _____ ☐ Video

☐ Drill ☐ Dermatome ☐ Arthroscope ☐ Staplizer ☐ X-Rays ☐ ESS Cart ☐ Other ☐ Nicolet   To _____

Hypo/Hyperthermia Unit
Type: _____ ECN # _____ Temp: _____

Frozen Section	Implants
1.	1.
2.	2.
3.	3.
4.	4.
5.	5.
6.	6.
7.	7.

Cultures	Specimens:
1.	1.
2.	2.
3.	3.
4.	4.
5.	5.
6.	6.
7.	7.

*POST OP SKIN CONDITION:

☐ Sutured ☐ Open ☐ Steristrip _____ X _____ ☐ Stapled X _____ ☐ Bovie Pad Site: _____

Dressings: ☐ Telfa ☐ 4 x 4's X _____ ☐ Kerlix X _____ ☐ Kling X _____ ☐ ABD ☐ Eye Pad ☐ Eye Shield ☐ Fluffs ☐ Bandaid ☐ Mastoid

☐ Tape ☐ Elastoplast ☐ Foam Tape **Cast Splints:** ☐ Volar ☐ Posterior ☐ Sugartong ☐ Side Bars

☐ Ace: _____ ☐ Sling ☐ Bennett Elev.

Comments

Discharge To: ☐ PACU ☐ OP ☐ ICU ☐ Hospital Room

VIA: ☐ Stretcher ☐ Bed ☐ RR Bed c̄ Side Rails Up   HOB: ☐↑ ☐↓

Wound Class: ☐ 1 Clean ☐ 2 Clean Contaminated

☐ 3 Contaminated ☐ 4 Dirty ☐ 5 Non Surgical

FIGURE 24.5   (*cont'd.*)

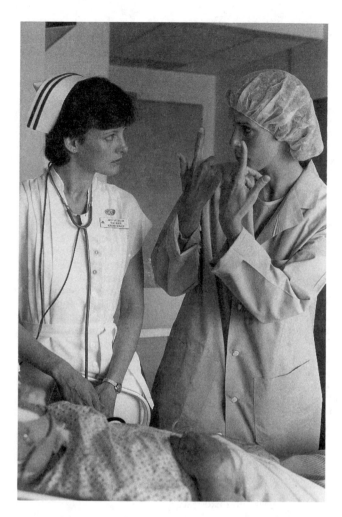

FIGURE 24.6.   The unit nurse and perioperative nurse evaluate Mr. Fischer postoperatively.

ily—contribute to evaluation of attainment of expected outcomes.

Like the other five components of the nursing process, evaluation is recurrent and cyclical. It is the thread that ties patient care together. Just as expected outcomes tell us where we are going, evaluation tells if we arrived at our destination. Without evaluation to judge its effectiveness, nursing care may not improve, and the patient's progress may remain at a standstill (Fig. 24.6).

Case Example
When evaluating the patient plan of care, the nurse compares the desired outcome criteria with the patient's actual response to care. The guides for measurement are the preoperative outcome statements given in the plan of care (Fig. 24.7). Expected outcomes for Mr. Fischer were formulated in earlier chapters. Here we evaluate success in meeting them.

One nursing diagnosis was a communication problem related to an altered airway, wired jaw, and tongue resection. The expected outcome was that Mr. Fischer would be able to communicate postoperatively. The following criteria could be used to evaluate the effectiveness of nursing care:

1. *Was Mr. Fischer able to communicate with the magic slate board? Factors influencing the attainment of this criterion would be his level of consciousness postoperatively; his ability to see, which would mean using his glasses; his orientation to time and space; and his physical strength. Could he hold the magic slate board, and were his hands steady enough to write legibly? The nursing record indicated that Mr. Fischer was able to use the magic slate board to communicate his needs on the second postoperative day.*
2. *Was Mr. Fischer able to use the nurse call bell? Factors that might influence this criterion could be his level of consciousness, his orientation to time and space, and placement of the bell within reach. Mr. Fischer was not confused, was awake the morning after surgery, and did not have any problems with using the nurse call bell. The bell was within his reach at all times when personnel were not at his bedside. This was documented in the plan of care.*
3. *Did Mr. Fischer use the finger codes for yes and no questions?*
4. *Did he respond on the telephone by tapping once for yes and twice for no in response to questions?*

Criteria that can be used to measure Mr. Fischer's understanding of his perioperative care prior to administration of preoperative medication might be that he:

1. *asks questions about his impending surgery.*
2. *describes the effect of surgery in own words.*
3. *expresses feelings of concern and fears regarding body image.*
4. *demonstrates turning, coughing, and deep-breathing exercises.*
5. *tells his family where the waiting room is located.*

Another expectation pertaining to intraoperative care was that Mr. Fischer would be free from neuromuscular complications 24 hours postoperatively. Because of the nature and length of the surgical procedure, the potential for damage to the neuromuscular system was greater than usual. Mr. Fischer was in the operating room approximately 12 hours. Criteria used to measure extent of outcome attainment might include but would not be limited to the following:

1. *No tingling sensation*
2. *No numbness*

INTRAOPERATIVE PLAN OF CARE
Mr. Ralph Fischer

Nursing Diagnosis	Expected Outcome	Plan	Implementation	Evaluation
PREOPERATIVE				
Knowledge deficit; lack of specific information regarding phenomena that might affect level of functioning	Patient will verbalize understanding of his perioperative care prior to administration of preoperative medications.	Provide explanations regarding each phase of perioperative period. 1. Preop: NPO, preop meds, IV line, shave, antiseptic scrub, where family can wait, approximate length of surgery, etc. 2. Intraop: EKG, BP, Foley catheter, possible blood transfusions, drains, jaw wiring, trach, etc. 3. Postop: ICU, possible ventilator, frequent suctioning, turning, respiratory therapy, pain meds, dressing change, etc.	• Specific information provided regarding the events surrounding the surgical procedure • Explanations given regarding expectations of the patient and family • Encouraged to express fears and anxieties • Patient explained his understanding of the surgical procedure and anesthesia • Preoperative instruction regarding postop care: 1–coughing, deep breathing, turning 2–pain 3–drains and tubes 4–IV 5–possible ventilator • Patient demonstrated turning, coughing, and deep breathing exercises.	The patient verbalizes understanding of his perioperative care prior to administration of preoperative medications. 1. Asks questions about his impending surgery 2. Describes in own words effect of surgery 3. Expresses feelings of concern and fears regarding body image 4. Demonstrates turning, coughing, and deep breathing exercises 5. Tells family where waiting room is located.
Communication, impaired; verbal, resulting from tracheostomy, wired jaw, and possible impaired anatomical structure (tongue)	Patient will be able to communicate postoperatively.	1. Teach patient to use magic slate and nurses call bell 2. Teach patient hand signals (one finger– yes, two fingers–no) 3. Ask patient yes and no questions whenever possible 4. Teach patient to communicate on phone by tapping on mouth piece.	Nurse conducted preoperative assessment • Rapport was established with patient and wife • Patient taught how to use alternative methods of communicating • Patient and wife return demonstrated use of fingers and phone messages.	The patient was able to communicate postoperatively 1. Write words on magic slate 2. Push nurse call bell 3. Use one finger for yes responses 4. Use two fingers for no responses 5. Tap on mouth piece of phone to respond yes or no to direct questions.
INTRAOPERATIVE				
Potential for neuromuscular damage due to required positioning and length of surgical procedure.	Patient will be free from neuromuscular complications 24 hours postoperatively.	1. Question patient preop re: any ROM limitations or neurosensory problems 2. Use positional devices on OR table to prevent pressure over bony prominences (i.e.	Operating Room: 1. Patient denied ROM limitations preoperatively. 2. Patient placed in supine position with egg crate mattress. 3. Foam pads on both elbows and heels.	The patient was free of neuromuscular complications 24 hours postoperatively 1. No tingling sensation 2. No numbness 3. No edema 4. No cramping 5. No pain or ache

FIGURE 24.7. Intraoperative plan of care, including preoperative, intraoperative, and postoperative nursing diagnoses, expected outcomes, plan, implementation, and evaluation for Mr. Fischer.

INTRAOPERATIVE PLAN OF CARE
Mr. Ralph Fischer (continued)

Nursing Diagnosis	Expected Outcome	Plan	Implementation	Evaluation
INTRAOPERATIVE (cont.)				
		flotation order mattress, egg crate, etc.) 3. Place foam pads on heels and elbows and consider foam ring under buttocks 4. Have rolled towel available for affected shoulder (prn) 5. Check with anesthesiologist and/or surgeon re: padding desired head and neck 6. Check with anesthesiologist and/or surgeon re: flexion of table or placement of blanket under popliteal space to lessen strain to lower back 7. After preliminary positioning ask patient about his level of comfort and adjust accordingly. 8. Prior to RR transfer check bony prominences and buttocks for discoloration, document findings and communicate abnormal findings to RR	4. Rolled towel placed under shoulder 5. Head and neck slightly extended. 6. O.R. table flexed to lessen strain on lower back during procedure. 7. Patient states he is comfortable. 8. Physical assessment when transferring to recovery room revealed no evidence of pressure areas or impaired skin integrity.	in joints 6. No swelling in joints 7. Flexion and extension of extremities 8. Abduction and adduction of extremities 9. No weakness 10. No stiffness
POSTOPERATIVE				
Respirations, alteration in due to tracheostomy	Patient will have patent alternative airway until tracheostomy is closed.	1. Intraop: have ABG kits available 2. Check with surgeon re: type and size of tracheostomy tube. 3. Notify recovery room if ventilator necessary 4. Have Ambu bag and oxygen tank ready on patient bed prior to transport	Operating Room: 1. Blood drawn for ABG and sent to lab. 2. Silastic tracheostomy tube size #7 inserted. Recovery Room: 3. Placed on ventilator per ET tube at 50% FlO$_2$, 1000 tidal volume, rate 12. 4. Ambu bag at bedside.	The patient's alternative airway was patent until tracheostomy closed 1. Presence of bilateral breath sounds 2. No gurgling or bubbling of mucus in trachea 3. Absence of crowing respirations 4. Absence of straining on inspiration

FIGURE 24.7   (cont.)

INTRAOPERATIVE PLAN OF CARE
Mr. Ralph Fischer (continued)

Nursing Diagnosis	Expected Outcome	Plan	Implementation	Evaluation
POSTOPERATIVE (*cont.*)				
		5. If jaw wired, have wire cutters available for recovery room	5. Wire cutters at bedside.	
Increased risk for postop (respiratory) complications due to history of bronchitis, history of smoking, exposure to environmental irritants	Patient will be free of respiratory complications 48 hours postop. 1. Infection 2. Atelectasis 3. Aspiration	1. Preoperatively teach respiratory exercises (coughing, deep breathing, turning). Have patient return demonstrate and state rationale. 2. Discuss altered breathing pattern with tracheostomy 3. Explain need for frequent suctioning 4. Due to increased risk of aspiration elevate head of bed per physician's orders and monitor closely for signs of respiratory distress during transport. 5. Monitor nasogastric tube for patency and return of gastric secretions.	1. Preoperatively the nurse conducted an assessment and taught the patient return demonstration. 2. Demonstrated altered breathing pattern. 3. Explained need for frequent suctioning. 4. Head of bed elevated immediately postop and until patient returned to nursing unit. Postop Unit: 1. Nasogastric tube to gravity drainage with scant amount of light green drainage. 2. Complaining of nausea and NG tube being uncomfortable. 3. Patient vomiting and aspirated secretions into lungs. 4. Physician notified.	The patient was free of respiratory complications 48 hours postoperatively 1. Presence of bilateral breath sounds 2. Free of rales or wheezes. 3. Scattered rhonchi for 8 days post-op. 4. Nonproductive cough. 5. Low-grade temperature for 3 days. 6. Free of chest pain. 7. Sputum questionable for *Pseudomonas* and *Escherichia coli*.

FIGURE 24.7   (*cont.*)

3. *No edema in lower extremities*
4. *No cramping*
5. *No pain or aches in joints*
6. *No swelling in joints*
7. *Flexion and extension of extremities*
8. *Abduction and adduction of extremities*
9. *No weakness*
10. *No stiffness*

Mr. Fischer denied any limitations of range of motion during the preoperative assessment. This was the baseline for comparing his response postoperatively. The nurse had observed during the physical assessment that he had trace edema bilaterally in the lower extremities. No other significant findings were recorded on the plan of care. Postoperatively, the patient record indicated that on the first and second postoperative days there was no evidence of edema. Beginning on the third postoperative day, however, trace edema was noted and recorded. Its presence was documented throughout the remainder of the hospital day.

Observations by physicians and nurses indicated that all the criteria were met. The edema was present upon admission to the hospital; it was not a negative response to care given. In evaluation, any baseline established on admission should be noted in the record, as well as the patient's present status.

Another of Mr. Fischer's problems was respiratory. Because he would have a tracheostomy, hemiglossectomy, and wired jaw, the expected outcome was that his alternative airway be patent until the tracheostomy was closed (Fig. 24.8). Criteria for evaluating continued patency of the tracheostomy tube were as follows:

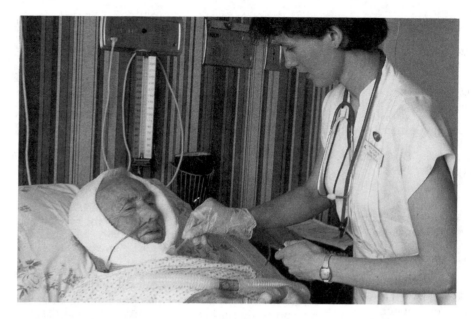

FIGURE 24.8.   Evaluation of patent alternative airway.

1. *Presence of bilateral breath sounds without rales, rhonchi, or wheezing*
2. *No gurgling or bubbling of mucus in trachea*
3. *Absence of crowing respirations*
4. *Absence of straining during inspiration or expiration*
5. *Arterial blood gas values within normal limits for Mr. Fischer*

In evaluating these criteria, the nurse noted that Mr. Fischer had some difficulty immediately postoperatively coughing up mucus from his trachea. He was suctioned frequently, and moderate amounts of secretions were obtained. He was taught to use the suction and was able to cough and suction himself when necessary. The record indicated that all the criteria were met; thus the alternative airway was maintained until the tracheostomy was closed.

Mr. Fischer had a potential for respiratory problems due to his history of bronchitis, smoking, and exposure to environmental irritants. The expected outcome was to prevent respiratory complications 48 hours postoperatively. Complications anticipated were infection, atelectasis, and aspiration. The criteria were:

1. *Presence of bilateral breath sounds*
2. *Free of rales or wheezes*
3. *Free of rhonchi*
4. *Nonproductive cough*
5. *Temperature same as preoperative baseline*
6. *Free of chest pain*
7. *Clear chest x-ray*
8. *Arterial blood gas values within normal limits*

Mr. Fischer aspirated gastric contents on the second day postoperatively. When reviewing the patient record to measure outcome attainment, the nurse found the following information:

1. *There was questionable right lower lobe atelectasis on the second postoperative day.*
2. *Mr. Fischer had scattered rhonchi for 8 days postoperatively.*
3. *No rales or wheezes were present, except on the fourth postoperative day when a few wheezes were detected in the right lower lung base.*
4. *The third day postoperatively, x-rays showed slight fluffy infiltrate in the right lower lobe.*
5. *Sputum was questionable for* Pseudomonas *and* Escherichia coli. *(Antibiotics were ordered specifically for these organisms.)*
6. *Mr. Fischer ran a low-grade temperature for 3 days postoperatively.*

Comparison of these data with the criteria indicated that the expected outcome was not met because Mr. Fischer developed respiratory complications due to the aspiration of gastric contents, which were present for 8 days postoperatively. The aspiration was due to vomiting created by gastric distention secondary to a nonfunctioning nasogastric tube.

REFERENCES

1. Saum, Margo F. "Evaluation: A vital component of the quality assurance program." *J Nursing Quality Assurance* 2(4):17–24, 1988.
2. Association of Operating Room Nurses. "Standards of perioperative clinical practice." *AORN Standards and Recommended Practices for Perioperative Nursing—1993*, pp. II:4–1 to II:4–4. Denver: AORN, 1993.
3. Association of Operating Room Nurses. "Patient outcomes: Standards of perioperative care." *AORN Standards and Recommended Practices for Perioperative Nursing—1993*. pp. II:7–1 to II:7–2. Denver: AORN, 1993.
4. Pelletier, Luc R., and Poster, Elizabeth C. "An overview of evaluation methodology for nursing quality

assurance programs." *J Nursing Quality Assurance* 2(4):55–62, 1988.

5. Milton, Doris. "Challenges of quality assurance program evaluation in a practice setting." *J Nursing Quality Assurance* 2(4):25–34, 1988.

6. Smeltzer, Carolyn H. "Evaluating a successful quality assurance program: The process." *J Nursing Quality Assurance* 2(4):1–10, 1988.

7. Inger, F., and Aspinall, M. I. "Evaluating patient outcomes." *NLN* October:197–205, 1987.

8. Yura, H., and Walsh, M. B. *The Nursing Process* 5th ed. New York: Appleton-Century-Crofts, 1988.

Suggested Readings

American Nurses' Association. "Task force on nursing practice standards and guidelines: Working paper." *J Nursing Quality Assurance* 5(3):1–17, 1991.

Carmody, Suzanne, Hickey, Patricia, and Bookbinder, Marilyn. "Perioperative needs of families." *AORN J* 54(3):561–567, 1991.

Ferguson, G. H., Hildman, T., and Nichols, B. "The effect of nursing care planning systems on patient outcomes." *J Nursing Administration* 17(9):30–36, 1987.

Gilette, Bonnie, and Jenko, Mimi. "Major clinical functions: A unifying framework for measuring outcome." *J Nursing Care Quality Assurance* 6(1):20–24, 1991.

Gordon, Marjory. *Nursing Diagnosis: Process and Documentation* 2nd ed. New York: McGraw-Hill, 1987.

Gordon, Marjory. "Toward theory-based diagnostic categories." *Nursing Diagnosis* 1(1):5–10, 1990.

Heggvary, S. T., and Haussmann, R. K. "The relationship of nursing process and patient outcomes." *NLN* August:29–37, 1987.

Lang, N., and Marek, K. D. "The policy and politics of patient outcome." *J Nursing Quality Assurance* 5(2):7–12, 1991.

Lower, M. S., and Burton, S. "Measuring the impact of nursing interventions on patient outcome." *J Nursing Quality Assurance* 3(1):27–34, 1989.

Marek, K. D. "Outcome measurement in nursing." *J Nursing Quality Assurance* 3(1):1–9, 1989.

McHugh, M. K. "Has nursing outgrown the nursing diagnosis?" *Nursing 87* 17(8):50–51, 1987.

Mitchell, Gail J. "Nursing diagnosis: An ethical analysis." *Image* 23(2):99–103, 1991.

Moritz, P. "Innovative nursing practice models and patient outcomes." *Nursing Outlook* 39(3):111–114, 1991.

Turner, Shirley J. "Nursing process, nursing diagnosis, and care plans in a clinical setting." *J Nursing Staff Development* September/October:239–243, 1991.

Wilson, Cathleen K. "Designing a quality assurance program evaluation: A process model." *J Nursing Quality Assurance* 2(4):35–44, 1988.

25

Improving the Quality of Patient Care

Integrating nursing quality activities with organizationwide quality improvement.

Quality improvement (QI) is an organization-wide philosophy and strategy for improving the delivery and outcome of patient care. It is based on the concepts of total quality management (TQM) and the belief that leaders and staff can improve systems and patient care by analyzing interdepartmental processes and establishing preferred patterns of care. The strategy is based on industrial models, statistical tools, and graphic representations of data (1).

The terms and concepts need not be overwhelming. Nor should the misconception that quality improvement activities mean more work keep perioperative nurses from exploring methods for improving the quality of care provided. In this chapter, quality improvement will be defined and differentiated from other quality activities (see Fig. 25.1.) The purpose and role of quality improvement in healthcare will become clear. Examples of how the concepts of quality-impact patient care will be provided.

Implementation of QI and development of indicators are truly at the cutting edge for healthcare organizations. This chapter will be introductory in nature but will provide a sound base in quality improvement as it relates to perioperative nursing practice.

The integration of nursing quality activities with the organizationwide quality improvement plan is essential. Healthcare facilities may differ in their approaches to implementing quality, but the concepts are sound and the results will strengthen the institution and improve services to patients.

QUALITY ASSESSMENT AND IMPROVEMENT

Why should nurses and healthcare organizations adopt quality improvement activities? The spectrum of benefits from implementing QI can be tremendous—from personal rewards to organizationwide improvement. Staff are empowered, through cross-functional teams, to develop critical paths or clinical guidelines for specific patient groups that delineate preferred care patterns. These teams establish thresholds that provide and reinforce practitioner-independent decision-making.

Data are collected and presented in such a way that opportunities to improve care can be identified. Patterns and trends can be easily interpreted and documented. Finally, both human and material resources are conserved. Conservation and the positive financial impact of QI are real for hospitals (2,3).

In addition to these benefits, QI is a required activity by the Joint Commission on Accreditation of Healthcare Organizations (JCAHO). The member organizations that are the constituencies of the Joint Commission believe that the philosophy and tools of QI can reduce the waste, rework, and needless complexity encountered in providing healthcare services.

Quality improvement or continuous quality improvement (CQI) is unique and different from quality assurance (QA) and quality control (QC). Quality assurance has traditionally been problem- and practitioner-focused and has entailed a case-by-case re-

Agenda for Change: A project undertaken by the Joint Commission to improve the processes and evaluation of patient care, standards development, and the survey process. A key component includes the development and field-testing of clinical indicators to be used nationally, with the eventual generation of nationwide performance data.

Cross-Functional Team: Consists of staff who perform different functions or tasks in the delivery of care to patients. Team representation is typically multidisciplinary and interdepartmental.

Important Aspects of Care: Care or service that is provided and is high-volume, high-risk, and/or problem-prone. Care can be identified as activities performed by staff, tests, procedure, diagnoses, or conditions. Care or service that is high-volume is performed frequently. High-risk care is care that could put patients at special risk if the care is: (1) underutilized, (2) overutilized, or (3) not provided correctly. Problem-prone activities or conditions are troublesome, difficult, and challenging.

Indicator; clinical or performance: Describes an event, outcome, or pattern of care for a specific target group of patients. The indicator has a numerator and denominator, with the latter being all patients at risk for experiencing the event or care pattern.

JCAHO; Joint Commission on Accreditation of Healthcare Organizations; Joint Commission: A nonprofit, private organization that develops standards in collaboration with healthcare professionals and others, surveys organizations, educates, and conducts research. The five member organizations are: American Hospital and Medical Associations, American College of Physicians, American College of Surgeons, and the American Dental Association.

Preferred pattern of care; algorithm; clinical guideline; critical path: A description of the ideal or preferred process of care for a specific group of patients with a given diagnosis, condition, signs and symptoms. May be a simple guideline or a very sophisticated, complex series of decision steps based on sequential activities, findings, or test results. Algorithms, critical paths, etc., are developed in teams by staff consensus and based on current knowledge, available technologies, patient characteristics, and other factors. Exceptions to these care patterns are identified as part of the development of these clinical guidelines.

Quality assurance; QA: Traditional method of evaluating the quality of care provided to patients. Typical methods include reviews of medical records, surgical cases, and blood and drug usage; infection control; risk management and utilization review. Usually focused on problems and practitioner performance issues.

Quality control; QC: Activities that a single department or service has exclusive responsibility for conducting, to ensure proper function of instruments, devices, etc., and the proper performance of tests, procedures, techniques. Examples: tourniquet calibration, patient positioning, sponge and needle counts, patient identification, medical device reporting.

Quality improvement, QI; Continuous quality improvement, CQI: An organizationwide belief and strategy that evaluates the interrelationships among administrative, clinical, and support services in the provision of patient care, with the purpose of improving processes and outcomes. Often based on the JCAHO Ten-Step Monitoring and Evaluation Model and the development and use of clinical indicators.

FIGURE 25.1.   Terminology related to quality improvement activities.

view of such data as surgical cases, medical records, and the use of drugs and blood products. Typically QA studies are centered on problem areas, and often focus on practitioner performance and decision-making rather than on systems of care delivery.

QI, in contrast, is based on the relationships among administrative, clinical, and support services in the provision of high-volume, high-risk, problem-prone care. Systems and processes are analyzed for these designated important aspects of care, and clinical indicators are developed and implemented. Indicator development is a multidisciplinary, interdepartmental, cross-functional team process that eventually results in the ongoing monitoring and evaluation of care.

Quality assurance is currently transforming into quality improvement; eventually traditional QA activities will be nonexistent. Instead, efforts and resources will be carefully focused on key conditions/diagnoses, clinical guidelines and outcomes, and their consequent improvement. Table 25.1 summarizes this transformation from QA to QI.

A cornerstone of QI is indicator development. Indicators are descriptions of processes or outcomes that are to be monitored for a given target group of patients. (Table 25.2 provides examples of quality indicators.) One of the key elements of the JCAHO's Agenda for Change is the development and use of a national set of clinical indicators (4,5). Hospitals will collect data on these indicators and transmit the information to the Joint Commission on a regular basis. In return, all healthcare organizations will receive a comparison of their performance with national data and on a case-mix and risk-adjusted basis. Ultimately a national database of performance indicators will be created and utilized—a truly revolutionary undertaking in healthcare.

INTEGRATION OF NURSING STANDARDS WITH QUALITY IMPROVEMENT

AORN's *Standards of Perioperative Clinical Practice* can be an integral part of quality improvement. In fact,

TABLE 25.1. Comparison of Quality Assurance and Quality Improvement

Quality Assurance	Quality Improvement
• Involvement of management level practitioners and staff • Oriented toward individual services/departments and their independent care delivery	• Involvement of every employee • Focuses on interrelationships among the administrative, clinical, and support services in the provision of care to specific groups of patients
• Problem- and practitioner-focused	• Emphasis is on high-volume, high-risk, problem-prone conditions, activities, tests, procedures, etc. • Primary focus is the systems and care processes related to these important aspects of care • Secondary use of information is the evaluation of practitioner performance
• Retrospective review of cases by select committees/staff	• Concurrent data collection • Ongoing monitoring and evaluation by cross-functional teams
• Independent studies of problem issues • Reviews: medical records, surgical cases, blood and drug usage, utilization • Infection control, risk management	• Development of indicators and thresholds of performance based on important aspects of care. Multidisciplinary consensus for preferred patterns of care
• Information and data reflect all cases, a specific sample, or problem issue	• Information and data depict a pattern or trend of care for a high-volume, high-risk, problem-prone event that staff/teams have agreed to monitor and evaluate, with specific intentions of improving care and identifying opportunities

they create the framework for identification of important aspects of care, and they are a connecting link to the development of cross-functional indicators.

The structure, process, and outcome standards for perioperative nursing prescribe the responsibilities, tasks/skills, and expectations required of perioperative nurses (6). To perform these activities and fulfill these standards, nurses often need the cooperation and skills of other healthcare professionals.

Administrative standards, for example, designate that perioperative nurses collaborate and coordinate effective interdepartmental relationships in order to achieve optimal patient care. Process standards explain that the nurse should consult with healthcare providers and others, make referrals, and ensure continuity of care. The results of care are identified as patient outcomes and are reflected in outcome standards.

To meet these standards and recommended practices, nurses rely on physicians to provide clear and timely orders, radiology and laboratory to provide reliable and accurate test results, pharmacy to provide correct medications and doses, and biomedical engineers to maintain safe and operable equipment. The list of nonnursing staff who support and cooperate with perioperative nurses to ensure that patients receive appropriate and quality care is long indeed. Practicing nurses can readily identify some of the frustrations and concerns that arise when other staff or services are not providing the "right" materials and information when they are needed.

This is the essence of quality improvement and indicator development: QI is an organizationwide activity. A high-volume surgical procedure, for example, may be identified and the process of care for these patients examined in terms of the continuity and coordination of care. Several services come together, identify the issues, achieve consensus on a best or preferred care pattern, implement the indicator/guideline, and monitor and evaluate care. A healthcare facility may have ten or twenty organizationwide indicators, where each service has a direct impact on at least two (possibly more) of the indicators that describe processes or outcomes.

Nursing standards are an integral part of QI. For perioperative nurses, the next step is evaluating how the implementation of these standards is related to the cross-departmental, multidisciplinary functions surrounding the care of perioperative patients.

The following section will discuss an approach to designing and implementing QI from the perioperative nursing perspective. The approach and examples provided are as descriptive as possible given the degree to which the Agenda for Change has progressed and the amount of information available that relates directly to healthcare experiences.

TABLE 25.2. JCAHO Field-Tested Indicators

These indicators have been developed by task forces and tested by several hundred hospitals across the United States. Indicators for areas not listed here are either being developed or field-tested, or have not yet been developed.

CARDIOVASCULAR INDICATORS

CHF PATIENT POPULATION
- Patients with a primary diagnosis with or without specific etiologies

Indicator Focus
- Monitoring patient's response to therapy

Indicator (Numerator)
- Patients with a principal discharge diagnosis of CHF with at least two determinations of patient weight and serum sodium, potassium, blood urea nitrogen, and creatinine levels

ONCOLOGY INDICATORS

ONCOLOGY PATIENT POPULATION
- Inpatients admitted for initial diagnosis and/or treatment of primary lung, colon, rectal, or female breast cancer

Indicator Focus
- Comprehensiveness of diagnostic workup

Indicator (Numerator)
- Patients with resections of primary colorectal cancer whose preoperative evaluation by a managing physician includes examination of the entire colon, liver function tests, chest x-ray, and carcinoembryonic antigen levels

Indicator Focus
- Symptomatic and/or palliative care

Indicator (Numerator)
- Systematic initial assessment of pain for all patients hospitalized due to metastatic lung, colorectal, or female breast cancer with pain

Indicator Focus
- Use of psychosocial support for patient followup

Indicator (Numerator)
- Referral to support or rehabilitation groups or provision of psychosocial support for female patients with primary breast cancer

Indicator Focus
- Patient education

Indicator (Numerator)
- Patients undergoing resection for primary colorectal cancer with enterostomy present at discharge who demonstrate understanding of enterostomy care and management instructions

TRAUMA INDICATORS

TRAUMA PATIENT POPULATION
- Patients with ICD-9-CM diagnostic code of 800 through 959.9 who either are admitted to the hospital, die in the emergency department (ED), or are transferred from the hospital or the ED to another acute care facility, excluding patients with the following isolated injuries: burns; hip fractures in the elderly; specified fractures of the face, hand, and foot; and specified eye wounds

Indicator Focus
- Use of blood products

Indicator (Numerator)
- Transfusion of platelets and/or fresh frozen

TABLE 25.2. *(continued)*

TRAUMA INDICATORS *(cont.)*
plasma within 24 hours of ED arrival in adult trauma patients receiving less than 8 units of packed red blood cells or whole blood

Indicator Focus
- Ongoing monitoring of trauma patients

Indicator (Numerator)
- Trauma patients with blood pressure, pulse, respiration, and Glasgow Coma Scale (GCS) documented in the ED record on arrival and hourly until inpatient admission to operating room or intensive care unit, death, or transfer to another care facility (hourly GCS needed only if altered state of consciousness)

Indicator Focus
- Airway management of comatose trauma patients

Indicator (Numerator)
- Comatose patients discharged from the ED prior to the establishment of a mechanical airway

Indicator Focus
- Timeliness of diagnostic testing

Indicator (Numerator)
- Trauma patients with diagnosis of intracranial injury and altered state of consciousness upon ED arrival receiving initial head computerized tomography scan greater than two hours after ED arrival

Indicator Focus
- Timeliness of surgical intervention for orthopaedic injuries

Indicator (Numerator)
- Trauma patients with open fractures of the long bones as a result of blunt trauma receiving initial surgical treatment greater than eight hours after ED arrival

Indicator Focus
- Timeliness of surgical intervention for abdominal injuries

Indicator (Numerator)
- Trauma patients with diagnosis of laceration of the liver or spleen, requiring surgery, undergoing laparotomy greater than two hours after ED arrival subcategorized by pediatric or adult patients

Indicator Focus
- Surgical decision-making for orthopaedic injuries

Indicator (Numerator)
- Adult trauma patients with femoral diaphyseal fractures treated by a nonfixation technique

Indicator Focus
- Clinical decision-making for femoral shaft fractures

Indicator (Numerator)
- Trauma patients with femoral diaphyseal fractures that are not associated with other injuries who do not receive physical therapy or rehabilitation therapy

INFECTION CONTROL INDICATORS

Indicator Focus
- Surgical wound infection

Indicator (Numerator)
- Selected inpatient and outpatient surgical procedures complicated by a wound infection during hospitalization or postdischarge

TABLE 25.2. *(continued)*

INFECTION CONTROL INDICATORS *(cont.)*
Indicator Focus
- Ventilator pneumonia

Indicator (Numerator)
- Ventilated inpatients who develop pneumonia

Indicator Focus
- Urinary catheter usage

Indicator (Numerator)
- Selected surgical procedures on inpatients who are catheterized during the perioperative period

ANESTHESIA INDICATORS
Indicator
- Patients developing a CNS complication occurring during or within 2 postprocedure days of procedures involving anesthesia administration, subcategorized by ASA-PS class, patient age, and CNS versus non-CNS related procedures

Indicator
- Patients developing a peripheral neurological deficit during or within 2 postprocedure days of procedures involving anesthesia administration

Indicator
- Patients diagnosed with an aspiration pneumonitis occurring during procedures involving anesthesia administration or within 2 postprocedure days of its conclusion

Indicator
- Patients experiencing an ocular injury during procedures involving anesthesia care

OBSTETRICAL INDICATORS
Indicator
- Patients with attempted vaginal birth after cesarean section (VBAC), subcategorized by success or failure

Indicator
- Term infants admitted to an NICU within 1 day of delivery and with NICU stay greater than 1 day excluding admissions for major congenital anomalies

MEDICATION USE INDICATORS
Indicator Focus
- Monitoring patient response

Indicator (Numerator)
- Inpatients receiving digoxin, theophylline, phenytoin, or lithium who have no corresponding measured drug levels or whose highest measured level exceeds a specific limit

Indicator Focus
- Monitoring patient response

Indicator (Numerator)
- Inpatients receiving warfarin or intravenous therapeutic heparin who also receive vitamin K, protamine sulfate, or fresh frozen plasma

Source: Joint Commission on Accreditation of Healthcare Organizations (4,5). Oak Brook Terrace, IL, 1992.

THE TEN-STEP MODEL

In 1984 the Joint Commission developed the Ten-Step Monitoring and Evaluation Model as a guide for assessing the quality of patient care (Table 25.3). The model reflects a planned, systematic, ongoing approach to evaluating patient care processes and outcomes (7). One of the key and challenging features of this model is the organization's development of indicators and thresholds based on their unique aspects of care. This section will discuss all 10 steps but will emphasize the "how-to" and examples of the most troublesome steps of the model, that is, indicator development and related issues.

Note that healthcare organizations can select any quality improvement model that meets the intent of the JCAHO standards. Many organizations have done so, and have done so successfully. It is important in any case to select a model that is meaningful and useful to leaders and staff, whether it be Deming, Juran, JCAHO, or some other model.

Once a model is adopted, its selection must be justified and its steps or strategy delineated and described. For example, the Ten-Step Model discussed here should be written as an organizationwide plan and guide for individual patient services.

Step One: Assign Responsibility

The healthcare institution's governing body and administration are ultimately responsible for organizationwide QA/QI activities. The director of each department or service is also responsible for the conduct of quality activities as it relates to the care the department provides. The nurse executive and other nursing leaders need to work with administrators to plan and conduct QI efforts.

The shape these efforts take depends on organizational structure, culture, and degree of involvement in QI or adoption of the CQI philosophy. What current communication mechanisms, committees,

TABLE 25.3. JCAHO Ten-Step Monitoring and Evaluation Model

1. Assign responsibility
2. Delineate the scope of care
3. Identify the important aspects of care
4. Identify indicators
5. Establish thresholds
6. Collect and organize data
7. Evaluate care
8. Take action
9. Assess actions and document improvement
10. Communicate organizationwide

Source: Joint Commission on Accreditation of Healthcare Organizations, Oak Brook Terrace, IL, 1991.

TABLE 25.4.   Scope of Care: Content and Example

	Patient Group	Related Nursing Care	Locations and Times of Care	Responsible Staff
Content	Kinds of patients • Major age groups? • Social characteristics that impact these cases? • Conditions/Diagnoses?	Kinds of care, tests, procedures performed for these patients?	Where and when does this care occur?	Personnel who perform and assist in the providing of this care • Physicians: specialties? • Nurses: specialties? • Technicians? • Technologists? • Other staff?
Example	Trauma patients • Accident • Domestic violence • Gang violence • Natural disaster	• Establish and maintain airway • Maintain fluids • Shock treatment	• Hospital OR 6 a.m.–6 p.m. 6 p.m.–6 a.m. Emergency only • Same-day surgery • Emergency area—24 hours • Clinic Mon.–Fri., 6 a.m.–8 p.m. Sat.–Sun., noon–5 p.m. • Postanesthesia care unit • Intensive care units	• Emergency physicians, residents • Registered nurses • Surgeons • Anesthesiologists • Technicians

and plans are already in place? Has the institution taken steps toward CQI, or is this an effort with roots in the nursing service?

Once the commitment to QI is made, staff should be assigned to assist in the effort. It is at the staff or clinical practitioner level where data collection often takes place, and where knowledge of the preferred care pattern or critical path is necessary for improving care.

Essentially, the assignment of responsibility should cover all tasks described in the Ten-Step Model. Who will serve on cross-functional teams? Who will collect, analyze, and report data? Who will design action plans and implement them? Who will report information so that staff and/or committees who need to know are knowledgeable?

Unlike QA, QI is an organizationwide transformation that impacts all staff in regard to their work and relationships with other disciplines and services. Educating and empowering staff are necessary parts of this process, but the degree to which QI is implemented, and on what timetable, depend on multiple factors. Some of these factors include the organization's culture, leadership knowledge of and commitment to QI, current organizational structure and communication patterns, and organization size and variety of services. These factors and the

design of a vision statement and QI plan are typically accomplished with the help of a consultant or quality-management consultation firm.

Step Two: Delineate the Scope of Care

Step Two is analogous to self-assessment of what services the healthcare organization provides and what types of patients it serves. Although it may seem simple and unnecessary, it will help in completing the next step, identifying the important aspects of care. Also, outside reviewers will need to understand the organization's scope of care, and this is a useful way to lay it out.

One way to approach this step is to develop a chart that lists the types of patients served, what services the institution provides to them, where and when these services occur, and who in nursing or other services provides this care (Table 25.4). If completing a table seems tedious, it may be helpful to write a narrative describing these components instead. Ideally, enough specifics should be provided so that an external healthcare practitioner from another city or state could walk into the institution, pick up the QI plan and, by reading the scope of care, understand the kinds of patients treated and the manner in which care is provided. The scope of

TABLE 25.5. Important Aspects of Care: Key Questions and Examples of Activities, Tests, Procedures, Conditions, and Diagnoses that Illustrate High-Volume, High-Risk, and Problem-Prone Categories

	High-volume	High-risk	Problem-prone
Key Questions	What is routine or common?	Would the patient be put at risk if this care were: • not provided when indicated? • provided when not indicated? • not provided correctly? What conditions place patients in a high-risk category, especially if treatment of their condition relies on care provided by perioperative nurses?	What procedures or patient conditions are particularly troublesome for staff and/or patients?
Examples of Procedures and Conditions	• Total joint arthroplasty • Open heart surgery • Cataract removal • Laparoscopic cholecystectomy	Care *not* provided when indicated: • Monitoring the patient receiving IV conscious sedation • Hypothermia blanket Care provided when *not* indicated: • Unnecessary surgery (tonsillectomy, C-section) • Indiscriminate use of antibiotics Test not provided correctly: • Operation of electrical equipment • Monitoring fluid intake/output • Positioning devices High-risk conditions from a perioperative nursing perspective: • Multiple system problems • Open heart procedures • Craniotomies	• Pediatric patients • Elderly patients • Multisystem problems

care should be a story about perioperative nursing in a particular environment, given the social and economic conditions as well as the available technologies and prevailing treatment protocols.

Step Three: Identify the Important Aspects of Care

Important aspects of care are those activities performed and conditions treated that are high-volume, high-risk, and/or problem-prone. As in Step Two, it may be helpful to create a chart of these categories of care (Table 25.5). From this information, the perioperative nurse and the cross-functional team can select issues for indicator development. In fact, Step Three can be examined at the perioperative nursing "department" level, and then key issues can be brought to the team for discussion and selection of indicator topics.

Important aspects of care are also those issues or activities that have the greatest impact on the quality

of patient care. High-volume procedures affect the largest number of patients for any specific group. For instance, what are the high-volume surgical procedures for (1) adults, (2) pediatrics, (3) males, (4) females, (5) Medicare patients, (6) females of childbearing age, (7) schoolage children—each major patient group in the facility's population?

Procedures or perioperative nursing practices are considered high-risk to the patient if they are (1) not provided correctly (involves a skill that requires special attention or a high level of skill), (2) not provided when indicated (care/procedures that may be underutilized), or (3) provided when not indicated (care/procedures that may be overutilized). High-risk care can be evaluated in terms of either specific kinds of care, or diagnosis or patient status.

Problem-prone care is care or procedures that are troublesome for the perioperative nurse, other staff, or patients. What kinds of care may be difficult to provide under certain circumstances? What care is difficult to provide because it's difficult to monitor

TABLE 25.6.   Components of Quality Perioperative Nursing Care

Appropriateness Does nursing care match what the patient needs at the time?	*Efficacy* Is the nursing care able to achieve the desired results?	*Safety* Is perioperative nursing care provided safely to patients and respectful of staff safety?
Continuity Is nursing care coordinated among healthcare practitioners and across services or functions?	*Efficiency* Is nursing care conducted in an environmentally and resource-sensitive manner?	*Timeliness* Is nursing care provided in a timely manner?
Effectiveness Is the nursing care provided/done correctly?	*Patient Involvement* Are patients and relevant support people informed about nursing care to the degree possible, and are they satisfied?	*Accessibility* Do patients receive perioperative nursing care when they need it?

patient status or interpret results? Is after-hours care more problematic because less experienced staff is providing it, or because the cases encountered are more severe? What care for a high-risk surgical group requires especially efficient and effective care that is coordinated among several services or disciplines?

The list of important aspects of care becomes the springboard for indicator development. Rather than evaluate all cases or a sample of cases, as in QA, QI pinpoints key patient care activities that impact the majority of patients or impose significant risk. These key aspects of care will be the basis of the indicators developed and monitored to improve care. Precious resources will be invested in these aspects, with the objective of preventing the need for problem-focused studies.

Step Four: Identify Indicators

Based on the important aspects of care identified in Step Three, the objective of Step Four is to select at least two procedures or conditions upon which to develop clinical indicators (8). Team input at this stage and onward is critical for several reasons: (1) to select issues that are cross-functional in nature, (2) to achieve consensus on each indicator's potential value for improving care and its worth in monitoring and evaluating care over a period of years, (3) to develop a realistic, relevant algorithm or care pattern, and (4) to examine data-collectibility factors and data interpretation issues.

Once an aspect of care has been selected, the next challenge is to identify quality of care issues concerning this procedure or activity. Table 25.6 lists the different components of quality nursing care that can be the focus of indicators. Any single indicator may need to address more than one quality component. The purpose here is to pose a question

such as, What about total joint arthroplasty patients? Is the concern appropriateness of care? Continuity of care? What exactly is the concern?

Once the issue is clearly identified, the next step is to compose the indicator statement. Indicators have a numerator and denominator. The numerator describes the patient target group and the process or outcome of concern related to this patient population. The denominator describes all patients at risk for experiencing the numerator process or outcome.

Some of the JCAHO field-tested indicators were listed in Table 25.2. What is the implied patient population at risk—the denominator description? Here are some examples:

1.
$$\frac{\text{Numerator}}{\text{Denominator}} = \frac{\text{Comatose patients discharged from ED prior to the establishment of a mechanical airway}}{\text{All comatose patients discharged from the ED}}$$

2.
$$\frac{\text{Numerator}}{\text{Denominator}} = \frac{\text{Adult trauma patients with femoral diaphyseal fractures treated by a non-fixation technique}}{\text{All adult trauma patients with femoral diaphyseal fractures}}$$

3.
$$\frac{\text{Numerator}}{\text{Denominator}} = \frac{\text{Selected inpatient and outpatient surgical procedures complicated by a wound infection during hospitalization or postdischarge}}{\text{Patients who have selected inpatient and outpatient surgical procedures}}$$

There are several issues worth noting here. First, the numerator must be clear and specific. What patients? What process of care or outcome? For instance, for the third example above, an individual hospital or team would designate exactly which surgical procedures would be monitored for wound infection. Note that the wound infection rate for all cases is not the issue. The issue is which surgical cases are of particular concern for the development of wound infection. Cases of concern are those in which care *can* be improved; that is, the infection rate is not largely dependent on factors outside the control of the perioperative nurse, such as patient/ case severity or the nature of the procedure.

Second, the ideal wording of an indicator statement should begin with "Patients who . . .". Note that the Joint Commission task forces have gotten more sophisticated in the wording of indicators. Early indicators may not have reflected the same degree of patient specification that will be expected as the indicators continue to be developed.

Third, note that indicators do not state that, "Patients should have care X," or "Patients will have care Y." Indicators are not standards. Indicators describe a specific group of patients who will be monitored and evaluated. The intention is often to set a preferred care pattern for certain patients but still allow for both discrepant cases and for independent practitioners to make judgments outside the preferred care pattern when appropriate. Is it not inevitable that patients for certain surgical procedures will develop infection no matter what type of care is given? Is it not possible that, for some reason, an adult trauma patient with a femoral diaphyseal fracture may not be treated with a fixation technique? This issue relates to threshold establishment in Step Five. Indicator development, however, includes looking ahead, not only to thresholds but to data collection and interpretation issues as well.

Fourth, an organization's indicators must be based on high-volume, high-risk, problem-prone activities. As a part of this process, organizations are required to consider the complete list of JCAHO field-tested indicators. These indicators are currently listed in an appendix of the JCAHO *Accreditation Manual for Hospitals* (4).

Finally, examples of clinical indicators beyond the JCAHO set are hard to find. Some examples are given in hospital case studies that have been published (3), while other examples come from personal consultation and work with individual institutions that are learning to create indicators. Table 25.7 lists some raw indicator statements prior to full team development and implementation.

TABLE 25.7. Examples of Unrefined Indicators Prior to Full Team Development and Implementation

- Same-day admit patients who have a delay in surgery due to absence of test results, x-ray, EKG, H & P, or lack of preparation by physicians (i.e., informed consent, epidural or anesthesia information, preadmission to hospital)
- Patients who have surgery in a supine position for 2 hours or longer and who develop neurological deficits in upper extremities
- Children between the ages of 6 and 12 undergoing tonsillectomy and adenoidectomy who arrive in the OR without lab results for PT, APTT, and platelet count, or who have abnormal results that are unresolved
- Patients who have procedures delayed more than 30 minutes due to unavailability of equipment
- Patients who are positioned with Modified Mayfield invasive positioning devices who develop lacerations at pin sites
- Diabetic patients having surgery whose blood glucose levels pre- and postop are not within normal limits
- Patients over 60 years of age who have femoral arteriogram that exhibit signs and symptoms of bleeding, hematoma formation, hypotension, dehydration, or renal function impairment within 48 hours postprocedure

Step Five: Establish Thresholds

After an indicator statement is composed, the next task is the establishment of a threshold for performance. The threshold should be somewhere between 1% and 99%. The underlying premise is that the threshold establishes when intensive evaluation of care will occur. As long as a threshold is met or not exceeded (depending on how the indicator is worded), review occurs on a regularly designated basis, usually quarterly. The threshold sets the trigger point for in-depth examination of the patterns and trends of care.

The concept and use of a QI threshold is different from the sentinel-event and review-every-case approach of QA. Sentinel events are serious events where the threshold would be 0% for occurrence. ABO transfusion reactions and deaths of elective surgery patients would be examples of sentinel events. On the opposite end, it is expected that there be 100% compliance with certain practices or standards of care.

Although sentinel events are important and need to be tracked and investigated, they do not provide the opportunities to improve care that QI indicators do. Sentinel events indicate that something went wrong, but what? Must an institution wait, so to speak, for a serious event to occur rather than develop a QI indicator that evaluates a care process and establishes an ideal clinical guideline geared to prevent the serious event? A well-developed indicator can provide data that help improve care by focusing on provider relationships and shared responsibilities.

If there are indicators developed that are assigned thresholds of 0% or 100%, they are often quality-control types of issues rather than multidisciplinary, cross-functional issues. For example, perioperative nurses already know to count sponges and calibrate medical devices prior to use. Tasks such as these are exclusively nursing and are under the nursing service's responsibility. These QC tasks or practices are important, but they are different from QI issues.

The establishment of a numeric threshold requires information-gathering and professional judgment. Healthcare organizations within a given geographic area may have the same indicator but different thresholds based on variances in case mix, treatment philosophy, and so on.

The threshold should be set in such a way that practitioners are allowed to step outside the preferred care pattern or critical path if it is appropriate to do so. The purpose of clinical indicators is to guide decision-making for the typical patient within a specific target group. Indicators are composed knowing that there will be exceptions to standards of care, discrepant cases, and random error. Healthcare professionals cannot be expected to deliver identical care to all patients with a specific diagnosis. Thresholds allow for some variation. Conceivably, thresholds could be set at 50% compliance for a given algorithm, or at 95%. A threshold may depend, for instance, on the care under discussion, the staff, and the state of the technology involved.

Table 25.8 identifies different ways to gather information on an indicator event. The team can evaluate the factors that may affect the rate of occurrence, such as those due to patient, practitioner, and organization. If possible, a retrospective review of cases is also helpful in establishing what baseline performance might be. Other sources of data are more difficult to locate because design and use of indicators in healthcare facilities is, as stated earlier, so new. With time the literature, professional associations, and societies will yield an increasing number of case studies and data sources.

It may be difficult to conduct any of the above reviews if the proposed regimen or algorithm is new or untried. In these cases, staff must use professional judgment in identifying a threshold. Regardless of how the threshold is established, the justification for it must be briefly written and documented. Table 25.9 is an example of this justification process.

TABLE 25.8. Methods to Establish an Indicator Threshold

Examine the factors that affect the occurrence of the indicator event.
- Patient factors: severity of illness, comorbid conditions, other patient-related factors (age, gender, ethnicity, disability)
- Practitioner factors: cognitive (knowledge level), skill (ability to perform task, hand–eye coordination), affect or sentiment toward patients, staff, protocols, policies and procedures, hospital philosophy
- Organizational factors: hospital culture, patterns of communication, traditions, characteristics of community served

Conduct a retrospective review regarding indicator occurrences over the past 6 months, year; whatever is deemed representative.

Review the literature, usually healthcare organizations describing their experiences with QI implementation.

Check other resources: hospital associations, professional organizations/societies.

Exercise professional and team judgment in selecting a threshold.

Once established, the threshold should remain intact—unchanged—for at least twelve months. This is also true for the wording of the indicator statement. The reasons for this are as follows: (1) a minimum of one year's worth of data is necessary to make informed decisions about indicator utility; (2) the essence of QI is ongoing monitoring and evaluation of an important aspect of care; and (3) given that indicator development is based on an important aspect of care and with team input, the indicator and designated threshold should possess significant value.

Step Six: Collect and Organize Data

Consideration of data collection and presentation methods often leads to at least some indicator revision prior to implementation. Are the numerator data collectible, easily retrieved? Who will locate the information and in what way will it be reported and translated into a graphic presentation?

Data collection should be conducted concurrently rather than retrospectively, if possible. Concurrent collection keeps staff and others directly involved in indicator performance alert and sensitive to the critical path or outcome being monitored and evaluated.

TABLE 25.9. Example of Indicator Development and Threshold Justification

Team Members:	Ellen Knight, RN, CNOR, perioperative nurse; Heather Kind, RN, CNOR, Director Surgical Services; Brad Skiller, MD, neurologist; John Welton, MD, orthopedic surgeon; Sam Pelter, physical therapist
Aspect of Care:	Care of patients having surgery for spinal instability
Indicator Focus:	Coordination of care to patients with neurological complications
Rationale:	Nerve root impingement is a potential complication that is preventable with appropriate care. This is a high-risk procedure.

Indicator:	Numerator:	Patients who have post-lumbar interbody fusion and who develop nerve root impingement associated with a bone graft
	Denominator:	Patients who have posterior lumbar interbody fusions (PLIF)

Factors Affecting Occurrence:

Patient: Lack of cooperation in wearing of brace
Variations in clinical pathology
Related disabilities
Nonunion of bone

Practitioner:
Surgical techniques
Referral to physical therapy
Coordination of care by healthcare team

Organization:
Organization of dialysis unit
Coordination of care with other services

Justification of threshold:
A review of the literature was conducted as well as a 6-month retrospective chart review. The medical and nursing staff, along with other team members, established a threshold of _____%. (Team should attach relevant data)

Initially, all cases may need to be counted. Whether all cases are counted or a representative sample is taken depends on the event or process being monitored. If it is a high-volume procedure, a sample may be sufficient. If it is a high-risk situation, perhaps all cases should be counted and evaluated.

Presentation of data should occur in some kind of pictorial fashion: histogram, pareto chart, scatter diagram, run or control chart, or other statistical method. The purpose here is to look for patterns and trends of care over a period of time. Once the applications of the tools or graphs are understood, staff can use a pencil and ruler or a sophisticated

software package to illustrate the data. The important thing is that the information be presented in a useful format so that the team can evaluate care (Step Seven).

Data collection and presentation techniques are important, and there are many issues concerning the "how-to." The references listed at the end of this chapter may be consulted, as well as others on the topic.

Step Seven: Evaluate Care

Care is evaluated based on the patterns and trends demonstrated by the diagrams or charts and in relation to the threshold. Evaluation of care is usually conducted by the team as a whole. In most instances, medical staff input is necessary. At a minimum, medical staff can establish criteria by which care can be evaluated by nonphysician practitioners. The degree of medical staff involvement depends on the nature of the indicator.

There is no direct correlation between quality of care and whether or not the threshold has been exceeded. Threshold establishment, as explained earlier, may not necessarily be well supported by the literature or past hospital experiences.

Documentation of data results and team interpretation are critical. Even if results seem unclear or unchanged from a previous quarter, this interpretation should still be noted.

Step Eight: Take Appropriate Action

Based on the evaluation the team discusses alternatives to improve care. Two hospitals with an identical indicator and identical data may decide to take two totally different plans of action. Action plan development depends on the perceived causes of the results as well as the healthcare organization's culture and established systems.

A decision to take no action can be as acceptable as development of a sophisticated, stepwise plan. It is important to document the reasoning behind the plan of action (or no action), determine who will implement the plan when it becomes necessary, and what the timeline will be for completion.

Step Nine: Assess Actions and Document Improvement

After plan implementation, the effectiveness of actions taken must be assessed. Should another plan be developed if the original plan is unsuccessful? If the plan has long-term goals, progressive assessment and documentation of evaluation should occur.

A part of documentation includes copies of memos sent to staff, educational sessions, revised policies or procedures, and so on. Individual staff, committees, and external reviewers should be able to follow the story behind every indicator and the sequence of events throughout the process.

Step Ten: Communicate Organizationwide

Many healthcare organizations have had to alter their committees and channels of communication to meet the intent of the quality improvement process. QI is a facilitywide commitment and evaluation of systems and care processes. To that end, indicators cross department and service lines in their prescription of critical paths or clinical guidelines. Multiple services and disciplines need to be aware of, informed about, and/or involved in indicator development and use.

A medical staff QA committee separate from other hospital QA/QI activities is probably not an effective mechanism. Many hospitals have instead established a QI council to orchestrate the various team issues and indicator development. Some have also set aside days on which teams present their indicators and results during monthly QI forums (3).

The goal at this step is, "Tell the people who need to know." The process analysis which typically occurs during indicator development often reveals the complexity of any given process, and all the different staff that impact the process as well. Thus staff and services that affect a particular patient care process "need to know" so that they can contribute to the improvement of care. In addition the performance of some indicators may be related to one another, making organizationwide communication even more crucial.

Compared to quality assurance, quality improvement is a far different approach to monitoring and evaluating patient care. It is an organizationwide philosophy and commitment to examining systems, interdepartmental, practitioner, and general staff relationships in providing care. It requires the creation of indicators that are unique to a healthcare organization's environment and services.

QI provides the perioperative nurse with the paradigm and tools to fully implement AORN standards, such as those in regard to practitioner collaboration and continuity of care. It provides the

method to solve common interdepartmental problems, and to create workable systems that ultimately serve the patient and improve the ability of perioperative nurses to provide optimal care.

REFERENCES

1. O'Leary, D. O. "Agenda for change initiatives: Setting the record straight (President's column)." *Joint Commission Perspectives* 11(2):2-3, 16, 1991.
2. Berwick, D. M., Godfrey, A. B., and Roessner, J. *Curing Health Care.* San Francisco: Jossey-Bass Publishers, 1990.
3. Joint Commission on Accreditation of Healthcare Organizations. *Striving Toward Improvement: Six Hospitals in Search of Quality.* Publication #CQI-104. Oak Brook Terrace, IL: JCAHO, 1992.
4. Joint Commission on Accreditation of Healthcare Organizations. "Appendix D." *1992 Accreditation Manual for Hospitals.* Oak Brook Terrace, IL: JCAHO, 1992.
5. "Medication use and infection control indicators complete alpha testing phase." *Joint Commission Perspectives* 11(5):5-7, 1991.
6. Association of Operating Room Nurses. *AORN Standards and Recommended Practices for Perioperative Nursing—1992.* Denver: AORN, 1992.
7. Joint Commission on Accreditation of Healthcare Organization. "Quality assessment and improvement." *Accreditation Manual for Hospitals.* pp. 137-143. Oak Brook Terrace, IL: JCAHO, 1992.
8. Joint Commission on Accreditation of Healthcare Organizations. *Primer on Indicator Development and Application.* Publication #RD300. Oak Brook Terrace, IL: JCAHO, 1990.

SUGGESTED READINGS

Byham, W. C. *Zapp! The Lightening of Empowerment.* New York: Harmony Books, 1988.
Crosby, P. B. *Quality without Tears, The Art of Hassle-Free Management.* New York: McGraw-Hill, 1984.
Duncan, R. P., Fleming, E. C., and Gallati, T. G. "Implementing a continuous quality improvement program in a community hospital." *Quality Review Bulletin* 17(4):106-112, 1991.
Eubanks, P. "The CEO experience—TQM/CQI." *Hospitals* 66(11):24-28, 32, 36, 1992.
Gottlieb, L. "Clinical guidelines and QM: A match made at HCHP." *Quality Connection* 1(4):3-5, 1992.
Joint Commission on Accreditation of Healthcare Organizations. *Transitions: From QA to CQI; Using CQI Approaches to Monitor, Evaluate, and Improve Quality.* Publication #QI-101. Oak Brook Terrace, IL: JCAHO, 1991.
McEachern, J. E., Schiff, L., and Cogan, O. "How to start a direct patient care team." *Quality Review Bulletin* 18(6):191-200, 1992.
Nolan, T. W., and Provost, L. P. "Understanding variation." *Quality Progress* (May 1990), pp. 70-78.
Plsek, P. E., Onnias, A., and Early, J. F. *Quality Improvement Tools.* Wilton, CT: Juran Institute, 1988.

Index

Note: Page numbers followed by **t** and **f** denote tables and figures, respectively.

403

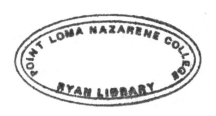

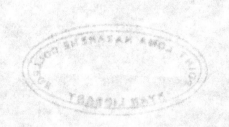